Contemporary Socio-Cultural and Political Perspectives in Thailand

Pranee Liamputtong
Editor

Contemporary Socio-Cultural and Political Perspectives in Thailand

Springer

Editor
Pranee Liamputtong
School of Public Health
La Trobe University
Bundoora, VIC, Australia

ISBN 978-94-007-7243-4 ISBN 978-94-007-7244-1 (eBook)
DOI 10.1007/978-94-007-7244-1
Springer Dordrecht Heidelberg New York London

Library of Congress Control Number: 2013958225

Printed on acid-free paper

Springer is part of Springer Science+Business Media (www.springer.com)

To my parents Saeng and
Yindee Liamputtong
who raised eight children amidst poverty

Acknowledgments

In bringing this book to life, I owed my gratitude to many people. First, the book would not have happened without the contribution from all authors who worked very hard to get their chapter to me. I would like to thank Esther Otten, a senior acquisition editor of Springer who saw the value of this book and worked to ensure that I was contracted to edit the book. I also thank Rosemary Oakes who helped reading through several chapters in this book. Rosemary has been a great support for my academic life since I have known her, and I deeply appreciate her help and support throughout these years too.

I thank my own families, both in Thailand and in Australia. This book is dedicated to my parents, Saeng and Yindee Liamputtong, who brought their children up amidst poverty in the south of Thailand. Without their wisdom and hardworking life, I would not have come this far. I also thank all of my siblings who are now all in Thailand. They have given me much support all these years that I have become an immigrant in Australia. Last, I thank my two daughters, Zoe Sanipreeya Rice and Emma Inturatana Rice, who deeply appreciate their Thai heritage and for their understanding of my working life that I have to perform on top of my mothering roles.

Contents

Contemporary Thailand: An Introduction

Pranee Liamputtong

1 Thailand at a Glimpse

Thailand, a constitutional monarchy, is located in Southeast Asia and has been known as the "Land of Smiles." Thailand was historically recognized under the name Siam (Wongtes 2000). The term Thailand was formally created in the early nineteenth century. Its capital city, Bangkok, was established in 1782, 15 years after Ayutthaya, an ancient city, was destroyed (Baker and Phongpaichit 2005). There have been many speculations about the origin of Thai territory and ethnicity. The Thais may have originated in some parts of China and the Malay Peninsula. There is also evidence to suggest that they may have come from the area that is now southern China (Phillips 2007). Today, there are still many Thai people living in southern China (Terwiel 1989; Baker and Phongpaichit 2005). In the late nineteenth century, Thailand expanded its borders to cover a large part of Southeast Asia. Additionally, Thailand has always been an independent country because it has never been colonized by any other nations (Einspruch 2007; Phillips 2007; Suwankhong 2011).

Thai culture, politics, and social systems have been influenced by many neighboring countries such as Malaysia, Indonesia, Cambodia, Laos, and Burma (Terwiel 1989). The Burmese used to live in the central and northern parts of Thailand. As a result, their religion, Theravada Buddhism, was adopted by the Thais. Between the eleventh and twelfth centuries, Cambodia spread its civilization through Southeast Asia, and this also has powerfully influenced the construction of Thai hierarchical society (Naemiratch 2004). As we have witnessed nowadays, Thailand has adapted the culture and religion of its neighboring countries to create a unique Thai culture (Phillips 2007).

P. Liamputtong (✉)
School of Public Health, La Trobe University, Bundoora, VIC, Australia
e-mail: pranee@latrobe.edu.au

Buddhism is the national religion of Thailand, with about 95 % of the Thais being Buddhists (Phillips 2007). However, people are free to follow any religion and practice. In some communities, it is possible to find Buddhist temples, shamanist and Chinese shrines, Muslim mosques, and Christian churches in close proximity (Wongtes 2000; Suwankhong 2011). As the majority of Thai people declare themselves to be Buddhist, Mulder (1985: 153) contends that Buddhism "is a way of life, an identity, and the key to primordial Thainess." Buddhism has had a deep influence on the Thai's modes of thinking and behavior. Buddhism, according to Mulder (1985: 132), is "the most visible and ubiquitous of Thai institutions." Several chapters in this volume will attest to this influence.

The social transition of Thailand has been marked by economic growth, population restructuring, social and cultural development, political tensions, and reforms in its national health-care system (Suwankhong 2011). This is clearly evident in many chapters in the volume. As a society, Thailand has been undergoing progressive development since the introduction of the National Economic Development Plan in 1961 (Naemiratch 2004). The First to the Third plans (1961–1976) were mainly centered on economic developments. The Fourth to the recent Tenth plans focused primarily on social and cultural development, population restructuring (1977–2011), and the improvement of health-care system (Bureau of Policy and Strategy 2007).

During the Asian financial crisis in the late 1990s, the Thai economy was badly affected. Thailand sought help from the International Monetary Fund (IMF) to help its economy recover. Thailand's economic woes returned between 2005 and 2007 (Wibolpolprasert 2007). It was at this crisis time that the "sufficiency economy" philosophy was created to give new direction for the country's development (Department of Foreign Affairs and Trade 2009; Suwankhong 2011). This philosophy has been promoted as a guideline to deal with economic crisis and social change. The economic crisis sounded the alarm to all relevant sectors of Thailand. In fact, Thailand attempted to reform its developing country paradigm, focusing on this direction since the Eighth National Economic and Social Development Plan (1997–2001). Participation of all sectors of society, especially at the grassroots level, is given priority because these sectors could create a balance between economic, social, and environmental development (Wibolpolprasert 2007). The sufficiency economy philosophy was also incorporated in the Ninth National Economic and Social Development Plan (2002–2006). Although Thailand is now applying the Tenth National Economic and Social Development Plan (2007–2011), it strongly combines those concepts to prevent negative effects from an imbalanced globalization development in the Thai economy and society. It is likely that this philosophy will be included in the next National Economic and Social Development Plan (2012–2016) because it could maintain the balance of economic, social, and environmental development (National Economic and Social Development Board 2008). This philosophy is discussed in several chapters of this volume.

When mentioning Thailand, most people will imagine the land as portrayed in the *King and I* movie, a country with beautiful temples, and for many people, clubs, bars, Thai women, gay men, and transsexual individuals. However, contemporary Thailand has changed dramatically from what is known to many people. Although we may still witness many traditional ways of life, contemporary Thailand is about changes and the immense impact of these changes on Thai people. Political situations such as coups and the recent Yellow and Red Shirts movements have been devastating. This internal political crisis has impacted tremendously on the life of Thai people and international relations between Thailand and other nations. Marked social and cultural changes have also occurred in Thailand. With this, we see new social movements and identities such as the rise of a new middle class and "lower" class groups and ethnic, gender, and gay movements. Social and health inequalities among Thai people continue to persist. These are captured in most chapters in this volume. Perhaps people still smile but there is much tension beneath the smiles of Thai people. I left Thailand about 30 years ago and I have also been going back home every year. Whenever I go back to Thailand, I could see the changes of Thai society, and more importantly, I could feel the tensions among Thai people, even among members of my own family who are also caught in the changing world of Thailand. These contemporary issues have not been captured in great depth in existing literature concerning Thailand. This book will fill this gap.

2 The Focus of the Book

This book has its focus on contemporary Thailand. The volume captures many contemporaneous aspects in Thai society. These are from social, cultural, and economic changes to the current political situations in Thailand. Chapters cover historical contexts to emerging issues in Thai society as well as range from social and public health concerns. The volume also includes issues concerning Thai people in general to those impacting on ethnicity, gender, social class, and sexuality. The volume offers comprehensive discussions regarding Thailand, its people, culture, and society from multiple angles as seen through multiple lenses. Due to a range of diverse issue covered in the volume, it is difficult to situate all chapters within a common conceptual framework. Thus, there is no appropriate common theory that pulls the chapters together in this book. I rely heavily on the contemporary perspective as a common theme of this volume. It must be noted that each chapter contains its own theoretical framework to which readers could refer.

There are too many books on Thailand and Thai people to list here. However, most of these existing books focus on a particular aspect of Thai society, for example, a political, social, cultural, historical, religious, gender, and transsexual perspective. For instance, Michael Connors' most recent book entitled *Contemporary Thailand: Politics, Culture, Rights* (2009) only focuses on the political aspects in contemporary Thailand. In his book, Connors explores the struggle for political order by examining four significant sites of contestation: monarchy, culture, rights, and the place of the Muslim South in the Thai nation. Apart from Connors' book, there has not been any recent book on Thailand that captures a full range of issues concerning contemporary Thailand as proposed in this volume. A search through Google as well as a library search does not provide any title that can compete with this volume.

This book was conceived when I attended and presented my work at the 11th International Conference on Thai Studies, in Bangkok in July 2011. There, I met many people who have their interests in Thai society and presented their work, which I found very fascinating. I made attempts to connect to many of them and those who were interested in presenting their work have now become contributors to this book. I am very grateful to all contributors who helped to make this book possible. Originally, there were more authors who had agreed to take part in the book, but for many personal reasons and work commitments, some were not able to deliver their work when the absolute deadline arrived. However, I believe that the contents of volume are still comprehensive and cover many fascinating contemporary materials in Thai society.

This book comprises five parts and contains 32 chapters. Part I includes chapters that portray contemporary sociocultural issues in Thailand. The first chapter in this part is about redefining "Thainess" and is written by Suwilai Premsrirat. In this chapter, Suwilai suggests that the notion of "Thainess" needs to be broadened to offer ethnolinguistic groups their own space within Thai political society on an equal basis so that they may be empowered to live a dignified life with security, justice, and opportunity. Willard Van De Bogart writes Chap. 2 on the Giant Swing and its significance to the religious culture of Thailand. In this chapter, Willard argues that the Giant Swing is one of Thailand's most well-known landmarks. What is less known about this historic landmark is its symbolic significance. Sophana Srichampa presents Thai amulets as a symbol of the practice of multiple faiths and cultures in Chap. 3. She points out that Buddhism is the religion of the majority of Thai people. But in Thai life, people's beliefs reflect multiple faiths and cultures. The value of amulets is an example of the influence of different faiths in Thailand. In Chap. 4, Saowapa Pornsiripongse, Kwanchit Sasiwongsaroj, and Pacharin Ketjamnong write about Buddhist temples from the perspective of a religious capital approach for preparing Thailand for an aging society. Thailand is experiencing a rapid increase in older population. The phenomenon has attracted the attention of various sectors in order to develop suitable guidelines to accommodate this situation. Mayumi Okabe, in Chap. 5, presents issues regarding community development and network construction among the Buddhist monks in northern Thailand. Mayumi examines how Theravada Buddhist monks have survived in the rapid social changes, which are the result of modernization in contemporary Thailand from an anthropological perspective.

Chapter 6, written by Adcharawan Buripakdi, presents an interesting contemporary issue in Thai society on hegemonic English, standard Thai, and narratives of the subaltern. This chapter addresses the status of English and Thai language related to the notion of Other – marginalized voices – in Thailand. The next chapter (Chap. 7) is about digital revolution and its discontents. It is about Thai "underground metal" scene and their love-hate relationships with new technologies and is written by Athip Jittarerk. Athip presents a case from a sector that also received enormous impact from this revolution, namely, "Thai underground metal scene," using the materials from his ethnographic fieldwork conducted in Bangkok from 2007 to 2011. Chapter 8 presents a fascinating work of Morakot Jewachinda Meyer on reimagining nationalism and nostalgia of the past in the contemporary Thai novel and its stage and screen adaptations. In this chapter, Morakot provides her analysis of the novel "*Thawiphop*" (Parallel Worlds) and discusses how it has been received in Thai society. Ratana Tosakul, in Chap. 9, presents issues relating to capitalism and the sufficiency economy in rural northeastern Thailand. She contends that since the 1980s, the notion of village sufficiency economy has been developed and endorsed by major institutions in Thai society. There is a hope that the adoption of this economic ideology and practice might eventually result in a sustainable village economic development.

Chapters in Part II discuss political situations in contemporary Thailand. It begins with an interesting chapter by Aim Sinpeng who writes about the party-social movement coalition in Thailand's political conflict, between 2005 and 2011. In this chapter, Aim seeks to address a gap between the literature about social movements and party politics by establishing a more systematic crossover understanding of the two fields. Following on from Aim's chapter on political party movements, Allan Lee presents his writing on "For king and country?: Thailand's political conflicts as dynamics of social closure" in Chap. 11. Allan argues that political conflicts in Thai society ought to be reexamined with an appreciation of the dynamics of social closure. The Yellow Shirts movement that emerged in the late 2000s is best understood as an attempt by various groups located in the middle stratum of Thai society to counter and contest their gradual economic, political, and social exclusion by the Thai state and elites. Chapter 12 is written by Pei-Hsiu Chen who discusses the vulnerability of Thai democracy with the main focus on coups d'etat and political changes in modern Thailand. In this chapter, Pei-Hsiu deals with Thai politics by delineating its type of regime, political culture, and elite politics. The coup d'etat in 19 September 2006 and the collapse of Thaksin regime are carefully examined in accordance with the analysis of political vulnerability in modern democratization of Thailand.

In Chap. 13, Serhat Ünaldi writes about politics and the city, paying particular attention to the protest, memory, and contested space in Bangkok. Serhat argues that the past years have seen a significant shift in the configuration of political space in Thailand, metaphorically and literally. He suggests that the rudimentary but progressive development of politics along programmatic and ideological fault lines between political and social groups has led to bitter contestations both within the political structure and in physical space. Moving away from political conflicts between parties in Thailand, Diane Archer, in Chap. 14, presents the politics of change in Thai cities focusing on the urban poor as development catalysts. She points out that low-income communities are playing an increasingly important role in city development, with consequences for civic participation and democratization of Thai grassroots.

Part III presents chapters that focus on ethnic issues in Thailand today. In Chap. 15, Sumitra Suraratdecha writes about language and cultural rights in the ethnic revival movement of the Black Tai in Khaoyoi, Petchaburi. The chapter addresses the notions of ethnocultural identity, language rights, stigma, prejudice, and discrimination in an educational sphere. Chapter 16, written by Matthew R. Juelsgaard, is about Lahu students in Thai schools, focusing on two Lahu sisters: Som and Noi. Teaching in an elementary school, Matthew observed that Lahu students encountered challenges different from those of their Thai peers. For both sisters, overcoming linguistic borders as well as socioeconomic constraints were significant aspects of their schooling experiences. The stories of these two Lahu women echo many of my personal experiences as a child growing up in a poor family in the south of Thailand. Chapter 17, written by Alexander Trupp, discusses rural–urban migration and ethnic minority enterprise, paying attention to Akha migrants. Over the last years, an increasing number of Thailand's ethnic highland minorities have moved to urban and tourist areas to enter self-employment. In this chapter, Alexander illustrates the evolvement of urban Akha souvenir businesses over time and space and explores the embeddedness of female Akha entrepreneurs in social networks and in the wider economic and political-institutional structures as well as the resulting chances and challenges. He also explores the strategies Akha migrants employ to become successful entrepreneurs by showing how they transform cultural and social resources into economic capital.

Part IV is concerned with gender and queer perspectives in contemporary Thailand. It commences with a very interesting piece of Kosum Omphornuwat who writes about learning to look good. It is about Thai women office workers and everyday consumption practices at work in Chap. 18. By arguing that consumption practices involve learning, in this chapter, Kosum explores how, through their engagement in the consumption of clothes and makeup, Thai women office workers learn to look good at work. Chapter 19 presents the work of Chantanee Charoensri who examines Thai daughters, English wives from the perspectives of a critical ethnography of transnational lives. Her chapter tells their story and reveals how the life trajectories of Thai women, as wives of Englishmen, have been deeply structured by a number of interconnecting forces beyond their control. However, at each stage in these trajectories, key qualities of the women's characters have played a pivotal role: characteristics of discipline, skill, and deep loyalty. In Chap. 20, Megan Lafferty and Kristen Hill Maher discuss the expat life with a Thai wife presenting Thailand as an imagined space of masculine transformation. In this chapter, they examine the narratives and circumstances of white western men living in Thailand to explore how their structural privilege plays out once they settle there. Their position and identity as western men generate not only social status but also a heightened sense of insecurity and social isolation. The narratives of the men illustrate some of the ways that they negotiate new forms of vulnerability and shifts in power by constructing themselves as neocolonial expats and masculine decision makers.

Chapter 21 discusses women NGOs movement for fighting against domestic violence by Suangsurang Mitsamphanta. In this chapter, Suangsurang shows that women's NGOs are groups of people who are concerned about the problem. Additionally, they have expended much effort in fighting against the problem. Many strategies are employed in their movement both in the private and public sectors. They finally managed to get involvement from the government. Andrea Katalin Molnar in Chap. 22 presents issues relating to women's agency in the Malay Muslim communities of southern Thailand. Andrea contends that women have invariably been described as victims in the literature on women's political participation in Southeast Asia. This discourse obscures women's agency. Andrea argues that women are politically engaged – whether through the formal political arena as politicians or through civil society as leaders and activists in social movements and NGOs. Women are agents of change and their political engagement makes significant impact on various human security issues including peace-building efforts in different parts of Southeast Asia. In her chapter, Andrea examines Malay Muslim women's agency in the conflict-torn Deep South of Thailand, focusing on civil society engagement.

Chapter 23 is written by Erin Kamler on trafficking and coerced prostitution in Thailand and pays attention to the reconceptualization of international law in the age of globalization. In this chapter, Erin argues that coerced prostitution, particularly in Thailand, should be regarded as a transnational rather than a local issue. She uses the migration practices of Shan ethnic community members as a case study to illustrate how cultural and economic push factors influence coerced prostitution. In Chap. 24, Monica Lindberg Falk writes about gender and Buddhism in the wake of the tsunami. This chapter deals, from a gender perspective, with the significance of Buddhism in the post-tsunami recovery process in small fishing communities in southern Thailand. It explores local adaptation strategies.

Witchayanee Ocha, in Chap. 25, presents the first fascinating chapter on queer perspective. This chapter forms a body of gender knowledge through the study of the emergent identities in Thailand's sex tourism industry that Thailand is becoming a well-known place for sex change operations. The chapter shows that bodies are plural and very diverse. There are not just two kinds of bodies. There are multiple kinds of bodies and lots of differences among them. The most important proposition of her paper is to revise gender concepts for a fuller understanding of "gender" in the world of technology. This clearly represents a challenge in current knowledge of "gender and development." In Chap. 26, Dredge Byung'chu Käng provides his writing on conceptualizing Thai genderscapes looking at transformation and continuity in the Thai sex/gender system. This is another fascinating chapter in this volume. In Thailand, Dredge suggests that genderscapes, or the terrain of gender and sexuality, continue to evolve quickly, with alternative genders proliferating. In this chapter, Dredge argues that genderscapes provide a provisional conceptualization of contemporary Thai gender and sexuality. In Chap. 27, the third gender as seen in Thai fiction is written by Jenjit Gasigijtamrong. There is a myth that Thailand is the haven of the third gender, be they lesbians, gays, bisexuals, or transgender (LGBT), although results from empirical studies regarding this issue remain inconclusive. Her chapter explores this topic in Thai language novels written in 1980s and early 2000s. Jenjit suggests that the third gender is mainly perceived and presented through the influence of a patriarchal idea. Being the third gender is not socially accepted; it is perceived as an illness that needs to be cured. Family influence or the way a person is raised is thought to be the main cause of such behavior.

The last part of this volume is dedicated to health issues in contemporary Thai society. The first chapter, Chap. 28, is on Theravada Buddhist temple taking care of people living with HIV/AIDS in Thailand and presented by Yoshihide Sakurai and Kazumi Sasaki. This chapter illustrates the case of social support by Wat

Phrabatnampu in Lop-Buri province, Thailand, from the perspective of social inclusion by the private sector in Thai civil society and the strategic usage of moral practice in Theravada Buddhism. They suggest that the case of Wat Phrabatnampu, regardless of being based on traditional Theravada Buddhism, could be considered a pioneering example of socially engaged Buddhism. In Chap. 29, Pranee Liamputtong and Somsri Kitisriworapan address the issues of authoritative knowledge and folk knowledge in antenatal care in contemporary northern Thailand. The chapter also presents the experience of pregnancy and antenatal care among northern Thai women. In this chapter, they conclude that to many Thai women, the cultural authority of biomedicine pervades. Despite several decades of campaigns for reproductive choices among women's movements, these notions are still problematic in Thai antenatal care.

Chapter 30 presents the work of Yongsak Tantipidoke on the moral aspect of local healing to show the process that morality can contribute to the effectiveness of healing. The chapter focuses on the story of two folk healers and analyzes how the healer associated his sensibility with the moral values in the local world and led to a starting point of a healing process, how sympathy and other related moral dispositions are called up in the process, and how the healer, through a healing process, becomes able to reify local moral values into practical humanized healing. The chapter then explores the outcomes of the healing process – power of virtue and merit – that can strengthen the effectiveness of healing. Dusanee Suwankhong and Pranee Liamputtong write about *phum panya chao baan* (local wisdom) and traditional healers in southern Thailand in Chap. 31. Thailand is now focusing on forming a sufficient health-care system by using local wisdom and traditional health resources. The use of local resources such as traditional medicine (TM) and traditional healers to share expenses can be cost-effective in increasing the good health of the Thai people. In the final chapter, Chap. 32, Atchara Rakyutidharm discusses issues regarding Thailand's NGOs and the Thai Health Promotion Foundation (THPF). She suggests that many Thai nongovernmental organizations (NGOs) and people's organizations (POs) willingly cooperate with THPF and other government agencies and business groups. The relationship as "collaboration" is not just only because the two parties gain benefit from each other but also because they have some things in common, particularly the vision, the concepts, and the approaches that they adopt in development.

3 Conclusion

Readers will see that the book captures many aspects of contemporary Thailand. Most chapters included in this volume are written using information from empirical-based and historical research. What we see in this book comes from real-life experiences of the writers and people, mostly Thai people, who took part in the research. Additionally, contributors are composed of both Thai and foreign scholars who have undertaken extensive research in Thailand. The book offers critical analyses of issues concerning contemporary Thailand as seen through the eyes of experts, both inside and outside Thailand. As I have anticipated, it is expected that this volume would be valuable to many readers who have your interests in Thailand and its contemporary sociocultural and political issues.

References

Baker, C., & Phongpaichit, P. (2005). *A history of Thailand*. Melbourne: Cambridge University Press.

Bureau of Policy and Strategy. (2007). *Health policy in Thailand 2007*. Retrieved July 6, 2009, from http://bps.ops.moph.go.th/HealthPolicy7.pdf

Connors, M. (2009). *Contemporary Thailand: Politics, culture, rights*. London: Zed Books.

Department of Foreign Affairs and Trade. (2009). *Country brief*. Retrieved July 6, 2008, from http://www.dfat.gov.au/GEO/thailand/index.html

Einspruch, A. (2007). *Countries of South-East Asia: Thailand*. Melbourne: Heinemann Library.

Mulder, N. (1985). *Everyday life in Thailand: An interpretation*. Bangkok: Duang Kamol.

Naemiratch, B. (2004). *Who is in control: The diabetic or diabetes? Lived experience of adults living with diabetes in Bangkok*. Unpublished doctoral dissertation, University of Queensland, Brisbane, Queensland, Australia.

National Economic and Social Development Board. (2008). *Summary the Tenth National Economic and Social Development Plan (2007–2011)*. Retrieved July 9, 2009, from http://www.nesdb.go.th/Default.aspx?tabid=139

Phillips, D. A. (2007). *Thailand: Modern world nations*. New York: Chelsea House Publishers.

Suwankhong, D. (2011). *Traditional healers (mor pheun baan) in southern Thailand: A contribution towards Thai health*. Unpublished doctoral dissertation, La Trobe University, Melbourne, Australia.

Terwiel, B. J. (1989). *A window on Thai history*. Bangkok: Duan Kamol.

Wibolpolprasert, S. (Ed.). (2007). *Thailand health profile 2005–2007*. Bangkok: The War Veterans Organization.

Wongtes, S. (2000). *The Thai people and culture*. Bangkok: Office of the Prime Minister.

Part I
Thailand and Current Socio-cultural Issues

Chapter 1
Redefining "Thainess": Embracing Diversity, Preserving Unity

Suwilai Premsrirat

1 Introduction

To be Thai is to exude the distinguishing qualities, behavior, and virtues of the Thai nation as encapsulated in the term "Thainess." For the nationalistic designers of the concept, at least, unifying the diverse, though not entirely disparate, cultural and linguistic varieties existing on the fringes of "Central" Thai society was a means to fashioning a sense of homogeneity that would serve the interest of the political elite in Bangkok at a time in the mid-twentieth century when colonial pressures threatened all borders of the country formerly known as Siam.

Today, many still regard the somewhat limited Thainess ideal as representing a single people with common traits. The significant diversity of language and culture is frequently ignored or misunderstood and this has resulted in marginalization for many and the gradual extinction of language and cultural heritage for some. But now, efforts are being made at a grassroots level, with considerable support from concerned parties outside, to restore pride and dignity to ethnic communities through language revitalization. It is hoped too that, as a matter of sensitivity and historical accuracy, Thainess will come to be redefined to encompass groups for whom the current erroneous definition does not fully fit and, in so doing, reflect the true cultural complexity that is, and always was, Thailand.

This chapter will discuss the language diversity in Thailand and how the indigenous communities and academics make a lot of efforts to reverse the language shift by preserving and revitalizing their threatened language in addition to improve the

S. Premsrirat (✉)
Resource Center for Documentation, Revitalization and Maintenance of Endangered Languages and Cultures, Research Institute for Languages and Cultures of Asia, Mahidol University, Salaya, Nakhon Pathom 73170, Thailand
e-mail: suwilai.pre@mahidol.ac.th

P. Liamputtong (ed.), *Contemporary Socio-Cultural and Political Perspectives in Thailand*,
DOI 10.1007/978-94-007-7244-1_1,

chronic underachievement in schools for the students in the border areas. This is especially for the Patani Malay-speaking students in the south which has led to cultural conflict and language identity issues that underlie the political unrest and violent situation in the area.

2 The Reality of Linguistic and Cultural Diversity in Thailand

Geographically, Thailand is situated at the center of Mainland Southeast Asia which is one of the most complex areas of languages and ethnicities in the world (with around 1,000 languages).

The linguistic diversity of Thailand is evident by the fact that with a population of 60 million, speaking more than 70 living languages, belonging to five language families: Thai (24 languages), Austroasiatic (23 languages), Austronesian (3 languages), Sino–Tibetan (18 languages), and Hmong–Mien (2 languages). Thai is the official/national language. Details can be found in Premsrirat and Others (2004) (Fig. 1.1).

The languages and the cultures they represent provide this region with a rich and rewarding diversity of ideas, philosophies, and values. To some people, cultural and linguistic diversity can be considered as a resource; to others, it is a problem. And to some, it represents a struggle for basic rights. Each consideration leads to the ways in addressing the diversity situation by either promoting and supporting or eliminating diversity as much as possible. It could also be seen as a right of the indigenous people that has to be protected.

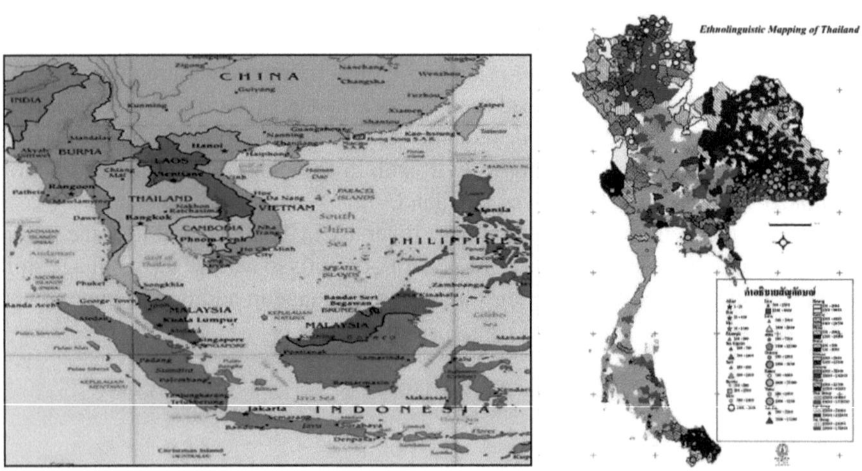

Fig. 1.1 Map of language diversity in Thailand at the heart of SEA

3 Language Endangerment Issue

World languages are now in crisis. The twenty-first century is an age of rapid change. Language loss, like the loss of biodiversity, is accelerating at an alarming rate. According to the estimation of linguists such as Krauss (1992), 90 % of world languages are facing extinction by the end of this century (or shortly thereafter) if nothing is done. The 10 % that seem to be "safe" are official/national languages or languages with political support. And at the moment, 50 % are not being learned by children. Languages in Thailand are facing the same fate. Ethnic minority languages, big and small, are not safe.

Globalization and nationalism are the main causes of the changes in the language ecology that lead to language shift and language loss. As for globalization, the global economy and sociopolitics and global culture influence the lives of most people. Even in remote areas, global communication, especially the powerful mass media, can reach into homes of people. Such media use global languages such as English or a national language. Nationalism too plays a role whereby national language and education policy determine or sculpture attitudes and values. For example, it heavily influences the speakers' negative attitudes about their ethnic language. The younger generation does not see the value of their ethnic language and increasingly choose to use the language of wider communication.

3.1 The Language Situation in Thailand at the Present Time

Ethnic minority languages in Thailand are declining (Fig. 1.2). The younger generation is becoming monolingual in Thai which is the official/national language. At least 15 languages are seriously endangered. They are small, enclave languages that are surrounded by bigger languages. They are Chong, Kasong, Samre, Chung (Sa-oc), So (Thavung), Nyah Kur, Mlabri, Maniq (Sakai), Lavua, Mpi, Bisu, Gong, Moklen, Urak Lawoi, and Saek. All major nondominant languages in Thailand are potentially endangered and show signs of contraction, especially in vocabulary and grammar such as Northern Khmer, Patani Malay, Mon, Lao *Isan*, and Kammuang (Premsrirat 2006a, b). Oral traditions such as folktales, poetry, and songs are severely endangered and are disappearing even faster than the spoken language itself. See also Chap. 15 in this volume.

Large language groups in border regions are not only facing the problem of language decline among the younger generation, but most also cannot access government services such as education or health. In general, ethnic minority peoples are considered, by outsiders, as slow and not likely to succeed in the modern development process. In some areas such as in Thailand's Deep South where the majority of the population are Muslim Melayu–Thai speakers, there is

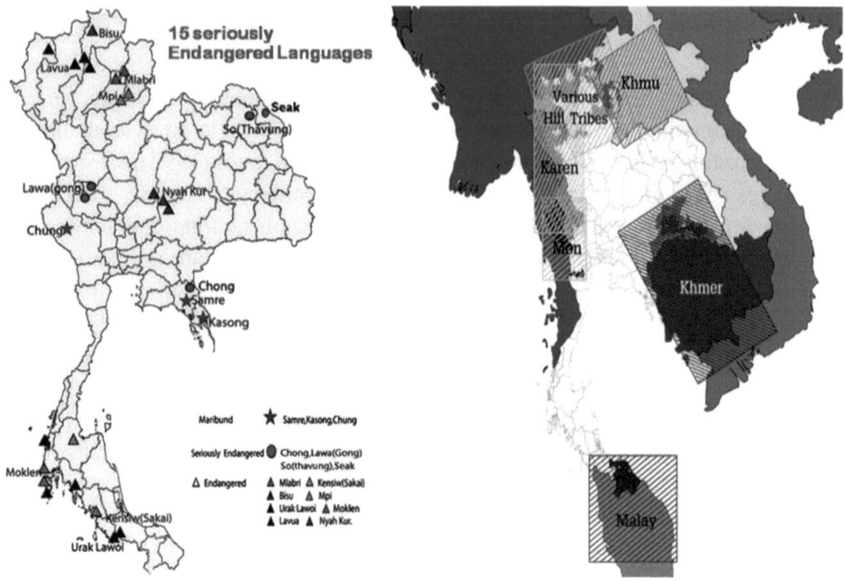

Fig. 1.2 Languages in crisis

resistance to many government services. The language identity issue and cultural conflicts are among the underlying factors which contribute to the violence and political unrest (Premsrirat 2008 and 2010).

According to the eight stages of Fishman's Graded Intergenerational Disruption Scales (GIDs), by which the degree of language endangerment can be identified, all languages in Thailand (large and small) with the exception of official language (standard Thai) are classified by Premsrirat (2007a) as being on the weak side for reversing language shift. Only Patani Malay, Northern Khmer, Lavua, and Mon can be put in stage 4 (strong side) if their tongue-based bilingual education, which is now being conducted as action research in formal school system, is accepted (Fig. 1.3).

3.2 *What Is Being Done to Slow Down the Death of Languages?*

There are several observations that I wish to make here. First, academics and language speakers are being encouraged to document as much as possible the language, culture, and oral traditions of languages at risk before they are lost forever. Second, the language speakers/ethnolinguistic communities are being encouraged to conduct language revitalization programs with technical support of academics (linguists, anthropologists, education experts, and so on) and with initial financial support from Thailand Research Fund (TRF) and other funding agencies. Last, the reconsideration of the national language policy to facilitate and support the use of ethnic minority languages along with the national language (Thai) and international languages (Fig. 1.4).

Weak side	**Stage 8**	So few fluent speakers that community needs to reestablish language norms; often requires outside experts (e.g., linguists) *[Kasong, Sumre, and Chung (Sa-oc)]*
	Stage 7	Older generation uses language enthusiastically but children are not learning it *[Chong, Lawa (Gong), So (Thavung)]*
	Stage 6	Language and identity socialization of children takes place in home and community *[Maniq (Sakai), Kensiw, Lua (Lavua), UrakLawoi, Moklen, Mlabri, Mpi, and Bisu]*
	Stage 5	Language socialization involves extensive literacy, usually including non formal L1 schooling or teaching L1 as a subject "Local Studies" in school *[Chong, So (Thavung), NyahKur]*
Strong side	**Stage 4**	L1 used in children's formal education in conjunction with national or official language *[Patani Malay, Northern Khmer, Lavua, and Mon]*
	Stage 3	L1 used in workplaces of larger society, beyond normal L1 boundaries
	Stage 2	Lower governmental services and local mass media are open to L1
	Stage 1	L1 used at upper governmental level

Fig. 1.3 Eight stages of language endangerment (levels of language vitality) according to Fishman's Graded Intergenerational Disruption Scale (GIDs)

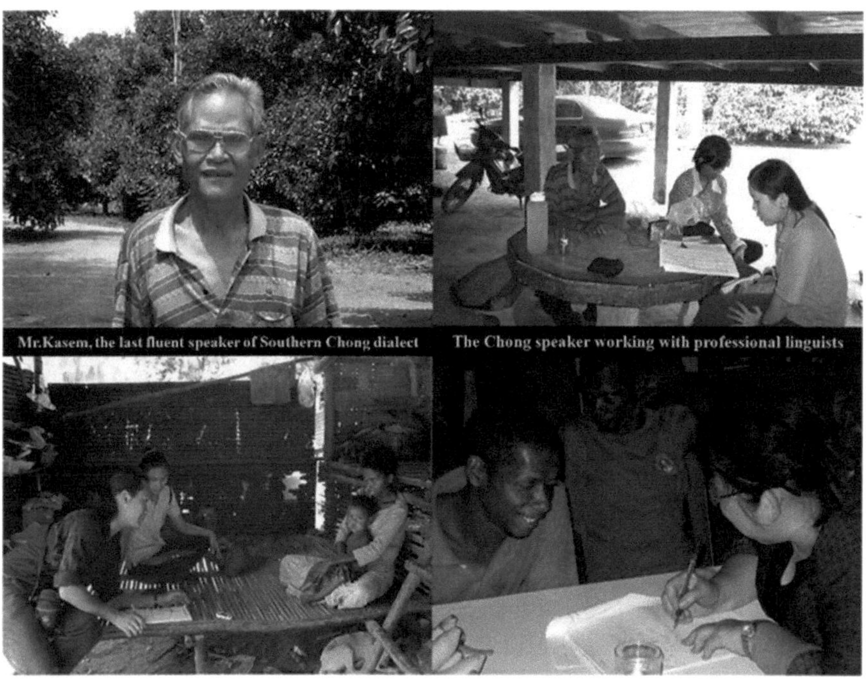

Fig. 1.4 Language and oral traditions documentation by linguists

4 Language Revival Efforts from Grassroots Communities and Indigenous Rights Movements (Focusing on Education)

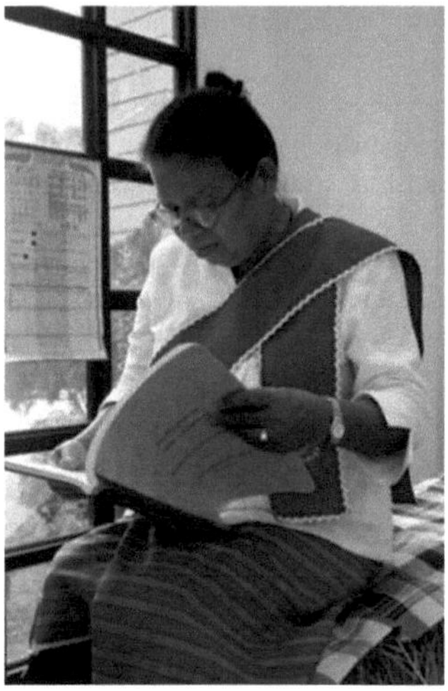

A Mon lady uses a vivid metaphor to describe the Mon language endangerment situation comparing it to a fruit which ***"is breaking off from the stem"*** and the language revitalization activity as ***"the last breath of the speakers."*** (Premsrirat 2007b)

Language revitalization is an attempt to provide a new domain of language use in order to increase the use of the language and the number of users. According to Crystal's (2000) six postulates to guide attempts of revitalization, an endangered language will positively progress if its speakers (1) increase their prestige within the dominant community, (2) increase their wealth relative to the dominant community, (3) increase their legitimate power in the eyes of the dominant community, (4) have a strong presence in the educational system, (5) can write their language, and (6) can make use of electronic technology. Since many ethnic minority languages (large and small in Thailand) have been classified as being potentially endangered at various stages, a group of linguists at Mahidol University have pioneered a cooperative program to preserve these languages. Endangered language speakers and communities will participate in language documentation and description as well as in the language revitalization and maintenance program. The focus is to put community members at the heart of revitalization efforts through involvement in almost all steps of the revitalization process such as orthography development, creation of local vernacular literature, collection of local knowledge, and instruction of the language to the next generation of speakers. This Mahidol Revitalization Model has been implemented with the cooperation of 22 language groups and the technical and moral support of the Mahidol research team (Premsrirat Forthcoming). The community-based language revitalization and maintenance model that has emerged from these efforts incorporates basic principles of reversing language shift (Fishman 1991), yet is sensitive to the distinct needs of each individual community. See also Chap. 15 in this volume (Figs. 1.5 and 1.6).

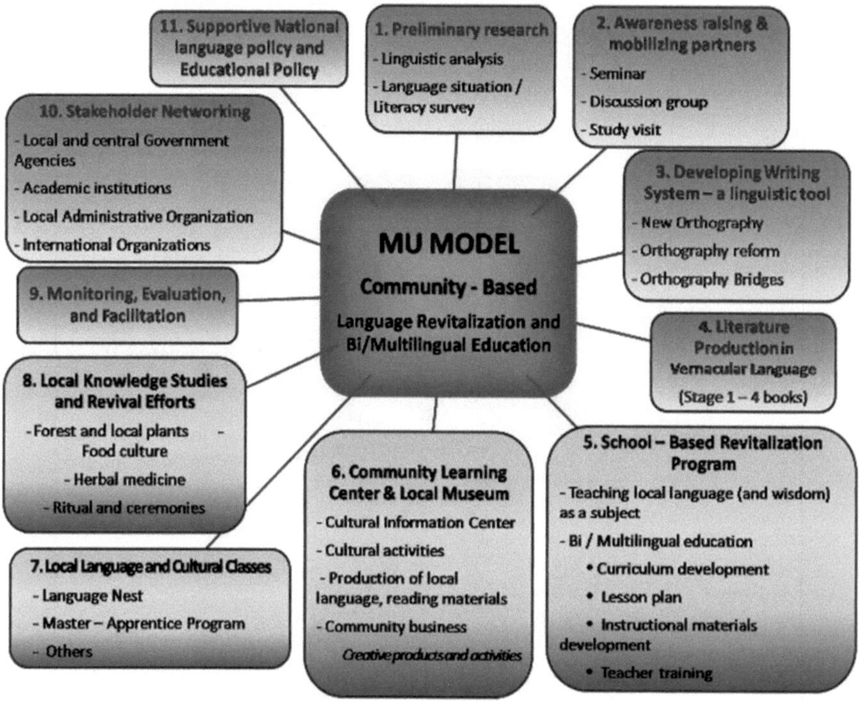

Fig. 1.5 Mahidol language revitalization model by Premsrirat (Forthcoming)

The model consists of 11 component activities which are adapted to utilize the best fit to the unique contextual needs of individual communities. The first step in the model is preliminary research, which consists of assessing the morbidity of a language in an area, surveying the literacy of the people, and performing a linguistic analysis. Once the linguistic situation is understood, awareness-raising activities such as seminars, discussion groups, and study visits are arranged to mobilize partners in the effort. After partnerships have been established, a writing system is developed for the language. With a writing system that has been deemed acceptable by the community, literature production commences; local authors create stories for big books, small books of different stages, and dictionaries that the language speakers compile themselves. The next step is to introduce the language into the formal school system. For small, seriously endangered languages such as Chong, Nyah Kur, and So (Thavung), the language is taught as a subject in local schools. This involves developing a curriculum and instructional materials, lesson planning, and teacher training. For the bigger language groups or languages that the children still speak such as Patani Malay, Northern Khmer, and Lavua, a mother tongue-based bilingual education is conducted in order to address the language identity crisis or cultural conflict and to raise students' levels of achievement in school. This form of language revitalization commences when the child first starts school. A way to

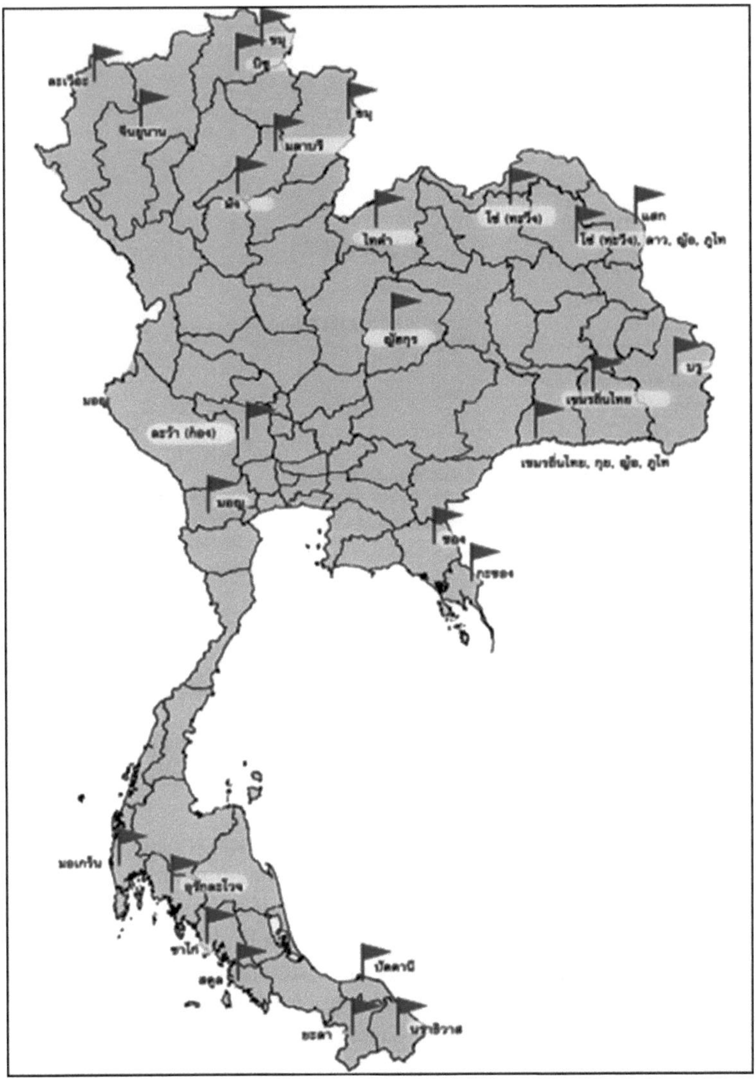

Fig. 1.6 Ongoing language revitalization efforts in 22 language groups

strengthen the presence of the language is through the establishment of a community learning center and local museum for the community at large. It serves as an information center for the public where cultural information can be provided, cultural activities and language classes can take place, production of new literature can occur, and community business can be conducted. Language nest may be set up for small children prior to kindergarten, as has been done among the Bisu and the Kasong (both severely endangered). Of fundamental importance is using the language to document local knowledge of forest plants for use in herbal medicine, for

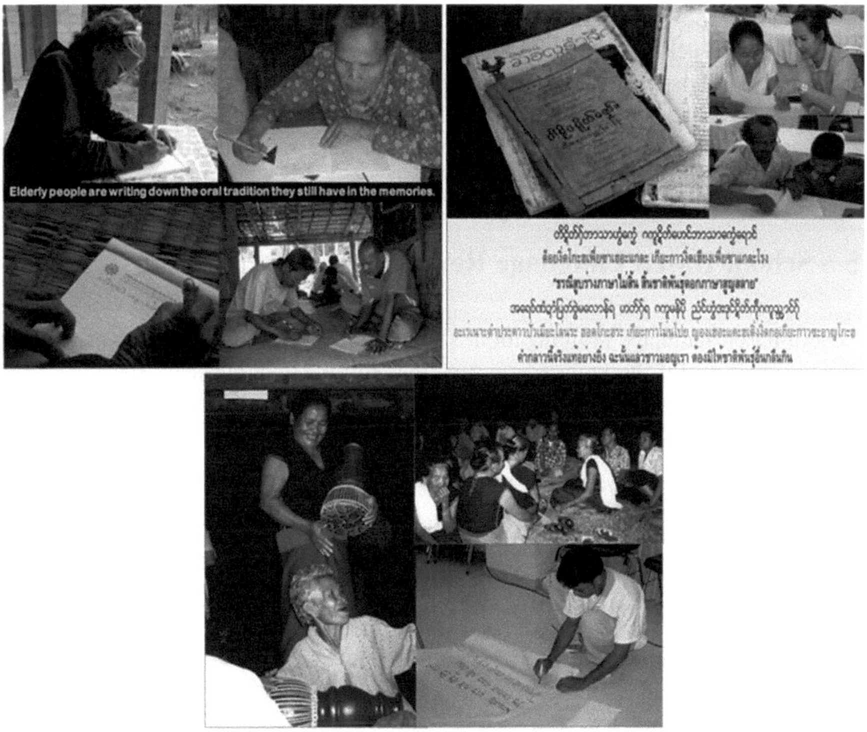

Fig. 1.7 Oral traditions are documented by the language speakers

rituals and ceremonies, and for food. All of these activities undergo continuous monitoring and evaluation, with facilitation as necessary. The eventual goal is to influence the national language and educational policies so as to guarantee that ethnic minority languages are protected and promoted alongside the national and international languages. Ultimately, it aims to ensure full government support for children’s rights “to an education in their own culture and provided in their own language” (United Nations Declaration on the Rights of Indigenous Peoples, Article 14 Section 3) (Fig. 1.7).

For unwritten languages, a writing system will be developed using a practical Thai-based writing system. The language speakers and linguists will work together to develop a writing system that is accepted and standardized (Premsrirat 2007c). For those with a traditional writing system, an orthography bridge may be needed such as Mon (Mae Klong), where a practical Thai-based orthography is used as a tool for studying the Mon script and Mon traditional writing system. Once they have practiced the writing system and have helped to develop it, they can write whatever they have in mind. They can write stories (stage 1–4 books), songs, poetry, personal experiences, and folklore. To be empowered to do these, the language speakers are happy and proud of their work. The dictionary can be compiled and the literature in local languages can be produced. The writing tools can also be used for recording oral literature from the elderly people such as stories and folktales, poetry, and local knowledge about herbal medicine. For those ready to offer an ethnic language class in school, teaching–learning materials will be produced in the local language. Those mentioned are attempts by the language speakers at the grassroots community and academics (mainly linguists).

5 School-Based Language Revitalization

School-based language revitalization is highly prestigious and a dream of the language speakers. Of the language groups that still have enthusiastic speakers, they would prefer to have their language taught in school as part of language revitalization program. There are two types of programs:

- Teaching Mother Tongue (MT) as a Subject (Chong, Nyah Kur, Northern Khmer, Mon (Ratchaburi))
- Teaching Mother Tongue-Based Bilingual Education (MTB BE) (Patani Malay–Thai, Northern Khmer–Thai, Mon–Thai, Lavua–Thai, Hmong–Thai)

Chong and Patani Malay have been selected as case studies to present two kinds of school-based language revitalization programs that involve strong participation of the language speakers and community.

5.1 Chong Language Revitalization Project (CLRP)

Chong is an indigenous language, spoken in Chanthaburi Province, Thailand. At present, there are about 2,000–4,000 speakers. It belongs to the Austroasiatic language family (Pearic branch) and is very famous for its four registers. There has been a rapid decrease in the number of speakers over the last 30 years. Chong people under 30 do not speak Chong. Thai is their first language. Only the older people use Chong in many situations.

The CLRP began with minor cooperation between Chong elders and Mahidol linguists with whom they had formed good relationships following earlier linguistic field work in the Chong area, where the Chong people were invited to join the Field Methods in Linguistic classes. The Chong people are aware that their language is declining. They also realize that their language can be written down and can be taught to other people as well as to their younger generation. They then joined hands with their Mahidol friends for language revitalization (Premsrirat and Malone 2006).

The pilot project began with community motivation and commitment. They then received financial support from the Thailand Research Fund (TRF) to conduct community-based research to solve the problem of language shift and to work on a language revitalization program. Apart from that, they received technical support (as well as moral or psychological support) from an academic institution (Mahidol University, network-linguists, and education experts).

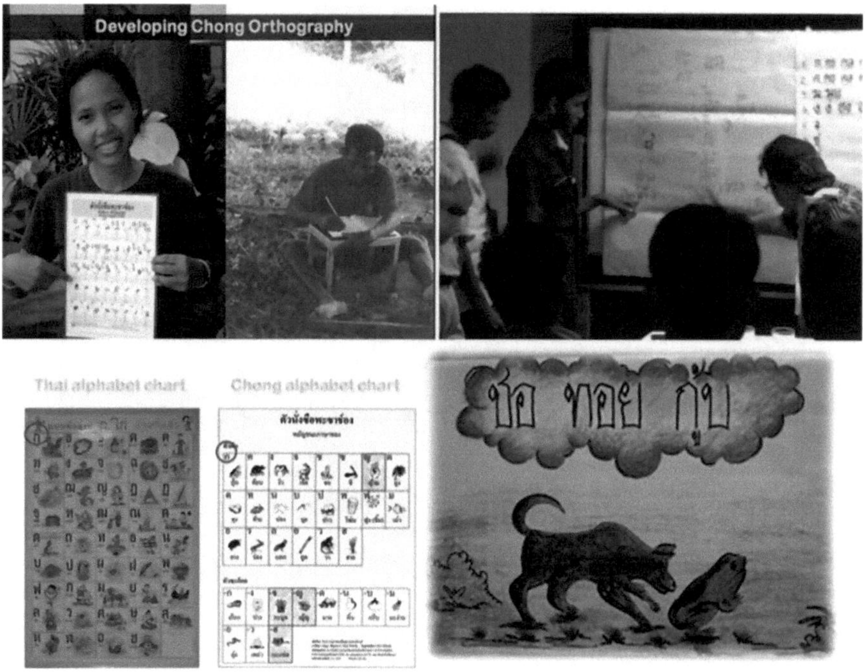

Fig. 1.8 Developing Chong orthography and producing literature in Chong language

Education is used as a tool for language revitalization. Since most ethnic minorities, like the Chong, want to have their language taught to their children at school, language documentation and language development are needed so that ethnic minority languages can be used in education as a tool for language revitalization. As part of the school-based language revitalization, a writing system for Chong was developed, and reading materials were produced. The Chong language is now taught as the subject "Local Studies" to students in three primary schools in the area. The CLRP includes orthography development, literature production, curriculum development, teaching Chong as a subject in school, and a Chong Community Learning Center for the community at large. Other ethnolinguistic groups with the same problem such as the Nyah Kur and the So (Thavung) use the Chong project as a model and adapt it for their own purposes (Figs. 1.8 and 1.9).

5.2 Patani Malay–Thai Mother Tongue-Based Bilingual Education Project in Southern Thailand

The Patani Malay (PM) language is spoken by more than one million Muslim–Thai people in southern Thailand living along the Thai–Malaysian border. In this area, language identity is an issue. It is believed to be one of the main causes underlying the political unrest and violence. The PM language is not officially accepted or used

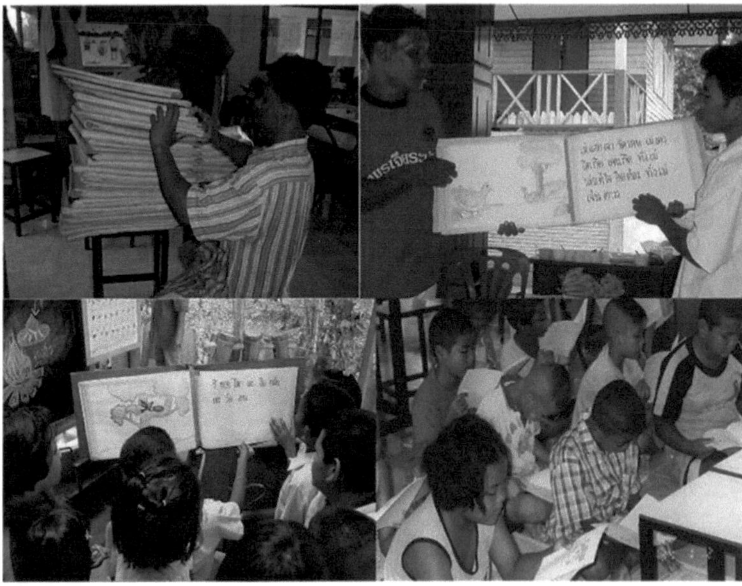

Fig. 1.9 Chong reading materials

in education. It is also declining as evidenced in urban areas of Narathiwat, Pattani, and Yala where a mixed language or creole is being developed and in Satun where language death is obvious. Another related big problem is chronic underachievement in schools. Children attend schools where Thai, the official/national language (but a language which is not their mother tongue), is the only medium of instruction and the content is not relevant to their local context. Because of this, the Patani Malay children scored the lowest in the national examinations given by the Ministry of Education. That means 35–40 % of the grade 3 students are still illiterate.

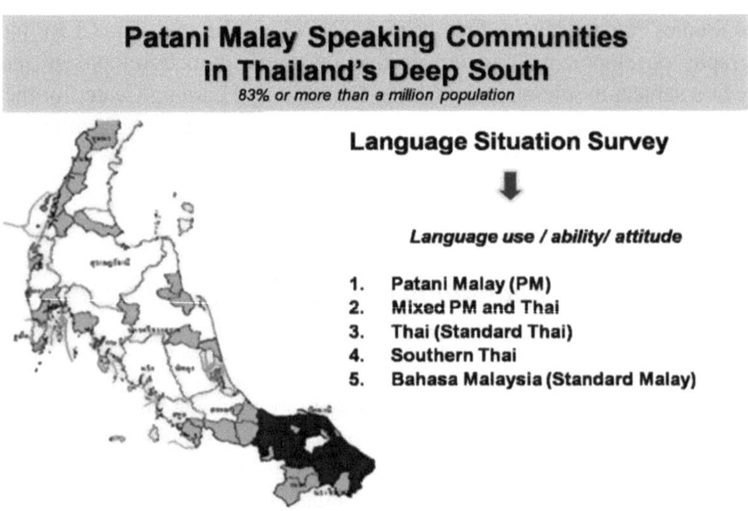

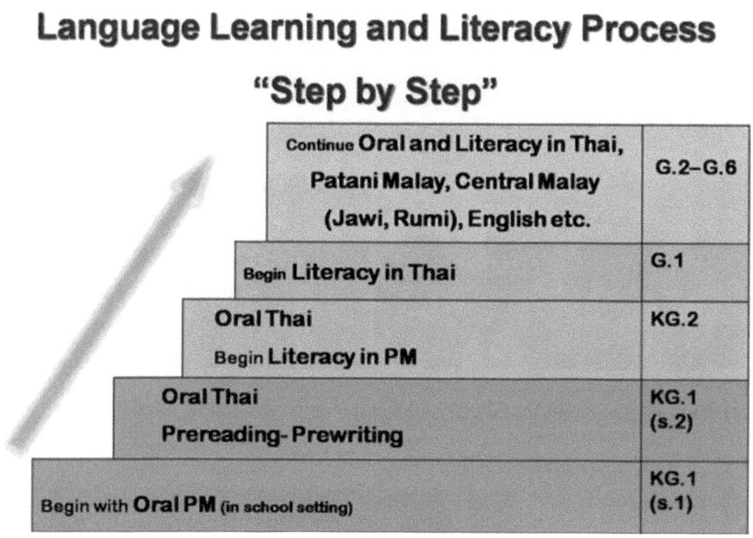

Fig. 1.10 Language learning and literacy process

A Patani Malay–Thai mother tongue-based bilingual education has been conducted as an action participatory research project in four schools in the southernmost provinces of Thailand (Premsrirat 2010). To address the problems of these learners, Mahidol University started a Mother Tongue-Based Education Bilingual Project in a selected Patani Malay community in southern Thailand, after the preliminary research such as the language situation survey has been done. The goals are to facilitate Patani Malay-speaking children to speak, read, and write well in both Patani Malay and Thai, to retain their Malay identity at the local level and Thai identity at the national level and to be able to live with dignity in the wider Thai society in order to foster true and lasting national reconciliation. The project was designed to develop the cognitive skills of the learners as well as their ability to use Thai as a language of learning in the later years of their primary education. The project adheres to the following principles of curriculum design: (1) academic development based on Ministry of Education standards coupled with the community's values and goals; (2) language development in a step-by-step process, starting with their mother tongue (Patani Malay) and gradually bridging to the official language (Thai), developing the four skills of listening, speaking, reading, and writing in both languages simultaneously; and (3) sociocultural development that helps the students preserve their local cultural identity as well as develop a national Thai identity (Figs. 1.10, 1.11, 1.12, and 1.13).

The Patani Malay–Thai bilingual project is being piloted in four primary schools in four southernmost provinces of Thailand where kindergarten 1 and 2 are taught first in Patani Malay, while the Thai language is introduced gradually. This approach will continue through primary grade six. The Southern Border Province Administrative Center planned to expand the project into 27 schools in the academic year 2012.

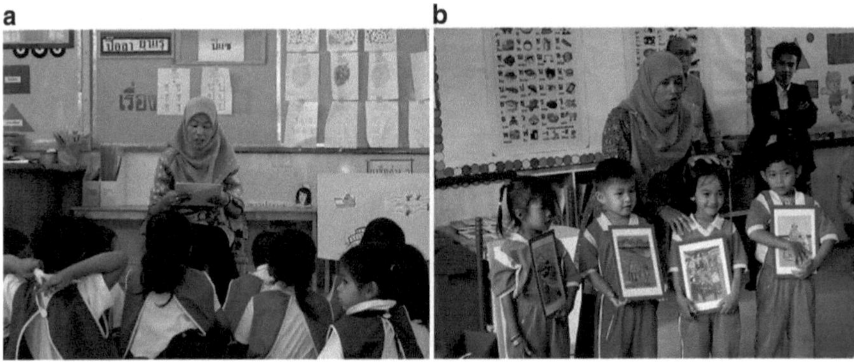

Fig. 1.11 (**a**) Listening to the stories from the community. (**b**) Telling picture stories

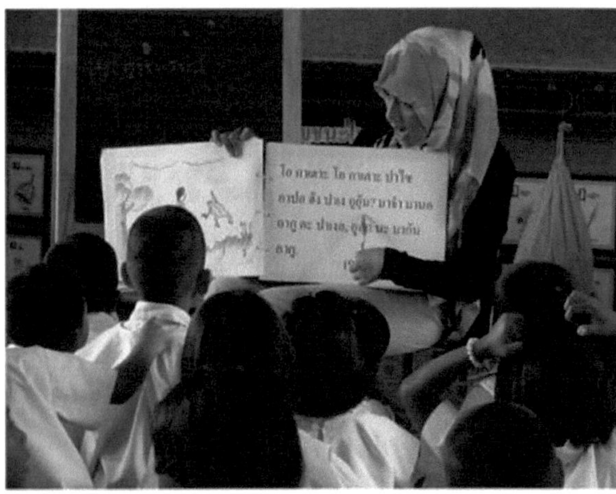

Fig. 1.12 Reading big books

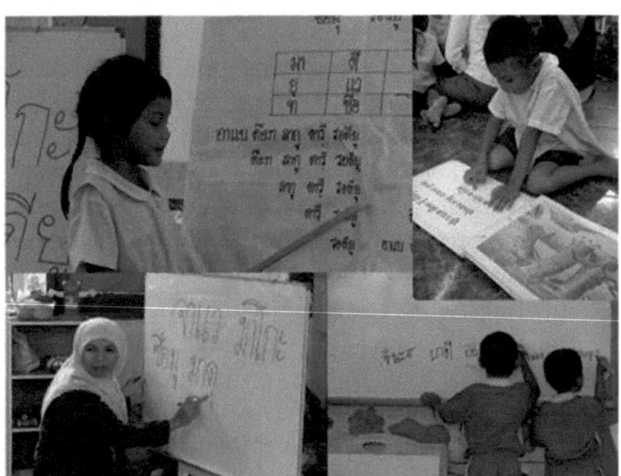

Fig. 1.13 Learning the four skills of listening (thinking), speaking, reading, and writing

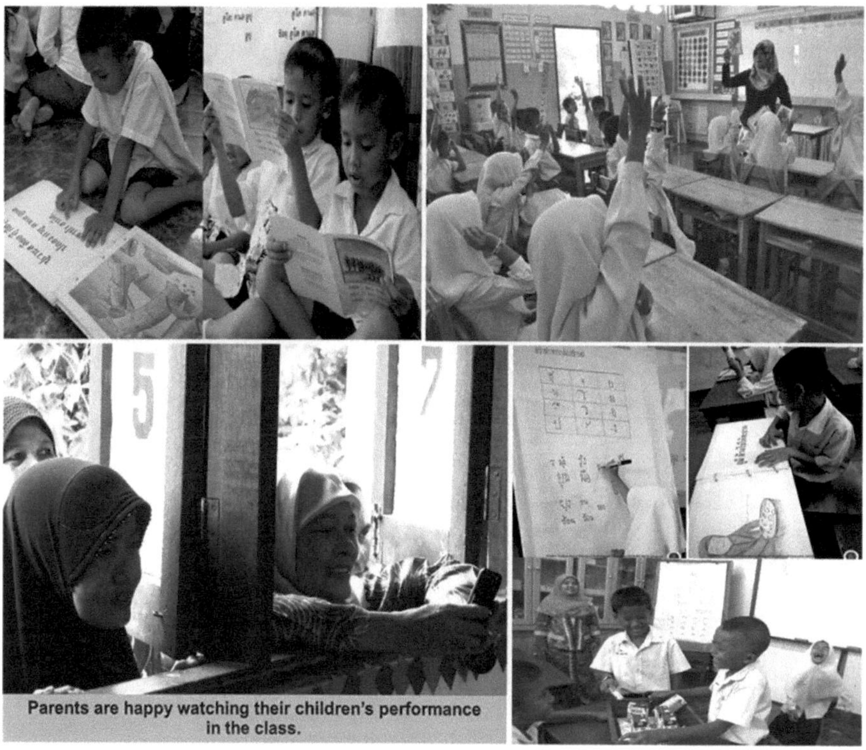
Parents are happy watching their children's performance in the class.

Fig. 1.14 Happy time at school

Comparing the test scores of learners of the Patani Malay pilot bilingual classes with the scores of learners belonging to control groups, it was found that the students in the pilot classes scored higher (avg. 72.14 %) than those belonging to the comparison groups (41.91 %). Furthermore, it was also observed that the learners in the pilot classes were happy, talkative, and creative. They loved going to school and loved reading and writing. The teachers were also happy and the parents were proud of their children (Fig. 1.14).

Two major factors which contributed to these positive results were local community support and a cooperative relationship between the schools and the community members ensuring that the projects are planned and implemented effectively. Multiple stakeholders, like local scholars and artists, religious leaders, school administrators, teachers, parents, academics, and other education officials, were given intensive workshops by Mahidol University to enable them to develop curriculum and teaching–learning materials which are culturally appropriate to the existing knowledge of the learners and still meet the standards set by the Ministry of Education, Thailand. The curriculum emphasizes meaning and understanding as well as accuracy and higher levels of thinking that will enable learners to know, to understand, to analyze, and to be creative in all types of learning activities.

Specifically, the community members and stakeholders were actively involved in the development of orthography, instructional materials, teaching methodology, curriculum design, and lesson plans, and most importantly in providing technical, financial, and psychological support.

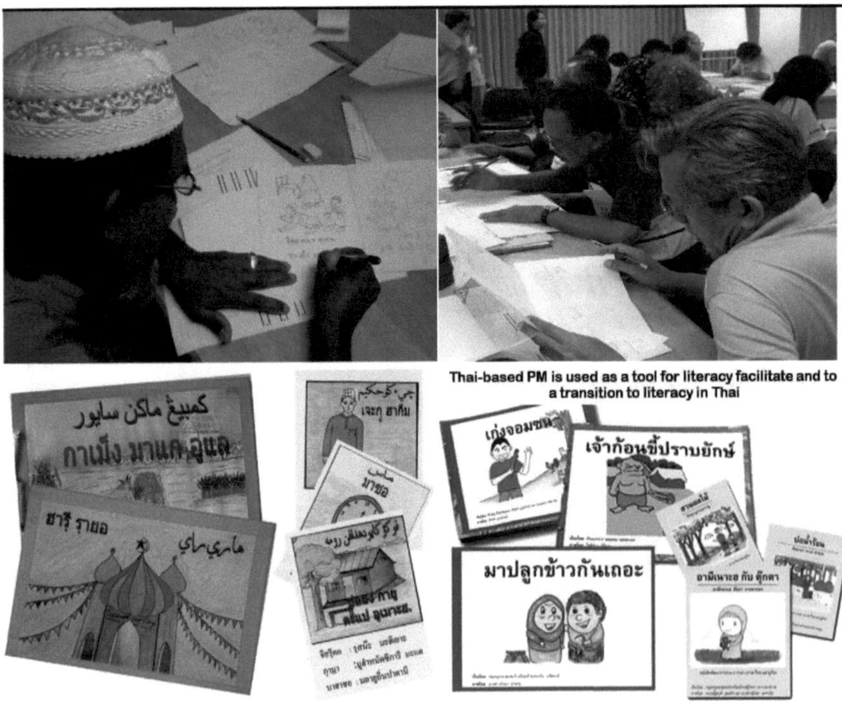
Thai-based PM is used as a tool for literacy facilitate and to a transition to literacy in Thai
มาปลูกข้าวกันเถอะ

The approach pioneered among the Patani Malay is seen as a model for other ethnic minority groups both large and small in Thailand and also among SEAMEO country members. MTB MLE is currently being used as a model for similar projects with various language groups in other parts of Thailand including hill tribe groups such as Lavua-speaking groups in the north and Khmer-speaking groups in the east.

6 International Responses

Language crisis is a global issue. Globalization and nationalism have contributed to the forced assimilation of diverse linguistic and cultural identities into the dominant culture. The reaction from grassroots communities and academics has been witnessed. The UN has responded by calling for the protection and preservation of language and cultural diversity through consecutive campaigns to raise awareness of this global issue. Some of the examples are UNESCO's declaration designating the 21st of February as International Mother Language Day. The UN declaration for

2008 as the "International Year of Languages" accompanied by a list of language-related projects, conferences, publications, and web forums dealing with such issues as language education, endangered languages, intercultural dialogue, indigenous knowledge, and language needs of handicapped persons. In the UN Secretary General's 2008 speech declaring the International Year of Languages, he called for immediate steps to protect and promote endangered languages and to ensure their preservation for the future generations. "The loss of these languages would not only weaken the world's cultural diversity, but also our collective knowledge as a human race" (Bun Ki-moon – UN Secretary General).

As for the basic education issue, there is a worldwide UN campaign in support of "Education for All" (EFA) in 2015, and the Millennium Development Goals (MDGs) provide ethnic minorities with the benefits derived from using the mother tongue-based education. In addition, *the United Nations Declaration on the Rights of Indigenous Peoples, Article 131* states "Indigenous peoples have the right to revitalize, use, develop and transmit to future generations their histories, languages, oral traditions, philosophies, writing systems and literatures," and *the United Nations Declaration on the Rights of Indigenous Peoples, Article 14* requires that "States shall, in conjunction with indigenous peoples, take effective measures, in order for indigenous individuals, particularly children, including those living outside their communities, to have access, when possible, to an education in their own culture and provided in their own language."

UNESCO (United Nations Educational, Scientific and Cultural Organization), UNICEF (United Nations International Children's Emergency Fund), and SEAMEO (Southeast Asian Ministers of Education Organization) also play active roles in promoting mother tongue-based education for ethnic minority children around the world to help them to succeed at school and be included within the larger society while still maintaining their heritage language and culture.

7 Redefining "Thainess": Embracing Diversity, Preserving Unity

In Thailand, globalization and nationalism have contributed to the forced assimilation of diverse linguistic and cultural identities into the dominant culture. The concept of "Thainess" was developed, defined, and has been periodically adjusted to the changing society by notable Thai intellectuals since the 1950s. The main purpose has been to support and maintain the centralized political regime and the hierarchical social structure. This ideology has had a profound influence on the Thai way of thinking and ideology of Thai society and culture (Satayanurak 2008). The practice of "Thainess" in its original senses which is mainly based on three things, the nation (ชาติ), the religion (ศาสนา), and the monarchy (พระมหากษัตริย์), normally refers to the Thai language which is the official/national language used to unify all people into one *nation*, with Buddhism as the *religion* of the majority, under the universal patronage of the *monarchy*. To be a

Thai is to speak Thai, to act or behave as a Thai, to be "good" like a Thai should, and to be educated and maintain one's socioeconomic status according to Thai values. Traits such as a friendly smile by Thais, as "*mai pen rai*" (not so serious) attitude and gentle, kind, and generous demeanor are all considered by Thais as characteristics of "Thainess." Other cultural markers for "Thainess," which people are generally aware of, are food, costume, dance, music, and the ubiquitous "*wai*," the Thai gesture for greeting and showing respect. Most people are happy and proud to identify themselves as Thai. These cultural markers, together with a consciousness of belonging to the same group, exemplify Thai identity and are generally accepted.

One positive aspect of "Thainess" is that one is able to move up the social hierarchy and be accepted doing so in the process. However, perhaps more important to its original adherents is that it can unify people of different ethnicities, languages, and cultures into a single nation. The use of the Thai language makes it possible for a common education curriculum to be promoted throughout the entire country. As a result, we can witness in Khmer–Thai areas, for example, Khmer elders, people who have joined the revitalization program, writing stories, songs, and poetry in Northern Khmer by using the Thai-based writing system. The identification of oneself as Thai, and the recognition and manifestation of Thai cultural markers, generally indicates an awareness and sense of possession of Thai identity. Notwithstanding this, a young Patani Malay-speaking man from Pattani may be happy and proud to be a Thai at a national level, but at the same time prefer to maintain his Melayu identity at a local level. So, although the promotion of the concept of "Thainess" has been very successful as far as its primary purpose of nation building is concerned, it has greatly contributed to the loss of language diversity among the 15 most endangered languages of Thailand and thereby focused attention on identity issues and cultural conflict among the large language groups in border regions such as the Patani Malay in southern Thailand.

With strife come solutions and there are now concerted efforts by grassroots communities to reverse this situation. With the technical support of academics, progress is being made in revitalizing and maintaining their language and cultural identity in various ways, including through education. Important methods used to this end include, first, the teaching of the ethnic language as a main subject such as those doing it among the Chong, Nyah Kur, Thavung, and smaller, seriously endangered languages facing the same problem and, second, the provision of mother tongue-based bilingual education to larger language groups, including Patani Malay, Mon, and Northern Khmer. To be able to cope with the complexity of a changing society, the notion of what is good for the nation and its citizens, and the required virtues for leadership, should be broadened. A multilingual/multicultural society should be envisaged and promoted to accommodate this undervalued cultural diversity. The notion of "Thainess" needs to be redefined to accommodate and maintain the language and cultural diversity of Thailand to offer ethnolinguistic groups their own space within Thai political society on an equal basis so that they may be empowered to live a dignified life with security, justice, and opportunity. Central to this is access to quality education and employment, to reinvigorate their cultural and linguistic identity. See also Chaps. 8, 15, and 32 for discussions on "Thainess."

8 Reconsideration of National Language Policy

Despite an attempt to guarantee the freedom of expression and non-discrimination on the basis of fundamental human rights, and an implicit recognition of the intimate connection between language and forms of cultural expression, the current national language policy is radically out of step with the realities of multilingualism. A national language policy that promotes a multicultural society and supports the use of ethnic languages in public life, education, and local mass media is crucial in order to meet the demands and needs of the various marginalized minority groups in Thailand. Such a policy will open up opportunities to positively exploit the variety of accumulated wealth and wisdom embodied within such unique cultures and linguistic histories and will provide sustainable public benefits in terms of both economic and security gains. It is hoped, therefore, that along with the promotion of Thai as the national/official language and languages such as English and Chinese as favored interactional languages, support for the use of ethnic languages belonging to the Thai and other language families, in public life, education, and the local mass media, is sorely needed to meet the demands and needs of ethnic minority marginalized groups. Such support will lead to sustainable public benefits in terms of both economic and security gains. In this way, Thailand will benefit from a language policy that strengthens the Thai language while preserving Thailand's ethnic minority/indigenous languages, encouraging Thais to learn strategic regional and international languages and ensuring information access for Thailand's blind and deaf communities. The recognition and respect that derives from truly interconnected and synergized communities will bring together Thais from all walks of life in true reconciliation, security, and happiness.

9 Conclusion

A dynamic and changing society demands a contemporary approach to interpreting and managing complex sociocultural issues. The notion of "Thainess," so effectively absorbed into the universal Thai psyche over more than 50 years, has undoubtedly been a cornerstone of nation building and creation of popular identity. It was also outstandingly successful in justifying and facilitating a centralized administration and validating traditional prejudices and social inequalities. Its significance today is diminished in its current, somewhat archaic, guise and a modern and more sophisticated understanding of what it means to be Thai is overdue: one that meets the hopes and expectations of all Thais and meets universal standards in terms of rights and opportunities. For some, this may require a substantive paradigm shift in perspective, but the potential rewards are unlimited. Reconciliation and capitalization of local knowledge and wisdom are just a start. Ultimately, the pride and confidence that comes from true recognition and respect for one's heritage, culture, and language is the optimal path to future unity, security, and a wealth of human dignity which goes to the heart of true Thainess.

References

Crystal, D. (2000). *Language death*. Cambridge: Cambridge University Press.

Fishman, J. (1991). *Reversing language shift*. Clevedon: Multilingual Matters.

Krauss, M. (1992). The world's languages in crisis. *Language, 68*(1), 4–10.

Premsrirat, S. (2006a). Thailand: Language situation. In K. Brown (Ed.), *Encyclopedia of language and linguistics* (2nd ed., pp. 642–644). Oxford: Elsevier.

Premsrirat, S. (2006b). History of Thainess. In *The new image of being Thai*. Nakhon Pathom: Institute of Population and Social Studies and Center for Peace Studies, Mahidol University.

Premsrirat, S. (2007a). Endangered languages of Thailand. *International Journal of the Sociology of Language, 186*, 75–93.

Premsrirat, S. (2007b). Revitalizing ethnic minority language. *Sangsaeng, 18*, 8–11.

Premsrirat, S. (2007c). Language situation and ethnolinguistic diversity in Thai society. *Journal of Language and Culture, 25*(2), 1–11 (In Thai).

Premsrirat, S. (2008). Language for national reconciliation: Southern Thailand. *EENET* (*Enabling Education Network*). Issue August 12, 2008. Accessed from www.eenet.org.uk

Premsrirat, S. (2010, November). *The role of MTB MLE in ECD and education: Experiences and challenges in southern Thailand*. Paper presented at MDGs conference. Accessed from http://www.seameo.org/LanguageMDGConference2010/presentations.html, UNESCO.

Premsrirat, S. (Forthcoming). Revitalizing ethnic minority languages. In S. Premsrirat, & D. Hirsh (Eds.), *Indigenous language revitalization: Insights from Thailand*. Peter Lang International Academic Publisher.

Premsrirat, S., & Others. (2004). *Ethnolinguistic maps of Thailand*. The National Cultural Commission of Thailand (In Thai).

Premsrirat, S., & Malone, D. (2006). Language development and language revitalization in Asia. *Mon – Khmer Studies, 35*, 101–120.

Chapter 2
The Giant Swing (*Lo Ching Cha*): Brahmanical Origins and Its Significance to the Religious Culture of Thailand

Willard G. Van De Bogart

1 Introduction

Stately, silent, motionless, and majestic are two towering teak wood pillars reaching to the sky in the center of Bangkok symbolizing a gateway to another time and another world. What was once a center piece for pomp and ceremony attended by kings and queens is now only a bare reminder of the once grand royal ceremony that invited the Hindu gods to visit earth.

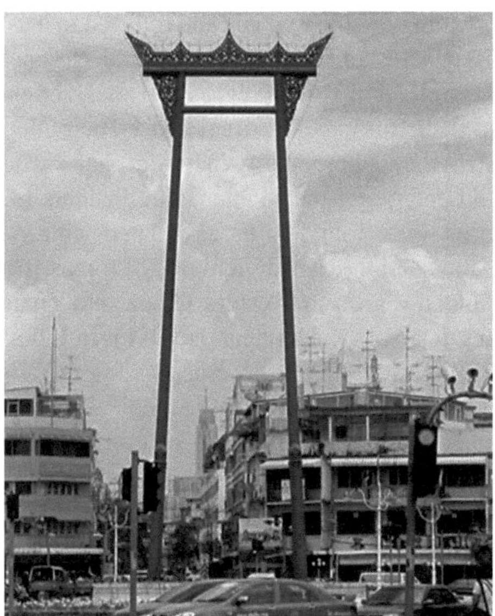

Giant Swing, Bangkok Thailand (Photo by Van De Bogart)

W.G. Van De Bogart (✉)
Language Institute, Bangkok University, Rangsit 12120, Thailand
e-mail: willard.v@bu.ac.th

P. Liamputtong (ed.), *Contemporary Socio-Cultural and Political Perspectives in Thailand*, DOI 10.1007/978-94-007-7244-1_2, © Springer Science+Business Media Dordrecht 2014

This is the Giant Swing, an enigmatic symbol that has been interpreted in many different ways but is for certain one of the most venerated historical sites in Thailand.

The origins of this stately historical landmark have taken me on a research adventure, much like a pilgrimage to a sacred site, causing me to wonder how in fact the humble swing became such a spiritual icon for the Nation State of Thailand. The many descriptions which are offered to explain what the swing is used for does not, as I have discovered, tell the whole story on how a swing could become Thailand's most important spiritual symbol with the exception of the emerald Buddha. Be that as it may, I believe that after reviewing the historical literature mentioned below and the current research related to swinging in the Hindu culture, a new appreciation for this landmark in Thailand will be gained.

2 Historical Perspective

Before I repeat any of the popular definitions of the Giant Swing, a short survey of the magical and spiritual uses of swings both ancient as well as in recent times is in order.

There have been a few other researchers who have also been curious about the origins of swinging. Most notable is James G. Fraser (1919) who wrote "Swinging as a Magical Rite," and Mircea Eliade (2004), who devoted extensive time researching how shamans used swinging in their rituals and referred to it as "Magical Flight." More recently, two Russian researchers (Sharapov and Nesanelis 1997) went to North Russia's Komi Republic and Tumen region and analyzed the theme of swinging used by shamans in their folklore and ritual texts. Their ethnographic research lends insight into the rhythmic perception in traditional worldview, as well as rhythm as a cultural and creational mechanism. The insights to rituals connected with the swinging motion were found to be associated with symbols of cyclical time, purification, sexuality, and the banishment of evil forces. The migration of the Akha tribe from the Yunnan region in Western China into Thailand brought with them their own swinging festival (Kacha-ananda 1971). In India, practically every region has an annual swinging festival, the oldest being in Orissa (Bhattacharya 2010) as well as references to swinging in the Vedic scriptures (Tandya Maha Brahmana, Vol. V, Chapter 1, Verse 10) of which we can take some clues and cover later to further our understanding of swinging.

Why swinging had been created by all these ancient cultures would take more space than this chapter allows, but there are certain features about swinging which can be discussed so that a clearer view of the act of swinging can be understood in the context of a cosmological framework.

Eventually, we will arrive at the doorstep of an ancient temple in Ayutthaya, Thailand, where a swing was offered as a gift to King Ramathibodi II, the 11th King of Siam (1491–1538), by two Brahman priests from South India (Van Vliet 1640). Let us first consider what swinging could represent and take our cues from Sharapov and Nesanelis (1997). These authors suggest that swinging originally came from an interpretive sense of the cosmos as it was seen by our earliest ancestors spread out before them in the heavens, but they did not have a developed language to communicate what the heavens meant or how to describe what it was they actually saw. The world must have appeared to our ancestors as some sort of magical symphony composed of all the elements in the natural world presented as a myriad of kaleidoscopic imagery. We could probably assume that the number of physical events which affected our earliest ancestors either caused them to become entranced by what they saw or extremely fearful of what they heard. Obviously, both forms of emotional responses were elicited by a reaction to the unknowingness of what constituted the makeup of the physical world. However, once our ancestors became accustomed to the repetition of these natural events, they then could be accepted and integrated into the existing social fabric. The symbolic significance of the phenomena of heavenly bodies is what eventually evolved into rituals and much later into religions. It was the inception of these natural phenomena into the cognitive framework of man's perceived world that prompted him to be very curious as to why stars and other celestial events moved in the heavens the way they did.

Obviously, this process of merging mind and heaven has been going on for thousands of years, as is evidenced by recent archaeological discoveries of fire altars, dated 3000 BCE, in the Harappan civilization (Feuerstein et al. 1995). Trying to imagine how events that were taking place in the heavens became part of everyday rituals for early civilizations may be difficult to understand. However, accepting the proposition that heaven and earth were connected in the minds of our early ancestors as one cosmocentric whole, which offered meaning and sustenance to their existence, then what we see today with rituals and ceremonies most assuredly originated from a time unknown; a time when language began and meaning was being developed.

Saraswati (1995: 1) suggests that the traditional vision of man is cosmocentric. In his introduction to the oral tradition, he states:

> Man is made up of four of five cosmic elements. The cosmic order that governs the dynamism of all reality, envelops human life, creates awareness, and signifies patterns of culture. As a result, the cosmic equilibrium is maintained both in nature and in culture. This primal vision is incontestable and fully integrated in two different but related traditions; the textual and the oral. The textual tradition offers a complete and systematic analysis of the universe. Reflections of the oral tradition are more concentrated in practice than systematic in analysis.

Within this oral or pretextual tradition, we can only imagine how the early personifications with nature were implemented within small tribal groupings. Since the origin of the swing is our main concern, we need to look at what the natural phenomena, comprised of the five elements, and the nature of being human have in common. What aspect to the integration of man and nature exhibit swinging? I pose a simple question of what exactly is swinging. What function was experienced initially in the hoary past which could be demonstrated by something suspended in the air only to be watched and witnessed moving with the wind? Clues to answering this question are many. Trees move in the wind, comets move across the sky, birds fly in the air, the breath moves in and out of the human body, the sun and moon move back and forth across the sky, and the heavens show a rhythmic oscillation with the stars. In a sense, everything in nature is swinging and nothing is static.

Swinging was a part of life, and the imaginings of nature's movements were built into the creation stories of these early oral cultures and eventually acceptance on how certain relationships of the forces of nature could be explained led to performing sacrifices and rituals.

Of the many phenomena that could be witnessed by our earliest ancestors, none could be more dramatic than seeing a solar eclipse or a comet streaking across the heavens with thunderous explosions in its wake. The water that fell out of the sky produced most all of the creation myths that were populated with gods who represented these sounds of thunder and bolts of lightning which most certainly caused fear and trembling and a deep respect for the forces of nature. But, it was in the evening, with no observable sun or moon that another sight unfolded, one which we of today still observe no differently than in times past, which is none other than the star studded canopy in the heavens.

This star-studded canopy is our template to work with as we try to understand how our ancient ancestors perceived the heavens. What kind of inner reflections of the universe were imagined when trying to formulate ideas and postulate concepts of existence? At this point, we have to consider the primal elements affecting those distant people in a time when only sensual data was experienced and from those assumed sensual impressions try to understand how a complex social order developed where obeisance to all these celestial phenomena took on a self-organizing principle on how people would interact among themselves and the world around them. This was the birth of a cosmocentric lifestyle where everything had meaning and was integrated into every aspect of daily living.

To offer an explanation on how swinging began from this cosmocentric worldview, I will suggest, as Saraswati (1995) states, that they originated out of this cosmocentric lifestyle, which permeated the early tribal cultures, and in an attempt to describe their world began with the natural forces comprising earth, air, fire and, water. When early man became conscious of his contact with nature, he personified the phenomena of nature (Chaubey 1998). These early cultures also created gods who became supernatural and have been part of all tribal and orthodox rituals up to the present day.

3 Tribal Swinging

3.1 Origins of Hook Swinging

Included in these cosmocentric cultures were stories and beliefs where a central pole or pillar would be installed in the center of the village symbolizing a connection between the upper world and the underworld thus establishing their center in the universe. How this central pole (stamba) and swinging (dola) were combined can be seen in the very ancient act of the charak-puja (Fig. 2.1), better known as "hook swinging."

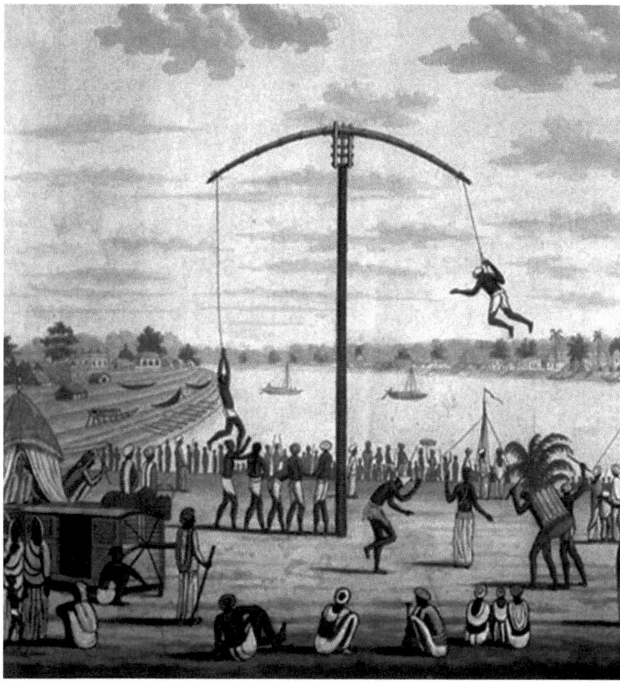

Fig. 2.1 Churruck Poojah on the banks of the Ganges by James Moffat, c. 1806

The relationship of hook swinging to the classical forms of swinging has not been discussed at great length in the literature. However, in 1914, a lengthy description of hook swinging was published suggesting it may be a direct link to an earlier form of human sacrifice (Powell 1914).

Sacrifice as a way to identify with the cosmic order was a way early humans could identify with the larger macrocosm and how the original cosmic man (Purusha) came into existence from out of the primordial waters where only the intention of existence was vibrating in the universe (Feuerstein et al. 1995). Anthropologists distinguish two streams of traditions in India called the "high" tradition which uses the legitimacy of the Vedic scriptures and the "low" traditions which are dependent on oral traditions and myths (Khubchandani 1995). Obviously, the Brahmins followed the high tradition and conducted rituals to the gods utilizing swinging which was not associated with bodily sacrifices. Both forms of swinging, aboriginal and caste, did exist side by side for centuries. But, the swinging performed by the lower tradition was a syncretic ritual combining both nature and man representing a cosmocentric worldview.

The liturgical and scriptural forms of swinging were created to have more access to the gods rather than be dictated by them. This is clearly demonstrated in the Thiruppavai and Thiruvempavai ceremony in Thailand where the gods are actually invited to come down to earth. The scriptures which show more direct access to the

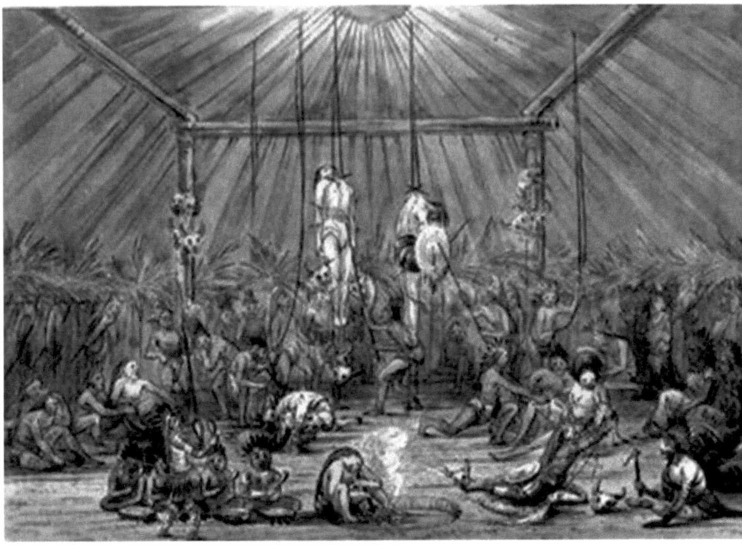

Fig. 2.2 Native American Indians in a Sundance suspension ritual

gods were associated with astronomy and the meaning given to the stars in order to explain creation which eventually became the origins of all the creation myths.

Two other forms of ancient swinging are worth mentioning briefly, one suspension swinging by the Native American Indians and the airborne swinging by the Akha tribe in Northern Thailand. I include these two types of swinging to show how placing the body in the air was an act of sacrifice and a form of ritual which seems to be pervasive in all tribal cultures most likely being reminiscent of a very ancient memory of some event that took place in the distant past. I will cover this aspect of an ancient memory and the symbols which can still be found related to ancient Hindu scriptures in the last section (Fig. 2.2).

Piercing the flesh and being suspended in the air was a sacrifice performed by the Native Americans in order to reach a trance state so as to receive spiritual guidance from the invisible spirits and a way to offer the physical body in exchange for a spiritual life (Campos 2010). The Sundance ceremony recognized the sun's new rise every day representing rebirth after a symbolic death. This is a clear example of how powerful the impressions of nature held over the minds of these native people.

3.2 *Ethnic Swinging in Thailand*

The Akha tribe in the north of Thailand installs four poles in the ground (Fig. 2.3), and by attaching a single cord at the apex they can swing out into the air.

The history of the Akha swing ceremony suggests that Appremiere, the Akha's god, created the world. The gods Umsa and Umyae were also created representing

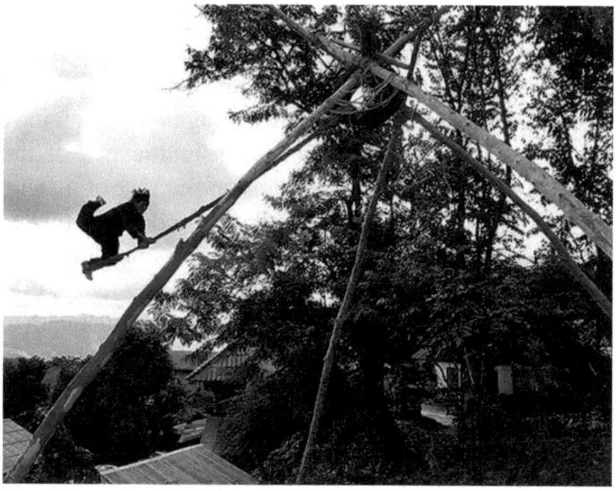

Fig. 2.3 Akha swing ceremony Chiang Rai Province, Thailand

the rain and sunshine. Theses gods were man and wife and had one son, Umsahyee, and one daughter, Umsahyeh. It is told that the swing ceremony was started by Umsahyeh to honor the godparents and assure plenty of rain and sunshine. All three depictions of the tribal swing exhibit a cosmocentric relationship to the natural forces (Kacha-ananda 1971).

4 Swinging in Ancient Temples of India

4.1 Archaeological Evidence for Swinging

The rural communities of the coastal and central areas of Orissa perform the Danda ritual devoted to the Shiva-Shakti cult; however, among the more orthodox Hindus, Durga or Devi is far more popular (Citaristi 1995). It is interesting to note that in these Danda rituals, self-punishments were performed whereby swinging was done upside down over burning ashes and known as the ritual of Ugra Pata. I mention this because burning coals will be made clearer when the archaeological research by Godbole (2010) is cited where he refers to meteors hitting the earth.

It is in the Eastern province of Orissa that we find the oldest swing ceremony dating as far back as the second century CE (Bhattacharya 2010). The name given to this swing ceremony is the Rajo (menstruation) which coincides with the summer solstice in the northern hemisphere. The ancient name associated with this ancient geographical area of India is Kalinga. Rajo (menstruation) is a 3-day "menstrual period" for mother earth and a date coincident with the Gemini asterism (*mithuna*). At the geo-location of Orissa, the Rajo is held on the second day where the sun touches the ecliptic with the Gemini asterism and is called *Sankranti* and is the main day of the swing festival. In this same geo-location, on the full moon during spring equinox the swing ceremony is called the "*Dola Purnima*." This full moon is in syzygy with central Orissa and is the location of the Lord Jagannath temple dated between the nineteenth and fifteenth centuries CE. At the Eastern gate of the temple is an engraving of a large ship in sailing mode, showing Kalinga, the great sovereign, sitting on a swing seat. The main significance of these two festivals in ancient Kalinga is that of the king sitting on the seat of a swing and traveling on a ship in the sacred temple. This makes the Rajo directly related to astronomical indicators giving us more clues that the swing has more symbolism associated with it than was initially recognized by earlier scholars, i.e., Gerini, Frazer, and Wales.

Another astronomical indicator at Lord Jagannath's temple is a carved relief of Nataraja (Fig. 2.7) which acts like a celestial compass (Fig. 2.8) (Bhattacharya and Nail 2008). The discovery was made by showing how *alpha Orioni*s (Rudra-star Betelgeuse) moves away from the ecliptic and celestial equator, now at 7° north of the equator. In 60 more years, Rudra will move south of the equator and be closer to *beta-Orionis* (Gouri -star Rigel) in the Gemini asterism as it begins to move north. This Hara-Gouri conjunction is how precessional movement brought these two stars together creating the concept of swinging. These findings and others came from noticing how the temple complexes at Bhubaneswar were built to reflect the position of the stars. In particular, the Parasurameswara temple acted as the center forming a star pattern (Taraka) formed by radial lines drawn out and connected to other temples in the area. A similar radial pattern could be found directly above in the heavens with *alpha Orionis* (Rudra-Beatleguese) being the center. The Orion constellation was, therefore, a very significant part of this temple complex in the *Siddhantic* (naked eye viewing) astronomy texts with *beta-Orionis* (Rigel) given the Puranic name of *Bana Raj*, meaning "King with Arrow." The relationship between Parasurameswara and Lingaraj temples is noteworthy. The star Sirius is called *Lubdhaka* and in the Siddhanta the consort of Rudra is *Lubdhaka*, which corresponds to the temple on the ground identified as Gouri, which is located directly next to Parasurameswara. Prior to the tenth century CE, Siva was the presiding deity of the Parasurameswara temple and would travel with a priestly entourage to the Gouri temple thus mirroring the Siddhantic connection of the stars of Rudra and Lubdhaka. This ceremony is still held today with a swing ceremony indicating its celestial origins. In fact, the most ancient Hindu temple art in Bhubaneswar depicting a swing is from the late eighth century CE and is in the Mukteswar temple (Fig. 2.4) as well as the elaborately carved Torana (arched gateway) used for swinging (Fig. 2.5). The swing at Mukteswar could have been used as a celestial reference for the movement between these two stars of Rudra and Gouri.

This being the case, it is entirely possible that the act of swinging was a way to travel the entire arc of heavens and also a way to understand the position of the stars. The swing could have acted as a celestial dial with the arms and legs of Lord Shiva (*Anirudha* – synonym of Siva) fixing a center place in the universe among the stars (much like the *Stamba*) but using *alpha Orionis* as the center. The swing would then symbolize the inclination of the ecliptic approaching and receding from the celestial equator mimicking the movement of Orion over time as well as the precessional cycle of 26,000 years, thus making Nataraja a candidate as a precessional marker.

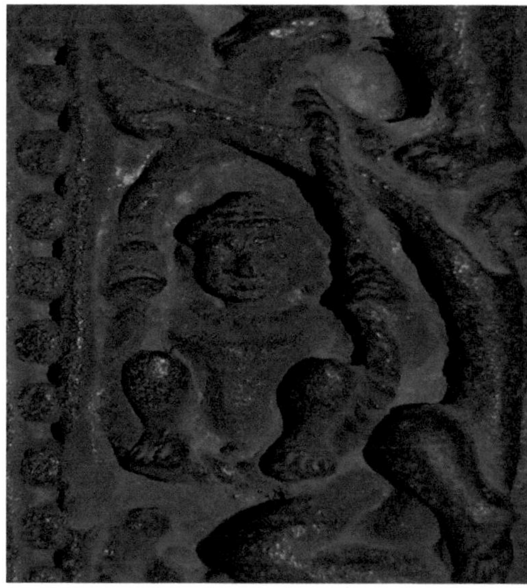

Fig. 2.4 Eighth century CE carving depicting swinging

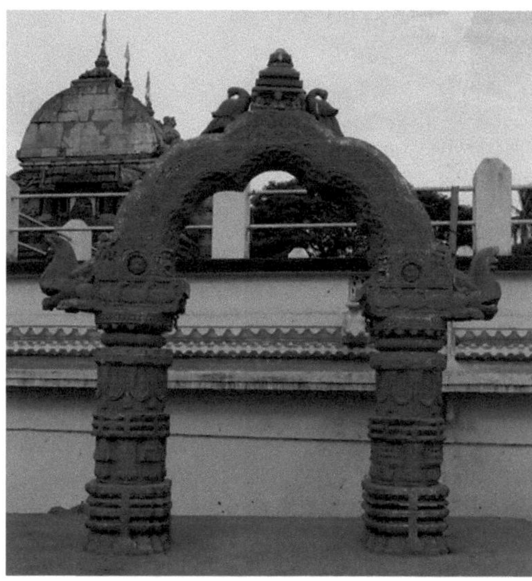

Fig. 2.5 Torana at Mukteswar temple

The Giant Swing Ceremony in Thailand, which invites Lord Shiva to earth once a year, shows a direct relationship to this ancient ceremony in Kalinga, India, where the center of the universe is symbolized by a swing. The name Taraka was taken from the *Thiruvachagam* and *Koyil purana* where it mentions the "Forest of Taraka" where Lord Shiva, in his Nataraja form, is said to have appeared on earth for the first time indicating the center of the universe. The star *Anirudha* (Siva) is the central member of the Orion constellation known as *Kalapurusha* (embodiment of time) giving the Nataraja its symbolic reference to other stars.

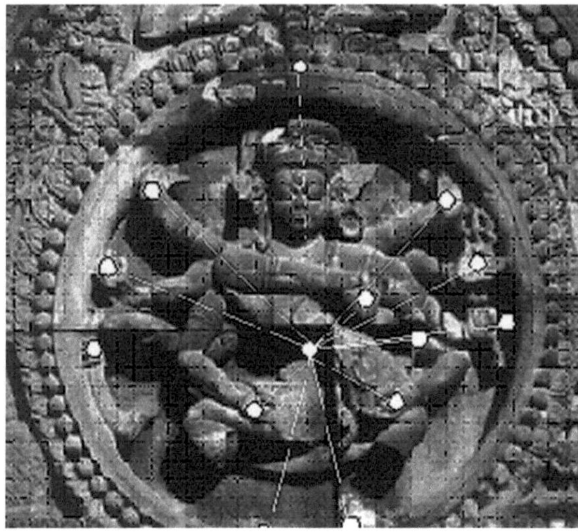

Fig. 2.6 Nataraja at Lord Jagannath temple with compass overlay

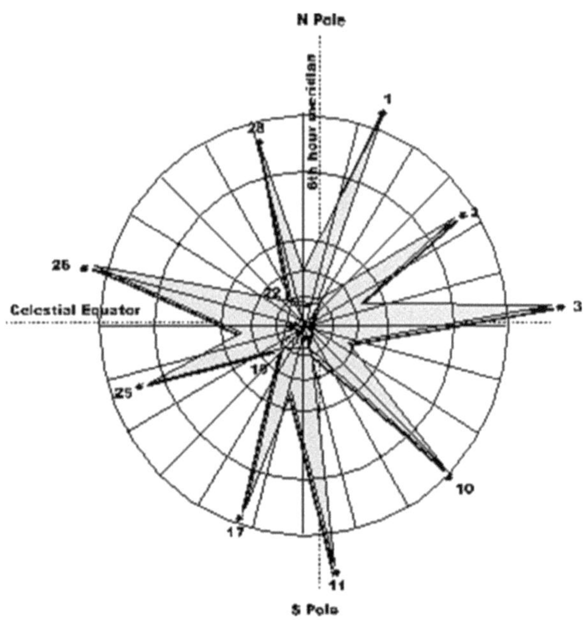

Fig. 2.7 Star pattern over compass

The term Taraka also means falling star indicating Shiva's footstep on earth was none other than a celestial citing. More on this aspect of a falling star will be covered later in the paper (Figs. 2.6 and 2.7).

The heights to which swinging became a significant part of the temple complexes in India is best shown at the Chittuldroog temple in Chamondee (Fig. 2.8). The three worlds of Hindu cosmology comprised of hell, heaven, and earth were always connected by a central pillar which can be seen at the tenth century Chittuldroog

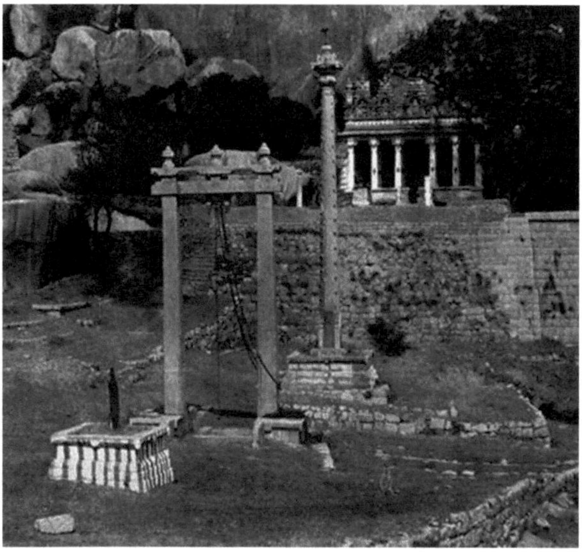

Fig. 2.8 Pillar and swing in the court of Chamundi Temple, Chitradurga

temple. Placed directly in front of the pillar is a swing carved from solid stone. By juxtaposing the swing next to the cosmic pillar is a significant indication to its inherent celestial symbolism. Similarly, a central pillar and swing were installed at the founding of the new capital of Bangkok. There can be no question as to the influence the Vedic swing ceremony had on how the Chakri dynasty would use both these Hindu artifacts to symbolize a relationship to the heavens as well as securing a way to communicate with the gods.

But, the Chamundi temple is not the only temple with a stone structure still standing indicating that swinging was a major part of the rituals and ceremonies of these ninth to tenth century temple complexes. The ancient Vitthala temple of Hampi in old Vijayanagara is a beautifully carved swing made from granite (Fig. 2.9). This swing is referred to as a *mandapa* with two cylindrical columns. Metal hooks attached to the beam above held a swing in which a sacred image was placed when it was removed from the Hoysalas (marriage hall) named Kalyana Mandapam when gods and goddesses were united on festive days. It is noteworthy to mention that there is a ceremonial avenue starting from the main temple gate where a chariot process takes place and the gods are transported to the swing. This is exactly what is meant by a "ship bound to heaven" which I will discuss further on.

4.2 Astronomical References to Swinging

Another example is the Hindola Torana at the Mala Devi temple in Gyaraspur (Fig. 2.10) built during the medieval period, in Madhya Pradesh. Mala Devi temple – sixteenth century – is constructed on the eastern slope of the hill. The temple

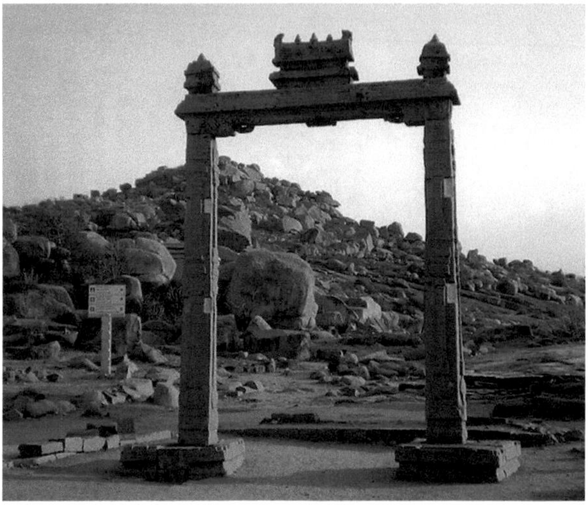

Fig. 2.9 Swing at Vitthala temple in Hampi

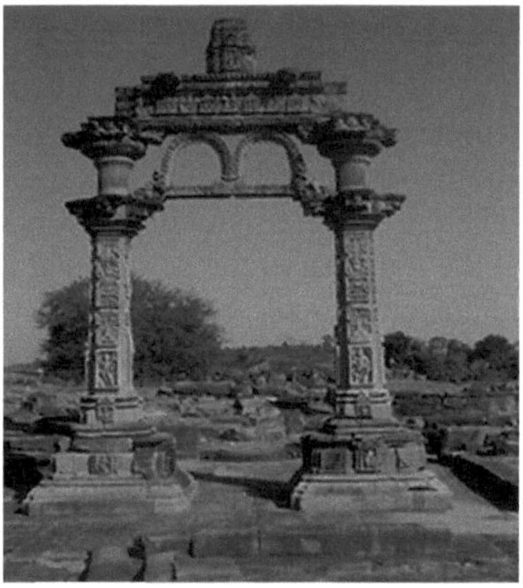

Fig. 2.10 Hindola Torana – Gyaraspur

is partly rock-cut and partly structural. The sanctum door jambs have Ganga, Yamuna, and other Hindu deities. Inside the sanctum are placed four Jain Tirthankar images, seated on padmasana. There is a sikhara above the sanctum, where Vaishnavi, seated on Garuda, is placed. What can we deduce from these symbolic deities? Most significantly is the river Ganga also referred as the celestial river or the Milky Way and Vishnu mounted on Garuda who is ready to take flight. The double arches sitting on top of the cross beam could very easily symbolize the swinging path of the stars during the long precessional cycle as (Allen 2008) has indicated on the planisphere diagram (Fig. 2.11) which also shows the celestial river (Ganga), Milky Way galaxy. Allen (2008) sees the study of precession as a study of time and represents the longest swing period which is the truly great swing across the heavens. The essence of oscillations, such as swings, is that they

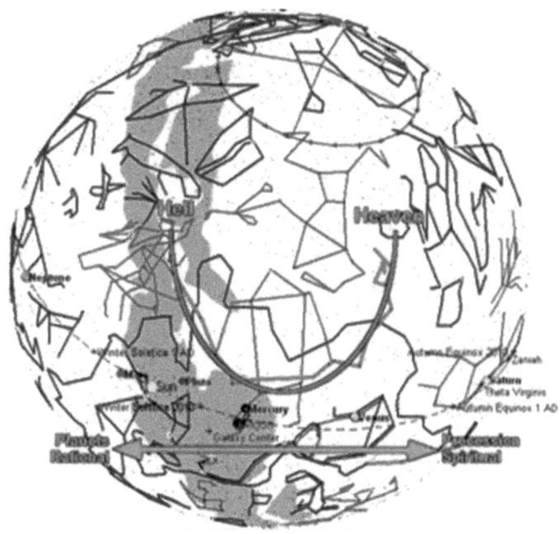

Fig. 2.11 Celestial gates (Allen 2008)

represent the return to origins. For Allen, the giant swing in the heavens symbolizes the restoration of the cognition of creative intent which is the same as (Reiser 1978) with his intent of creation.

5 Swinging Mentioned in Tamil Lyrics

Accompanying rituals were human sounds which are now classified as chants, mantras, and songs (Staal 1996: 191–362). The integration of all these elements are beyond the scope of this chapter, but the seeds for the origin of swinging most certainly comes from these primal observances and enactments of human behavior through sound.

Much later on in the evolution of tribal cultures, the oral traditions were translated into written form. This process of human sounds leading to a meaningful exchange of language for communication took thousands of years to develop. The symbolism is quite extensive when we approach the pathways of the gods with their descent to earth and return to their heavenly abode, which has been a recurring theme in all cosmogonic myths. In Indian music, we have terms signifying going from a low pitch to a high pitch (Aarohanam) and from a high pitch to a low pitch (Avarohanam) (Ramaswamy 2010). In the Dasaavataara stotram mentioning the Matsya Avataaram (Vishnu as fish), the interpretation is as follows:

> ChaDaa Dola AarOha sadOhaLam bhagavatha
>
> The ebb and flow of the waves of the Ocean seemed to be a swinging cradle that soothed and almost lulled Him into a comfortable reverie (Ramaswamy).

The word avatara is taken from this descending pitch to symbolize the gods coming down to the earth. Krishna is the eighth avatar of Vishnu and is always placed in a swing in many fertility rites throughout India. And all these rites have been well described in the Upanishads. English translations of Carnatic lyrics by (Dasu 2010) from the composer Annamacharya provides us with these lyrics relating to the swing.

In this song, alara chanchala maina – madhyamAvati – Adi describes symbolically the cycle of creation as the divine sport of the Almighty. He visualizes the swing as the cosmos with Dharma as base:

> Oh Lord, You shine in all souls and also in the air we breath. The transient nature of creation is your divine leela and splendor. It is the divine swing.
>
> The dawn and dusk are mountain-like pillars and the sky itself is beam across, bearing the swing-like cosmos.
>
> The Vedas are golden chains holding the swing safely. The seat of the cradle is Dharma. It is indeed an amazing swing.
>
> The panoramic clouds enhance your brilliance, shinning like a blue mountain. The clouds are your ornaments.
>
> Beautiful women feared that the cosmos would tilt but they continue to push the swing swiftly. The scary movement of the swing made you embrace your consort. The celestial women found your delight and happiness in the swing. It is a rare feast to Brahma and other celestials to worship you. The magnificent Lord of Venkatadri is extremely delighted with the swing.

Venkatadri is in reference to a hill which was a seat of the worship of Vishnu near the temple of Tirumala in Tirupati. When Vishnu incarnated as Krishna it inspired Saint Andal, 1 of 12 *alvars* (saints) of India, to write her 30 Thiruppavai stanzas in the seventh century CE of which the last two are chanted at the Giant Swing Ceremony in Bangkok. The significance of the Giant Swing Ceremony to be called the Thiruppavai can only be appreciated when the meaning of these stanzas are put into perspective as being composed by Sri Andal the quintessence incarnation of Sri Bhumi Devi the Divine Consort of Sriman Narayana (Swamy 2010; Padmanabhan 1999).

When a marrying couple is seated on a swing, it is called Oonjal or Oonchal. During the Jhulan Yatra festival, people celebrate the divine love between Lord Krishna and Radha (Fig. 2.12). Songs are sung when the bride and groom swing for the first time on a decorated swing. This is not simply a ritual but a divine message to be one with nature. All throughout India, the swing ritual praises Vishnu or Krishna. These are two translated stanzas by (Ramachander 2010: 1 on blog):

> After erecting the magical pillars of red coral,
> After hanging the hooks made of emerald,
> On the very pretty swing made of nine gems,
> Abhimanyu and Vathsala, please swing.
>
> One side swung by Indra and his wife Sasi,
> And another side swung by Lord Shiva and Parvathi,
> With the accompaniment of Veena played by Dumburu and Narada, Please swing along with Sri Ranga Natha

6 Perspectives on the Meaning of Swinging

The swing referred to as a "ship bound for heaven" was mentioned by Eilade (1958: 103) and is found in the Tandya Maha Brahmanas. The chariot pulled along the ceremonial avenue at the Vitthala temple in Hampi was also a ship bound for heaven

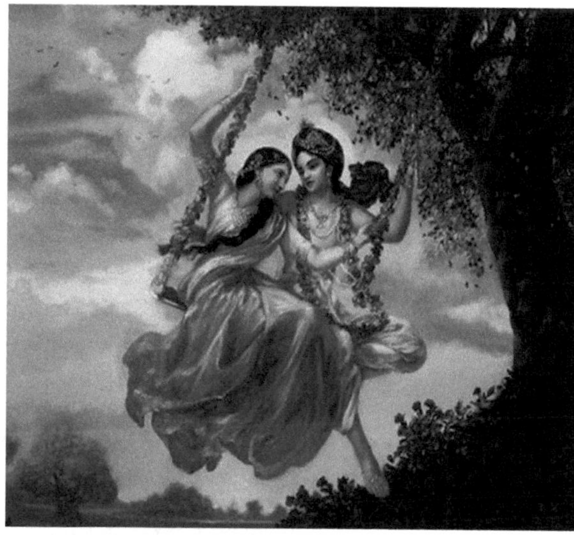

Fig. 2.12 Lord Krishna and Radha

as it was transporting the gods out to the swing to travel among the stars. A more complete interpretation of this ship sailing across the Milky Way is expressed by Gerini (1892: 39) who states that

> In the cosmogonies where the sky is held to be a liquid mass or celestial ocean (something like the 'waters that are above the firmament') as in the Egyptian, all planetary bodies and stars – personified as gods or animal deities- are floating on it and sailing across in it boats.

The celestial story becomes even more interesting when we consider that a ship is carved on a wall at Lord Jagannath temple in Orissa carrying a swing on its deck, which can be none other than a ship sailing (swinging) on the eternal ocean. Gerini (1892) located the ship on the Hindu planisphere in the seventh Nakshatra (*Punarvasu*) which is identified as the same ship where Vishnu took on the image of a fish (*Matsya*). It is here that there are two rivers which Gerini explains are on the northern and southern parts of the Hindu planisphere forming the Milky Way and are called the *Akasa Ganga* (perennial sky stream). It is at either end of these rivers that there are two gates. The southern gate is the one through which Vishnu and Shiva pass through to visit the human world during the swing ceremony. This celestial drama is demonstrated in (Fig. 2.13) where on either side of the planisphere a dotted line is shown connecting the gates of man and the gates of gods. Recognizing how our earth aligns with the sun and the galactic center was a reason why the ancients held rituals and built monuments so as to harmonize with the universal will and movements of the heavens (Hedke 2008).

On January 11, 2011, the gates of the gods were directly above in the heavens and the Giant Swing Ceremony in Bangkok, held on the second lunar month, was the time when the gates of Kailash were opened by the royal priest at the Devasthan Bosth Brahman temple inviting Shiva and Vishnu to visit earth. Slowly, a more complete picture of the hidden cosmology behind this ancient ceremony of swinging was beginning to fall into place.

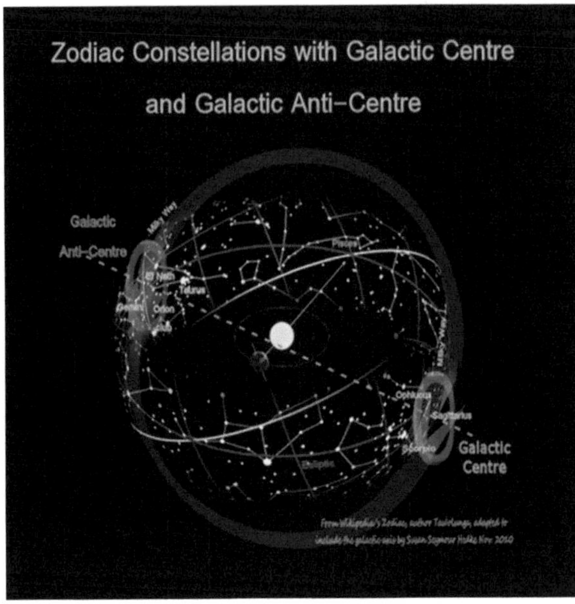

Fig. 2.13 Galactic axis – northern and southern gates (Susan Seymour Hedke 2008)

Eliade (1958) explains how solstice rites mentioned in the Mahavrata were composed by Sivaistic ascetics and would have priests (hotrs) placed on swings referred to as the breaths of *prana*, *yvana*, and *apana*. Likewise, shamans also partake in some form of flying or swaying of their body under the influence of mind-altering substances (Whitten 2007) similar to the ancient Soma ritual that included the ingestion of Ephedra (Lamberg-Karlovsky 2002). Ephedra is the well-known substance used in the drink of the gods called "amrita" and was used in these same rituals by the Sivaistic ascetics to reach the abode of the gods, and residues of it have even been found in the fire altars at Harappa.

The recent discovery of a Harappan script containing an unusual spiral image next to a unicorn has been uncovered by Godbole (2010). The Harappan scripts are still largely undeciphered, but there is no question there where symbolic references being made to various aspects of their civilization leading many scholars to believe they did possess a spoken language (Parpola 2005). Rituals where reference to swinging has been recorded in the Vedas that reflect celestial events have been interpreted by Godbole (2010) who associates this "starfish script" (Fig. 2.14) with a spiral image produced by a comet when it enters earth's atmosphere (Fig. 2.15). Godbole interprets the Vedic scriptures to emphasize his beliefs and, as a chemist by training, analyzed the faience (coatings on the Harappan seals) to determine that they were made from a clay-like substance whose composition was altered due to these meteor impacts. His discovery has led to a new interpretation of the Vedic verses revealing they were eyewitness accounts of celestial phenomena.

The Mahavrata is a very ancient tradition with much of its meaning having been lost. However, in the first and fifth chapters of the *Aitareya Aranyaka* of the *Rig*

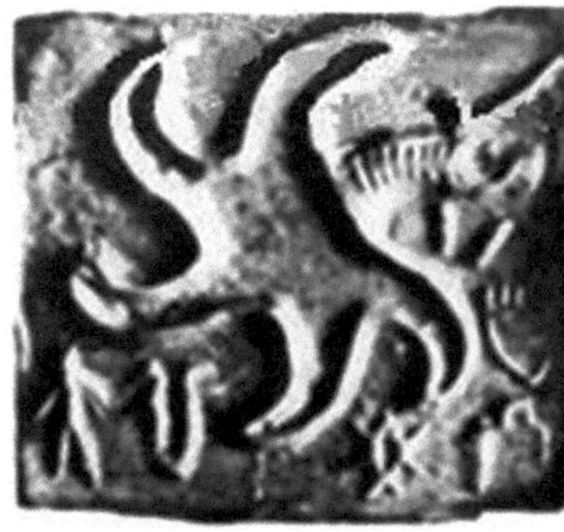

Fig. 2.14 Harappan seal - 2000 BCE

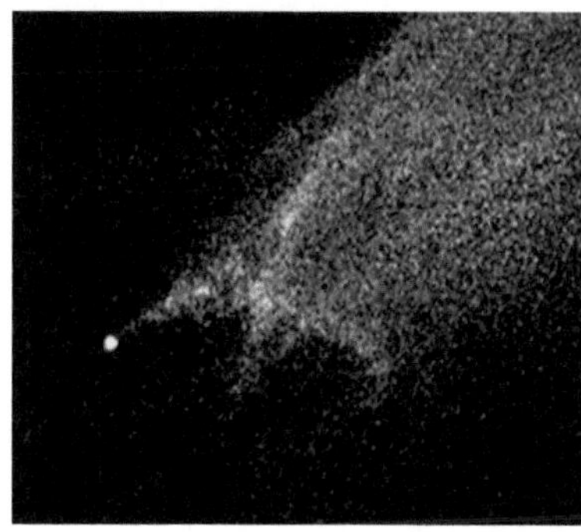

Fig. 2.15 Asteroid – NASA Jan 29, 2010

Veda there is a detailed description of the Mahavrata rituals where Godbole explains how the "*Hotra*" sits on the swing and chants. In *Aitareya Aranyaka* (1.2.3) there is an explanation of the swing:

> "They ask, why is swing a swing?" he, who blows is the swing.

Then in *RgVeda* (7.87.5) mentions the swing as quoted:

> On him three heavens rest and are supported, and the three earths are there in six-fold order.
> The wise King Varuna hath made in heaven that Golden Swing to cover it with glory.
> He swings forward in these worlds and then a swing is a swing.

The interpretations Godbole (2010) offers are very extensive and worth reading. Another example offered is where the wise King Varuna (who comes from the sky in a golden swing) and the Falcon (which represents Indra) are symbolic of celestial objects. And from *RgVeda* (10.178) called the "*Tarkshya Sukta*" which is chanted to avert evil astral bodies. There is not enough space to cover all these translations, but they show how new interpretations of the Vedas are a direct result of comparing geological, astronomical, and Vedic scriptures as a way of seeing history though the eyes of the ancient sages who only knew of their universe from a cosmocentric view point as was mentioned earlier.

It was the work of two British astronomers who had researched the roles giant comets play to develop a new theory of "coherent catastrophism" (Napier 2010). Our solar system periodically passes through the orbit of the Taurid belt of asteroids, as it is doing so in our present era, which can eventually cause debris to enter the inner solar system. These findings are what led Godbole (2010) to infer differently on the soil samples analyzed by researchers such as Sana Ullah (Cook 1994) in and around the Mohenjo-Daro region in the Indus Valley. The seal in Fig. 2.11 containing a spiral-like shape is what Godbole claims is the depiction of an eyewitness account of a meteor. The image NASA's Hubble space telescope captured lends credence to Godbole's assertion.

7 Interpretations of the Giant Swing in Thailand

We finally arrive at the point in this chapter where we can now look upon the Giant Swing in Bangkok with a little more understanding of why it is held in such high esteem as one of Thailand's most venerated icons. Brahmanic influences are undoubtedly the source for the idea of swinging as a ceremonial ritual, and throughout India these rituals go by many names: Dolatsava, Jhula Yatra, Jhoola, Oonchal, Onnchilla, the well-known Hindola which takes place in the month of Shravan, and finally the Rajo swing festival in Orissa.

The Giant Swing Ceremony in Bangkok was originally 1 of 12 royal ceremonies held in each of the months of the Thai lunar calendar in the Sukhothai Kingdom and officiated over by Brahman priests. Therefore, we are on safe ground when we compare the meaning of this swinging ritual held once a year in the Tamil lunar month of Margazhi with the Giant Swing Ceremony in Bangkok. And when we begin to look more closely at what is taking place in the swinging ritual, it will be possible to also speculate, with some degree of certainty, the symbolic significance that the Giant Swing represents for Thailand. Interestingly, it was only in 1931 that any definitive description of the swinging ceremony held in Thailand was first made available to the outside world (Wales 1931: 238–255). Although Wales considered the main reason the swing ceremony took place was to reflect the sun's passage in the sky, that view now can be seen as not being the only symbolic function, but in fact the swing ceremony represents much more than just a solar passage. The other author to offer his description of the Giant Swing Ceremony was Gerini (1895) whose interpretation was somewhat different than Wales, prompting Wales to discard them in favor of his own solar interpretation. So, let's look at these two authors' comments as they are the only two authoritative interpretations on record for the meaning of the Giant Swing Ceremony in Thailand.

If we consider the new interpretations from Godbole (2010) with a comet impacting the earth around 3100 BCE and read the Vedic verses with these celestial phenomena in mind, we find that the solar reference can be equated with a comet and not the sun as Fraser (1919), Wales (1931), and Gerini (1895) had implied. Fraser was the first to mention that in the RgVeda, the sun is called "the golden swing in the sky" claiming it helps us understand Vedic rituals by showing how a priest sat in a swing and touched, with the span of his right hand, at once the seat of the swing and the ground. In doing so, Fraser goes on to say that "the great Lord has united himself with the great lady; the god has united himself with the goddess" (p. 280). This explanation is where Wales took his cue for the solar interpretation of the swing because Fraser offers the explanation that the author of the Vedic scripture meant to indicate that the sun had reached the lowest point on its course closest to earth. Fraser takes his information from (Griffith 1891).

Wales quotes the same passage in his description of the swinging festival, but uses a reference to Fraser rather than the original translation by Griffith. Wales's interpretation for the Giant Swing Ceremony, as being identified as a sun ceremony, is based on three assumptions. His first is that it takes place during the winter solstice; secondly, the swing goes from East to West, the same direction as the course of the sun; and, thirdly, the circular dancing around the base symbolizes the revolution of the sun. Wales also adds that the swing ceremony was intended to force Lord Surya (sun god) to fulfill his function.

Gerini (1895) states exactly the same as Wales, but does so 35 years earlier mentioning that it is a solstice festival and that the swinging and dancing represent the revolution and birth of the sun. He also mentions that the swing goes from East to West in the direction of the course of the sun. So far, Gerini is saying exactly the same as Wales but doing so in 1895. Gerini also makes an association with the Hindu Dola Yatra festival admitting that the significant features of the meaning of the swing were lost in India's legendary past. Where Wales disagrees with Gerini is when Gerini makes the association of the swing ceremony representing the churning of the Ocean of Milk affected by the gods. Both of these interpretations are made from a familiarity with Hindu mythology available at that time and were the only descriptions available to the outside world. If we consider Godbole's interpretation we find ourselves needing to consider an entirely different scenario for the meaning of the Vedic scriptures. Quoting from the Mahavrata ceremony, Godbole (2010: 9) offers this interpretation:

> The swing is made from the wood of an Umbar tree. It is supported by erecting two poles in the ground. The right to occupy the seat is only that of the Hotra. He approaches the swing, sliding like a serpent and puts his chin on the seat of the swing. Then he uses his hands to grip the ropes of "darbha" and assumes a sitting posture. While taking swings he is supposed to keep one foot hanging down so as to brush the ground as the swing descends, however, he is not allowed to touch the ground with both the feet simultaneously.

Godbole asks the question what is symbolized by this *Hotra* swinging in from above, sliding one foot on the ground, and then swinging upwards again. His interpretation comes from RgVeda 10.120 and believes it symbolizes the birth of the terrible one and the destruction he caused indicating an awe inspiring fleeting Falcon (comet) with the *Hotra* climbing on the swing, sliding like a serpent (moving in the air) and begins taking swings. He touches the ground with one foot symbolizing speedy movement or bright celestial objects approaching or even occasionally touching the surface of the earth. This interpretation is very close to Fraser's mentioning: "The great Lord has united himself with the great lady, the god has united himself with the goddess" (p. 280).

If we seriously consider the geological record indicating a meteor impacting the earth in 3100 BCE or earlier and also associate these events with Godbole's interpretation of the Vedic scriptures, we can then begin to see how the language stemming from a cosmocentric world view is full of poetic metaphors providing us with new insights as to why swinging was held in such high regard. The swing then could also be looked at as a bright burning comet streaking and crisscrossing against the sky, touching the earth and causing reverence and obeisance to its awesome power and presence. These celestial events were recognized as actions fostered by the gods prompting sacrifices and offerings which would last for thousands of years to come in order to appease their wrath and ask for their blessings. Many of the rituals which are performed today are done so without any cognizance of the fact that they were spawned at the inception of witnessing ancient celestial events, which I contend, are still embedded in our collective memories allowing the swinging ceremony to still be faithfully performed and imbued with the same sacred intentions that were held in the past.

I could easily offer the thought that these celestial events were not a onetime happening in the heavens, but repeated themselves cyclically throughout the millennia. To quote Eliade (1954: 3):

> If one goes to the trouble of penetrating the authentic meaning of an archaic myth or symbol, one cannot but observe that this meaning shows recognition of a certain situation in the cosmos and that, consequently, it implies a metaphysical position.

If I could offer my opinion about the return of these "bright ones" from the depth of space, as related to the winter solstice of 2012, I would say that our archaic memories are causing the alarm and the concern worldwide concerning a natural cataclysm whether from a comet, earthquake, or volcano. For if in fact the Vedic Falcon returns (Mayan Quetzalcoatl), he will surely bring about a similar fate as witnessed and recorded by our ancient ancestors in myths and star lore the world over.

8 Witnessing the Thiruppavai/Thiruvempavai

Understandably, after researching the meaning of swinging rituals worldwide, especially in India, attending the Giant Swing Ceremony on January 11, 2011 in Bangkok, it gave me an exhilarating feeling knowing I was entering a very ancient realm and would be witness to how Brahman priests communicated with the gods. From my first impressions of this royal ceremony gained from reading the account that Wales (1931) provided to witnessing a symbolic sacrifice which I understood was done to appease the gods as Godbole (2010) had indicated caused me to feel as if I had been caught between an ancient world of sensual imaginings, mythic musings, and a rational world seeking answers attending a Brahmanical ritual. The difference between my Western mindset and that of an Eastern mindset could not have been more apparent. On the evening of January 11, the mythical gates of Kailash were opened by Phra Rajaguru Vamadevamuni, and Lord Shiva was invited to visit earth for 10 days.

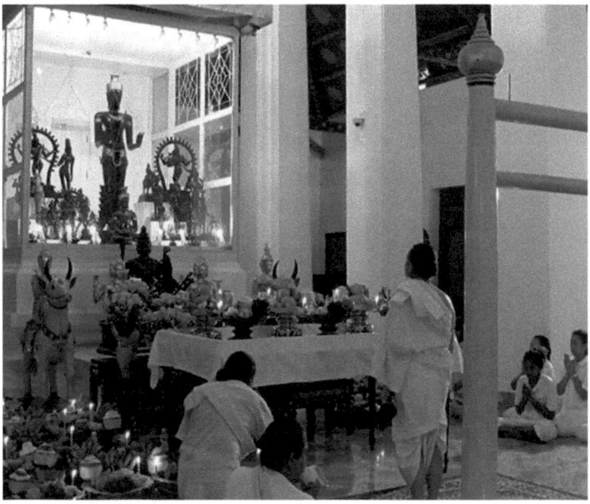

Fig. 2.16 Raja Guru opening the gates of Kailash

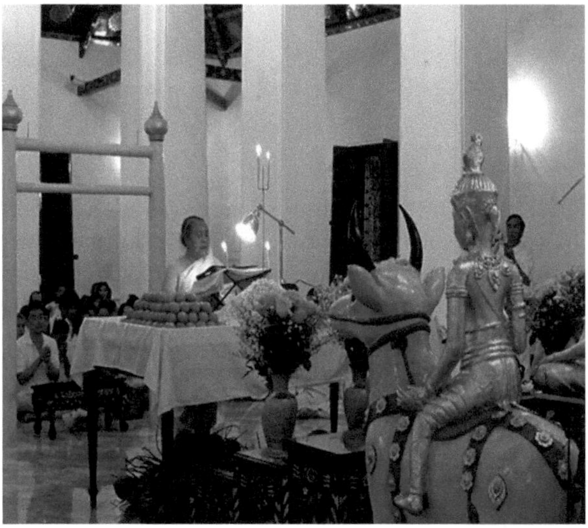

Fig. 2.17 Raja Guru receiving Lord Shiva

The auspiciousness of this ceremony dedicated to the Hindu gods made me realize how ingrained these ancient beliefs still hold sway over the spiritual foundation of the Kingdom of Thailand. The gods Lord Surya, Lord Chandra, Goddess Ganga, and the earth goddess were invited in the early morning hours as shown in (Fig. 2.16), and in the evening Lord Shiva was invited to visit earth (Fig. 2.17). Lord Ganesh was also invited to earth, but this ceremony, which is similar to inviting Lord Shiva, was done in a separate temple dedicated to Lord Ganesh. And although the King was not observing this most auspicious event as in times past, prayers were still

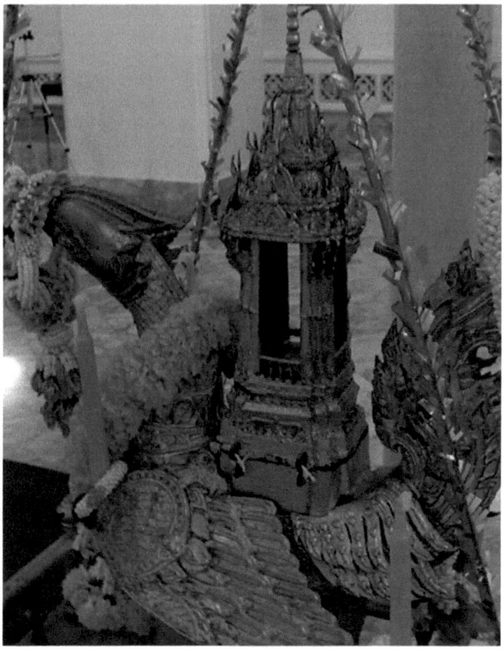

Fig. 2.18 Hamsa with shrine for the gods

offered to the royal family. There was no ceremony around the giant swing; however, smaller swing posts installed inside the Devasthan Bosth Brahman temple were used to suspend Hamsa (Brahma's mount) where small replicas of the gods are placed in a shrine on his back and swung in a gesture to return the gods back to Mt. Kailash when the moon was full (Fig. 2.18). Incidentally, the full moon in the previous month was a full eclipse connected to Lord Shiva as it took place in the constellation of Mrigashira to the north of Orion in the antelope's head and considered by Hindus to be the most important celestial event in the 26,000-year cycle of the great year (Frawley 2010).

It takes many hours of preparation by the Raja Guru before the swinging actually takes place lending an atmosphere of sanctity which could only be achieved with all the ritual details needing to be attended to for preparing the gods for their journey back to Kailash. This is a very rare ceremony to see because the final sending of the gods does not happen until the very early hours of the morning shortly after midnight. When the swing begins its movement, the conch shells are sounded and chanting lasts for over an hour. This then is the very crucible of the swing ceremony in the early twenty-first century, but what is a very reduced ceremony compared with the pageantry that accompanied the Giant Swing Ceremony in the past still has the accoutrements of a ceremony that fixates on exact procedures which have been mastered by the royal priest to give to the gods a welcome and a departure fitting the most austere refinements of respect for the sacredness of these deities.

9 Discussion and Conclusion

The journey from the beginning of time when speech was first being formulated in the recesses of our ancestors minds to a small replica of Lord Brahma's mount carrying the miniature replicas of the gods on its back to return to the sacred mountain, covers a span of time lasting at least a quarter turn of the great year of some 26,000 years. The only evidence of civilizations existing prior to this time are stone megaliths and monuments scattered about the surface of the planet and under coastal waters (Hancock 1998). What I have covered in this chapter is a story of devotion to nature mimicking the forces impacting the earth leading to poetic expressions that have been forever saved in rituals and monuments which has led to the idea that our ancestors were guided by the stars and personified them with names and actions through verse and song giving us a clue to our shared heritage. By the time the swing reached the ancient city of Sukhothai, with King Lithai in the early thirteenth century to ancient Ayutthaya in the early seventeenth century with King Ramathibodi II and then King Rama I in 1784 in Bangkok, the swing transformed itself many times but it was still honored as a sacred way to pay homage to the gods. This could not be shown more dramatically than at the elaborate ritual performed at the Devasthan temple on the full moon of January 20. And as mentioned above, although King Rama IX (Maha Bhumibol – the present King of Thailand) was not in attendance, prayers for his well-being and the Kingdom of Thailand were still offered. If we are to learn from what has been left on this earth reminding us of our celestial heritage, then the wisdom that is transmitted through the ritual, which uses the swing as a metaphor to communicate with the gods could, therefore, be considered a direct link to understanding our shared mythologies. And now that we are at the threshold of another moment in time when the great year once again returns to its starting point and is about to begin another long swing of the ages, it would be prudent to listen and give respect to that wisdom that has been given to us, which is embedded in the ancient swinging rituals still being performed in Thailand and across all of India attracting millions of devotees who set out on their annual pilgrimages (Fig. 2.19).

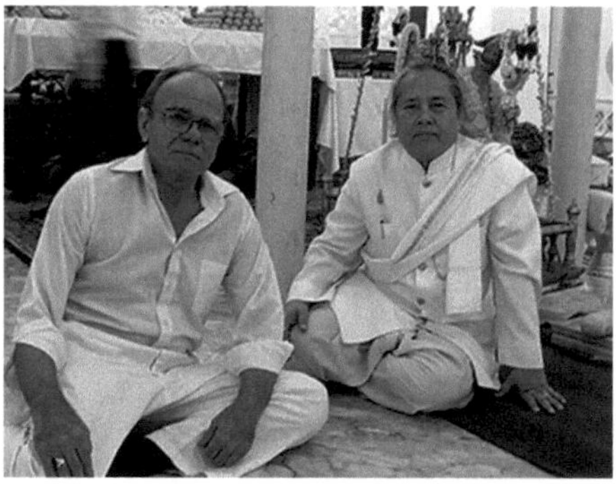

Fig. 2.19 Author with Raja Guru Jan 20, 2011

Acknowledgments Special thanks goes to Phra Rajaguru Vamadevamuni, Royal Priest, Office of the Royal Household for the monarchy of Thailand, for allowing me to participate in the annual swinging ceremony. A special thanks also goes to Dr. Chirapat Prapandvidya, Assistant Professor and Advisor, Sanskrit Studies Centre of Thailand, for all his archaeological work on the inscriptions relating to Brahmins coming to Thailand. In India, I am indebted to the honorable Dr. Sachidanand Sahai for his council and guidance for supporting my research; Dr. Deepak Bhattacharya of Orissa whose research on the Rajo and studies at Bhubaneswar temple contributed greatly to the historical use of the swing in ancient India; Ravindra Godbole of Pune, India, with his providing a translation of his work on the Meaning of the Vedas which uncovered important insight into Harappan use of the clay seals; Rush Allen on astronomical insights; Susan Seymore Hedke for her diagrams of the heavens; and to the many who corresponded with me and contributed papers leading to a more complete understanding of swinging.

References

Allen, R. E. (2008). *Taputapu-atea marae*. Retrieved July 12, 2012, from: http://www.siloam.net/index.html

Bhattacharya, D. (2010). *Rajo: The swing festival of Kalinga (India)*. (C/o Sri Radha Krishna, Kedar Gouri Road, Bhubaneswar, India – 751002). Retrieved January 15, 2013, from: http://ebookbrowse.com/rajo-swing-festival-kalinga-india-pdf-d111595766

Bhattacharya, D., & Nail, P. C. (2008). Archaeoastronomy of Nataraja. [Art history and archaeology]. *Indian Journal of History and Science, 43*(3), 411–423.

Campos, T. (2010). Sundance – Suspension rituals of Native American tribes. *Suite*, 101. Retrieved January 5, 2013, from: http://www.suite101.com/content/sundance--suspension-rituals-of-native-american-tribes-a300945

Chaubey, B. B. (1998). Origin and evolution of Vedic rituals. *Journal of the Ananthacharya Indologiea Research Institute, 1*(1), 17–23.

Citaristi, L. (1995). *Danda ritual: Five elements* (Prakriti series, Vol. 1, Chapter 17, Delhi, India, IGNCA). Retrieved January 15, 2013, from: http://ignca.nic.in/ps_01020.htm

Cook, G. (1994). *An Harappan seal at Berkeley*. [Archaeology]. Wisconsin archaeology reports: From Sumer to Meluhha: Contributions to the archaeology of South and West Asia in memory of George F. Dales, Jr, 3.

Dasu, D. R. (2010). *Sangeeta sudha*. Retrieved from January 15, 2013, from: http://www.sangeeta-sudha.org/annamacharya/vol2/a.html

Eliade, M. (1954). *The myth of the eternal return: Cosmos and history* (2nd ed.). New York: Princeton University Press.

Eliade, M. (1958). Yoga: Immortality and freedom (2009 ed.). Princeton: Princeton University Press.

Eliade, M. (2004). *Shamanism: Archaic techniques of ecstasy*. Princeton: Princeton University Press.

Feuerstein, G., Kak, S., & Frawley, D. (1995). *In search of the cradle of civilization*. Delhi: Moyilal Banarsidass.

Frawley, D. (2010). *Winter solstice 2010*. Retrieved from January 15, 2013, from: http://www.facebook.com/pages/Dr-David-Frawley/180761044927

Fraser, J. G. (1919). *The dying God*. London: MacMillan.

Gerini, G. E. (1892). *A retrospective view and account of the origin of the Thet Maha Ch'at ceremony* (2nd ed.). Bangkok: Sathirakoses-Nagapradipa Foundation.

Gerini, G. E. (1895). Festivals and feasts (Siamese). In *Hastings encyclopaedia of religion and ethics* (Vol. V, p. 885). New York: Charles Scribner's Son

Godbole, R. V. (2010). *The meaning of Vedas* (S. S. Phadke, Trans.). Marathi: Deshmukh and Company (Pvt.) Ltd.

Griffith, R. T. H. (1891). *The hymns of the RigVeda* (Vol. III). Bernares: E.J. Lazarus.
Hancock, G. (1998). *Heaven's mirror: Quest for the lost civilization*. New York: Crown Publishing Group.
Hedke, S. S. (2008). *The Galactic Centre*. [Lulu on-line publisher]. Retrieved January 15, 2013, from: http://www.lulu.com/shop/susan-seymour-hedke/the-galactic-centre-2012-and-the-great-waves-coming-in-december/paperback/product-6297844.html
Kacha-ananda, C. (1971). The Akha swing ceremony. *Journal of the Siam Society, 59*, 120–128.
Khubchandani, L. K. (1995). *The supernatural in nature: Sindhi tradition* (Vol. 1). New Delhi: D.K. Print World.
Lamberg-Karlovsky, C. C. (2002, February). Archaeology and language: The Indo-Iranians. *Current Anthropology, 43*(1), 63–88.
Napier, B. (2010). *Bill Napier*. Retrieved January 2, 2011, from: http://www.bill-napier.com/research.html
Padmanabhan, C. (1999). *Tiruppavai*. Retrieved January 2, 2011, from: http://www.tiruppavai.net/about_us.html
Parpola, A. (2005). *Study of the Indus script. 50th ICES*. Retrieved January 2, 2011, from: http://www.scribd.com/doc/33521988/Study-of-the-Indus-Script-Special-Lecture-Asko-Parpola
Powell, J. H. (1914). "Hook-Swinging" in India. A Description of the Ceremony, and an Enquiry into Its Origins and Significance. Retrieved August 15, 2013, from: http://www.jstor.org/stable/1254904.
Ramachander, P. R. (2010). *Aaadeer Oonjal*. Retrieved January 2, 2011, from: http://translation-sofsomesongsofcarnticmusic.blogspot.com/2010/10/aadeer-oonjal.html
Ramaswamy, S. A. (2010). *Dasaavataara Stotram of Swami Desika*. Retrieved January 2, 2011, from: http://srivaishnavam.com/stotras/dasavatharam_meaning.htm
Reiser, O. L. (1978). *The intent of creation: Man's search for cosmic meaning*. Lakemont: CSA Press.
Saraswati, B. (1995). *Prakriti: The integral vision* (Vol. 1). New Delhi: Indira Gandhi National Center for the Arts.
Sharapov, V. E., & Nesanelis, D. A. (1997). *Theme of "Swinging" in Shamanism and Folk Culture*. Retrieved August 15, 2013, from http://www.elore.fi/arkisto/2_97/sha297.html
Staal, F. (1996). *Ritual and mantras: Rules without meaning*. New Delhi: Motilal Banarsidass.
Swamy, B. (2010). *Sri Andal's Tirup-pavai*. Retrieved January 2, 2011, from: http://namperumal.tripod.com/TPMain.htm
Van Vliet, J. (1640). *The short history of the kings of Siam* (L. Andaya,Trans.). Bangkok: The Siam Society.
Wales, H. G. Q. (1931). *Siamese state ceremonies*. London: Bernard Quaritch, Ltd.
Whitten, N. E. (2007). *Soul vine shamanism*. Retrieved December 11, 2010, from: http://polarfinearts.com/cgi-bin/cgiwrap/magician/htmlos.cgi/PFA_2009/SVS_FILES/

Chapter 3
Thai Amulets: Symbol of the Practice of Multi-faiths and Cultures

Sophana Srichampa

1 Introduction

Before the influence of Brahmanism-Hinduism and Buddhism to Siam, local Thai people believed in spirits. In the reign of King Ashoka Maurya, under the leading of Sona and Uttara in the third century B.C., Buddhism settled in the area known as Nakhon Pathom, about 50 km from Bangkok (Lochan 2006: 189). After King Ramathibodi I's establishment of Ayutthya as the center for his kingdom in 13 A.D., he accepted Khmer culture which was influenced by Indian civilization. Brahmanism has mantra and deities, whereas Buddhism has the Buddha image and monks. Therefore, local beliefs are mixed with Brahmanism and Buddhism in Thailand.

It is crucial to provide some definitions here. Belief, according to Srinivas and Kutumba Sastry (2007: 67), is "a kind of feeling that makes an individual accept something as true even when there is no conclusive evidence. In epistemology, a belief is considered to be a claim to knowledge. However, it is not a mere opinion. Beliefs can be true or false. Epistemologists make a sharp distinction between belief and knowledge. The latter presupposes the former, but not vice versa. Belief is also defined by many epistemologists as a mental state or state of mind… According to scholastics, belief is nothing but faith or opinion lacking evidence." An amulet is something carried or worn as a charm against evil (Crowther 1995: 37; Moore 2009: 45).

S. Srichampa (✉)
Research Institute for Languages and Cultures of Asia, Mahidol University, Salaya, Nakhonpathom 73170, Thailand
e-mail: sophana@gmail.com

P. Liamputtong (ed.), *Contemporary Socio-Cultural and Political Perspectives in Thailand*,
DOI 10.1007/978-94-007-7244-1_3,

2 Thai Beliefs

Human beings' beliefs are related to nature, which affect life positively and negatively in ways that could not be explained in the past. Therefore, people are afraid of unseen or unexplained phenomena. They tried to secure themselves by carrying a small thing with them, which gradually became a sacred amulet.

Thai people have a variety of beliefs which are accommodated by different rituals. Beliefs in Thai society can be classified as follows:

2.1 Buddhist Beliefs

- Triratana: Thai people believe in Triratana, a core Buddhist Dhamma principle.
- Karma law: Thai people believe in "do good get good," "do bad get bad." No one can avoid it.
- Reincarnation: Human and animals reincarnate because of their deeds which are related to Buddhist principles.
- Law of nature: Buddhism does not believe in the existence of any god, the creator of the world. It believes that it is governed by Law of Nature, known in Pali as Niyyaama, the regulator, or the Law of Nature. There are five kinds of law, namely, the Law of Kamma (Action), the Law of Season (Utu), the Law of Seed (Bija), the Law of Consciousness (Citta), and the Law of Dhamma (States, i.e., natural happenings such as earthquake and flood). These five laws regulate the different happenings, things, and events of the world.
- Heaven and hell: Some Buddhists believe that there is heaven and hell when we are still alive. People who suffer for their survival are like being in hell, but people who have happy lives are in heaven. Moreover, many people believe that after death, there is heaven in the sky for the good people and hell, underground, for bad people.

2.2 Superstitious Beliefs

Thai people believe in mysteries which cannot be proven by science. It can be divided into two types:

1. Magic beliefs: Old scripts written as content are believed to be powerful and mysterious. When it was pronounced to be a magical formula, then it is believed to be sacred or magic. These beliefs faded away in this modern era because of the advance of science and technology.
2. Amulet beliefs: Beliefs in natural things such as iron and tiger tooth which can protect people from accident.

2.3 *Sacred Thing Beliefs*

This belief has been part of Thai life since the old days, and the sacred things include the Buddha images, images of respected monks, and spirit houses.

2.4 *Deity Beliefs*

Beliefs in unseen things which are more powerful than humans. This cannot be easily explained in a scientific way.

2.5 *Astrological Beliefs*

Astrology is believed by all classes in Thai society through fortune-tellers. This depends on astronomy. The horoscope is taught and can be a profession in Thai society (Suntaree 1991; Phra Paisal Visalo 2012).

3 Background of Amulets

Natural things are used to create amulets such as /lèk lǎj/[1] "a kind of miraculous iron believed to melt like gum when heated by a candle and characterized by its quality of rendering the owner invulnerable", /k^{h}ǎw kwaːŋ khút/ "ungrown deer horn," /k^{h}îəw mǔː tan/ "pig tooth," /k^{h}îəw sɯ̌ə/ "tiger tooth," and /kluəŋ t^{h}ǎw wan/ "a species of vine" (Thaphra 2010: 21, 14, 244). Other sacred constructed ores such as bronze, nine kinds of metal, seven kinds of metal, and five kinds of metal are made for protection from danger.

---

[1] In this article, the Thai names of amulets are transcribed by the International Phonetic Alphabet (IPA) which is divided into consonants, vowels, and tones.

- Initial consonants in Thai are 44 scripts, 21 sounds: ป /p/, ผ,พ,ภ /p^{h}/, ม /m/, บ /b/, ฝ, ฟ /f/, ฏ, ต /t/, ซ,ศ,ษ,ส /S/, ฐ, ฑ, ฒ, ถ,ท, ธ /t^{h}/, ณ, น /n/, ฎ, ด /d/, ก /k/, ข,ค, ฆ /k^{h}/,ง /ŋ/,อ/ʔ/, ห, ฮ /h/, จ /tɕ/, ฉ, ช, ฌ /tɕ^{h}/, ร /r/, ญ, ย /j/, ว /W/, ล, ฬ /l/.
- Final consonants are of 8 forms: ม /m/, ญ,ณ,น,ร,ล,ฬ /n/, ง /ŋ/, บ,ป,พ,ฟ,ภ /p/, จ,ช,ซ,ฌ,ฎ,ฏ,ฐ,ฑ,ฒ,ด,ต,ถ,ท,ธ.ศ.ษ.ส /t/, ก,ข,ค,ฆ /s/, ย /j/, ว /W/ and /ʔ/ when the word with a short vowel has no final consonant.
- Vowels: There are short and long vowels as follows: -ะ /a/, -า /aː/, -ิ /i/, –ี /iː/, -ุ /u/, -ู /uː/, เ-ะ /e/, เ- /eː/, แ-ะ /æ/, แ- /æː/, -ึ /ɯ/, -ื /ɯː/, เ-อะ /ɣ/, เออ/ɣː/, โ-อะ /o/, โอ/oː/, เ-าะ /ɔ/, -อ/ɔː/

  There are three diphthongs: เอีย/ia/ เอือ /ɯa/ อัว /ua/
- Tones: There are five tones: mid-tone (no tone mark), low tone (เอก ̀), falling tone (โท ̂), high tone (ตรี ́), and rising tone (จัตวา ̌).

3.1 Types of Amulets

In Thailand, there are ten types of amulets:

1. Natural things: Soil is made as rishi or /naːŋ kwàk/ "an ancient lady in a hand-palm downward" and made sacred.
2. Stones: These include stones, ore, gold, silver, or mixed metals.
3. Plants: Parts of a plant such as root, bulb, resin, leaf, flower, and fruit.
4. Animals: Parts of an animal such as nail, tusk, horn, bone, and eye.
5. Human: Parts of the body such as a tooth of ancestors, tooth of a respected guru, and bones of well-known Buddhist monks.
6. Wax
7. Water: Water can be changed to various forms. It can be made sacred water from Buddhist rituals.
8. Oil
9. Paper, cloth, and string.
10. Drawings and pictures: Drawing called /jan/ "magic designs or letters placed or inscribed on a piece of cloth or metal plate." Figures of animals from Himmaphan[2] such as /kʰót cʰa sǐː/ "a mythical animal with the body of a lion and an elephant's trunk," /râːt cʰə sǐː/ "lion," elephant, Garuda, and Naga which are believed to have supernatural power including god and giant pictures. These things should be made with miraculous power before using (Phayakharanon 2010: 10–13).

3.2 Ways of Using Amulets

There are various ways that amulets can be used:

- Strapping: Amulets put around head, waist, or arm.
- Wearing: Amulets worn around neck, head, arm, finger, and so on.
- Implanting: Implant amulets such as /tə krùt/ "a magic jewelry," charms, or amulets of rolled brass, inserting into the skin of people.
- Keeping in the mouth: An amulet is kept in the mouth as a little ball such as a sacred wad and a small amulet (Thaphra 2010: 2).

---

[2] The Himmaphan forest is said to be located on a mountain range of 84,000 peaks; many writers have suggested that it is corresponded to the Himalayas, a geographical location in India where the stories are originated from. It has influenced storytelling for religious purposes of both Hinduism and Buddhism (http://vnuriya-streams.blogspot.com/2010/05/himmapan-forest.html).

3.3 *Forms of Amulets*

Amulets are made in the following various forms:

- Male: Amulets in male forms are --/**rák jom**/ "a small pair of boys in a small bottle;" /kumaːn tʰɔːŋ/ "a gold baby boy;" rishi, an old man; and /**cʰuː cʰók**/ "a greedy Brahman character."
- Female: Amulets in female form such as /**mæ̂ː naːŋ kwàk**/ "an ancient lady in a traditional costume sitting with both legs tucked back to one side by beckoning a right hand-palm downward," /**mæ̂ː pʰoː sòp**/ "Goddess of rice," /**mæ̂ː sɯ́ː**/ "a guardian spirit of child," and other female forms.
- Animals such as tiger, elephant, cow, turtle, crocodile, and snake which are believed to be Bhodhisatavas who will become the Buddha (Thaphra 2010: 2).

3.4 *Levels of Amulets*

There are also three levels of using amulets:

- High-ranking amulets which are used on the upper parts of body from head to waist and have been blessed by sangha.
- Low-ranking amulets such as /**palàt kʰìk**/ "a small image of penis to be hung at the waist."
- Hanging amulets such as flag with fish, grasshopper, and bird figures (Ibid:5).

4 Why Do Thai People Make Amulets?

As mentioned above, Thai people including many monks have mixed concepts of local beliefs, Brahmanism-Hinduism, and Buddhism. They only have to "believe" in whatever or whoever they respect, and then "faith" will be increased. Moreover, many Thai people prefer to depend on and request the Buddha image and other sacred things for their achievements. Therefore, an amulet is an alternative choice for any Thai believers to worship and receive blessings. Some kinds of amulets are popular from time to time, and they are reproduced many times and sold for a good price. In fact, amulets can help the country to increase GDP informally up to 50 % (Akhara-serani 2010: 2).

The purposes of making amulets are for the three advantages:

- Prosperity: Nowadays, the society is consumeristic and materialistic. People use amulets by pronouncing an incantation over a power for selling well or slapping on the selling objects in the store when receiving a big bank note from the first customer. It is like a wealth charm.

- Mercy and love: Some people want mercy and love from others. They may carry amulets with them and pray for them to help. Anyone who is single, he/she will finally satisfy with his/her love. Any couple who cannot get along well can do the same, and they will be satisfied. It is like an attraction charm.
- Safety from any danger: Some people wear or carry amulet(s) for their safety from any dangers. They are amulets for protection (Phayakharanon 2010: 12–13).

There are many places in Bangkok selling amulets, but the big center is located at Phantip, Ngamwongwan. There are markets for selling old and new Buddha images and pseudo-Buddha images. The most famous amulet affecting GDP is Jatukham Ramathep which yields sales of about 20,000 million baht per annum. Other related business such as advertisements of Jatukham Ramathep could earn more than 300 million baht (Radomsithiphat 2010: 131). Making a new series of Buddha images or any amulet creates many new jobs for local people. Nowadays, selling the new Buddha image for charitable work is also popular because it touches the faith of Thai people.

In terms of language used in selling the Buddha images including other sacred things, Thai people do not use /k^hǎːj/ "sell" or /sɯ́ː/ "buy" but use /c^hâw/ "rent" instead because it sounds softer than selling and buying the sacred things, despite it means buying or selling.

In this chapter, the amulets in animal shapes, which are found to be the most frequent of the collected data from secondary sources and are believed to be sacred, will be examined in terms of language, faith, and culture.

5 Thai Amulets

Thai amulets make use of animals which are symbolized according to their characteristics as follows:

5.1 A Tiger Shape

A tiger symbolizes power which makes other people scared and respected. There are amulets made in a tiger body from a tiger tooth and from a wild pig tooth as follows:

- **/k^hɪ̂əw sɯ̌ə (NP) + tan (Adj.)/ > NP** which is made from the tooth of a tiger. It symbolizes "impenetrable, invulnerable." The tooth is sculptured as a tiger body.
- **/k^hɪ̂əw mǔː (NP) + tan (Adj.)/ > NP** which is made from a wild pig's tooth. There are two kinds of tiger's tooth used for sculpture of a tiger amulet: a solid tooth and a hollow tooth. They symbolize "superpower and protection from danger."

The respected monks who create these amulets perform a sacred ceremony. Those who possess this amulet are expected to behave properly and rightly. Otherwise, this amulet will disappear from that person.

The tiger shape can be conceptualized as A (NP) = power and protection from danger.

5.2 A Lion Shape

A lion symbolizes power which makes other people and animals scared.

- /**kraj sɔ̌:n râ:t chə sǐ:**/ Its structure is NP+NP. It is described by Phraya Sri Sunthon Woharn (cited in Thaphra 2010: 26) that it has white skin, mouth, and tail with four red feet. It is the most powerful animal and is scary to humans and animals. It is sculpted from a white elephant tusk. The tusk should be taken from an elephant pierced in a rut in a tree or fallen in the forest.
- /**sǐŋ**/ "lion" or simha is a NP. The Indians initiated placement of a pair of simha in front of the steps of religious places such as Elephanta Cave near Mumbai and distributed this concept to Indonesia and Cambodia. Thailand was influenced by Cambodia.

Belief in simha power is for religious protection. But the simha should be made sacred and contain yantra (magic words/symbols) such as "ta-to-bodhi-satto-raja-singha-ca-man-hit-thi-ko; ta mat-thang-pa-ka-sen-to sat-tha-a-ha" (Thaphra 2010: 30) or any amulet to control the stable and permanent power of simha and then set up as simha statue.

Nowadays, simha is a type of handicraft for selling as a souvenir which is made of brass, resin, stone, or wood. Both foreigners and Thai buy them for Buddhist room decorations at home.

Simha has been known as a sacred thing for less than 10 years. It was built and made sacred for wearing as a locket. The worshipers should offer the simha flowers and pray regularly, including gaining merit by helping the public—simha will then bless the doers to be happy and prosperous without any obstacles.

The lion shape can be conceptualized as A (NP + (NP)) = power, happiness, and prosperity.

5.3 A Cow and a Buffalo Shape

This amulet can be made of mixed metal, wax, and bamboo called /**wuə t^{h}ə nu: k^{h}wa:j t^{h}ə nu:**/. Its structure is composed of two NPs conjoined together. This amulet has the power to protect against the evil spirits.

The mixed metal amulet is made from metals including some elements from the dead person and the coffin such as a nail from the coffin and a coin from the mouth of the dead mixed with tin and bronze. The sacred scripts are put in a cow or bison form. This type is considered to be the first class.

The wax cow is made from wax covering the face of the victim of a violent death mixed with its hair, the eyes of a civet, and the eyes of a vulture, all burnt and then mixed with the ash from cremation. Honey is put into it and molded as a cow or buffalo, pronounced with a magical formula to it. It is the second rank.

The bamboo oxen are the third rank which is done by cutting the bamboo once with the praying of Namo Tassa (showing humble respect to Lord Buddha). The bamboo is then woven into the head of a cow shape.

The cow and buffalo shapes can be conceptualized as A (NPs) = power to protect from evil ghosts.

5.4 A Fish Shape

The amulet is made by metal in the form of a bream called in Thai **/tə p^{h}iən/**. It is decorated with gold leaves or a silver color, and it is called **/pla: təp^{h}iən t^{h}ɔːŋ pla: təp^{h}iən ŋən/** "gold and silver fish." Its structure is composed of two conjoined NPs. Some famous guru did not mold the fish shape, but only cut a flat metal shape as a magic fish design.

The Thai name of fish /tə **p^{h}iən/** is a fresh water fish which is known for its skilful and active living. Older people use its shape as a trademark because the last syllable of its name **/p^{h}iən/** is homophonous with a Thai word "เพียร" **/p^{h}iən/** "diligent, studious," making reference to as doing business diligently. The guru monks put some magic on the amulet and made it sacred by some magic letters. Therefore, this kind of fish symbolizes "fortune, luck, and mercy." The merchants prefer to worship this amulet in the shop by sticking gold leaves on the fish shape or hanging garlands around it.

The fish shape can be conceptualized as A (NPs) = fortune, luck, and mercy.

5.5 A Bird Shape

There are three kinds of bird shapes:

5.5.1 /sǎː rí kaː/

Which is NP as its structure. Sarika is the name of a bird which can sing sweetly and rhythmically. Some people feed it for its singing. It symbolizes "charm, mercy, and popularity." There are three kinds of Sarika:

1. **/sǎː rí kaː lín t^{h}ɔːŋ/** which is NP as its structure which means "gold tongue Sarika" by putting sacred letters at the tongue tip or upper teeth with the controlled words to such a person.

2. **/kʰîː pʰɯ̂ŋ sǎː rí kaː/** which is composed of two NPs which mean "wax Sarika": Mix scented oil into the wax and make it sacred by some magic for mercy and then rub on the lips of the ones who believe.
3. **/sǎː rí kaː lǒŋ rák/** which is a clause and its structure means "fall in love Sarika": Sculpture wood, tusk, or mold powder as **/sǎː rí kaː/** shape (male and female) and put together with **/kʰîː pʰɯ̂ŋ sǎː rí kaː/** in a small box.
4. **/tə krùt sǎː rí kaː/** which is composed of two conjoined NPs which mean "amulet of rolled gold and silver strips inscribed with sacred letters /náʔ/" rubbed with **/kʰîː pʰɯ̂ŋ sǎː rí kaː/** "wax Sarika" and strung around waist or the wrist.

The **/sǎː rí kaː/** shape can be conceptualized as A (Cl, NP(s)) = charm, mercy, and popularity.

5.5.2 /nók kʰûm kanfaj/

/nók kʰûm or nók kʰúm/ is a kind of bird that lives in the bush or in the field. It cannot fly but can shift to avoid its enemy. It is not eaten by farmers because it is believed that it was a Bodhisattva of Lord Buddha who could stop the fire from his truth. **/nók kʰûm kanfaj/** this kind of bird protects people from fire which has a syntactic structure as a clause. There are three kinds of **/nók kʰûm kanfaj/:**

1. A mold /nók kʰûm/ made by earth or metal
2. Drawing /nók kʰûm/ on the cloth or paper controlled by yantra
3. Writing with an iron stylus as /nók kʰûm/ shape

Any bird of this kind should be controlled by sacred words.

This bird can protect people from fire or stop fire or change the direction of wind. Those who worship and pray for yantra of /nók kʰûm/ at home should not be careless in terms of using electric equipment or anything dealing with fire.

/nók kʰûm kanfaj/ shape can be conceptualized as A (Cl) = protect from fire.

5.5.3 /pʰəjaː kʰrút/

"Garuda" is a kind of sacred animal. Its structure is NP. It could fly very fast and had strong power. The Indians believe that it has the same power as a god. It could disguise itself as a human.

Garuda is a vehicle of Narayan or Vishnu Mahadev. Garuda has a shape like a bird with a half-human, half-bird figure. It has hands with a bird body shape. In Thailand, a Garuda is called /sù ban/ and we accept the ancient Indian concept through the Khmer as the king is a part of Phra Narayan. Garuda is used as the seal of the king on various materials of the king, the king's utensils for sovereign ranking such as a flag called /tʰoŋ məhaː raːjaː/ "a flag of Maharaja," or a seal called /pʰrá kʰrút pʰrâː/ (Wattanamahat 2004: 77–78).

The Thai government who serves the king for administration uses Garuda as a symbol. Any activities of both the Thai people and foreigners in Thailand who have given positive outcomes for the country are also offered the use of the Garuda symbol in front of their buildings for their honor.

There are three types of Garuda:

- **/kʰrút jút nâ:k/** "Garuda stops Naga." Its structure is a clause—Garuda arrests Naga with two hands and the closed talons of its feet. The body of Naga becomes the frame line between Garuda's wings and legs which is a beautiful shape. It was a marker of King Rama II.
- **/kʰrút ram/** "dance Garuda." Its structure is a clause—Garuda's end of both wings is raised up above its head. This was originated from Khmer art. It was a marker of King Rama VI. It is said that this shape is comparable to the eagle shape of the west.
- **/kʰrút bin/** "fly Garuda." Its structure is a clause—Garuda spreads the wings as if it flies without raising its two wings up. It was a marker of King Rama VII.

As Garuda is a sacred animal, it is constructed as an amulet for protection from danger and enemies, and it represents prosperity because it relates to kings. The believers may offer flowers regularly. People should be careful not to post the Garuda image directly to other people's homes because it will cause danger to them.

Garuda shape can be conceptualized as A (Cl) = strong power of protection.

5.6 An Elephant Shape

/cʰá:ŋ ʔera:wan/ a white elephant with three heads. Its structure is NP. In India, it is considered as a vehicle of Indra God who can go anywhere with lots of power. It can destroy the earth easily. Its nature is like other elephants, to not harm anyone first. But it will respond to those who attack it.

The biggest museum of **/cʰá:ŋ ʔera:wan/** is at Samut Prakan. Many Thai people worship it as a sacred thing and believe in its power. The founder of the museum produces small amulets for the believers to rent and take back to worship at home.

The elephant shape can be conceptualized as **A (NP) = power.**

5.7 A Snake Shape

Naga or **/nâ:k/** is a semidivine being, half human and half serpent. The Indians were the first group who worshipped the big snake Naga. They considered it to be an ancestor of snakes. However, Naga is involved in Buddhism such as a place for

Lord Buddha to sit above it while protecting him from sunshine and rain which is the model of Buddha image for a person who is born on Saturday called /paːŋ nâːk

Naga is a constituent of Buddhist architecture in Thailand by building a single-headed or seven-headed Naga with its body along the way to vihara.

Naga is not only a powerful protector, it also provides wind, rain, and fertility. Naga is built as an amulet for blessing success and protecting places and property from danger. There are various types of Naga:

- **/nâːk kîəw/** is a clause in terms of syntactic structure. This amulet has two Nagas embracing each other. It is made of soil or metal. It blesses for mercy especially for a couple which is called **/nâːk sǒmpʰoŋ/.**
- **/nâːk ʔaː rák kʰǎː tʰûə paj/** "a Naga for general protection" is a clause in terms of syntactic structure. It has a shape of Naga not higher than 5 in. placed in front of a car. It is made from soil or metal.
- **/nâːk ʔaː rák kʰǎː sətʰǎːn tʰîː/** "a Naga for place protection" is a clause in terms of its syntactic structure. It was built higher than 5 in. and placed outside a building for protection from evil things. The destiny of the owner of the house should be checked to see whether it is suitable to have this type of Naga or not. If it is not suitable, that person and family may not have a normal life.
- **/nâːk fâw sáp/** "Naga protects property" is a clause in terms of syntactic structure. Its shape is not bigger than 12 in. It is built for property protection (Wattanamahat 2004: 85–94).

The Naga shape can be conceptualized as A (Cl) = mercy, protection.

5.8 A Pig Shape

The Chinese concept toward pigs is positive because they love to eat its meat and fat. It is a useful animal. The pig is the last zodiac symbol of the Chinese system. It symbolizes the end, satisfaction of action, and success. It also conveys peace, rest, and home. The Chinese word for house invents the word for pig as a combination. Pigs bring good luck.

Thai also was influenced by Chinese concepts. Thai considers that pigs eat all the time. It shows prosperity and fertility, and so it is linked as an amulet. It is made of metal—gold, silver, and bronze—called **/mǔː məhǎː moŋ kʰon/** "super luck pig" which is NP and **/mǔː jan pæ̀ːt thít/** "eight directions yantra with a pig" which is NP. Moreover, a wild pig is sometimes made as an amulet too, such as **/pʰra jaː mǔː pàː kʰâːp kæ̂ːw/** "king of wild pig holds a glass in the mouth" which is a clause.

The pig shape can be conceptualized as A (NP, Cl) = prosperity and fertility.

5.9 A Goat Shape

Goats are known in Thai society because they are fed by Hindus and Muslims. A goat is a foolish animal, but it symbolizes fertility. It was a valuable animal in the ancient trade for exchanges. It can earn a living with an easy life. The goat is a popular amulet in Thailand. It is a personal amulet for people who are born in the goat zodiac sign. It is made of elephant tusk or animal bones.

There are famous amulets such as **/pʰǽʔ lŭəŋ pʰɔ̂ː ʔàm/** "goat of vulnerable monk Am," from Rayong Province which is the oldest and most famous. Its syntactic structure is NP. **/pʰǽʔ râːt cʰə kʰru/** "Goat of Purohit" which is NP. It was built in Ayutthaya Province from the skeleton of an elephant with sacred letters beneath its body which focuses on luck and prosperity.

There are other places making the goat amulet by using metal and wood. (Wattanamahat 2004: 155–160).

The goat shape is conceptualized as A (NP) = fertility.

5.10 A Monkey Shape

Hanuman is one member of the outstanding team of Ram for snatching Sita away from Longka Island in Ramayana.

For the Thai people, the monkey is a sacred animal which is involved in Thai superstition since the Rattanakosin period. There are various shapes of monkeys such as sitting monkeys holding a pole, a stick, a knife, or a trident. Examples of the amulets called **/liŋ lom/** "Nycticebus cinereus" which is an NP, **/liŋ lom soŋ kʰrɯ̂əŋ jài/** "this kind of monkey has an elegant dress." Its structure is a clause. It symbolizes mercy and prosperity. It was made from metal.

The monkey shape is A (Cl, NP) = mercy and prosperity.

5.11 A Shape of Gecko

/túk kæː mə hǎː lâːp/ "Great luck gecko." Its syntactic structure is NP. The ancient Thai considered geckos to be a sacred animal which symbolizes happiness and fertility. Only in a fertile environment can we see the gecko and can hear its cry many times, which is good for habitats in that area.

There are divinations when geckos cry; for example:

- If it cries only once, the hearer may lose money or things unwillingly.
- If it cries three times, people in that house will be happy with prosperity.
- If it cries four times, it may cause a bad event, such as a person in the house feeling sick immediately, or people quarreling, or an accident with fire happens in the house.

- If it cries five times, the owner will be in trouble with some unexpected event.
- If it cries seven, nine, or ten times, it means that the people in the house are lucky. Life will be prosperous.
- If the gecko cries from 6:00 in the morning until 6:00 in the evening, the hearer and people in the house will get good news.
- If it cries from 6:00 in the evening to midnight, it will be both good and bad news. If it cries after midnight until 6:00 in the morning, it will be fake news.

The gecko is built as an amulet from soil. It can protect people from ghosts and black magic as well as bringing prosperity into the house. Those who worship a gecko amulet should perform merit regularly to the monk who built that amulet. Sweet juice with dessert is offered regularly to a gecko amulet then the worshiper will be successful in his/her desire (Wattanamahat 2004: 270–275).

The gecko shape can be conceptualized as A (NP) = happiness, fertility.

5.12 A Shape of Lizard

The lizard is a sacred animal which symbolizes luck **/cîŋ còk sɔ̌ːŋ hǎːŋ/** "two-tailed lizard" which is an NP. The lizard blesses with luck, and it is not done easily. The one who wants to make it should be an expert in meditation and insight contemplation. The two-tailed lizard is useful for good sales with more money and mercy. It is used by some groups, and sacred letters are applied.

Moreover, an amulet which is made from baking a two-tailed lizard and framing it for carrying is one of the ugliest amulets in Thailand. Therefore, people suggest that it should be made from other materials such as soil, wood, or metal. Some make a lizard shape with nine tails called **/cîŋ còk kâw hǎːŋ/** which is NP. Another type is mixing three types of lizard in one coin called **/cîŋ còk ʔàt^{h}ə t^{h}ít/**, which is composed of two conjoined NPs, which means "lizards on the octagon dias" by making a combination of lizards in one coin: a pair of lizards for mercy, two tails of a lizard for luck and money, and a long-tailed lizard for good business with yantra in another side of coin. This coin is not strictly used for wearing only. It can be put in a purse and made into a key ring (Wattanamahat 2004: 276–279).

The lizard shape can be conceptualized as A (NP) = luck, well purchasing.

5.13 A Frog Shape

A frog symbolizes fertility and is called **/kòp məhǎː lâːp/** "the luckiest frog." Its structure is NP. It is made from soil with a herb called /wâːn/ in a locket size. Some temples make them by candle wax and paint them with color.

The frog shape is conceptualized as A (NP) = fertility.

5.14 A Conch-Shell Shape

A conch shell is a sacred animal. Asura stole Veda from sleeping Brahman. God Vishnu followed and disguised himself as a conch shell and hid beneath the sea. The God took Veda from the conch. Therefore, all conches are considered sacred. A conch is used for Abishek ceremony for the highest blessing.

In Thai concepts, there are two types of conch: A conch with a turned right bottom or circumambulatory is used for pouring sacred water in all holy ceremonies. The conch with the turned left bottom is used for pouring water to remove inauspicious things.

Some monks construct this amulet with mixed masses and make it in a conch shape and size with a sacred ceremony. It is worshiped by placing it on an altar or putting it in sacred water. There are some types of names such as **/pʰráʔ mə hǎː sǎŋ moŋ kʰon/** "a superb auspicious conch" and **/pʰráʔ sǎŋ càk kæ̂ːw cin daː mə niː/** "gems conch," which are NPs (Wattanamahat 2004: 302–307).

The conch shape is conceptualized as A (NP) = auspicious blessing.

5.15 A Shape of Spider

The shape of a spider while spinning a web symbolizes diligence and cleanliness. It is used for customer attraction in trading. It can be made from soil, carved wood, or molded in metal. It is called **/mæːŋ mum dàk sáp/** "a spider traps treasures" which is a clause in terms of syntactic structure. It is made in a locket shape.

There is **/mæːŋ mum phét cʰə kʰâːt/** "killing dead spider" which is NP + NP or **/mæːŋ mum jon/** which is an NP "a bandit spider" for property protection. It is made by black magic. This type of spider can notify the owner when there is fire or flooding by awakening the owner (Wattanamahat 2004: 311–320).

The spider shape is conceptualized as A (Cl, NP) = customers' attraction, property protection.

5.16 A Wasp Shape

A wasp shape is made from wood, alloy, and other metals with sacred letters called **/tɔ̀ː ŋən tɔ̀ː tʰɔːŋ/** "silver and gold wasp" which is NPs in terms of syntactic structure. The nature of the wasp is to be diligent **/tɔ̀ː ŋən tɔ̀ː tʰɔːŋ/**. This means an increase in money. It is made from rare parts of jewelry and herbs mixed together with the sacred incantation into a locket size.

The wasp shape is conceptualized as A (NP) = prosperity.

6 Conclusion

The concepts of making amulets as animal shapes vary according to the background of the creators. Most are originated from the local Thai faith. Some are influenced by other cultures and religions such as Indian and Chinese cultures, Hinduism-Brahmanism. However, creating amulets is not taught in Buddhism. But, it is the syncretism of cultures and faiths in Thailand. One positive concept of worshipping the amulets is that the worshiper should behave well and make merit (do good things for others). Moreover, he/she has to offer some specific things to such respected amulets regularly. This means that they have to have faith, respect, and care.

In terms of the economy, the production of amulets involves several sectors in society which can create many jobs. In some periods, this can also increase the country's economy. In terms of animal shapes, syntactic structures, and faiths, they can be summarized as presented in the following table:

The NP structure is the most frequently found in the above analysis. Power and prosperity have the same highest frequency, mercy and fertility have the second highest, protection is the third, and happiness and luck are the least frequent. It reflects that Thai people who believe in amulets need their help for greater power and prosperity which are more difficult to achieve by one's own capacities. It may take time and effort. If there is a magic power to help them to have more confidence, they may achieve it faster. Indeed, it shows that Thai people depend on superstition more than their own karma.

Summary of the animal shapes, syntactic structures and faiths

Animal shapes	Syntactic structure	Faith
1. Tiger	NP	Power
2. Lion	NP+(NP)	Power, happiness, and prosperity
3. Cow and buffalo	NPs	Power to protect from evil ghost
4. Fish	NPs	Fortune, good luck, and mercy
5. Bird		
/sǎː rí kaː/	Cl, NP(s)	Charm, mercy, and popularity
/nók k^{h}ûm kanfaj/	Cl	Protect from fire
Garuda	Cl	Strong power of protection
6. Elephant	NP	Power
7. Snake (Naga)	Cl	Mercy, protection
8. Pig	NP, Cl	Prosperity and fertility
9. Goat	NP	Fertility
10. Monkey	Cl, NP	Mercy and prosperity
11. Gecko	NP	Happiness, fertility
12. Lizard	NP	Good luck, well purchasing
13. Frog	NP	Fertility
14. Conch	NP	Auspicious blessing
15. Spider	Cl, NP	Customers' attraction, property protection
16. Wasp	NP	Prosperity

Abbreviations: *A* animal, *NP* noun phrase, *NPs* noun phrases, *Cl* clause

References

Akhara-serani, N. (2010, August 19–20). *Inaugural speech in the seminar on 'Amulets: Buddhist culture in Suvannabhumi'*. Organized by the National Discovery Museum Institute and the Centre of Folklore Research, Faculty of Arts, and Thai Studies Institute, Chulalongkorn University.

Crowther, J. (1995). *Oxford advanced learner's dictionary of current English* (5th ed.). Oxford: Oxford University Press.

Lochan, A. (2006). Thailand. In *The encyclopedia of the Indian Diaspora*. Singapore: Editions Didier Millet.

Moore, B. (Ed.). (2009). *Australian concise Oxford dictionary* (5th ed.). Melbourne: Oxford University Press.

Phayakharanon, C. (2010, August 19–20). *Amulets in Thai society*. Proceedings of the seminar on 'Amulets: Buddhist Culture in Suvannabhumi' (pp. 12–13). Organized by the National Discovery Museum Institute and the Centre of Folklore Research, Faculty of Arts, and Thai Studies Institute, Chulalongkorn University.

Phra Paisal Visalo. (2012). *Spiritual materialism and the sacraments of consumerism: A view from Thailand*. Retrieved August 5, 2012, from http://www.visalo.org/englishArticles/consumer.htm

Radomsithiphat, W. (2010, August 19–20). *Markets of talismans*. A paper presented in the Seminar on 'Amulets: Buddhist Culture in Suvannabhumi'. Organized by the National Discovery Museum Institute and the Centre of Folklore Research, Faculty of Arts, and Thai Studies Institute, Chulalongkorn University.

Srinivas, K., & Kutumba Sastry, V. (2007). *A concise dictionary of philosophy*. New Delhi: D.K. Printworld Ltd.

Suntaree, K. (1991). *Psychology of the Thai people: Values and behavioral patterns*. Bangkok: National Institute of Development Administration (NIDA).

Thaphra, S. (2010). *The most outstanding of Siamese amulets*. Bangkok: Saengdao Publishing House.

Wattanamahat, K. (2004). *Auspicious animals and amulets*. Bangkok: Sangsan Book, Ltd.

Chapter 4
Buddhist Temple: A Religious Capital Approach for Preparing Thailand Toward the Aging Society

Saowapa Pornsiripongse, Kwanchit Sasiwongsaroj, and Patcharin Ketjamnong

1 Introduction

An increase in the aged population is a global phenomenon occurring in both developed and developing countries due to lower birthrates and longer life expectancy. The United Nations forecast that, from 2015 to 2020, the number of global populations aged 65 years and over would surpass that of the populations under 5 years old for the first time. The number of older persons would increase 2.5 times in 2050. This situation was different in 1950, when the number of the population under 5 years old was three times as much as that of the elderly population (The United Nations 2010). Additionally, it was expected that in 2025 the entire Asian region would become an aging society, with East Asia becoming one faster than Southeast Asia (The United Nations 2006).

As for Thailand, the population structure indicates that the country has become the aging society since 2005, with an increasing rate of population over 60 years old of 10 % (National Statistical Office of Thailand 2008a). The number of the aged people increased from 6.3 % in 1970 to 10.3 % in 2005 (National Statistical Office of Thailand 2008b). This number was forecast to increase 25.2 % in 2030 (Office of the National Economic and Social Development Board 2007).

Due to the change of the population structure, Thailand has been categorized in a "second-wave" country in the global aging society. It took the country only 30 years to increase its aged population from 9.40 % in 1990 to 16.8 % in 2020. Comparatively, it took a developed country approximately 70–100 years to attain this proportion, almost 10 years faster than what the United Nations had forecast. This means that Thailand has very little time to prepare its personnel and systems to accommodate the increasing aged population (The United Nations 2002).

S. Pornsiripongse (✉) • K. Sasiwongsaroj • P. Ketjamnong
Research Institute for Languages and Cultures of Asia, Mahidol University, Salaya, Puthamonthon, Nakhon Pathom 73170, Thailand
e-mail: lcsps@mahidol.ac.th; kwan7chit@yahoo.com; iamtooktik@gmail.com

P. Liamputtong (ed.), *Contemporary Socio-Cultural and Political Perspectives in Thailand*,
DOI 10.1007/978-94-007-7244-1_4,

An increase in the aged population has a direct impact on socioeconomic situations and national administration, because when the aged population increases, the ratio of working population taking care of the aged population will decrease. In 1990, the ratio was 10 to 1 (the burden rate of the aged population was 0.12). In 2020, it is forecast to be 4 to 1, or the burden rate of 0.24 (National Statistical Office of Thailand 2008b). Such a change has a direct effect on the GDP, savings, investment, and state service provision regarding social security, health, and welfare to the aged population. As a consequence, population structure change to the aging society has attracted the attention of policy makers, academics, and the business sector. Thailand has continuously improved the quality of life of older persons. It started from the 1997 Constitution, leading to the issuing of the Elderly People Act in 2003 and the second National Older Persons Plan (2005–2021). The focus is on preparing the population to become quality elderly people, improving their health, providing a social protection system, managing development work, developing personnel, and compiling and developing knowledge related to the elderly (National Commission on the Elderly 2011). Furthermore, the government designated the preparation of Thailand toward the aging society as a strategy in the 11th National Social and Economic Development Plan (2012–2016) (Office of the National Social and Economic Development Plan Board 2011).

Increasing numbers of older persons, changes of status and roles of the elderly from caregivers to dependants, and changes of family patterns and number of children per family have altered the relationship between caregivers and the elderly. In the past, family played a significant role in caring for older persons; however, the state sector has now been playing a more important part, bringing about a principal policy in encouraging communities, community organizations, neighbors, and volunteers to participate more in taking care of the elderly (Foundation of Thai Gerontology Research and Development 2007, 2008, 2009, 2010). Nevertheless, previous work on older people focused mainly on providing welfare. Even the 2003 Older Persons Act is welfare oriented (Thawlayaphothi 2008), emphasizing physical welfare and neglecting spiritual well-being of the elderly. Physical changes and loss of family and work-related roles directly affect mental/spiritual health of older persons. The 2006 report of the Gerontology Institute revealed that the Thai elderly suffered from depression the most. Thailand has possesses rich religious capital, and it should be utilized for better spiritual health of the elderly. The faithfulness to religion of older persons should be used as their spiritual refuge, which would positively affect their spiritual health and well-being (Ketpichayawathana et al. 2000; Intersoll-Dayton et al. 2001).

Buddhist temples are considered as a large social capital of the country because a temple exists in almost every community, playing various roles in the society from the past until the present (see Chaps. 5, 24, and 28 in this volume). It is a place for Buddhist relations and a social network of the faithful, bringing about the norms of trust and reciprocity as well as civic engagement. It is an essential factor for the success of the livelihood of an individual (Coleman 1988; Putnam 1993), creating a sustainable relationship network (Putnam 1993; Field 2003) and affecting other kinds of capitals. Therefore, social capital is a collective phenomenon and dispensable in the future

(Light 2004). State and other agencies have provided older people with social welfare and physical assistance at a certain level. However, their spiritual assistance has not been given a priority. It is thus recommended that the religious institution be utilized to take care of the spiritual well-being of the aged, so that the country's transition to an aging society may be smoothly done.

This chapter examines the plausibility of utilizing religious institutions to look after the spiritual well-being of older people who have rapidly been increasing in number. A social capital approach has been used to analyze the institution in conjunction with past and present roles of temples, beliefs, and faith of Buddhist followers in compliance with Buddhist principles. Other considerations include temple capital (venue, personnel, finance, and relationship network) and previous policies and work of state agencies related to the elderly. What roles should temples play in caring for the spiritual well-being of older people that are not against Buddhist discipline, and which aspects of temple potential should be equipped, so that they are prepared to accommodate an aging society?

2 Buddhist Temples as the Religious Capital of Thai Society

Social capital refers to a network of social relationships at the individual and group levels, a norm of exchange and mutual trust. The capital provides returns to individuals or groups and facilitates efficiency of social development by encouraging collective collaboration (Putnam 1993; Field 2003). Putnam (2000) theorizes that collective faith of social members is the most important aspect of social capital. He regards religion as a part of social capital, and religion plays a crucial role in establishing social capital. The social capital concept regards a social network as valuable (Field 2003). Social capital is composed of various kinds of capitals, including financial, physical, human, and cultural (Light 2004). The functions of social capital are bonding social capital, bridging social capital, and linking social capital (Putnam 2004; Woolcock 2004). See also Chaps. 14 and 17 in this volume.

Religious or spiritual capital is a part of human capital, which is developed simultaneously with socioreligious behavior in an attempt to understand religious motivation, input, and outcome. The social capital approach tries to understand the impact of religions on lives, such as work, volunteerism, economic development, and public participation.

Berger and Hefner (2003) are interested in religion as a social capital. They define social capital as power, influence, knowledge, and disposition of individuals by being group members. Religious capital is a part of social capital, referring to power, influence, knowledge, and disposition from participating in religious institutions. Sociological evidence indicates that religion is a part of social capital. Two-thirds of groups in America form a network of churches, which are community based and encourage volunteerism. For instance, religious institutions provide people with opportunities to meet, share their experiences, and make good things happen. Church members are willing to donate their time and money to support their churches. Over 50 billion dollars is donated to the church, three times higher than for education and five times higher than for health organizations. Additionally, religion provides career training to poor people (Coleman 2003). Attending church is related to an increase in volunteer activities (Wilson 2000). Religious belief influences the definition of volunteerism. Those with religious experience have a public mind toward their communities (Wuthnow 1994).

The discussion of this chapter is based on the concept of social and religious capitals, viewing that Buddhism is an important social capital[1] in Thai society. The capitals include financial capital, referring to the capital for developing, supporting, and organizing religious activities of the temples. Physical capital includes places for monks to conduct religious activities: ordination hall, chapel, pavilion, auditorium, and library. Human capital is composed of monks and laypeople. Cultural capital consists of Buddhist teachings, and religious capital refers to beliefs and faith in Buddhists on Buddhism, temples, and monks. These capitals create a relationship network, trust between followers and the temple, a norm of practice, and religious activities, participation, support, and ownership. These capitals are an alternative to prepare Thai society toward the aging society.

3 Buddhist Paradigm on Well-Being

The majority of Thai people are Buddhists, and Buddhist teachings therefore influence their perspectives, thoughts, and beliefs. The teachings also play a crucial part in cultivating their values, personalities, and livelihood. Furthermore, they are both social rules and a device for socialization (Paonil 2003). Buddhism also influences people's perspective on the world, life, health, sickness, and death. Sickness is viewed as a natural phenomenon of life, but living a life should not be pointless. Health must be properly taken care of to minimize sickness and to lengthen our lives for continuous Dharma practice. If sickness cannot be controlled, it will become chronic or even fatal, which is not regarded as a loss. However, this phenomenon should be taken into serious consideration in order to understand the truth of nature, so that we should be cautious and do more good deeds in order to prevent this phenomenon from causing us suffering.

Buddhism categorizes sickness into two main groups, physical and mental, with the latter outweighing the former. Therefore, Buddhist teachings focus on building spiritual immunity or empowerment to prevent spiritual ailments. When it happens, the focus is on treatment, that is, eliminating it. Nevertheless, Buddhism views that body and mind must reciprocally exist together as a single entity. Spiritual practice for complete elimination of suffering or ailments is based on the practice of creating awareness on laws and truths of nature: all things are subject to the three

[1] Social capital is in line with the five components of Buddhism, namely, the Buddha, religious doctrines, religious rituals, religious building structures, and religious followers.

characteristics of existence,[2] namely, impermanence, conflict, and soullessness. Understanding this ultimate truth has positive effects on physical and spiritual well-being (Payutto 2001: 75–76).

Healthcare and sickness prevention under the Buddhist paradigm is based on monitoring one's mind. Religious practices will enable one to gain an insight on the truths of all things, so that one would not feel so attached to oneself, one's body, or belongings that one suffers or becomes psychologically sick (Paonil 2003). Therefore, Buddhist teachings are valuable to apply to older people, so that they are able to accept changes, both physical and social, in order to live a happy old life.

3.1 Buddhism and the Meaning of the Elderly

Buddhism defines older people not in terms of age but as those with intelligence and specialization enough to teach the young. They must be role models and lead a peaceful, calm, and happy life. They must be well rounded and respectable. Old age is a time to find spiritual peace, to make merit, to meditate, to be content in the quiet, and to renounce worldly possession to their children, so that they are able to attain spiritual insight and to teach others (Buddhadasa Bhikkhu 1987).

Moreover, the aged should be familiar with calmness and free mind, neither happy nor sad, and understand the ways things are. This means that there is no love, no anger, no hatred, no excitement, no jealousy, no conflict, and no worry.

A good older person in religious view must be able to accept physical deterioration, depend on himself when he/she can, and be most satisfied with his/her assigned responsibilities. Such a person is religiously regarded as a perfect and happy older person (Buddhadasa Bhikkhu 1987). Continuously maintaining the social role and relationship of the elderly would make them feel worthy, honorable, and happy. At the same time, religious beliefs and faith would enable them to accept changes, leading to better well-being.

Besides being physically healthy, older people must be spiritually sound and understand the principle of impermanence, conflict, and soullessness. This principle would help them to accept changes more readily.

3.2 Buddhism and Health of Older Persons

As for Buddhism and the quality of life of the aged, temples should play a spiritual role by teaching the principles to be integrated into their lives during this transition period, so that their lives can be happy, meaningful, and worthy. Conducting

---

[2] Impermanence is a transitional state of existing, decaying, and disappearing. Conflict is a state of frustration for attempting to maintain ephemeral entities, and soullessness is the actual state of entities that cannot be controlled (Payutto 2001).

religious activities is regarded as preparing the final phase of their lives (Busayawong and Thaengphet 2007). It is also suggested that well-being is related to frequency in listening to sermons at the temple. Awareness of the value of Buddhism, mindfulness, and secludedness are positively related to life satisfaction of the aged (Wongsit 1998). It is, therefore, recommended that older people should participate in religious activities to enhance their well-being (Itabashi et al. 2010).

In addition to being a place for monks to practice and spread Buddhist principles, a temple is a center of community activities, strengthening the relationship between the temple and laypeople, particularly the elderly group (Wongsit 1998). Factors attracting the aged to the temple include spiritual suffering, faith, family tradition, fear of death due to ailments, being sick of worldly conditions, and interest in Dharma. Furthermore, the temple has created a new role for older persons as patrons and caregivers of the religion, temples, and monks (Santhawachart 2009). It is also suggested that the social role of the elderly is most expressed through religion orientation (Kamonpornpichit et al. 2005).

Studies on the relationship between religion and health of older people have attracted more attention in the West, with over 1,200 topics (Benjamins 2004). It has been found that religion affects health promotion, disease prevention, and different awareness levels of health as well as death in general (Koenig et al. 1999). Moreover, religion also affects stroke (Colantino et al. 1992), hypertension (Koenig et al. 1998), health-related depression (Wink et al. 2005; Nooney and Woodrum 2002; Schwadel and Falci 2012), osteoporosis (Pressman et al. 1990), and immunity system (Koenig et al. 1997). Religiosity will increase when people get older and are more involved in religious activities (Pargament and Park 1997). Faith in religion affects stress levels when people become older. Idler and Kasl (1992) revealed that participating in religious activities could direct levels of body work. Religious practices positively affect physical and spiritual health (Ellison and Levin 1998).

Religion is beneficial to the well-being of older people. Benjamins and Buck (2008) revealed that religious practices and faith in religious teachings could predict the levels of self-assistance (physical movement) of the aged. Beliefs, faith, and religious practices were found to be linked to good health behavior (Ellison and Levin 1998). There are numerous studies on the relationship between religion and mental health. It has been revealed that participating in religious activities has affected the levels of wellness, hope, optimism, self-worth, problem-solving capabilities, stress, and restlessness.

Those involved in religious activities encounter less or shorter depression which directly impacts physical well-being (Koenig et al. 2001). They also have better physical and mental health than those not participating in religious activities (Koenig 1998; Levin 1998). In Japan, religion also encouraged the Japanese elderly to help members of their social network, particularly male elders (Krause et al. 1999).

The influence of religion on health increases with older age (Koenig et al. 1998). It was found that faith had more influence on the wellness of people over 75 years than on those aged 55–74 years. The impacts of religion on health include being a mechanism to create indicators on social support and health behavior; being reinforcement for positive psychological conditions such as faith, hope, and inner peace;

strengthening the drive to seek or maintain positive health behavior; and being influential on health (Oman and Thoresen 2002).

In Thailand, there have not been many studies on Buddhism and health. Most are taken from oral accounts from direct experience of individuals. For instance, one person said that Dharma improved her health and meditation calmed her mind, lessened her worries and made her fall asleep faster, improving her overall health. Walking meditation was beneficial to her health in many respects (Paonil 2003).

From the above literature review, it can be concluded that religion affects longevity, better health, and the reduction of chronic diseases. Religious faith and participation in religious activities have brought about improved wellness, hope, optimism, self-worth, and lower levels of depression and stress of older people. Buddhism also emphasizes self-reliance, satisfaction with one's responsibilities and acceptance of change. Consequently, work involving the aged should be based on these truths, and Buddhist principles should be used as a guideline in developing the well-being of older persons in conjunction with other social welfare work. Besides its principles, Buddhism is composed of its teachings (cultural capital), rituals (social or religious capital), facilities (physical capital), and personnel (human capital). These capitals can be used to support the improvement of overall well-being of older people. It is thus imperative to revise previous state work on the aged to find out whether and how much the religious institution had been incorporated.

4 Work on the Elderly in Thailand

One way to consider how much the country lays importance on older people and guidelines to treating them is through legal entities and mechanisms concerning the aged. Since Thailand became a democratic society with the monarch as the head of state in 1932, up to 2012, there have been 18 volumes of the constitution.[3] The 1991 volume (the fifteenth) was the first to have a passage about the elderly.[4] However, older people are viewed negatively and are categorized in the same group as the physically challenged, a social burden that the state must assist (Thawlayaphothi 2008).

Since 1997, Thailand has legally recognized the importance of older persons. The 1997 constitution (the seventeenth) was the first to issue an act about the elderly separate from that of the disabled.[5] It designated older persons with insufficient

[3] Due to frequent political coups d'état in the country, constitutions have been redrafted and amended.

[4] The mention of the elderly in the charter was partly from the pressure of the World Assembly on the Aged, held in Vienna, Austria, in 1982. The assembly defined an older person as an individual with the age of 60 years and over.

[5] The issue was in response to the UN Assembly on December 16, 1991. Member countries were obliged to specify national principles and goals on the elderly and to incorporate them into their national plans.

income for subsistence as being eligible to state assistance, and the state must provide welfare to the elderly, the poor, the disabled, and the underprivileged in order to improve their quality of life and to make them self-reliant. The 2007 constitution (the eighteenth) provided right protection and assistance to the aged. Additionally, the state must arrange savings for the public and state officers in their old age.

The 1997 constitution brought about the Older Persons Act in 2003, the first and only one specified for the elderly. The aims were to protect and provide assistance to older people with insufficient income and to establish the Older Persons Fund to provide financing for the protection, promotion, and support for the aged. Nonetheless, the act was merely concerned with state social welfare, not meant to accommodate the new population structure with an increasingly larger number of aging population. Simply depending on financial support from the state is inadequate to prepare for the aging society of the country (Thawlayaphothi 2008).

Since the legal system regards older people as dependants requiring special care and assistance, previous and current policies[6] and work have mainly been based on welfare. State care and welfare for the aged have been categorized into institutional, family, and community levels.

4.1 Care of the Elderly at the Institutional Level

Care of the elderly at the institutional level refers to the state carrying out or managing assistance for older people and viewing them as invalid. For welfare operations, 13 welfare centers for the aged were established nationwide, accommodating 1,112 people; 12 welfare development centers for older persons, accommodating 1,169 people; and 113 social service centers and long-stay homes for the aged operated by the private sector and public organizations (Foundation of Thai Gerontology Research Development 2009). Additionally, a 300-baht monthly allowance was provided to poor or neglected older persons.[7] As for assistance, a state-sponsored fund for the aged was established to support various projects related to the elderly and to provide public services and benefits to them. It can be seen that religion was not incorporated into this state-initiated assistance.

---

[6] The Second National Elderly Plan (2002–2021) focuses on five issues, namely, preparing the population for the quality elderly, promoting health of the elderly, social safety net of the elderly, managing development work and developing personnel related to the elderly, and processing and reinventing knowledge on the elderly (National Commission on the Elderly 2011).

[7] The policy was implemented in 1993. It was raised to 500 baht in 2002, but not covering all older persons. In 2009, the policy covered every older person, except those already receiving fringe benefits from state agencies. In 2011, the tier system was implemented: those aged 60–69 years get 600 baht, 70–79 years get 700 baht, 80–89 years get 800 baht, and 90 years and over get 1,000 baht (Foundation of Thai Gerontology Research Development 2009; Bureau of Empowerment for Older Persons 2011).

4.2 *Care of Older People at the Family and Community Levels*

State welfare provision to the aged has not been sufficient compared with the rapidly growing number of elderly. As a consequence, the state has encouraged family and community to participate in caring for older persons. The state established policies for the family and community to implement. Instances of this collaboration include visiting volunteer projects, friends helping friend volunteers, home healthcare centers, older persons clubs, community welfare funds, multipurpose community centers for the aged, temple service centers for the elderly, and temples as health promotion centers[8] (Foundation of Thai Gerontology Research and Development 2009). Despite getting family and community involved, the state's perspective remains the same: viewing them as dependants requiring assistance from various sectors.

It is noted that religious institutions have been involved in the implementation at the community level. However, most of the focus is on the physical capital of the temples. Buddhist teachings for developing the spiritual well-being of the elderly have not been much implemented.

5 Temples and the Aging Society: Practical Possibility?

Buddhist temples have been an integral part of the Thai society. It can be said that the life of a Thai person is closely connected to the temple from birth to death. Temples are an easily accessible social capital and should be used to care for the spiritual well-being of older people.

5.1 *In Line with State Policies*

Thai society has become an aging society faster than the developed countries have. Within a time span of three decades, the ratio of aged population has almost doubled (The United Nations 2002). Therefore, the country has had little time to prepare for this demographic phenomenon. The state has realized that it is not able to handle the situation alone. Hence, families, communities, organizations, and social networks have been encouraged to take care of older people. As a social organization existing throughout the country and a place for spreading Buddhist teachings, using temples to care for the aged is appropriate and possible.

---

[8] It is designated that a temple is a place for supplementary activities of monks and laypeople. A temple carrying out health promotion activities must have the following five elements: having clean buildings and environment; conducting religious practices and sermons; having qualified monks and activities that promote healthcare; conserving traditions, arts, and culture; and having community members participating in development activities.

5.2 In Line with the Concept of Socially Engaged Buddhism

A temple is a community center that plays many social roles. It is an educational center for children to be educated religiously and academically. It is a welfare institution for poor children to live and be educated; a medical center to heal the sick by using folk wisdom[9]; a shelter for travelers; a club for community members to interact, relax, and seek knowledge; an entertainment venue during festivals; a court to reconcile conflicts and family problems; a cultural center collecting artifacts; an inventory storage for villagers to borrow; an administrative center for villagers to hold meetings; a religious place to conduct rituals; and a place to learn Buddhist principles (Sirintharo et al. 1982). Consequently, the temple playing a role in caring for the spiritual well-being for the aged is in line with the concept.

Nevertheless, there has been a controversy as to whether Buddhism is meant for personal salvation or for others. Critics on the concept of socially engaged Buddhism include Ven. Buddhadasa Bhikkhu, Ven. Payutto, Ven. Phaisan Wisalo, Sulak Siwalak, Weera Somboon, Ven. Thich Nhat Hanh, H.H. the Dalai Lama, Ven. Dr. Rahula, Thomas Freeman Yornall, and Marshall White (Naracheto 2010). It has been unanimously concluded that Buddhist principles are meant for the ultimate benefits of mankind. The duties of monks cover religious practices for personal salvation, preaching others to overcome suffering, and applying the teachings to help laypeople overcome their daily suffering (Sirikanjana 1996). Additionally, monks are obliged to spread the teachings and help guide the correct development of society. Monks cannot exist without support from lay society, and at the same time, they are a part of the community empowerment process (Chiamphaw 1986; Wasi 1997; Naracheto 2010). One challenge for the Buddhist institutions is what roles they will play to ensure a smooth transition for Thailand into an aging society.

5.3 In Line with Belief and Faith

Faith in Buddhist teachings has brought about core values of Thai society (Paonil 2003). The temple is a spiritual center of laypeople (Sirintharo et al. 1982; Khongphet 1991; Santhawachart 2009). Monks are spiritual leaders and center of collaboration, since they are believed to be spiritually pure, intellectual leaders, and altruists (Chiamphaw 1986). In addition, the temple is a model for cleanliness, tranquility, and enlightenment, because it is a center for morality, ethics, customs, traditions, and cultures of localities. Monks have a close relationship with their followers, especially as spiritual guides for the aged to lead a moral life. With beliefs

[9] The health relationship between the temple and laypeople is in the form of welfare, in order to ease physical and mental suffering. It is in line with a Buddhist principle that monks can provide treatments to the sick, provided that no monetary cost is imposed, a gesture of giving practice. The 1992 Monks Act also states that monks can perform their duties within the framework of religious disciplines. It is not immoral or against the disciplines.

and faith in the religion, the temple becomes a venue for older people to interact and share their experiences, knowledge, and information. During the Buddhist Lent, old people would stay overnight on Buddhist holy days to observe the precepts and overcome the loneliness of staying home alone when others go to work, a means to strengthen their relationship networks (Busayawong and Thaengphet 2007).

International studies have revealed that faith and religious practices affect longevity and reduction of stress, depression, and severity of illness. In Thailand, studies have found that people aged 65–69 years conducted religious activities at the temples the most and more so among those involved in agriculture. Temples can create activities for the aged to participate in, which offer a new identity and role for them, enabling them to maintain their roles and social relationship. These activities make them feel strong and useful to others, creating a sense of prestige and self-worth. Spiritually, temples should be able to play a part in changing the rhetoric from "the elderly as a social burden" to "the valuable and honorable older persons." As a consequence, the temples as a community organization should collaborate with the state sector in preparing for the aging society.

5.4 In Line with the Definition of the Healthy Elderly

Buddhism views older persons not as those who are old but as those who accept the principle of cause and effect of all things in the universe and understand the impermanence, conflict, and soullessness principles. That is, they accept physical changes and self-reliance, are satisfied with their roles and duties, and are physically and mentally healthy. Old age is a valuable period of life, and older people are able to contribute greatly to their families and society: a perfect time of life. Faith in Buddhism would enable the elderly to accept changes of all things, and the temples with monks preaching Buddhist principles should be the most suitable agency.

5.5 Physical Facilities

Almost every village in the country has a temple. At present, there are 37,057 temples nationwide. Each temple is divided into religious quarters and living quarters for monks.[10] The temple is a public place for everyone to conduct religious ceremonies or secular activities of the community. There is no need for new investment, and what is required is improvement of the facilities, so that they are suitable for the aged and others (Sasiwongsaroj et al. 2012). Furthermore, most temples have maintained a natural and peaceful environment suitable for spiritual practice (Table 4.1).

[10] The walled temple ground is divided into two sections: the religious quarters, where religious ceremonies are held and building structures located, and the monks' living quarters (Phayakharanon 2004).

Table 4.1 Number of temples nationwide by regions

Regions	Number of temples	Percentage
Bangkok	425	1
North	8,809	24
Central	2,984	8
Northeast	17,906	48
East	1,865	5
West	1,878	5
South	3,244	9
Total	**37,075**	**100**

Source: National Office of Buddhism (2011)

5.6 Personnel

According to the National Office of Buddhism (2011), there were 291,116 monks nationwide. From a survey on the readiness of the temples for the aging society from 867 development-oriented temples nationwide, it was found that secular education of monks ranged from primary school to doctoral degree and 64.1 % held the highest religious studies. Furthermore, 81.1 % were keen on spreading Buddhist principles to the elderly and 58.5 % on disseminating secular knowledge to older people. Monks are also able to encourage the elderly to participate in learning activities on a regular basis. Moreover, they are able to motivate the aged to become inquisitive, an example of lifelong learning (Pornsiripongse et al. 2012).

5.7 Budget

Temples do not receive budgetary support from the state for religious operations. However, from interviewing five abbots in the North, it was revealed that budget did not pose any problem in carrying out religious and social activities, since financial support was from public donations (Pornsiripongse et al. 2012). Temples with abbots who are knowledgeable, development oriented, and are able to solve community problems will attract more donations from their faithfulness (Srithanyarat and Darikanlert 2010). As for work related to older people, Wongsit (1998) suggests that abbots attempt to convince the elderly to participate in activities. If community members have faith in the abbots, temple-based activities tend to become successful. Faith brings about human capital, including monks, laypeople, and villagers, willing to help. It will also bring in financial capital and cultural capital, which temples could mobilize for further development.

5.8 Creating a Network with Other Agencies

In attempting to solve social problems in the past, many agencies focused on the temples as they viewed that temples were social capital with potential. Consequently, temples have collaborated with various agencies in carrying out activities based on either their interests or state policies, such as healthcare and health promotion of the elderly. Such an activity was conducted by a temple whose abbot or monks provided treatments to sick villagers and older persons (Chanket et al. 2008; see also Chap. 28 in this volume). For temples in collaboration with external agencies according to state policies, the cooperation is in the form of temple area use. For instance, the Ministry of Public Health established community health centers, the elderly clubs, and centers for health promotion in temple grounds. The Ministry of Education established centers for non-formal education and career training centers. The Ministry of Social and Human Resource Development established service centers for the aged. Collaboration with these state agencies is in line with temple needs. It was revealed that many abbots would like their temples to become centers for public activities rather than as places for religious activities per se (Srithanyarat and Darikanlert 2010). With the view of attracting laypeople into the temples and returning benefits to communities, temples have welcomed projects of various agencies, because they have areas for activities and for maximum use. As a consequence, if a temple is interested in working for older people, collaboration with external agencies is possible, since these agencies have already perceived the capabilities of the temples.

6 Preparing Temples for the Aging Society

From the above discussion, it is noted that Buddhist temples have been prepared to become involved in accommodating an aging society. Nevertheless, during the past three decades, Thai society has become more modern and sophisticated. There are new social institutions taking over the roles of the temples. Education has been transferred to schools and universities. Hospitals have been in charge of medical treatments, and museums are in charge of collecting and displaying cultural artifacts. Therefore, temples can no longer respond to social needs as in the past. Some are no longer community centers. Since the institution has not conducted the function of cultivating moral and ethic ground to young children, many people are distant from religion, do not understand Buddhism, and do not see the use of having a religion (Payutto 1970).

Temples have also been encountering other problems. One is that fewer people are ordained for a long period of time. Many are ordained for 1 or 2 weeks, not an entire Lent.[11] Some are ordained when they are old due to having no one to look after them or having other purposes besides studying the principles (Payutto 1970). The result is that there are fewer qualified monks who can conduct religious practices and social work. This situation is in line with a survey conducted by Pornsiripongse and others (2012), revealing that over half of the temples surveyed had one to ten monks and over 70 % had fewer than ten monks who had been ordained for 5 years. The other is that monks do not have sufficient secular knowledge. The Theravada sect has prospered due to mutual support between monks and laypeople. Monks should possess

[11] The Lent is a period of 3 months, starting from the 15th day of the waxing moon of the eighth lunar month to the 15th day of the waxing moon of the 11th lunar month.

both religious and secular knowledge. Monks restricting themselves in religious arena without learning about the modern world would not be able to connect the religious world with the modern secular world (Wisalo 2009).

Faith in Buddhism and regular religious practices are beneficial to preventing and lessening the severity of ailments. To prepare the temple as temple-based health promotion of the elderly (Holt and McClure 2006), it is advisable to solve the problems currently encountered by the temples. The following are some guidelines to prepare the temple for the aging society.

6.1 Brainstorming About Older People

It is not uncommon for temples to have the elderly carrying out religious practices. Temples should focus more on old age and the principles of cause and effect as well as the three characteristics of existence. When older people understand and accept the principles as universal truths, they will be prepared for changes in life, making their lives worthy and happy. What should be done is to get more older people to come and encourage those taking care of grandchildren at home to come to the temple while they are still physically strong. Monks should highlight study findings about the benefits of religious practices and participation in religious activities as a means to persuade the aged. Nowadays, many older persons suffer from various chronic ailments, such as diabetes, hypertension, high cholesterol, and heart disease. These people feel hopeless and depressed because they think that they will never be able to overcome these diseases (Pornsiripongse 2007). It is thus imperative to brainstorm with other temples, local organizations, and other agencies to promote the mental and spiritual health of the elderly.

6.2 Various Means of Operations

Operational means to promote healthcare for older persons should be various and flexible due to different contexts of temples. Some have sufficient physical capital with communities willing to fully cooperate with the temples. Others have qualified abbots, and many are ready in every aspect. Therefore, patterns of operation should be varied according to the local context.

6.3 Collaborating with Communities and Temple Networks

It is recommended that temples utilize participatory management principles to deal with work related to older people. Monks alone cannot handle the job because many temples do not have sufficient number of monks and/or many monks are not qualified. It is thus necessary to work with communities and a network of local temples. Working with other communities, agencies, organizations, temples, and laypeople does not mean competing for the same job but rather cooperating for public benefit. Local organizations should support temples in terms of publicity, budget, advice, and suggestions. Regarding the shortages of monks, temples should work in the form of a temple network because different temples have different strengths and levels of preparedness.

6.4 *Improving Religious and Secular Knowledge of Monks*

Secular knowledge is a base and a means for religious knowledge (Wisalo 2009). Monks who are able to promote the well-being of the aged and provide them with a spiritual refuge must have profound religious knowledge as well as secular knowledge. With new and interesting teaching techniques, they will be able to effectively link the realities of secular society with Buddhist principles.

6.5 *Improving Temple Environment*

In addition to building structures in the temples, what should not be overlooked is a cool, clean, and peaceful natural environment within the temple grounds. A suitable temple environment will facilitate and improve the religious practices and atmosphere for the elderly.

7 Conclusion

To prepare for a rapidly increasing aged population, the state must prepare spiritual support for older people in addition to providing them with social welfare. In this respect, Buddhist temples should be involved, as they already organize religious activities on a regular basis, but without focusing on any particular group. Temples have to respond to community needs in general. In the face of an aging society, more focus should be on those in the elderly group. Temple problems should be solved and their potential enhanced in order for temples to promote the spiritual well-being of the elderly effectively and efficiently.

References

Benjamins, M. R. (2004). Religion and functional health among the elderly is there a relationship and is it constant? *Journal of Aging and Health, 16*(3), 355–374.

Benjamins, M. R., & Buck, A. C. (2008). Religion: A socio-cultural predictor of health behaviors in Mexico. *Journal of Aging and Health, 20*(3), 290–305.

Berger, P. L., & Hefer, R. W. (2003). *Spiritual capital in comparative perspective*. Spiritual capital research program. Philadelphia: Metanexus Institute.

Buddhadasa Bhikkhu. (1987). *Dharma for the elderly. Dharma speech for the elderly group from Lampang on 22 March 1987*. Retrieved February 19, 2012, from: http://www.youtube.com/watchtv=5dYXwJXfwXY

Bureau of Empowerment for Older Persons. (2011). *The government policy for older persons*. Retrieved January 25, 2012, from: http://www.oppo.opp.go.th/pages/download/download.html

Busayawong, C., & Thaengphet, S. (2007). *Role of temples in social well fair arrangement for the elderly in rural Northern area*. Retrieved January 10, 2012, from: http://www.nrtnet.com/images/main_1297470640/p2.pdf

Chanket, R., Limpananon, J., & Patrakan, P. (2008). *Integration Thai traditional medicine into modern medicine health service systems*. Bangkok: The War Veterans Organization Publishing.

Chiamphaw, W. (1986). *Role of Buddhist monks on moral training and educating the youth*. Unpublished thesis, Faculty of Graduate Studies, Mahidol University, Thailand.

Colantino, A., Kasl, S. V., & Ostfeld, A. M. (1992). Depressive symptoms and other psychosocial factors as predictors of stroke in the elderly. *American Journal of Epidemiology, 136*(7), 884–894.

Coleman, J. S. (1988). Social capital in the creation of human capital. *The American Journal of Sociology, 94*(Suppl.), S95–S120.

Coleman, J. S. (2003). Religious social capital: Its nature, social location, and limits. In C. E. Smidt (Ed.), *Religion as social capital: Producing the common good* (pp. 33–49). Waco: Baylor University Press.

Ellison, C. G., & Levin, J. S. (1998). The religion health connection: Evidence, theory, and future directions. *Health Education & Behavior, 25*(6), 700–720.

Field, J. (2003). Civic engagement and lifelong learning: Survey findings on social capital and attitudes towards learning. *Studies in the Education of Adults, 35*(2), 142–156.

Foundation of Thai Gerontology Research Development. (2007). *Elderly situation report 2007*. Bangkok: Tee Que Pee Ltd.

Foundation of Thai Gerontology Research Development. (2008). *Elderly situation report 2008*. Bangkok: Tee Que Pee Ltd.

Foundation of Thai Gerontology Research Development. (2009). *Situation of the Thai elderly 2009*. Bangkok: Tee Que Pee Ltd.

Foundation of Thai Gerontology Research Development. (2010). *Elderly situation of the Thai elderly 2010*. Bangkok: Tee Que Pee Ltd.

Gerontology Institute. (2006). *A survey and study of the elderly health in four regions of Thailand*. Nonthaburi: Agricultural Cooperative Assembly of Thailand.

Holt, C. L., & McClure, S. M. (2006). Perceptions of the religion-health connection among African American church members. *Qualitative Health Research, 16*(2), 268–281.

Idler, L., & Kasl, S. V. (1992). Religion, disability, depression, and the timing of death. *The American Journal of Sociology, 97*(4), 1052–1079.

Intersoll-Dayton, B., Saengtienchai, C., Kespichayawattana, J., & Aungsuroch, Y. (2001). Psychological well-being Asian style: The perspective of Thai elders. *Journal of Cross-Cultural Gerontology, 16*, 283–302.

Itabashi, S., Chompikul, J., Keiwkanka, B., Sowattanagoon, N., & Trukulsri, S. (2010). Life satisfaction of the elderly in Phukhiao district, Chiyalhum Province, Thailand. *Journal of Public Health and Development, 8*(2), 123–124.

Kamonpornpichit, P., Thawprayoon, W., & Wathinsunthorn, M. (2005). *Role and relationship among temples, monks and Thai elderly*. Research report. Nonthaburi: Bureau of Health Promotion, Department of Health, Ministry of Public Health.

Ketpichayawathana, J., Sangduanchai, J., & Angsuroch, Y. (2000). Happiness of Thai elderly. *Journal of Gerontology and Geriatric Medicine, 1*(3), 21–28.

Khongphet, A. (1991). *Study of need of the elderly in academic activities for lifelong learning education*. Surindra: Surindra Rajabhat University.

Koenig, H. G. (1998). Religious attitudes and practices of hospitalized medically ill older adults. *International Journal of Geriatric Psychiatry, 13*(4), 213–224.

Koenig, H. G., Weiner, D. K., Peterson, B. L., Meador, K. G., & Keefe, F. J. (1997). Religious coping in the nursing home: A bio-psychosocial model. *International Journal of Psychiatry in Medicine, 27*(4), 365–376.

Koenig, H. G., George, L. K., Hays, J. C., Larson, D. B., Cohen, H. J., & Blazer, D. G. (1998). The relationship between religious activities and blood pressure in older adults. *International Journal of Psychiatry in Medicine, 28*(2), 189–213.

Koenig, H. G., Kvale, J. N., & Ferrel, C. (1999). Religion and well-being in later life. *The Gerontologist, 28*(1), 18–28.

Koenig, H. G., McCullough, M. E., & Larson, D. B. (2001). *Handbook of religion and health*. New York: Oxford University Press.

Krause, N., Dayton, B. I., Liang, J., & Sugisawa, H. (1999). Religion, social support, and health among the Japanese elderly. *Journal of Health and Social Behavior, 40*(4), 405–421.

Levin, J. S. (1998). Religious factors in aging, adjustment, and health: A theoretical overview. *Journal of Religion and Aging, 4*(3/4), 133–146.

Light, I. (2004). Using social capital to help integrate planning theory, research, and practice: Social capital's unique accessibility. *Journal of the American Planning Association, 70*(2), 145–151.

Naracheto, P. Y. (2010). *Concept of socially engaged Buddhist*. Bangkok: Mahachulalongkornrajavidyalaya University.

National Commission on the Elderly. (2011). *Second national plan for the elderly (2005–2021)*. Bangkok: Teappenwanit Publishing.

National Office of Buddhism. (2011). Database of the national office of Buddhism. Retrieved April 21, 2012, from: http://www.onab.go.th/index.php?option=com_content&view=category&id=77&Itemid=298.

National Statistical Office of Thailand. (2008a). *Thai elderly 2008: Perspectives and reflections from statistic*. Bangkok: National Statistical Office of the Prime Minister.

National Statistical Office of Thailand. (2008b). *Report on 2007 survey for the older persons in Thailand*. Bangkok: Thana Press.

Nooney, J., & Woodrum, E. (2002). Religious coping and church-based social support as predictors of mental health outcomes: Testing a conceptual model. *Journal for the Scientific Study of Religious, 41*, 359–368.

Office of the National Economic and Social Development Board. (2007). *Summary the tenth national economic and social development plan (2007–2011)*. Bangkok: Office of the Prime Minister.

Office of the National Economic and Social Development Board. (2011). *Summary the eleventh national economic and social development plan (2012–2016)*. Bangkok: Office of the Prime Minister.

Oman, D., & Thoresen, C. E. (2002). Does religion cause health?: Differing interpretations and diverse meanings. *Journal of Health Psychology, 7*(4), 365–380.

Paonil, V. (2003). *Buddhist paradigm: For health and healing in Thailand*. Nonthaburi: Health Systems Research Institute.

Pargament, K. I., & Park, C. L. (1997). In times of stress: The religion–coping connection. In B. Spilka & D. N. McIntosh (Eds.), *The psychology of religion: Theoretical approaches* (pp. 43–53). Boulder: Westview Press.

Payutto, P. A. (1970). *Buddhism and present Thai society*. Bangkok: Siwaporn Ltd.

Payutto, P. A. (2001). *Dharmma* (1st ed.). Bangkok: Social Science Association of Thailand.

Phayakharanon, J. (2004). *Encyclopedia for the youth*. Bangkok: Dansutha Publishing.

Pornsiripongse, S. (2007). *A model development on holistic health care for people with diabetes*. Bangkok: Thai Health Promotion Foundation.

Pornsiripongse, S., Sasiwaongsaroj, K., Burasith, Y., Ketjamnong, P., & Kusakulrat, N. (2012). *Religious institutions and preparing for an aging society*. Unpublished report. Salaya: Research Institute for Languages and Cultures of Asia, Mahidol University.

Pressman, P., Lyons, J. S., Larson, D. B., & Strain, J. J. (1990). Religious belief, depression, and ambulation status in elderly women with broken hips. *The American Journal of Psychiatry, 147*(6), 758–760.
Putnam, R. D. (1993). The prosperous community: Social capital and economic growth. *The American Prospect, 4*(13), 1–11.
Putnam, R. D. (2000). *Bowling alone: The collapse and revival of American community*. New York: Simon & Schuster.
Putnam, R. D. (2004). Using social capital to help integrate planning theory, research, and practice: Preface. *Journal of the American Planning Association, 70*(2), 142–192.
Santhawachart, S. (2009). *Practicing dharma for developing the body and mind of the Thai elderly people*. Unpublished thesis, Faculty of Political Science, Chulalongkorn University, Bangkok.
Sasiwongsaroj, K., Pornsiripongse, S., Burasith, Y., Ketchamnong, P., & Kusakulrat, N. (2012). Buddhist temple: The well-being space for the aged in Thailand. *Journal of Population and Social Studies, 20*(2), 2–19.
Schwadel, P., & Falci, C. D. (2012). Interactive effects of church attendance and religious tradition on depressive symptoms and positive affect. *Society and Mental Health, 2*(1), 21–34.
Sirikanjana, P. (1996). *Buddhism and soul of Thai society: Research issues on religion and culture*. Bangkok: Mahachulalongkornrajavidyalaya University.
Sirintharo, P. S., Wasi, P., Soongsumran, S., & Siwarak, S. (1982). *Role of the temples and future of Thai monks*. Bangkok: Kretthai Publishing.
Srithanyarat, W., & Darikanlert, L. (Eds.). (2010). *Procedure knowledge management and synthesis of health promotion hospital: Guideline for the elderly services*. Bangkok: Sahamitre Printing and Publishing.
Thawlayaphothi, N. (2008). *Elders in Thai law*. Retrieved April 21, 2012, from: http://www.krisdika.go.th
United Nation. (2002). *World population prospects: The 2002 revision*. Retrieved April 18, 2012, from: http://www.earth-policy.org/images/uploads/book_files/outnotes.pdf
United Nation. (2006). *World population prospects: The 2006 revision*. Retrieved April 24, 2012, from: http://www.un.org/esa/population/publications/wpp2006/WPP2006_Highlights_rev.pdf
United Nation. (2010). *World population prospects: The 2010 revision*. Retrieved April 21, 2012, from: http://esa.un.org/unpd/wpp
Wasi, P. (1997). *Monk and social up date*. Bangkok: Moh Chaoban Publishing.
Wilson, J. (2000). Volunteering. *Annual Review of Sociology, 26*, 215–240.
Wink, P., Dillion, M., & Larson, B. (2005). Religion as moderator of the depression health connection: Findings from a longitudinal study. *Research on Aging, 27*(2), 197–220.
Wisalo, P. P. (2009). *Thai Buddhism in the future: Trend and solution for the crisis*. Bangkok: Komon Keemthong Foundation Publishing.
Wongsit, M. (1998). *Study of community readiness to take care and service the elderly: Qualitative research* (Institute Report No. 263). Bangkok: College of Population Studies, Chulalongkorn University.
Woolcock, M. (2004). Why and how planners should take social capital seriously. *Journal of the American Planning Association, 70*(2), 183–189.
Wuthnow, R. (1994). *Producing the sacred: An essay on public religion. Public expressions of religion in America*. Urbana: University of Illinois Press.

Chapter 5
Beyond Localities: Community Development and Network Construction Among the Buddhist Monks in Northern Thailand

Mayumi Okabe

1 Introduction

The study on which this chapter is based examines how Buddhist monks have survived in the rapid social changes that have resulted from modernization in contemporary Thailand from an anthropological perspective. The study focused on the recent phenomenon of network construction among Theravada Buddhist monks in the country with particular attention to the case of the "Community Development Monks' Network in Northern Thailand (*khru'akhai phra nak phatthana chumchon phak nu'a*)," which was founded in Chiang Mai in 2001.

In Thailand, many Buddhist monks have recently engaged in social work such as road improvement, credit unions, buffalo banks, care for HIV/AIDS patients and treatment for drug addicts, and environmental conservation. However, the areas of work in which they engage now range widely throughout the country. Social engagement among monks might seem to be no longer something out of the ordinary. See also Chaps. 24 and 28 in this volume.

These monks have been called *phra nak phatthana* or development monks since NGO-led alternative development became influential in Thai society in the late 1970s. The term *phra nak phatthana* describes monks who have a strong interest in the affairs of this world or social engagement. It may also imply that development monks are far different from an ideal image of Theravada Buddhist monks, who devote themselves to ascetic practices in pursuit of otherworldly goals or enlightenment.

However, Theravada Buddhist monks not only have played many roles in religious rituals and ceremonies; they have also been inevitably involved in worldly affairs in

M. Okabe (✉)
Research Fellow of Japan society for the Promotion of Science,
National Museum of Ethnology, Senri Expo Park 10-1, Suita,
Osaka 565-8511, Tokyo, Japan
e-mail: mayumixokabe@gmail.com

P. Liamputtong (ed.), *Contemporary Socio-Cultural and Political Perspectives in Thailand*,
DOI 10.1007/978-94-007-7244-1_5,

local communities. For example, these roles include practicing traditional knowledge on astrology and herbal medicines, giving advices to the villagers on naming infants, introducing migrant works, and arbitrating on family or village conflicts. The roles of these monks can be paradoxically derived from the very fact that they ordain as world renouncers. The question is: Why should we make different the monks who engage in worldly affairs or community development as "development monks" from the other monks?

In the field of development studies, most existing studies on development monks appreciate their roles with morality and values against the capitalist system from an idealistic and policy-oriented viewpoint of alternative development (see Wasi 1988; Phongphit 1988, 1996). Sociological studies on the monks who engage in community development discuss their social position from a macro-viewpoint focusing on political and economic transformation in contemporary Thailand (Suksamran 1977, 1988; Laptananon 1986, 2007; Phisitphanphon and Prasandi 1991).

Such former studies, either development studies or sociological studies, see "development monks" not as a discourse but as an entity. "Development monks" are not any sect, or *nikai*, but a category which was formed gradually through the development discourses in contemporary Thai society. It may be more considerable that the social engagement among monks and development discourses have been resonant with each other. Hence, this study considers that it is more important to have a viewpoint to examine the controversy over social engagement among the Theravada Buddhist monks than ask who is or is not the "development monk."

2 Theoretical Frameworks: Controversy Over Social Engagement Among the Theravada Buddhist Monks

There have been some previous studies that identified this kind of controversy over social engagement among monks. Whether monks have a positive or negative opinion toward such engagement depends on their position within the Sangha hierarchy, their educational background, and their distance from the central administration (Tambiah 1976; Suksamran 1981). Some believe that it is risky for monks to engage too much in worldly affairs because such matters will cause suspicion among the villagers if they interpret the monks as being political in nature or inconsistent with popular Buddhism (Mulder 1973). These arguments were put forth soon after the Thai government launched a number of projects to dispatch Buddhist monks to rural areas for engagement in community development activities on a local level under close cooperation with the Sangha since the middle of the 1960s.

Within anthropological research, there has not been much discussion about how the Buddhist monks have experienced community development in the contested opinions toward monks' social engagement in contemporary Thailand from the viewpoints of the monks themselves. Even a handful of anthropological works carried out by Darlington (1990, 1997, 1998, 2003a, b) has focused only on the outstanding "development monks" practices in community development in Northern Thailand.

There are many interests on the relationship between them and laypeople in each local community but not so from a broader context. This is the point that research on social engagement among the monks is crucial because the issue further raises the need to reconsider the politics of identity in relation to monks in this broader context of increasing fragile and rapidly globalizing modernity in contemporary Thailand.

My study also sought to focus on the communality, which had been created by Buddhist monks and among "development monks" in particular. Although extensive networks among Buddhist monks have been constructed in Thai society lately,[1] few previous studies have investigated the phenomenon. How should we approach this new trend seen among monks in recent years?

Let me start to explore the studies of Tambiah, who initially analyzed the relationship between religious practice and social structure within a local village in northeastern Thailand and then investigated the relationship between religion and politics in a modernized state (Tambiah 1970, 1976). In the latter study, Tambiah (1976) also referred to a network of monks to explain their high mobility between temples, often from rural areas to urban areas, with a special quotation from a classic article by Wyatt (1966). Following on from Wyatt's point of argument, Tambiah explains that high mobility among monks results from their pursuit of better educational opportunities, which also enhances their value as human resources by improving the social status they will have in the event of disrobement. In line with Wyatt's argument, Tambiah points out that vertical connections such as the master-disciple (*luksit-acan*) or senior-junior relationship observed in temples is quite significant for individual monks. When a monk moves to and settles at a temple, he may depend upon a senior monk from the same village.

On the other hand, horizontal relationships such as those between ordination associates are not as significant to them and may be described as fragile connections (Tambiah 1976). This argument has considerable meanings, as it focused on the networks among Buddhist monks and highlighted the significance of vertical relationships for them. However, careful observation of the practices of monks in recent years shows that these development monks do not totally conform to Tambiah's views. That is to say, they seem to actively try to construct horizontal relationships among themselves.

Why, then, should they attempt to construct such networks despite also being members of the Sangha, which acts as their traditional community? What kind of communality can be observed within this type of network among Buddhist monks? Through analysis involving the case of the "Community Development Monks' Network in Northern Thailand," this study focused on the new phenomenon seen among the monks and examined how they have survived in the rapid social changes that have resulted from modernization in contemporary Thai society by seeking to create a new communality.

[1] For example, the *Sekkhiyatham* group (*klum Sekkhiyatham*) was originally founded in 1989 among development monks in northeast Thailand with the total support of Sulak Sivaraksa and "Inter-Religious Committee for Development" by Sulak's initiative. Then the leader of *Sekkhiyatham* group is Phra Phaisal Visalo.

3 The Sociohistorical Process of Network Construction Among the Monks: The Case of the "Community Development Monks' Network in Northern Thailand"

3.1 Data Collected from the Author's Fieldwork

The data examined here are based on my continuous fieldworks in Chiang Mai City and its suburbs since October 2004.[2] In the city itself, research was mainly conducted to collect elementary data on the "Community Development Monks' Network in Northern Thailand" at the office of the *Phothiyalai* Institute (*Sathaban Phothiyalai*), which is located in the compound of temple Suan Dok (*Wat Suan Dok*) in Chiang Mai City.[3] Sometimes when the monks and lay staffs of *Phothiyalai* Institute went out to the other temples in Northern Thailand for their activities, I followed them to carry out participant observations.

Meanwhile, in the suburbs, research was mainly conducted to record the life history of a particular young monk at temple D (*Wat D*) in Doi Saket District, Chiang Mai Province, who made special efforts toward the construction process of the network, as a part of intensive fieldwork for the author's PhD thesis. To date, further additional research has also been intermittently conducted in the form of interviews with monks in other provinces[4] of Northern Thailand who have also made special efforts toward network construction.

3.2 Network Construction: Two Case Studies

3.2.1 Case One: Monk I's Experience

A number of important episodes should be noted in considering how the Community Development Monks' Network in Northern Thailand was founded. Here, let us look at the individual experience of one young monk at *Wat D* in Doi Saket District,

[2] My fieldwork can be divided into three periods as follows: (a) preliminary research in Chiang Mai City and around Northern Thailand for the 5-month period from October 2004 to March 2005; (b) intensive fieldwork in Doi Saket (a suburb about 20 km far from, Chiang Mai City) for the 13-month period from May 2005 to May 2006; and (c) additional research intermittently conducted to date.

[3] These elementary data are obtained both by conducting personal interviews with people related and by collecting original publications such as Muangmit's report book (Muangmit 2004).

[4] These monks are based in the provinces of Chiang Rai, Phrae, Nan, Lamphun, Lampang, and so on.

Chiang Mai Province, first. Monk I,[5] who moved from Wiang Haeng District in Chiang Mai Province, has dwelled at *Wat D* for over 20 years. Monk I is a Shan monk and has no relatives in the local community around *Wat D* at the beginning of his move there. He decided to move to this temple from a small temple in Wiang Haeng, where he was ordained as a novice, to pursue higher educational opportunities at the religious school founded at *Wat D*.[6] After the abbot there (Monk P[7]) was assigned to the position of head of the Doi Saket District Sangha, he (Monk P) became too busy with administrative work than before. Now he had to attend administrative meetings of the provincial Sangha as a representative of the district Sangha. As a result, Monk P had less time to spend on community development activities by himself as he did before, and instead Monk I gained a variety of opportunities to engage in community development, especially health-care activities such as treatment for HIV/AIDS patients and home visit projects. As Monk I's eager involvement in community development deepened, he was also increasingly invited to seminars and meetings on HIV/AIDS held by NGOs in Chiang Mai, around Northern Thailand and in Bangkok.

At one seminar in Chiang Mai City, Monk I encountered an unexpected question from a lay participant, who asked: "Where are monks working on the HIV/AIDS issue? We have all risen up to combat it, but we don't know where or how many monks are engaged in solving these problems." He was the only monk there, and although he did his best to respond to his/her question, he was unable to give a clear answer. This experience became quite meaningful because it highlighted the lack of

[5] In this study, a proper noun such as a person's name is written in an assumed name for the purpose of protecting one's privacy.

Monk I (40 years old) was born in Shan State of Myanmar in 1973 and then moved across the Myanmar-Thai border to settle in Chiang Mai's Wiang Haeng District. Soon after elementary school education, he was ordained as a novice in Wiang Haeng. With the relative's support, he moved to *Wat D* in 1989 soon after junior high school education. Although he graduated from and entered into the master course at Mahachulalongkorn Buddhist University, Chiang Mai Campus, he finally did not obtain the master degree because he did not submit the thesis.

[6] At that time, *Wat D* was becoming famous for its practical education for young novices and high ratio of successful Pali examinees. The school for novice education of *Wat D*, which was founded in 1977 by Monk W on the model of Wat Buppharam in Chiang Mai City, boasted of the most numbers of successful Pali examinees in Chiang Mai Province for 3 years during 1986–1988.

[7] Monk P (68 year old) was born in Nan Province of Northern Thailand in 1945. He was ordained as a novice and a monk in Nan and then moved to Wat Buppharam in Chiang Mai City to pursue educational opportunities. Since that time, Monk P has been one of the disciples of Monk W, who has discharged his duty as the abbot of Wat Buppharam.

In fact, Monk W has been famous for a variety of his community development activities around Chiang Mai and Doi Saket in particular from an early period in the 1970s (Gosling 1981, 1983). He had been the head of Chiang Mai Provincial Sangha of *Maha nikai* for a long time until 2009. The case of Monk W indicates a quite interesting point that there were two outstanding Buddhist monks active in the field of community development in Chiang Mai, one Monk W of *Maha nikai* and the other Phra Thep Kavi of *Thammayut nikai*. See Wonguthai's master thesis for the details about Monk P and Darlington's work for Monk W (Darlington 1990; Wonguthai 1999).

ways to link monks and those working on the HIV/AIDS issue and opportunities for them to exchange information on their work.

After this episode, Monk I started to make contact with other monks he knew who had worked to provide HIV/AIDS care around Chiang Mai City and had them introduce other monks to him so that he could become acquainted with them. He was able to contact a large number of monks in this way, thereby gradually expanding the network of such individuals in terms of both geographical spread and the variety of issues in which they are involved.

3.2.2 Case Two: Monk K's Experience

At the same time, there was another episode in Northern Thailand, specifically in Chiang Mai. Monk K[8] was the key person here. In 1997, when Thailand's newly revised constitution was adopted, many groups of laypeople gathered in front of Chiang Mai Provincial Office from rural and remote mountainous areas where land problems had been caused by the development policy of the Thai government in order to demonstrate against the constitutional revision. Four Buddhist monks who were invited by the demonstrators performed religious rituals and spoke for both sides—the government and the people—in the hope of solving the problems in a nonviolent way. After the demonstration calmed down, these monks gathered repeatedly to discuss the problems faced by the people—especially impoverished farmers—and what they could do to solve them. Monk K took the leadership and founded a small group of individuals, naming it "Monks for the Poor (*phrasong phu'a khon con*)."

These two cases along with the individual and the social experiences of the monks around Chiang Mai prompted the formation of a single movement in Northern Thailand. Monks and laypeople gathered twice for meetings at *Wat D* in 1999 to discuss various aspects of their community development activities and also came together at *Wat H* in Nan Province for a meeting to introduce themselves to each other and exchange opinions on such work. About 150 monks attended this meeting and confirmed plans to found a group of them in the near future. They also organized a small committee at *Wat Suan Dok* in April 2000. The monks held a meeting at *Wat D* with more than 100 attendees from all over Northern Thailand and finally founded the Community Development Monks' Network in Northern Thailand in March 2001.

---

[8] Monk K passed away on July 2011. He was born in Tak Province. He was a Lisu. He ordained as a monk in Tak 1992 and soon moved to *Wat Sri Soda* in Chiang Mai City the next year. He kept going back and forth to Tak and *Wat Sri Soda* often and then had dwelled at *Wat Sri Suphan* in Chiang Mai City. During his study at Chiang Mai University, he got to know many people who were interested in NGO, and he also started his community development activities in his own village and around in Tak for a few years. He was selected as Ashoka fellow and had many connections with development agencies. Finally, he was disrobed in 2004.

4 Sharing Interests on Community Development Among the Monks Beyond Localities

4.1 *Structural Aspects of the Network*

From its foundation, the Community Development Monks' Network in Northern Thailand upheld the ideal of fostering the abilities of monks involved in community development work and set the following as its purposes:

1. To improve the abilities of development monks involved in development-related activities in Northern Thailand
2. To support and encourage development activities conducted by individual monks, groups of monks, and local organizations
3. To increase the awareness of monks in administrative positions within the Sangha and related institutions as well as laypeople in regard to the development activities of monks
4. To advocate new directions and models of community development based on Buddhist Dhamma

This network has no firm membership except a small committee of about ten young monks and an advisory board consisting of a few senior monks and laypeople.[9] Monk B performs the role of the network's representative. Accordingly, it is difficult to know exactly how many monks are in the network. Each time the committee plans a meeting or an event, it is difficult to specify the number of people who will attend.

Meanwhile, the administrative duties of the network (such as making contact with monks, arranging their transportation, and dealing with paperwork) are performed by the *Phothiyalai* Institute, whose office is located on Mahachulalongkorn Buddhist University's Chiang Mai campus within the compound of *Wat Suan Dok* in Chiang Mai City. Monk B serves as the head of the institute and is also vice-principal of the university.[10] Approximately, there are ten staffs, including monks and laypeople, working at the institute's office. When the committee arranges small meetings of the network, they are often held at the institute's office or in an open area of the campus. Thus, the network maintains close relationships with both the *Phothiyalai* Institute and Mahachulalongkorn Buddhist University.

4.2 *Collective Activities*

The main activities of the Community Development Monks' Network in Northern Thailand are based on holding seminars and meetings to report the latest news and exchange information on their community development activities. Also, "members"

---

[9] Monk I is a committee member, and Monk P, the abbot of *Wat D*, is an advisory board member.

[10] Monk B has been released of this post and has been a lecturer at the university since 2011.

sometimes visit other member monks throughout Northern Thailand to provide encouragement for their activities and cultivate friendships.

The aims of such discussions, which are accumulated through a variety of opportunities of its activities, are to share individual and concrete knowledge and experience based on the monks' social engagement in each local community and also to exchange opinions on general and discrete subject of social engagement among monks in contemporary Thailand. Thus, the discussions in the network seem infinite which enable the monks to produce practices reflexively when return to each temple and local community.

Moreover, the *Phothiyalai* Institute regularly publishes a magazine called *Phothiyalai* Magazine (*Culasan Phothiyalai*) to publicize its activities. It sometimes includes special features in interview articles introducing individual members of the Community Development Monks' Network in Northern Thailand and their activities in each local community. Accordingly, it can be said that the publication also plays a certain role as a public relations magazine for the network itself.

Here, I will show a scene of the meeting held at temple A (*Wat A*) in Nan province on August 25–26, 2005. The participants were about 40 monks from at least four provinces[11] in the north and seven laypeople from *Phothiyalai* Institute. Monk N, the abbot of *Wat A*, served as the host of the meeting on that day. Some participants who were highly interested in Monk N's activities[12] tried to make contacts with him and visit his office within the compound of *Wat A*. This shows that activities of the network in a form of meetings can also be informal opportunities for the monks to become acquainted with others who share the interests in community development.

On the first day, the meeting was opened with Monk N's remarks, and then Monk B, the head of the network, started to explain the aims of the meeting. According to his explanation, the meeting was regarded as a meeting to mark the 5th year of the network and review the past activities thoroughly. Until that time, the network seemed to have countless activities carried out by individual monks all over Northern Thailand named as a "network." However, for the future, the network will let the monks coordinate the translocal zones which are set up according to the topics (HIV/AIDS, environment, the young or the aged, credit unions, and so on). Most of the participants were in a full agreement with such proposal of Monk B. Then they divided the whole Northern Thailand into six zones and appointed the leaders for each zone. After that, seven monks made the presentations on their development activities in each local community.

On the second day, they confirmed the contents of the first day's discussion at the beginning and then started honest and informal discussion on their community development activities. Some senior monks, such as Monk A from Fang District and

[11] The participants' list of this meeting indicated 28 monks from 4 provinces: Chiang Mai (10), Chiang Rai (1), Phrae (2), and Nan (13). The numbers inside (·) means the number of monks. At this meeting, the author founded about 40 monks including the 28 monks referred above.

[12] He is highly famous for his earnest forest conservation activities such as "ordination of tree" (*buat ton mai*).

Monk S from San Sai District, both in Chiang Mai Province, gave their talks on the difficulties that they have confronted in community development activities and showed how to overcome these difficulties.

In their messages, it was underlined that "As we ordained, the monks have been dependent upon villagers for everything to eat, wear and live in. So, we monks have to repay them. The villagers' hardships, which might occur from a lack of 'solidarity (*samakkhi*)', are also ones of us. The monks have to be engaged themselves to solve problems of the "community (*chumchon*)." Many other monks, especially young monks, listened to their talks with high interests and exchanged their opinions about some concrete cases of the villagers' problems in each local community.

In fact, these messages seem not to be an original way of thought created by the monks of this network. Rather, they have been gradually expanded throughout Thailand. What is significant is that the monks obtain the opportunities not only to share the individual and concrete knowledge and experience of community development works but also to access the discrete and general discussions. Here, it can be found that a new communality based on sharing the interests about community development beyond localities has emerged among the monks.

5 Discussion and Conclusion: Consideration of a "Network" Among the Monks

The results of examining the case of the "Community Development Monks' Network in Northern Thailand" can be summarized as outlined below.

Firstly, the sociohistorical process of the network's construction can be traced back to two particular cases along with involving monks' experiences in Northern Thailand. Monk I inherited the idea that monks should work for society from senior monks—Monk P and Monk W. Here, we can see that the vertical relationships connecting monks within a temple still have a fair level of significance for them, as previously pointed out by Tambiah (1976). However, as discussed in Sect. 3, the two cases of Monk I and Monk K highlight the point more than Tambiah.

That is, Monk I encountered cutting feedback from lay participants at an NGO seminar on HIV/AIDS in Chiang Mai. This experience prompted him to feel an urgent need to construct a "network" among the monks who share a close interest in social engagement in Northern Thailand. As part of this process, the monks involved in community development came together to exchange and share experiences and difficulties arising from their individual development activities.

Another case demonstrates that many monks became aware of the need for making a "network" of the monks involved in development activities in each local community. Monk K, one of the most active monks in the process of its construction around Chiang Mai, and a few leading monks tried to foster relationships with other monks who were interested in this sphere from all over Northern Thailand. The relationship between individual monks here is based not on vertical relationships within the temple or the Sangha but on non-vertical or horizontal relationships by sharing similar interests.

Secondly, what kind of communality can be observed within this type of network among Buddhist monks? This question can be answered by considering its activities, which mostly involve holding meetings and seminars and sometimes also being active in arranging tours for the observation of monks' activities to provide encouragement. These activities create opportunities for monks to share individual and concrete knowledge and experience based on the monks' social engagement in each local community and also to exchange opinions on general and abstract subjects of social engagement among monks in contemporary Thailand. When they return to each temple and local community, these activities of the network seem to enable the monks to produce practices reflexively.

Thus, monks belonging to the network are engaged individually in community development based on the local context of temples and communities and have also started to build another communality among individuals who share close interests in community development beyond localities. This communality is based on horizontal relationships among the monks, which is in contrast to the vertical relationships whose importance was previously emphasized by Tambiah.

Finally, a number of related questions arise (although there is insufficient space to discuss them here): What is the significance behind the formation of horizontal relationships between monks who share similar interests in contemporary Thai society? How do monks engage in their practices between the horizontal and vertical relationships seen today? These research topics, which have arisen from the present study's investigation of network development among monks, require further consideration about the identity politics of monks in the context of increasing fragile and globalizing modernity in the world.

Acknowledgments An early version of this chapter was presented at the 11th international conference on Thai studies held at the Siam City Hotel, July 26–28, 2011. I would like to express my special gratitude to all the attenders, especially a few questioners who helped to stimulate my thought on this chapter.

References

Darlington, S. M. (1990). *Buddhism, morality and change: The local response to development in Northern Thailand*. Unpublished PhD thesis, University of Michigan, Ann Arbor, MI, USA.

Darlington, S. M. (1997). Not only preaching: The work of the ecology monk Phrakhru Pitak Nantakhun of Thailand. *Forest, Trees and People Newsletter, 34*, 17–19.

Darlington, S. M. (1998). The ordination of a tree: The Buddhist ecology movement of Thailand. *Ethnology, 37*(1), 1–16.

Darlington, S. M. (2003a). Buddhism and development: The ecology monks of Thailand. In C. S. Queen (Ed.), *Action dharma: New studies in engaged Buddhism* (pp. 96–109). London: Routledge Curzon.

Darlington, S. M. (2003b). Practical spirituality and community forests: Monks, ritual, and radical conservationism in Thailand. In P. Greenough & A. Lowenhaupt Tsing (Eds.), *Nature in the global south: Environmental projects in South and Southeast Asia* (pp. 347–366). Durham: Duke University Press.

Gosling, D. L. (1981). Thai monks in rural development. *Southeast Asian Journal of Social Science, 9*(1–2), 74–85.

Gosling, D. L. (1983). Redefining the Sangha's role in Northern Thailand: An investigation of monastic careers at five Chiang Mai wats. *Journal of Siam Society, 71*, 89–120.

Laptananon, P. (1986). *Botbat phrasong nai kan phatthana chonnabot*. Krungthep: Sathaban wicai sangkhom, Chulalongkon mahawitthayalai.

Laptananon, P. (2007). *30 Phrasong nak phatthana den nai phak Isan 2546–2547*. Krungthep: Sathaban wicai sangkhom, Chulalongkon mahawitthayalai.

Muangmit, K. (2004). *Kansu'ksa lae phatthana sakkayaphap khu'akhai phrasong: koroni su'ksa phra nak phatthana chumchon phak nu'a*. Sanapsanun doi Sathaban Phatthana Ongkorn Chumchon.

Mulder, J. A. N. (1973). *Monks, merit and motivation: Buddhism and national development in Thailand*. DeKalb: Center for Southeast Asian Studies, Northern Illinois University.

Phisitphanphon, N., & Prasandi, S. (1991). *Thamniap phrasong nak phatthana phak isan*. Krungthep: Sathaban wicai sangkhom lae phatthana, Mahawitthayalai Khon Kaen lae sathaban wicai phutthasat Mahachulalongkorn ratchawitthayalai.

Phongphit, S. (1988). *Religion in a changing society: Buddhism, reform and the role of monks in community development in Thailand*. Hong Kong: Arena Press.

Phongphit, S. (1996). *23 Prasopkan kan thamngan kiaokap rok et phak nu'a khong Thai*. Krungthep: Krasuang Satharanasuk.

Suksamran, S. (1977). *Political Buddhism in Southeast Asia: the role of the Sangha in the modernization of Thailand*. New York: St. Martin's Press.

Suksamran, S. (1981). Religion, politics and development: The Thai Sangha's role in national development and integration. *Southeast Asian Journal of Social Science, 9*(1–2), 54–73.

Suksamran, S. (1988). A Buddhist approach to development: The case of 'development monks' in Thailand. In L. T. Ghee (Ed.), *Reflections on development in Southeast Asia* (pp. 26–48). Singapore: Institute of Southeast Asian Studies.

Tambiah, S. J. (1970). *Buddhism and spirit cults in northeast Thailand*. Cambridge: Cambridge University Press.

Tambiah, S. J. (1976). *World conqueror and world renouncer: A study of Buddhism and polity in Thailand against a historical background*. Cambridge: Cambridge University Press.

Wasi, P. (1988). Sasontham kap kanphatthana muban. In S. Phongphit (Ed.), *Thitthang muban Thai*. Krungthep: Samnakphim Muban Thai.

Wonguthai, C. (1999). *Botbat phrasong nai kan songkhro chumchon panha rok et: koroni su'ksa Phrakhru Sophonpariyattisuthi Wat D changwat Chiang Mai*. Unpublished master thesis, sataranasu'k sat, Mahawitthayalai Chiang Mai, Chiang Mai, Thailand.

Wyatt, D. K. (1966). The Buddhist monkhood as an avenue of social mobility in traditional Thai society. *Sinlapakon, 10*(1), 41–52.

Chapter 6
Hegemonic English, Standard Thai, and Narratives of the Subaltern in Thailand

Adcharawan Buripakdi

1 Introduction

English has spread so pervasively that it is fostered into the rest of the complex world as an international prestigious brand. Within this construct, how English has become an international language is not because of a utopian ideal, but by virtue of its political and ideological construct (Pennycook 1994). Such a political establishment, accordingly, has a monumentally ideological impact on people in the means in which they think and behave. Presently, the status of English, the language "on which the sun never sets" (Crystal 2004: 10), has been still maintained, promoted, and marketed through a system of both material and institutional structures, namely, the World Bank and IMF or International Monetary Fund (Phillipson 1992). With this discursive power, people find it difficult to resist the promotion of English as "natural, neutral, inevitable and beneficial" (Pennycook 1994: 6).

The growth of English has major cultural, educational, and political implications. To deal with the political aspect of English, language users need to study English and how it works in different kinds of cultural forms and also across cultures. Also, to better understand about the global rise of English and its role English played out in any context, we need to look at English through its local milieus rather than through a priori assumptions about imperialistic effects (Pennycook 2000). In this way, in order to come at a clearer understanding about English usage and local languages in Thailand, English should be viewed from Thai contexts, since it can never be removed from the historical, social, cultural, economic, or political contexts in which it is used.

The study on which this chapter is based examines status of English in relation to Thai language and other competing discourses through the lenses of language

A. Buripakdi (✉)
School of Liberal Arts, Walailak University, 222 Thaiburi,
Tha Sala, Nakorn Si Thammarat 80160, Thailand
e-mail: ajarngob@gmail.com

P. Liamputtong (ed.), *Contemporary Socio-Cultural and Political Perspectives in Thailand*, DOI 10.1007/978-94-007-7244-1_6, © Springer Science+Business Media Dordrecht 2014

users—one foreign and nine local participants—living in Thailand. This chapter aims to describe how the informants conceptualized these discourses. The contribution of this study is to provide a better understanding about the status of English, Thai, and other emerging aspects related to the sociolinguistic position of English in Thailand.

2 English in Thailand

English has become increasingly crucial both in local and global contexts. Thailand is an example of the linguistic phenomenon of adopting and using the English language to serve her own sociolinguistic will, contexts, and functions. As the passage below describes:

> The Thai nobility recognized early on the importance of English not just as an intellectual interest, but as a vehicle for communicating with countries which threatened to arrive as colonizers. English was used by the Thai people to protect their independence and as a vehicle for absorbing modern ideas and technology into the country. (Masavisut et al. 1986: 205)

Historically, the first contact with English in Siam (the former name of Thailand) took place in the reign of King Nang Klaw (1824–1854) when American missionaries were assigned to teach the language to young children of noble birth (Aksornkool 1980: 72). Later, the policy makers during the reign of King Mongkut (1851–1868) (Masavisut et al. 1986) realized the tremendous adversity of not knowing English—the language of the invader. Out of fear of a colonial power and a wave of change, English was therefore inevitably and politically introduced to the royal palace. From that situation, English, at the beginning, was learned on a restricted basis by royal family members and elite groups of Siamese. In later reigns, English was reluctantly promoted outside the palace. English ultimately became accessible to middle-class Thais in the reign of King Vajiravudh (1910–1925).

From the beginning of the twentieth century, Thailand has gradually been experiencing a new paradigm shift regarding English. Thais used English "mainly with other non-native speakers of English, and only to a lesser extent with Native speakers" (Foley 2005: 6). In recent decades, English has been used by people at all levels of Thai society, from government leaders to bar girls, to fulfill their own objectives (Masavisut et al. 1986). Although the use of English in Thailand is restricted as Standard Thai dominates the domestic scene (Rappa and Wee 2006), among 11 optional foreign languages, English is regarded as the most significant one in Thailand (Wongsothorn 2000). Now English, the language of Thailand abroad (Foley 2005), becomes a symbol of modernity (Huebner 2006). Indeed, the deep penetration of English in Thai society is reflected through its political agenda, which Thai people might seem unaware of.

3 Conceptual Frameworks

3.1 Neutral English

The laissez-faire or the modernist position on the global role of English is underpinned by the ideology that English is a functional device for pragmatic purposes. English, in this view, is a lingua franca or the language of globalization par excellence (Bamgbose 2003). This apolitical approach to language is the most common line of English within the field of English language teaching and applied linguistics (Pennycook 2001). Within this mindset, English is constructed, reconstructed, and internalized as apolitical (Crystal 1997) or as "natural, neutral, and beneficial" (Pennycook 1994: 7). The debate about this claim is on the rise worldwide (e.g., Pennycook 1994; Phillipson 1992). Central to this framework is the assumption that English is an instrumental tool—an aid to help language users develop themselves and to have an economic advantage. The pivotal belief of this economic progression argument is that learning English equates with an economic growth.

The modern thinking that English is merely an instrument is widespread. Within this construct, English with the universalism profile has been softly marketed as the prestigious brand of the language through English learning and teaching (ELT) worldwide. The problem with this position, however, is that it is mistaken and unhealthy. Simply put, this position dodges "all the crucial concerns around the global use of English, and buys into the apoliticism of applied linguistics and Teaching English to Speakers of Other Languages (TESOL)" (Pennycook 2002: 38). The view that English just happens to be in the right place at the right time (Crystal 1997) turns out to be especially problematic when "the seductiveness of this English position makes its social and political naively dangerous" (Pennycook 2000: 109). Besides, such a view of English as lingua franca terminally consigns English to "the level of a technical language stripped of expressive and aesthetic characteristics and denuded of any critical or self-conscious dimension" (Said 1994: 369).

Learning or using English, in fact, does not just mean learning or using a foreign language but "unconscious implantation of the Anglocentric attitudes or the perspective of the dominant race in the native's mind" (Tripasai 2004: 11). English not only held a hegemonic position but was also designated as the sole official language and viable choice for modern education. The underlying ramification of this glorification of English as the language of the skies and the seven seas (Bolton 2004) is a powerful imperial construct of English.

In effect, the hidden agenda of this instrumental construct is that English is politically and economically av form of colonial control. Based on the argument of economic progression, Pennycook (1994: 22) claims that the underlying goal of the promotion of global English was to "protect and promote capitalist interests." Indeed, in this neutral message, this selling point of English appears to serve economic and political purposes only. As Tollefson (2000: 8) remarks, "at a time when English is widely seen as a key to the economic success of nations and the economic well-being of individuals, the spread of English also contributes to significant social, political, and economic inequalities." Undoubtedly, another acute problem of this instrumental English domination is the production of an English language industry around the world. As a consequence of the colonial discursive construct, the neocolonial ideology remains even stronger today (Pennycook 1994, 1998; Phillipson 1992).

In the cultural pluralism paradigm, English grows from many roots. As Rushdie (1982: 8) contends, "the language needs to be decolonized, to be made in other images, if those of us who use it from positions outside Anglo-Saxon cultures are to be more than 'Uncle Toms.'" The interaction of localism and globalism becomes more increasingly complex and multifaceted than we have imagined. It has led to remarkable changes in the spaces of economics, politics, and culture around the globe. Can Thailand ignore this emergent tendency?

3.2 Standard Culture

The hegemonic construct of language use, for any language, is concerned with standardization construct. Refined version of the language, or, for example, Standard English, is linked with being rational, moral, civilized, and intelligent, whereas the vulgar version or non-Standard English varieties were seen as irrational, emotional, materialist, and imprudent (Joseph 1987). This standardization construct also echoes Bourdieu's (1991) notion of symbolic domination and symbolic power. These unequal power relations can result in symbolic violence. According to Bourdieu (1991: 170), symbolic violence takes place "when individuals mistakenly consider a standard dialect or style of speaking to be truly superior to the way they themselves speak, rather than an arbitrary difference afforded social significance."

Within this construct, some people attempt to maintain this symbolic power of English in workplaces by conforming to its standard form. Essentially, the motivation for this practice is the belief in the eloquence of Standard English that functioned as "a mantle of power" and increased "personal standing" (Joseph 1987: 43). This practice reflects that Standard English held ideological, economic, and political power which "project one's practice as universal and common sense" (Fairclough 2001: 27). Set into a global perspective, this powerful construct of the standardization discourse is resonated in Bhatt's (2001: 414) contention:

> Standard English ideology seems only to reproduce socio-economic inequalities as it privileges only those who have access to its possession, leaving others disenfranchised. Thus, the struggle between Cockney and Standard English, between African and General American English, or between English and Hindi in India, or English and Filipino in the Philippines, is indeed a struggle between competing economic interests: Standard English serving the elite and native language serving mainly the working class.

After all, in this discourse of standardization and the linguistic utopian construct, the dominant discourse has an association with "goodness"—the quality of language users that becomes so natural, desirable, and venerated.

4 Narrative Inquiry

This chapter presents the status of English and other competing discourses from the voices of ten informants from school, media, and professional contexts. Table 6.1 summarizes the participants' profile.

This qualitative study employed a multi-method approach. To delve into the participants' voices, data collection was drawn from five modes: everyday conversations (1 informant), telephone conversations (2 informants), face-to-face interviews (4 informants), English literacy autobiography (1 informant), and Facebook's online chat room (2 informants). All of these methods aimed to explore how the participants perceived their English in relation to Thai and other competing discourses. Details of data collection will be described as follows:

1. Daily conversations. Dialogues between the researcher and the participant, Tang, were kept in a field note over time when the relevant issues emerged.
2. Face-to-face interviews. I sent an invitation letter via email and snail mail to the informants. Then, the interviews with Saijai, Ladda, Kampol, and Pim took place at the informant's offices and a coffee shop in downtown Bangkok.
3. Online discussion. I purposively sent an inquiry to the participants via "message" box of Facebook. Then the dialogues among the participants, Kim and Chai, and myself took place.
4. Telephone conversations. In fact, the two participants, Kati and Pong, were recruited in this project by chance. One day, one of the students of mine made a call to seek an advice about his internship problem. From the dialogue on that day, I considered this case very interesting. Thus, their views were noted and reflected in this study.
5. English literacy autobiography. This participant, Pan, took one of my classes. Having a conversation with him and observing him in class struck my interest. Therefore, he was invited to participate in this project. His assignment was to write an English literacy autobiography to reflect upon his English learning since early ages.

Table 6.1 Participants' profile

Participants	Profession	Language use	Affiliation
Saijai	Novelist, poet	Thai, English	Bangkok
Kampol	Business columnist	Thai, English	Bangkok
Pim	Business journalist	Thai, English	Bangkok
Ladda	Environment journalist	Thai, English	Bangkok
Tang	Chinese instructor	Mandarin, English, Thai	Nakornsrithammarat
Kim	English instructor	Thai, English	Mahasarakham
Pan	Student	Thai, English	Nakornsrithammarat
Chai	Project consultant	Thai, English	Bangkok
Kati	Student	Thai, English	Phuket
Pong	Student	Thai, English	Krabi

The language of communication in the field is both Thai and English. This depended on the participants' free choice. Overall, the interviews, the online discussion, and conversations lasted between 90 and 120 min. The interviews and the discussion on Facebook were conducted only one time while the telephone and face-to-face conversations were conducted three times.

Data analysis was based upon a grounded theory approach (Strauss and Corbin 1998). The focus of analysis was an examination of the participants' self-positioning in relation to English, Thai, and other competing discourses. A categorization system was a significant discourse-analytic tool for text analysis. Emphasis in conceptualization of the coding process was placed on research device building, reconceptualization, interrogation, and analysis of raw data under investigation (Coffey and Atkinson 1996).

5 Narratives of the Subaltern

Over the course of this study, the participants expressed different perspectives toward the English and Thai language. The informants, in one way or another, situated themselves or sometimes were located by others as subalterns. In this chapter, I refer subalterns to the oppressed or those who are socially placed in a marginal position. That is, the majority of the participants showed a marginalized position toward their English and Standard Thai. Their attitudes were greatly influenced by discursive construct of standard language ideology and economic forces to use Standard English or Standard Thai. All of the participants developed discourse of negative construction of self that exemplified how they located themselves in an unfortunate position. They illustrated not only a deep-seated inferior self-image in relation to English. Some compared and contrasted a deficit status of their English competence with Standard English varieties, namely, American English. Others were evaluated by people through the myth of Standard Thai.

The following section presents the narrative of the self-marginalization of the participants.

5.1 They Don't Expect You to Go Off Like Singapore English

Saijai, a native of Thailand, is a renowned poet and a novelist. Her literary work is mainly in Thai; some are in English. She spent a high school year in a convent school in Penang, Malaysia, where she learned to appreciate English taught by Irish nuns. Saijai revealed that this early literacy background made her strict with what she called King's English, which the nuns "drilled into her head everyday." Thus, this is the reason why she held a strong view toward the use of Standard English. Her English educational background in Penang, as she described, framed her attitude into the dominant construct of Standard English. In response to her stance, Saijai recalled her educational history:

> Because when you're taught by the nuns, the nuns taught you the perfect English. They don't expect you to go off. They don't expect you to go off like Singapore English, like they say 'come come, don't shy, come sit like that, you know. They don't expect you to do that. So I'm very strict with my grammar.

Here, King's English or Standard English seemed to be located at a higher position than other varieties. In Saijai's opinion, it appeared that even Singapore English was perceived with relatively lower status than King's English. This historical statement rationalized her assent toward the form of Standard English. As such, Saijai affirmed: "I will try to write King's English as much as I can."

5.2 You Have to Make It Look English, Not Thai

Pim is a business columnist of English newspaper in Thailand. She strongly supports the use of Standard English at her workplace. Her reflection clearly demonstrates how non-Standard English varieties are trivialized. In response to a question about her language ideology, she stated:

> I'm writing for professional, for executives, for business in high ranking, people in high level. Then I also write mainly for international people to read. That's why you know they don't want to read something that they don't understand although they very appreciate on Thai. But when you write in English, you have to make it English. Don't make it look Thai.

With such strong belief, Pim put herself in Standard English mode in order to "upgrade" her English, as she further argued:

> My boss keeps saying you have to make it looks like what you see in Wall Street Journal and Financial Time, very professional newspapers of the world. So, I have to upgrade my working to have a very high standard.

5.3 A Writer of a Beautiful Essay Must Be Educated from Abroad

Ladda is an environmental journalist writing for an English newspaper in Thailand. Most of her articles illustrate how she has tried to bring voices to the powerless in Thai society. Her attempt is echoed in her statement: "In this mainstream media, what I've tried to do is speaking up on behalf of marginalized groups in Thai society." This passage implies that Ladda did not want to surrender her voice to mainstream thinking. However, in terms of language use, Ladda learned that in practice she needed to negotiate with dominant discourses and authority of the newspaper editors. She mentioned that when her English was edited, it was adjusted to fit into a Standard English rule of usage. Regarding her stance in language ideology in general and writing in particular, she succinctly put it: "When we come across a beautifully written essay, we tend to assume that a writer must grow up or be educated from abroad."

5.4 *My English Is Like a Country Song; I Still Can't Make It Classical*

Kampol is a business columnist working and residing in downtown Bangkok. His work is both in Thai and English. Taking his lower position toward Standard English, Kampol devalued his English. The reflective statements illustrated a deep-seated inferior self-image and how he located himself in a subaltern position. In light of this, he compared and contrasted a deficit status of his English with the imagined Standard English. One of the prominent statements related to such poor competence was the belief that incapability to speak perfect English or Standard English was a marker of lower intelligence and prestige. Kampol remarked:

> My English isn't perfect. I worry about my English a lot.... My English is too simple, not that sophisticated, uneducated, something like that.... Speaking about Thai English, I've noticed for example *Khun* [Mr.] Anan's English. I think his English is so beautiful, classy and sophisticated, but mine isn't. I think my English is at a lower class level compared with his English. (Translated from Thai)

Kampol was obviously aware and concerned with the fact that neocolonialism in Thailand has been deeply rooted and affected Thai ways of life. On the one hand, he raised the issue of brainwashing and the deep impact of Eurocentric ideology on Thai people. On the other hand, Kampol's positive responses in line with the Standard English variety were reflected from time to time. He expressed: "If one's written language is beautiful, we tend to assume that the person is smart. I think my English is too simple, not that sophisticated. My English is like a country song. I still can't make it classical."

5.5 *When I Speak English, They Respect Me More than When I Speak Thai*

Tang, a native of Taiwan, has been teaching Chinese in a Thai university for almost 8 years. She is a colleague of mine. Fluent in Thai, Tang has tried to fit in Thai mainstream culture by learning to converse to local people in Thai. She, however, felt that her attempt was not welcomed by the locals. She observed that when she spoke Thai, the locals did not welcome her like when she spoke English. Her fluent communication in the local language did not give her any privileged position in Thai society.

Thus, she gradually learned that whenever she needed Thais to socially accept her, Tang switched to use English although she did realize that many of those locals could not speak or understand English at all. Her remark about the status of English is noted: "I just don't understand Thais here at all. I know that they don't even speak English or understand English. But when I speak English, I feel that they respect me more than when I speak Thai." From Tang's experience, language ideology played out in a complex way. English discourse was compared with Thai along a discourse continuum. In some of Thai people's minds, according to Tang, Thai discourse, in comparison with Standard English, seemed to have a secondary status.

5.6 *People with the Perfect English Accent Are Always Selected*

A native of the Northeastern Thailand, Kim is now an English teacher and a doctoral candidate. He shared his two episodes of linguistic discrimination based on nonnative accents. These were situations when his English-Thai accent was not fully accepted and his English was evaluated based on the native-speaker-like accent, not the message.

> It was the situation in some classrooms of mine or some international conferences in Thailand where I was a MC. Thai audiences or participants in those conferences tend to appreciate the native like accent, which is true I agree because I used to be one of them too. But I am always polite and like to pay attention to listen to speakers with a strong English Thai accent. Most of people I know might be slightly swallowed to swiftly judge someone's overall English competence by the accent they can mimic. For me, this can be termed "unfair."

Another incident sheds light on the professional language use context in relation to linguistic prejudice. Kim addressed how the power of the native-speaker ideology of "perfect English accent" played out in a job market. He wrote:

> There are always some demands of native speaker's accent, such as in the language school or in the high class social events. People with the perfect English accent and pronunciation are always selected. The less skillful ones are marginalized like second-class citizen.

5.7 *You Were in Symptom of* Thinglish *(Thai English)*

A fourth year English major student, Pan, felt frustrated to negotiate his English discourse with the expectation of his American teacher. In his journal, he expressed his miserable feeling of being judged by Standard English. Calling himself a rural boy, Pan wrote:

> For the first time I was not happy with studying English in university because I envied some friends who were smarter than me. I folded myself to live alone and read the grammar book

> a lot. I went to work with teacher (foreign one) and tried to speak with them but I had to be shocked because the teacher told me you were in symptom of *Thinglish*. For the first time, I didn't understand what the *Thinglish* is. But, after that I had chance to study Thai study subject that taught about *Thinglish* too.

Grounded in native-like accent justification, Pan reflected two episodes that caused low-self-esteemed feeling when his accented English was compared with Standard English. He also mentioned the contrastive picture of those who speak Thai with an accent. As he made a remark, "I always find this surprising. When foreigners speak Thai, we think they are so cute even though they made grammatical mistakes. But when we Thais speak mistakes in English, we think it's a shame. We feel insulted so badly." In addition to speaking, Pan addressed anxiety: "I lose face about English. I'm very poor about listening skill. Sometimes, I don't understand the accents and I can't response the question suddenly. I must take my breath to prepare the answer because I'm afraid that it will be ungrammatical."

5.8 I Had No Confidence and Good English to Spend with Them

Chai is a native of the southern Thailand, holds a BA in English, and is now working in downtown Bangkok. He recalled his two incidents of situational English usage that made him feel depressed and stigmatized:

> Once that I have welcomed my debater friends from international Bangkokian students, they all have an excellent English like native. They spent their good English all time when they were together with no exception and yes, they sometimes talked Thai to me as I had no confidence and good English to spend with them. Another one is when I interned at AMCHAM where all native speaker and Thai having an excellent English. At that circle, they all were having a good chat. They laughed. They asked. They talked. But not me as I just could pretend to understand them. Who knew? I just did catch not over ten words of their conversation so badly.

5.9 We Failed Because They Said We Speak Thai with an Accent

An outgoing from Phuket, Kati was a fourth year English major student. In the last semester, she was on an internship mission for one semester. This was a requirement of the English program. Therefore, she and her classmate, Pong, decided to choose a public relation company in Bangkok as their destination. Both dreamed to be a great PR. They went through an oral interview. However, their first application for an intern failed. They did not pass it. Kati shared reason:

> It's really funny. We really want to work in this PR department so badly. We did an interview. I think I did a good job. Pong did so too. We're so confident. But we failed. They said

we speak Thai with an accent. They need someone who can speak Thai fluently like *kon-krung-thep* (Bangkokians). We have to accept this. We can't speak Standard Thai but *thongdaeng* (accented Thai). This is too bad!

6 Discussion and Conclusion

One of the central phenomena emerging from the result is the interaction of power, discourse, position of authority related to dominant discourses along a continuum of discourse hierarchy. The participants' reflections on their understandings toward their English and Standard Thai captured a paradox in negotiations and power relations. A number of theoretical and ideological emerged from my results. At this point, three major concerns pertaining to the global proliferation of English are worth articulating: (1) the global English hegemony in Thailand, (2) discourse of self-marginalization, and (3) mythology and stereotype.

6.1 The Global English Hegemony in Thailand

The most salient research finding was that English use in Thailand was deeply embedded in a colonial construct within the political and economic hegemony of Western Anglophone powers. This result validates the notion that English language usage is never apolitical and is always involved in global inequality and imposition of ways of thinking (Phillipson 1992; Pennycook 1994). The way most of participants conceived of Standard English in relation to Thai and Thai people viewed Standard Thai unveiled the powerful construct of Standard form of discourse hidden in language use.

The participants' voices confirm that "the sociolinguistic reality of actual language use is less important than the symbolic assertion of cultural and political separateness which is embodied in the designation of English as the sole official language" (Markee 1993: 351). This colonial construction of the mind illustrates the unfortunate consequence of the cultural politics of promotion of English (Pennycook 1994, 1998; Canagarajah 1999). This chapter has reflected how the hegemonic position of English is unconsciously and consciously constructed and enacted by the participants.

6.2 Discourse of Self-Marginalization

Central to this English hegemony construct is the classic colonial production of an inferior Self and a superior Other. Manifestations of the discourse of self-marginalization refer to the way in which language learners on the periphery yield their voices and visions to the center and maintain marginalizing relations with English through an "us-them" mentality (Kumaravadivelu 2006). Finally, this uncritical acceptance of those on the periphery toward the dominance of the native speaker or the Eurocentric norms results in legitimizing their own marginalization.

This study demonstrates that some participants who conformed to the Standard English or Standard Thai and also those who were around with the participants viewed the world from the perspective of colonial subjects. They placed themselves marginally in the discourse hierarchy in relation to the dominant discourse and Western ideology. Moreover, some created a colonized image of nonnative language user and non-Western writers as inferior Self and the construction of the Standard English and Standard Thai as the superior Other. The premise that the West or the Western ideology or the *Bangkokian* or the capital ideology was more advanced and sophisticated was deeply situated in the minds of some participants and those of people around them. The hierarchical assumptions of discourse reflected in this study reaffirmed that these informants had low self-esteem, even put down their own discourse, and are put down by others.

For example, Ladda hoped that one day her opinion pieces could be published in the way she wanted to without sacrificing her voices to her editors. Kampol, who evaluated his English as "low class, too simple, not sophisticated, and uneducated," made these remarks about the root of the marginalizing social relationships in Thailand: "I think after all it's about perception. This is how most Thai people perceive of English. We have a perception that if one's written language is beautiful, we tend to assume that one is smart."

The discursive production of self-marginalization reflected the interconnectedness of language, power struggles, and social class. In case of Tang, whenever she needed Thais to socially accept her, she chose to switch to use English although she did realize that many of those locals could not speak or understand English at all. Tang realized that these people tended to regard English superior than Thai. The power relation between dominant English and local discourse, Thai, were in place. Besides, Pim and Ladda resonated their struggle to be accepted by their English newspaper editors. In order to be published, their writing needed to be conformed to the newspaper's policy that preferred dominant Standard English to non-Standard English varieties.

Besides, Pan's episode of "my teacher says my English has a *Thinglish* symptom" reflects an inferior position when his accented English was compared with Standard English. Lastly, the story of Kati and Pong captured a phenomenon of marginalization in urban areas of Thailand. Working as interns in Bangkok, both learned how *Bangkokians* (*kon-krung-thep*) stigmatized countryside people (*kon-ban-nok*) by judging them from an accent. Unable to speak Standard Thai fluently, both southerners unfortunately failed an interview for a job. Their accented Thai became a footnote of an outsider or Other.

I argue that this construct is embedded in ideological and political positions toward English and Thai discourse. Canagarajah's (2002: 256) work could be used to problematize this phenomenon. He contends that "native speakers' norms of identity and proficiency disempower learners with a sense of inadequacy." Therefore, no matter what scenarios regarding imperial constructs of English take place, the most serious effect of English hegemony is the "colonization of the mind." Simply put, "you glorify English and its culture while stigmatizing and devaluing your own language and culture. It may sound a bit too extreme, but you are enslaved to English and its culture" (Tsuda 1997: 24–25).

6.3 *Mythology and Stereotype*

In this study, English hegemony and self-marginalization were maintained through discursive construct of mythology and stereotype discourses. Regarding language myths, the informants made stereotypical statements pertaining to language ideology and language use. Over the course of data collection, the participants mystified language usage. For example, as Pim put it, "English is universal language. So English is the language that is understood by people from every country." The second scenario maintaining English hegemony was through discourse of stereotype employed against nonstandard language varieties (Bhabha 1990; Bourdieu 1991). Basically, the point some participants made was loaded with linguistic prejudice about privileging Standard English over non-Standard English varieties. They legitimized the higher status English varieties such as American English but disregarded Singapore English (*Singlish*). In this way, stereotyping results in fixated form of representation, as Milroy and Milroy (1991: 3) put it:

> Even though public discrimination on the grounds of race, religion and social class is not publicly acceptable, it appears that discrimination on linguistic grounds is publicly acceptable, even though linguistic differences may themselves be associated with ethnic, religious and class difference.

Additionally, this stereotyping discloses a deep and pervasive underlying prejudice against not only accented English but also accented Thai or non-Standard Thai. As presented in the participants' narratives, this manifestation played out around the linguistic discrimination in the job market. This biased discursive process indicates that English seems to prevail everywhere yet it seems not equal to everyone (Holborow 1999). In this respect, Ladda addressed the issue of prejudice toward non-Standard English varieties. As she put it, "When we come upon poor or a strange kind of English writing, we are likely to think that it was written by Thais." Her observation illustrated that this stereotypical discourse dies hard. Eventually, it seems that such a discourse might keep buoying up the hegemonic position of English in Thailand.

To conclude, this chapter has addressed the status of English and Thai languages related to the notion of Other—marginalized voices—in Thailand. It has presented narratives of nine language users from educational and media contexts in Thailand. Although these people engaged in different language use situations, the episodes of their experiences coincidently and interestingly echo the same phenomenon—the marginalized positions in Thai society. The salient research finding presented thus far is that language use in Thailand—the nation that is never colonized by any country during a colonization era—is embedded in a colonial construct. These conceptualizations of English concerning Thai by the participants demonstrate the impact of English in the construction of colonial discourse not only in their written works but also in their minds.

The research findings presented thus far theorize the cultural and ideological domination of English and standard ideology and most significantly the powerful construct of postcolonial English in Thailand. Most of the participants were linguistically, culturally, and professionally marginalized within hegemonic mainstream discourses—Standard English and Standard Thai. Suffice it to say that colonial power still imposes its presence and potency in the participants' minds even though Thailand has never been a colony of a European nation.

7 Implications

This study has taken a small yet critical step in exploring English status in relation to Thai language. It probes into the theoretical understanding of sociolinguistics in Thailand. To a certain extent, the dominant discourse of English and Standard Thai describes the phenomena of linguistic hegemony, power relations, and postcolonial identity. Needless to say, this inquiry offers an interesting invitation to delve into this line of research. The study is of paramount importance for understanding power relations including the fundamental inequality of discourse, language use, and postcolonial English in Thailand.

This chapter suggests that language, ideology, and power are intertwined. It not only has offered a great deal of critical insights into the sociolinguistic context of Thailand, but it also has allowed us to better understand the theoretical, conceptual, ideological, and power-related concerns of English hegemony and standard language. This research opens up future studies to explore the status of the global English paradigm and language use in Thailand. Interestingly, it seems that more questions are raised than answers given in exploring the ongoing complex relationship between language use and postcolonial power in Thailand.

Acknowledgments My deepest gratitude goes to my respectful informants who provided me the input and allowed me to learn a great deal from them over the course of the project. Also, I would like to express my appreciation to the reviewer and the editor, Professor Dr. Pranee Liamputtong, for inviting me to write this chapter. It is such an honor to be part of the great team and contribute to this remarkable volume.

References

Aksornkool, N. (1980). *EFL planning in Thailand: A case study in language planning*. Unpublished Ph.D. dissertation, Georgetown University.
Bamgbose, A. (2003). English in language policy and planning. *World Englishes, 22*(4), 419–431.
Bhabha, H. K. (1990). *Nation and narration*. New York: Routledge.

Bhatt, R. M. (2001). Language economy, standardization, and World Englishes. In E. Thumboo (Ed.), *The three circles of English: Language specialists talk about the English language* (pp. 401–422). Singapore: UniPress.

Bolton, K. (2004). World Englishes. In A. Davies & C. Elder (Eds.), *The handbook of applied linguistics* (pp. 367–396). Malden: Blackwell.

Bourdieu, P. (1991). *Language and symbolic power*. Oxford: Polity.

Canagarajah, A. S. (1999). *Resisting linguistic imperialism in English teaching*. Oxford: Oxford University Press.

Canagarajah, A. S. (2002). Reconstructing local knowledge. *Journal of Language, Identity, and Education, 1*(4), 243–259.

Coffey, A., & Atkinson, P. (1996). *Making sense of qualitative data: Complementary research strategies*. Thousand Oaks: Sage.

Crystal, D. (1997). *English as a global language*. Cambridge: Cambridge University Press.

Crystal, D. (2004). *The language revolution*. Cambridge: Polity.

Fairclough, N. (2001). *Language and power* (2nd ed.). London: Pearson Education.

Foley, A. J. (2005). English in … Thailand. *RELC Journal, 36*(2), 223–234.

Holborow, M. (1999). *The politics of English: A Marxist view of language*. London: Sage.

Huebner, T. (2006). Bangkok's linguistic landscapes: Environmental print, codemixing and language change. *International Journal of Multilingualism, 3*(1), 31–51.

Joseph, J. E. (1987). *Eloquence and power: The rise of language standards and standard languages*. London: Pinter.

Kumaravadivelu, B. (2006). Dangerous liaison: Globalization, empire, and TESOL. In J. Edge (Ed.), *(Re-)locating TESOL in an age of empire* (pp. 1–26). New York: Palgrave Macmillan.

Markee, N. (1993). Symposium on linguistic imperialism. *World Englishes, 12*(3), 335–373.

Masavisut, N., Sukwiwat, M., & Wongmontha, S. (1986). The power of the English language in Thai media. *World Englishes, 5*(2–3), 197–207.

Milroy, J., & Milroy, L. (1991). *Authority in language: Investigating language prescription and standardisation* (2nd ed.). London: Routledge.

Pennycook, A. (1994). *The cultural politics of English as an international language*. Essex: Longman.

Pennycook, A. (1998). *English and the discourses of colonialism*. London: Routledge.

Pennycook, A. (2000). English, politics, ideology from colonial celebration to postcolonial performativity. In T. Ricento (Ed.), *Ideology, politics, and language policies: Focus on English* (pp. 107–119). Amsterdam: John Benjamins.

Pennycook, A. (2001). *Critical applied linguistics: A critical introduction*. Mahwah: L. Erlbaum.

Pennycook, A. (2002). Turning English inside out. *Indian Journal of Applied Linguistics, 28*(2), 25–43.

Phillipson, R. (1992). *Linguistic imperialism*. Oxford: Oxford University Press.

Rappa, A. L., & Wee, L. (2006). *Language policy and modernity in Southeast Asia: Malaysia, the Philippines, Singapore, and Thailand*. New York: Springer.

Rushdie, S. (1982). The Empire writes back with a vengeance. *Times, 3*, 8.

Said, E. W. (1994). *Culture and imperialism*. London: Vintage.

Strauss, A. L., & Corbin, J. M. (1998). *Basics of qualitative research: Techniques and procedures for developing grounded theory* (2nd ed.). Thousand Oaks: Sage.

Tollefson, J. W. (2000). Policy and ideology in the spread of English. In J. K. Hall & W. Eggington (Eds.), *The sociopolitics of English language teaching* (pp. 7–21). Clevedon: Multilingual Matters.

Tripasai, P. (2004). *Debating Anna: The textual politics of English literature teaching in Thailand*. Retrieved August 2, 2008, from: http://www.aare.edu.au/04pap/tri04046.pdf

Tsuda, Y. (1997). Hegemony of English vs. ecology of language. In L. E. Smith & M. L. Forman (Eds.), *World Englishes 2000* (pp. 21–31). Honolulu: University of Hawaii Press.

Wongsothorn, A. (2000). Thailand. In H. W. Kam & R. Y. L. Wong (Eds.), *Language policies and language education* (pp. 307–320). Singapore: Time Academic Press.

Chapter 7
Digital Revolution and Its Discontents: Thai "Underground Metal" Scene and Their Love-Hate Relationship with New Technologies

Athip Jittarerk

1 Introduction: After the Great Digital Divide

A specter is haunting the music industry—the specter of piracy. All the powers of old music industry have entered into a holy alliance to exorcize this specter: major labels and indie labels, Sonny Bono and Metallica, British rocks stars, and American pop-dance queens. Now in 2012, it could be said that digital music piracy has tremendously changed the way people consume music and the music industry itself. We could see this change around the world, at least where ordinary people could possibly establish a high-speed Internet connection. It is quite clear now that within the reach of the high-speed Internet connection, CDs, and other tangible media that contains music are now artifacts of the past or at least they are now collectors' items rather than general commodities as they used to be.

It is generally said both among the public and the music industry that piracy contributes to the decline of CDs sales in the 2000s, and it is reasonable for the music industry to take action. In the USA, where the struggle of the music industry is most intense, there has been a constant struggle to end piracy from digital right management (DRM) to mass suing of digital pirates. Recently, the attempt to pass controversial Stop Online Piracy Act (SOPA) from late 2011 can also be said to be part of this over decade struggle which fails to "improve" the situation of piracy. SOPA threats to civil rights cause a public outcry that lead to a mass "blackout" of various websites, leaded by Wikipedia, on January 19, 2012 which is now considered to be the largest scale of Internet protest since its existence. Hence, the attempt to "stop online piracy" is no small issue at all, and we have to note that one of the largest supporters of this legislation is the US music industry. Why is music piracy a bad thing?

A. Jittarerk (✉)
Pathum Thani, Thailand
e-mail: athipj@gmail.com

P. Liamputtong (ed.), *Contemporary Socio-Cultural and Political Perspectives in Thailand*, 111
DOI 10.1007/978-94-007-7244-1_7, © Springer Science+Business Media Dordrecht 2014

Most of the public discourses on music piracy come from the music industry from a simple demonization of piracy as a kind of "theft" to more seemingly scientific calculation about the job and economic losses caused by piracy. In the industry point of view, piracy is always bad, but what are the other stakeholders' points of view? There are few studies that address the issue, and most of them just came out recently and addressed it just indirectly. The data in these studies are also not quite conclusive about other stakeholders' points of view about piracy. So currently, there are no other clear voices about piracy apart from the music industry.

My position in this chapter is to investigate this issue from the information I gathered from the research I conducted in Bangkok from mid-2007 to early 2010 in Bangkok's "underground metal" scene.[1] In the field, I always see both musicians and other scene members expressing different attitudes toward piracy or even inconsistently at times. However, as the research progressed, what I found is that I cannot single out piracy from the new musical production situation brought about by the widespread usage of digital recording and the distributing of music and related information through social network websites. At the first place, this may sound too complex, but my point here is that we cannot just ask people about their attitudes toward piracy without asking their attitude about the whole new musical world that, what I call "digital revolution," brought about. People may subjectively say they do not like or even oppose piracy while, objectively, they enjoy all the by-products of piracy without knowing that all they enjoy will not be possible without piracy. So, the new and more appropriate question is about the attitudes of the people toward this whole new musical world brought about by piracy and other aspects of digital revolution.

2 Backgrounds: The "Negative" Impact of Digital Revolution, Music Industries, and Piracy Studies

My initial question about the merit of piracy in general is shaped by the public discourses on piracy and what I would like to call here "piracy studies." I will elaborate here why most, if not all, studies miss the aspect of the piracy question that I found in the field.

Coming to the level of the research, piracy is, most of all, an economic question. What I mean here is that there are possibilities of other aspects of piracy to be researched, such as ethics, but most of them that come out are based on economic questions which make the researches quantitative in nature. The reason here is quite simple when we look at the major sponsors of these researches which are the music

[1] Scene here refers to the site where the music production and consumption took place. I initially use the term "field of cultural production" to refer to what I refer to here as "scene" in previous work for different emphasis. For more details of the research, see Jittarerk (2011).

industries.[2] The music industry in the USA as well as most part of the developed world sponsored this kind of research to focus on economic losses of a particular industry due to piracy. The aim of the research is to demonstrate to the public and interest groups how bad piracy is and sometimes they have clear political implication to support some laws or state policies to combat piracy. The number of job losses and the number of CD sales losses are highlighted in this kind of research which many times came out as an annual report or factsheet of the music industry and other copyright-related associations.[3]

The industry-sponsored kind of piracy research dominated the study of piracy throughout the 2000s. However, in 2011, more academic types of research came out. *Media Piracy in Emerging Economies* (Karaganis 2011) is a multi-authored volume that has a number of researchers to research on the piracy situation in various developing countries. What is significant is that this research is a very first comprehensive multidisciplinary study on piracy that is not sponsored by the copyright-related industry, and it is also the very first English publication to show various aspects of piracy in some of the third world countries. The broad scope of this research ranges from the relationship between the international trade agreement and local legal aspect of copyright infringement to the social life of piracy on the streets. Different chapters focus on different aspects of piracy. Nevertheless, music piracy is one of the constant topics that each chapter always contains.

The interesting parts of this research are the parts that directly intend to argue with the validity of the previous researches sponsored by the industry. The overall arguments that are relevant here are that *Media Piracy* has said that the industry-sponsored research data are mostly unreliable and the ones which use reliable data tend to overstate the negative impact of piracy (Karaganis 2011: 1–73). The basic mistakes those studies made are the overstatement of economic loss originated by piracy. *Media Piracy* points clearly again and again that these researches tend to maximize the calculation of loss by multiplying the number of pirate copies with the actual sale price. This is based on the assumption that every pirate copy implies one actual sale loss. This is a questionable assumption that is even dropped by later industry-sponsored researches.[4] However, the bigger mistake about these losses claim is the inconvenient fact that piracy does not reduce the overall consumption in the whole economic system at all. This means that the losses from piracy in a particular sector must also mean the gains in other sectors.

---

[2] I later found out that this kind of industry-sponsored research should be complemented with the academic research about piracy from the economist (these works are reviewed in Dejean 2009). These economic researches are quite quantitative in nature as industry-sponsored piracy studies. Two kinds of research asked the same question; they just conclude qualitatively different, and both leave the structural transforming impact of piracy untouched. (Anyway academic research that reaches a similar conclusion as industry-sponsored research, but with less moral overtones, also exists (see Liebowitz 2006).)

[3] This kind of research is generally available for downloading in the website of the copyright industry interest groups. For example, see http://www.ifpi.org/

[4] Later research use, for example, production cost instead of sale price which make the calculated loss dropped tremendously.

To put in a more technical term, the question is "what are substitution effects created by piracy?" This is a very complex question that requires a detailed and elaborate answer for each particular case that one might not be able to expect on a macro study of piracy. We will not know clearly how reduction in consumption in the intensively pirated sectors, such as music, movies, software, and computer games, would result in the increase in consumption in which sector unless we conduct a more detailed study on this specific issue, and I have not seen any research that has taken this path.

Nevertheless, in the musical sector, it is widely believed from late 2000s that the large part of the budget shift away from CDs consumption more or less goes to the concert consumption (Karaganis 2011: 43). The data that supports this belief is the tremendous growth in the total concert industry revenue about the time that the record sales decline. The more empirical connection about this causality does not exist yet, but if we accept this connection, the way to evaluate the total economic merit of piracy is to measure the increase in the concert revenue with the decrease in the sales of records. If the two have about the same amount, we can initially conclude that the budget shift is just within the music industry from the recording music sector to the live music sector.

However, are things this simple? Even the weights of the two are the same, the point that the calculation misses is the issue of the distribution of musical income.[5] To put it simply, even if the revenue of the concert industry increase about the same as the decrease in the recording industry revenue, the potential recording income loss of a particular artist does not necessary mean that he will automatically gain that income by playing at the concert. From the current situation, it is more likely that the potential record income loss of the newer musicians goes to the pocket of the older superstars and concert organizers.[6] Nevertheless, it is still too simplistic to rush to the conclusion that this lower income distribution among musicians is "bad" even among the musicians themselves. As I mentioned earlier, the whole issue for the musician is not about piracy, but it is about the whole new world the digital revolution brought into being against the old world. If we want to really evaluate the merit of piracy based on the people point of view, we have to investigate their attitudes toward this new world. However, what is this new world? I would like to confidently say that people engaged in different music genres in different places and times will perceive this new world differently and I have no intention here to propose a general theory of this new musical world that could be applied across place and time. Instead, I shall explain the overall impacts of the digital revolution based on the given local situation.

---

[5] Income distribution is a very basic issue in development economics which research from any industry normally neglect.

[6] This seems to be true since there are data that suggest that in the period of increasing total concert revenue in the USA, the number of the concerts and concert attendance is actually decreased. What made the total revenue increase is the rising concert ticket price, and this makes the concert industry revenue concentrated in the smaller amount of concerts than the previous period. See Krueger (2005).

3 "Productive" Impacts of the Digital Revolution

When I was in the field, I learnt that piracy is always something of a spectral quality. People know it exists, but no one wants to talk about it openly. But, as I make the diachronic comparison between the scenes in the 1990s and late 2000s, it is clear that piracy[7] changes the way people consume and make music. As the CD sales decline, specialized heavy metal record stores faced the similar fate as other record stores in Thailand's capital city.[8] They closed down one after another continuously. The independent heavy metal music labels existed before the advent of piracy closed their operations one by one.

These are the worst dreams possible for the people from the 1990s who are not familiar with the digital technology. The closing down of the record stores means that there would be no place to buy heavy metal records and interact with other "metalheads."[9] The closing down of the labels means that there would be no metal records being released by those records. In short, this is a disastrous destruction of the ways of the 1990s to maintain the scene and to keep underground metal music being produced.

While this "disaster" would make a perfect sense in the 1990s, the situation is much more complex in the late 2000s. Now, the distributive and interactive functions of the heavy metal record stores are transferred to small "underground" heavy metal shows and social network websites.[10] The recording financing functions of the music labels are now in the bands' own hands because of the reduction of minimum recording cost due to the affordable prices of digital recording devices. If we want to judge the quality of the scene based on the number of the bands producing heavy metal music and the shows devoted to heavy metal music, the late 2000s is far from dystopia of underground metal music. The time can even be best described as the

[7] Or rather new form of piracy since the Thai hard rock/heavy metal scene in the past is no stranger to cassette piracy. In fact, cassette piracy is really the main material that created the scene in the first place (Jittarerk 2011).

[8] Normally, the scene member refers to the music they related to shortly as "metal," since they have to distinguish different subgenres such as heavy metal, thrash metal, death metal, black metal, power metal, and gothic metal. However, in this work I do not want to emphasize on the subcategorization of "metal" music, and I will use "heavy metal," the generic term for outsider, throughout.

[9] "Metalhead" is an internationally common term to refer to the member of contemporary heavy metal subculture or scene. This term is sometimes used in Thai context. However, the scene members understand the term even if they do not use it.

[10] The term "underground" is used in the scene frequently by the member both among themselves and to outsiders for referring to the name of the scene. We have to note that the scene is not "underground" in the sense that the musical activity is illegal, but in the sense that it is outside "mainstream." This is true for Thailand where the scene has always been outside the radar of the authority. The term underground is also used as an adjective such as "underground metal" to signify that heavy metal music is outside mainstream. It has to note that although there are some heavy rockers in "the mainstream," which could be seen in public media, these heavy rockers are never counted as part of the underground scene and their music is not part of "metal" in the scene member's perspective.

highest point of the scene since it started to exist.[11] There are more bands than ever which produce more music and having more shows than ever. The origin of the situation is what I called digital revolution where piracy only plays a negative part to free more time and take more money from the people so these resources can be shifted toward musical production instead of consumption. Here, I shall return to the question raised about "what are substitution effects created by piracy?" I will look at "substitution effects" in the broadest sense, which is not limited to just substitute consumptions but also substitute productions. I will also answer it by comparing the behaviors of the members of the scene in the 1990s that I interviewed and the behaviors of the members of the scene in the late 2000s who saw in the field, or, in short, by comparing the pre-piracy people with the post-piracy people.

3.1 The Rise of Digital Recording and Its Impacts

Digital technology has transformed many cultural production sites in the late 2000s, and one of the sectors that received this impact of digital technology is the musical sector. Not only digital musicians specialized in synthesizers are benefitting from the technology, but those producing music in the rock music tradition of recording live instruments also receive lots of impacts from digital recording. In the 1990s, analog recording is the rule of making the rock recording. The cost of building the studio is practically unaffordable for the lay musicians. It would probably cost a million, if not millions of baht to create the recordable studio in the 1990s. I cannot gather the rental rate of the commercial studio at the time, but there is an interview which indicated that the recording of the very first underground metal album in Thailand, released in the mid-1990s, costs 200,000 baht (Donpheebin 2008). We also have to note that his is the cheapest recording because it was initially meant to be only the demo recording, so the quality of the recording is not quite good when compared to commercial recording of the time.

Now, the situation is much different. The musicians in the late 2000s I interviewed did not have to invest a large amount of money for recording compared to the 1990s. The bands that finance their own recording in the commercial studio in the late 2000s might have to invest only 20,000 baht for all the recording and mixing process to get their tracks ready for the album.[12] Looking only at the price, this is ten times cheaper than the 1990s recording.[13] Examination of the quality of the tracks shows

---

[11] There are conflicting opinions about the beginning of the scene (Jittarerk 2011).

[12] The bands I have talked to have various ways of recordings. Those who record their music at home might invest for their audio interface, use pirated musical software to program drums, and have lower cost of production than 20,000 baht. Still, some richer musicians use more budget than 100,000 baht for their recording, but I would say that this is quite a rare case that also astonished other musicians when I told them.

[13] If we include the impact of inflation between the mid-1990s and late 2000s into calculation, this gap would even be larger.

that they are considered better than 1990s underground recording because of the clarity of the instruments.

This kind of recording is possible because the rehearsal studios around Bangkok adopted digital recording and extended their business to include recording service in the mid-2000s. The digital recordings of these studios provide a budget alternative for the musician who wants to make a recording in the late 2000s. It makes sense to assume that the price is affordable since the recording budget 20,000 baht is shared among band members as all the bands I interviewed asserted. Given that the average number of most metal band is four members,[14] the average cost of recording per member for each album recording is 5,000 baht per member. The price is affordable for sure since it is less than the cost of the musical instrument the members have to use in playing live.[15]

The affordability of recording makes the bands' recordings compulsory for the promotion of the band and to get the show.[16] The bands have to present themselves through the bands pictures and their music in public places where they can meet the show organizers and fans. This is where social network sites come into the picture.

3.2 The Rise of Social Network Sites and Its Impacts

There is more reason than financial issue that 1990s bands have to rely on recording labels. It is distributional issue. Not only is it almost impossible for a band to finance an album recording in the 1990s, to get the music being heard is equally difficult. Cassette tape was the dominant vessel of music in the 1990s. Music had to be put in cassettes to be sold and heard. Producing cassettes in the 1990s required more investment than bands could afford. So, there was a need for finance from the label.

In 1990s cassette regime, 100,000–200,000 cassettes sale for each album is considered a loss even for the indie labels of the time (Sukosol Klapp and Potisaratana

[14] Most underground metal bands in Bangkok consist of 3–5 members which is the same as metal bands elsewhere in the world as far as I know. The variation of the members is mostly due to the number of guitarists in the band (can be either 1 or 2) and whether the vocalist is playing any instrument or not.

[15] The minimum instrument necessary for playing live for a band is the guitar and a distortion effect, the bass guitar and the double-bass drums pedal, and snare drum. The total price of all the instruments is more than 20,000 baht for sure. I would assert that people who could afford to buy these instruments could also afford the recording cost in the late 2000s.

[16] There are some bands trying to get a record deal in the period I study, but they are the minority. Most bands accept the situation of no label existing to give them a deal and making a recording on their own budget. However, there are not many albums recorded in this period. Most, I would say 70–80 %, recordings that came out in the late 2000s are either demo or EP consisting of not more than 5 tracks. This is a big contrast with the 1990s recording that more than 90 % of recording is album recording. This shift from album making to demo and EP making is interesting and needs more discussion I cannot properly give here.

2008). But, the best-selling underground metal cassettes could reach only about 70,000 copies.[17] This creates a big loss of investment to most labels who signed underground metal bands which either eventually bankrupted them or made them get rid of all underground metal bands from the label.

The whole situation starts to change in early 2000 when CD sales start to decrease and finally the whole recording business reach a similar situation. One of the famous Thai popular song composers from the biggest Thai label claimed in 2011 that, in the past, the sales less than 500,000 copies was a disaster, but now, if any record can sell more than 10,000 copies, it is something to celebrate.[18] The sales of contemporary underground metal decrease similarly. For all that I know from the field, the best-selling underground metal album that reached the highest sale in the late 2000s cannot even reach 2,000 copies, and normally any record of underground metal bands cannot even sell more than 1,000 copies. For the bands that I know, it took them many years and lots of effort to sell all 500 copies of the album.[19]

Even the recording cost is much cheaper in the late 2000s. This is still not a good situation to invest in metal bands. The bands now have to finance their own recording as mentioned above. However, what replaced the old way of getting music out to the public via tangible media such as cassette and CD is the Internet. When I started conducting the research in 2007, I could say that 95 % of the bands had their band pages on www.myspace.com.[20] On the show, I participated bands even announce their Myspace addresses on stage.

Myspace basically provides everything that bands need to promote themselves on the Internet.[21] Bands can upload their songs and their pictures on the site to show on their pages and they can even customize their page to fit their image. Myspace is also the site where bands, their friends, their fans, and show organizers interact. Bands post the advertisement of their latest releases on each other's profile. Show organizers find new bands for their show via Myspace and invite them to play. When the show poster comes out, it is normal for both the organizer and bands to put the

---

[17] Estimated from one of the widely known Thai underground metal album which is Donpheebin's second album *Sen Tang Sai Morrana* (*The Way of Death*) (see Donpheebin 2008).

[18] The composer's name is Nitipong Hornak. He claimed the number on the news show "*Joh Kow Den*" (Investigating Hot News) of Channel 3, which is a public TV channel, on January 19, 2011.

[19] Actually the album is also used in the practice known as "trading" which is exchanging album with foreign metal band via mail. This chapter is too short for discussing the detail of transnational CD exchange which provides more outlet of the CD produced in various locations. Only a faction of bands in Bangkok have this practice, but the practice creates a connection that both brings foreign underground metal to play a show in Bangkok and makes Bangkok's underground metal bands get the show abroad.

[20] I actually encountered more than 100 bands in the field, both online and offline. I found only one band that has no Myspace page. But it has its page on another social network site—Multiply.

[21] By late 2009, Myspace is quite obsolete as almost all interactions between bands, organizers, and fans move to Facebook. But, the overall functions are quite the same. Bands still promote themselves through Facebook pages, organizers post the show posters around various "walls" in Facebook, and fans still interact with bands, or even band members, in their pages or personal accounts.

poster out as their profile picture and when other scene members see the poster they go to the show for support. Finally, we reach the most important component of the scene, the show.

3.3 The Rise of the Shows and Its Impacts

The show is the most important component of underground metal scene. Some bands in the scene even heading toward playing in the show while they are still playing only cover songs of famous foreign metal bands. It has to be noted that an underground "show" is different from what is called "concert." In the Thai language, *concert* generally means a big commercial concert, normally in a big hall or a stadium. However, when scene member refer to what is equal to underground "concert," they will use *ngarn taidin*. *Taidin* means underground, literally under the ground, and *ngarn* generally signifies a trade fair or exhibition. As far as I have heard, the scene members never refer to the underground "show" as "concert" and referring to the show as concert signifies the nonmembership of the scene.

Underground shows in Bangkok mostly took place in small pubs around Bangkok that have 100–300 capacity. The organizers normally rent the place in daytime and use the pub's instrument that is used for their nighttime live music, namely, the microphones, the amplifiers, the drums set, the mixer, and the PA. Normally, the pub will not be selling anything at the daytime show and will not allow any drink to enter the door. The common picture of the underground show is the scene members, and even the bands, getting drunk in front of the pub.

The profitability of organizing the show is quite mysterious for most of the scene members or even the bands. However, I also did a research with the organizers and even organize the show with the group of "friends" I find in the field.[22] I can assert that it is quite impossible to make any profit in the late 2000s show and in the early 2010s the situation is getting economically worse.

I know from talking with various pub owners and organizers that the rental price of the pub for a show normally ranged from 15,000 to 25,000 baht. The average ticket price for all the shows of all Thai bands was about 150 baht in 2007. At that time, the shows that get the most people in the beginning of the field is "metalcore"[23] show, which is trendy music at the time. It might get 200 ticket sales at most for the 25,000 baht venue. This means 5,000 baht profit at most for each show. The less trendy shows of "old school heavy metal"[24] in the same period and same venue could not even get 100 ticket sales. This means a loss of more than 10,000 baht.[25]

---

[22] The group is called "Bangkok Thrash" and still organizing a yearly thrash metal show.

[23] Metalcore is this sense is a music that is a mixture of 1990s' New York style hard-core punk music and early 2000s' Swedish style death metal. The subgenre is very popular in the USA in the mid-2000s and its popularity came to the underground scene in Thailand shortly.

[24] The term normally means heavy metal subgenre that emerged in the 1980s in the USA and UK.

[25] The rough calculation of this profit and loss is based on the assumption that most of the show did not get additional revenue from the sponsors. But if they had a sponsor, each sponsor tended to give few thousand baht only, and all Thai band shows normally do not get more than 1–2 sponsors.

As time passes, metalcore is slower sliding out off the trend and the show also gets less than 100 sales in a matter of few years.[26] This situation reflects the general situation of the underground show in the late 2000s. Every show attracts not many people and keeps making loss. In my opinion, the key cause of this situation is that shows keep increasing constantly in the late 2000s. As shows increase, if there are no additional scene members and the present scene member did not attend more shows, the number of attendance and ticket sales of each show seems to inevitably decrease.

What is quite strange for me is that in the period the ticket price for each show seems to decrease too. In 2007, the normal price range is between 150 and 200 baht, but by 2010, the normal price range is between 100 and 150 baht. This reduction is price may originate from the price competition between organizers. However, even where there is the reduction is price there is no significant increase in demand for attendance and the result is disastrous for those who cut their ticket price down.

Even if there is no significant demand for watching the show, there is a constant demand in playing in the show. I notice that new bands keep entering the scene since the first day of my research and it does not seem to have stopped. It may be a too big question for this chapter to speculate why people keep producing this unprofitable music. However, if we assume that this drive to make underground metal music is relatively constant for the last 20 years, we may see clearly that the digital revolution is the precise structural condition that brought the whole situation. There are always people who want to make underground metal music; digital revolution just enables them to do so in the late 2000s. This leads us to the last point of evaluating digital revolution from the musician's point of view.

4 To Pay or to Be Paid, That Is the Question: Digital Underground vs. Traditional Underground

Nowadays, shows keep increasing to the extent that some organizers collect some money from the bands participating in the show to finance the show. This musician paying to play instead of playing to be paid situation might be weird in the first place, but it is the very logical outcome when the organizers of the shows are keeping on making losses at the same time as more bands are willing to play.

The pay to play problem is scandalous in the scene for a while in late 2010 to early 2011, and there was even an online campaign against the organizer who organized the show this way. The campaigners even tried to organize the show where "good" bands can play without having to pay any money. The issue finally faded away. The organizer who collected money from musicians when organizing the show disappeared from the scene and the campaigners who tried to give a good band a free chance to play also disappeared without their show being organized. But, the whole monetary issue points the gap that separates two generations of musicians.

[26] I observed this in 2009, not more than 2 years since I entered the field.

Getting money from underground musical activities or not is the issue that marks the generation gap of the pre-digital revolution musicians and post-digital revolution musicians.[27] Even if I mention how unprofitable underground music used to be in the 1990s, the musicians of that generation still expect to be paid for their unprofitable musical work. The labels mostly are not able to pay them and end up with bitter relationships toward musicians who accused them of cheating and ripping off.[28] Even if the label does not exist as an active component of the scene, the musicians of this generation have the tendency to request the paying fee from the organizer and normally when they know they will not get paid, they will refuse to play. It is interesting to note that the musicians of this generation are normally acting as "professional" musicians in the sense that they act the same way as those living by playing music even if they're not. It is quite understandable since musicians of this generation tend to have gained money from their musical activities for at least some part of their lives, so they continue the same monetary demand even if the whole scene is making losses.

The post-digital revolution generation of musicians tends to be accustomed to not being paid for their musical activities. As I have said above, this generation has to finance their recording on their own and actually some of them have to organize their own show. This is the generation that is normally investing in their musical activity not finding the investors to invest and take risk for their musical activities as previous generations. Furthermore, given that this generation mostly starts playing shows in the mid-2000s, in general, they have no experience of being paid for playing in a show.

When it comes to the evaluation of the current situation, both generations see the current situation of the scene differently. Even the members of the older generation who appreciate the productive impact of digital revolution to be appropriated by them look at the situation of the whole scene negatively in various ways. Some members of this generation still keep complaining about "piracy problems" that destroy the whole label system which in fact destroy the appropriate system of making the music, where the duties of the musician are composing songs, rehearsing, and recording, leaving everything else to be the duty of the label. Many musicians of the generation are quite happy with the opportunity that digital technology provides,

---

[27] Of course, there are shades of differences and exceptions. The two categories could be read only as Weberian "ideal type." It is also noted that sometimes the attitudes of the pre-digital revolution musicians exist in post-digital revolution musicians too, but this is rather a marginal phenomena to reject the generation-based explanation of the difference in attitudes. Furthermore, this kind of exception can be explained by the transference of attitude through association between some parts of the musicians of both generations.

[28] This is quite a complex and sensitive issue. There are some interviews that bands accused labels of ripping off (Donpheebin 2008) and the 1990s musician I talked to told me disappointingly that he "never got any money" despite "a lot of records being sold." So far as I know, most of "underground" metal label that are accused of "ripping off" tend to not have any signed contracts, and it is impossible to know the deal between the bands, or some members of the bands, and the labels. Given the fact that labels tended to make losses when they released an album, it is unclear whether they really "rip off" or not.

but they say disappointingly that newer bands have great technological possibility to produce albums but fail to produce anything more than an EP with few songs. Some even go so far to say that now it is too easy to be in a band and to play a show today to the extent that the whole scene is flooded with bands that do not have musical quality, especially in terms of musical skill. They add that it would be better if there are fewer bands on the scene with better quality of music enough to deserve to be paid for their show.

Normally, the newer generations have a different attitude toward the current situation of the scene. They do not see competition at all among bands and they are very supportive of new bands being formed. They view the show as a place for a band to improve to be a better band not the place where only the best bands in the scene share the stage. This generation looks at the digital technology very positively. Most of them acquire new music by downloading[29] and distributing their music through the Internet.[30] They have no problem with the bands having to finance recording themselves or even having to make a recording themselves. Actually, when some bands make recordings themselves, they are proud to take the role of the recording engineer and producer of their own album. In short, they see that digital technology change the scene in a good way.

In summary, it is not possible to conclude that the whole musical community have positive or negative evaluations about the total effect of digital revolution in general or even piracy in particular. Even most of the musicians agree that newer digital resources give more possibility to create music, not everyone agrees that it is good that this possibility is available to everyone, and this complicates the evaluation of piracy which is a major component of this revolution.

5 Conclusion: Technophilia or Technophobia? Yes, Please

Some people believe that Internet access can be separated from piracy, and this is a heated political debate of today about whether the measures are abolishing online piracy would equal the destruction of the Internet or not. As far as evidences around the world goes, Internet access always goes hand in hand with piracy. I do not see that it is appropriate to separate the current "piracy problem" from the overall impact of Internet connection, and since it is digitization of data that is a crucial link of both, the analysis should also include the digitization aspect. The systematic connection of the three aspects is what I call "digital revolution" and I have analyzed it through this chapter.

[29] This does not mean that this generation of musicians does not buy CDs at all. Buying CD and other merchandises becomes more like a duty to support other bands rather than the only way to get the music to be listened to as in a previous era.

[30] This does not mean that most of the bands give their music for free but means that they at least make their music available for streaming on the Internet.

In short, for underground metal bands in Bangkok, digital revolution makes what is previously unaffordable unnecessary and make what is previously necessary affordable. The traditional way of analog recording and getting music distributed through traditional distribution channels that was unaffordable for a band is now unnecessary. The new digital recording and digital distribution of music make what is previously unaffordable production and distribution of music available for every individual band. Piracy first brought the old intermediaries such as labels and record stores down. Digital recording provides an alternative way for making the recording independent from label's investment on recording. Internet connection provides both distribution channel and interactive functions gone with the record stores closing down. The new production situation drives more bands to emerge in the scene creating more music, but at the same time, more production of music drives the profitability of each producer in the whole scene down. The merit of the situation depends on the background and perspective of the beholders in the scene. The pre-digital revolution generation sees things getting worse as unqualified bands flood the scene and qualified bands do not get the payment they deserved. The post-digital revolution generation sees things getting better as there are more people who are serious enough about metal music playing in more and more bands, making records and improving themselves by performing in the shows.

It might all be too easy to finally conclude that the merits of piracy after all depend on perspective, but it is necessary since the public discourse keeps on asserting that piracy is some kind of absolute moral issue. This clash on perspectives about piracy brings it back to political issue where it always belongs. Piracy is no small issue in 2012. It becomes a highly politicized issue as the copyright industry is trying to regulate the Internet. Even if the battle started a long time ago, this might be the first period in history that the majority starts to feel that they are in the midst of the battle and, as good Weberian academic, I might have no task other than shedding some light on this politicized battle.

References

Dejean, S. (2009). What can we learn from empirical studies about piracy? *CESifo Economic Studies, 55*(2), 326–352.

Donpheebin. (2008). *Donpheebin: 25 Kanvela Soonumfah Soopadindow*. Unknown place of publication: DPB Publisher. [In Thai]

Jittarerk, A. (2011). *The birth and transformation of the field of metal music production in Thailand from 1970s to 2010s*. Unpublished MA thesis, Department of Sociology and Anthropology, Thammasat University, Bangkok, Thailand. [In Thai]

Karaganis, J. (Ed.). (2011). *Media piracy in emerging economy*. New York: Social Science Research Council.

Krueger, A. B. (2005). The economics of real superstars: The market for rock concerts in the material world. *Journal of Labor Economics, 22*(1), 1–30.

Liebowitz, S. J. (2006). File sharing: Creative destruction or just plain destruction? *Journal of Law and Economics, 49*(1), 1–28.

Sukosol Klapp, K., & Potisaratana, T. (2008). *Bakery & I*. Bangkok: A book Publisher. [In Thai]

Chapter 8
The *Thawiphop* Phenomenon: Reimagining Nationalism in a Contemporary Thai Novel and Its Stage and Screen Adaptations

Morakot Jewachinda Meyer

1 Introduction

In the late nineteenth-century Britain, Alice – the famous children's book character created by Lewis Carroll (2006) – enjoys time galore in the fantasy world down the rabbit hole and in the looking-glass house. Across the Indian Ocean in the late 1980s, Thailand witnessed the debut of *Maneechan* or *Manee*, the protagonist of the novel *Thawiphop* (Parallel Worlds). A beautiful young lady, *Manee* uses a standing mirror to travel back and forth between the present and the fantasized past of Thailand or Siam as the country was known before 1939. After her adventures in the fantasy world, Alice comes back to her house and presumably goes on to enjoy her life in the British Empire of her times. By contrast, *Manee* never returns from her final sojourn in the parallel world. She makes a conscious decision to live her life in the fantasized past of the mid-nineteenth-century Siam, where she has developed genuine love for *Dhep*, a young noble who works in the royal foreign affairs service. *Manee*'s and *Dhep*'s relation, however, cannot be reduced to romantic love; they are also bound together by their passion for defending the nation from the encroachments of Western imperialism.

This chapter offers a textual and contextual analysis of *Thawiphop* and its adaptations. Scholars have so far shown little interest in the novel and its various stage and screen versions although *Thawiphop* has been widely acknowledged for its significance in revealing certain aspects of contemporary Thai social and cultural life. Chaochuti (2009, 2012) offers literary criticism and a psychoanalytical account of the novel and one of its adaptations, the film *The Siam Renaissance* Harrison (2010) also studies this picture along with other productions by Thai directors released between the mid-1980s and the early 1990s. She argues that these

M.J. Meyer (✉)
Pridi Banomyong International College, Thammasat University (Tha Prachan Campus), Prachan Road, Pranakorn, Bangkok 10200, Thailand
e-mail: morakot.j.meyer@gmail.com

P. Liamputtong (ed.), *Contemporary Socio-Cultural and Political Perspectives in Thailand*, 125
DOI 10.1007/978-94-007-7244-1_8, © Springer Science+Business Media Dordrecht 2014

works represent ways of constructing Thainess through presentations of the West. *Thawiphop* and its various adaptations have nevertheless remained understudied, in particular as regards their relation to middle class identity.

Winichakul (2011) suggests in passing that *Thawiphop* and its cultural practices may be the most prominent examples of the promotion of "Thai royal-nationalist history" in popular consciousness. In particular, according to Winichakul, they reflect a persistent myth surrounding the Thai nation and its independence that extols the kings of the Bangkok Era (1782 to the present) as saviors who rescued the nation with their diplomatic talents from falling into the hands of Western powers. A close reading of *Thawiphop*, however, discloses that the novel does not simply reinforce the "official" line that the kings of Siam/Thailand are to be credited with this success as Winichakul claims. Instead, the novel portrays and celebrates upper-class and middle-class elites as preservers of the nation's integrity.

I argue that the Thai public's consumption of *Thawiphop* in its various versions reveals a new terrain of interrelation between forms and practices of entertainment, on the one hand, and the dynamism of nationalist culture in modern Thailand, on the other. The novel and its adaptations are products of wider developments in Thailand during the late Cold War and the following two decades. *Thawiphop* takes Lewis's legendary books *Alice in Wonderland* and *Through the Looking Glass* (2006) as its inspiration and becomes itself a mirror of the Thai middle class's identity[1] and of the interaction of middle-class Thais with national, regional, and global developments. At the same time, the *Thawiphop* phenomenon shows that the culture of nationalism is not exclusively fostered by state power. Entertainment also provides sites for negotiating nationalism (Holdsworth 2010; Lam 2012; Smith 2000; Schlesinger 2000; Story 2010; Inglis 2005), especially through representations of the past (Bhabha 1990).

2 The Emergence of *Thawiphop* as a "Looking Glass"

In the last three decades, no other novel received as much praise in Thailand as *Thawiphop*. Social and political developments in the country as well as the impact of regional and international changes help to explain why the novel has never lost its appeal for the Thai public.

Thawiphop is the work of female novelist Wimol Siriphaiboon (2008), who is best known by her pseudonym Tamayanti.[2] The novel has become a part of Thai popular culture through a rather traditional channel. The weekly literary magazine *Sakulthai*[3] (Thai Family or Thai Nation) printed the work chapter by chapter shortly before it was published as a book in 1987. *Sakulthai* was launched in 1954 and

[1] On the construction of class identity, see Thompson (1968) and the contributions to the volumed edited by Lopez Ricardo and Weinstein (2012).

[2] Note that Wimol has also used a number of other pseudonyms.

[3] Other popular literary magazines include *Banggog*, *Kwan Ruan*, *Ying Thai*, and *Satrisan*.

gained popularity with the growth of new middle class in the following decades. The magazine served as an affordable and accessible means of entertainment targeted at educated urban women.

From its first publication in *Sakulthai*, *Thawiphop* proved immensely popular with female readers of all ages from the upper and lower middle class, both in Bangkok and in the provinces. Since its original release, the novel has been republished more than 15 times. As a novelist, Tamayanti is a master of her craft. In *Thawiphop*, she tells the story of an individual love using a "Thai way" of expressing emotions through short conversations and narration. The novel continues a literary tradition that combines love stories with historical narratives of the Bangkok Era seen through the eyes of women. The genre was pioneered by Kukrit Pramoj's *Four Reigns* (2007), first published in the daily newspaper *Siamrat* in 1953. *Thawiphop*, however, also departs from the model set by the *Four Reigns*. Kukrit's work follows the tradition of royal chronicles and traces the development of the country through successive reigns. It emphasizes the centrality of royal power as a source of physical and emotional well-being for the female protagonist, a traditional wife and mother living her life in a domestic sphere. *Thawiphop*, by contrast, does not emphasize the role of the kings and features a female protagonist who has the desire and ability to take action in order to shape the nation's destiny.

The differences between Kukrit's and Tamayanti's novels reflect a transformation in what I propose to call "the emotional culture of Thai nationalism," which capitalizes on widespread nostalgia while changing in tandem with the development of the Thai entertainment industry. The late 1980s saw a renewed interest in the consumption of the past through entertainment, which has continued ever since. This fascination with history has coincided with the global boom of retro consumption in areas such as music, design, advertisement, and film (Brown 1999).

Thawiphop tells a humorous and witty love story with a happy end and a positive outlook. These features suit Thai audiences, which favor comedy and lighthearted content and show less interest in "art for society."[4] This preference results from the political culture of the Cold War and the Indochina Wars when Thailand identified itself with the democratic West even though the country itself lacked democracy (on this latter point, see Baker and Phongpaichit 2002; Wyatt 2003). Even after the wars, government infringements of free speech and the media promoted a flourish of entertainment evoking a life free of serious cares and conflicts (Siriyuvasak 1998; Wyatt 2003).

In spite of this overall conservative tone of entertainment, love stories and cheerful plays leave authors and artists some room for political commentary and innovation, for making fun of power and society, and for reproducing, reinterpreting, and shaping "Thainess" and ideas of the nation (see also Chap. 1 in this volume). Tamayanti makes use of this maneuvering space. The plot of *Thawiphop* uses familiar elements to address the unfamiliar. Through a story of romantic love, a critique of present conditions can be made in a lighthearted way.

---

[4] A new category of artistic creativities which became popular after the student uprising on October 14, 1973, a revolution that ended 14 years of military rule.

The popularity of *Thawiphop* inspired Cherd Songsri, a well-known Thai film director, to produce a movie based on the novel in 1990. Cherd's ambitious project and its selective cast gave a short fresh breath to the waning Thai film industry, which had lost out to Hollywood and the rise of the television (Jiratikorn 2003). In 1994, army-run Channel 7 broadcasted a TV version of *Thawiphop* produced by Dara Video. Possibly, this adaptation was the first to reach a wider rural public because the channel used a new transmission technology that extended the availability of its signal to much of the national territory.

In the aftermath of the 1997 financial crisis, *Thawiphop* came to life once again. In 2004, Bangkok Films released *The Siam Renaissance*, a new adaptation of the novel for the silver screen. A year later, a company called Scenario launched a musical play based on *Thawiphop* at the new Thailand Cultural Centre in Bangkok. In 2011, Scenario's play was put on stage again at Rachadalai Theatre in Bangkok, where it was performed 42 times between June 29 and August 7. In the same year, Channel 7 ran a new serial adaptation of Tamayanti's novel realized by Dara Video. The two 2011 versions of *Thawiphop* are inextricably linked with the Thai-Cambodian conflict and military clashes over border areas claimed by both countries.

The novel *Thawiphop* and its on-screen and on-stage adaptations have become sites of open discussions among writers, producers, and their readers and audiences about their fears, their dreams, and their interactions with domestic, regional, and global changes. In other words, *Thawiphop* has become a phenomenon in which sociocultural, economic, and political changes intersect with nationalism and entertainment.

3 The Thai Wonderland "Through the Looking Glass"

While *Thawiphop* and its adaptations focus on the Siamese past of Thailand, they also offer a brief glimpse of the present, more precisely the social conditions in Bangkok from the late 1980s to 2011.

The novel and its adaptations cast aspersions on the fast speed of modern life. In the original version, *Manee* tells *Dhep* that she lives in Bangkok in 1986. The narrative of her life in and between the parallel worlds portrays conditions in the capital as cheerless, notwithstanding the modern lifestyle and the impressive cityscape with its skyscrapers. The cars and bustling streets of Bangkok represent the anxiety caused by the high speed of modern life.

The restlessness of the middle class is another point raised by *Thawiphop* and its adaptations. It is a local response to the unprecedented process of globalization that drastically changed Thailand beginning in the 1980s (Baker and Phongpaichit 2002). *Manee*'s life in 1986 unfolds mostly in her home but also in her car as she is rushing home through the streets of Bangkok. *Manee* is obsessed with staying home or getting home so as to be in front of her standing mirror in time for catching the unpredictable moment when the gateway between the two worlds is opened for her.

The passage through the mirror does not simply denote a chance of refuge from the present, but signifies a strong belief in the power of the middle class who can seek and seize opportunities and deal with the uncertainties brought about by global changes and turbulences. The opportunities of passing between the two worlds are rare, however, and exclusively reserved for *Manee*, who stands for middle-class women more generally. This gender aspect of *Thawiphop* is linked with the increasing opportunities and numbers of women in higher education, a development that began in the 1960s (Wyatt 2003).

The novel and its adaptations also highlight the power of motherhood. Possibly, the promotion of Queen Sirikit as the mother of the nation has contributed to the prominence of this issue in the various versions of *Thawiphop*. In an effort to foster national unity through social service, the National Council on the Social Welfare of Thailand decided in 1976 that the queen's birthday on August 12 should be observed as mother's day in the kingdom – a practice that has continued ever since. On the occasion of her 53rd birthday in 1985, the queen herself suggested that "the growth of the nation flows from motherly love" (Matichon, August 13, 1985).

Thawiphop echoes the concern about the erosion of traditional family ways that underpin the official discourse on motherhood. At first glance, *Manee* may seem to lead an enviable life. In the charming house that she calls her home, maids attend her every need. *Manee*, however, feels unhappy, lonely, and melancholic much of the time because her father's career as a diplomat makes a normal family life difficult. She is often separated from her parents, and the big and elegant house looks empty. While *Thawiphop* vividly evokes motherly love as a source of emotional comfort and security for *Manee*, the novel also shows that the power of this love is threatened by modern life.

The dangers evoked by the original *Thawiphop* in 1986 have undermined *Manee*'s family in *The Siam Renaissance*, produced by Bangkok Film in 2004. The film presents *Manee*'s mother as a powerless, sad-looking woman, who is suffering from her divorce. This somber view no doubt reflects the impact of the Southeast Asian financial crisis of 1997, which severely affected daily life.

In *The Siam Renaissance*, *Manee*'s impotent mother stands for the shock and hopelessness of the middle class who were overwhelmed by the economic downturn. Unlike other adaptations of *Thawiphop*, the film does not present the belief that only motherly love can save the family. Instead, it gives more prominence to *Manee*'s father, a character who plays a marginal role in other adaptations. The creators of the film portray him as a historian rather than a diplomat. Therefore, he is familiar with the parallel world to which *Manee* is moving. Although he loves his daughter, he finds it difficult to express his feelings for her because of his marriage problems. One of the last scenes shows *Manee*'s parents holding one another's hands as a gesture of overcoming their personal conflicts and consoling one another over the loss of their daughter to the world of the nineteenth-century Siam. However, the shot focuses on the woman's hand with two plain golden rings on one finger, a symbol of widowship or separation. Unlike other adaptations of *Thawiphop*, the film does not present the belief that only motherly love can save family.

4 The Siamese Wonderland "Through the Looking Glass"

After some journeys to the past, *Manee* becomes more and more estranged from her existence in modern Thailand while growing ever more bewitched by life in the late nineteenth-century Siam. The present evokes nostalgia for the past, more precisely an awe of Siam under King Chulalongkorn. But, this nostalgia goes hand in hand with what Aeusrivongse (1993) calls "a new middle-class cult of worshiping Chulalongkorn" as a father of prosperity, a new view of the monarch that emerged in the late 1980s. The *Thawiphop* phenomenon reveals how the identity of the middle class and their nostalgia for the past are connected through the construction of gender roles and the interpretation of political conflicts.

4.1 Nostalgia and the Construction of Gender Roles

In *Thawiphop*, the tale of the parallel world attributes the progress of Siam to the wisdom and hard work of women as represented by *Manee* and *Dhep*'s mother *Sae*. *Sae* signifies the idea of "mothering the nation," whereas *Manee* stands for the modern women who first appeared in Thai society in the 1960s. These two characters demonstrate conflicting ideas of gender roles held by Thai middle-class women and men alike. Modern schooling and the experience of work outside of the household empower middle-class women to realize their potentials and to assert their rights beyond traditional social practices and expectations. At the same time, however, women are still tied down by traditional roles in the family, which are sustained by the conservative discourse on motherhood and family as essential elements of Thainess and as foundations of the Thai nation.

Although first articulated in the 1980s, the idea of "mothering the nation" results from a social trauma dating to the preceding decade, which led to nostalgia for an imagined "Thai family." The 1976 massacre at Thammasat University hit hard at the very essence of Thainess, which was believed to stand for a peaceful and harmonious way of life anchored in Buddhist principles, in particular, in the Buddhist prohibition of killing. In this view of Thailand, students were considered *dek* (i.e., children or young people) of the big family constituted by the Thai nation. The killing of students in the 1976 massacre exposed this vision as mere propaganda and caused a social trauma in the country.

In the 1980s, Thailand enjoyed political stability and economic prosperity, achieved by a political compromise between the monarchy, royalists, the army, businessmen, and the middle class. This compromise resulted in a semi-democratic system, which was established at the beginning of the decade and shaped by the government of General Prem Tinsulanonda (1981–1988) (see also Chaps. 10, 11, 12, and 13 in this volume on political issues in Thailand). Prem's rule not only had to address various challenges in international politics, the question of national unity, and social problems, it also had to deal with fears of a loss of identity in the face of the new culture and lifestyle that came with globalization and economic growth.

These fears led to efforts by the government to promote Thainess. In this context, highlighting the decline of the "Thai family" served as a rallying cry for fostering a renewed sense of Thainess and unity. In 1986, the Bangkok daily *Matichon* published a series of stories portraying supposedly good and warm families, all of which represented the lifestyle of the middle class.

From 1990 to 2011, new social and economic anxieties of the middle class sustained the nostalgia for the "Thai family" and fostered support for the idea of "mothering the nation." The affluence and confidence of the middle class had increased with the rapid economic growth of the 1980s. As a result, the military met with a middle-class uprising when it attempted to usurp power in 1992. The uprising set the country back on the track of democratization and led to the rise of civil society (Baker and Phongpaichit 2002). The 1997 financial economic meltdown in Asia, however, prevented Thailand from settling down. From 2001 to 2006, the premiership of Thaksin Shinawatra escalated existing conflicts of interest between the country's old and new elites. Although Thaksin had been elected and reelected by large majorities, a military coup toppled his government in September 2006, ostensibly because he was corrupt and pursued policies that were undemocratic, too capitalistic, and directed against the monarchy. The new military regime sponsored a new constitution that places serious limits on democratic rule and was adopted in a controversial national referendum in 2007. The figure of Thaksin has become the focal point of a conflict that pitches discontented poorer groups of mainly provincial voters, the so-called Red Shirts, against parts of the affluent middle class in Bangkok who are willing to support restrictions on the democratic process or even authoritarianism in order to defend their interests. Confrontations between these groups had taken place before September 2006 and returned with renewed force between late 2008 and the first half of 2010. In April and May 2010, military crackdowns ended massive Red Shirt protests[5] in Bangkok at the cost of 94 lives. The persistent opposition and demonstrations against the authorities and the army demonstrated the discontent of those who were disenfranchised by the 2006 coup and demanded that their political rights be restored. In this period, violence seemed ubiquitous, and the military crackdown on protesters in May 2010 exacerbated social tensions and political divisions. See also Chaps. 10, 11, 12, 13, and 14 in this volume.

Against the backdrop of these developments, the world of the nineteenth-century Siam evoked by *Thawiphop* appeared far more pleasant and attractive than Thailand's troubled present. In particular, motherly love and care provides life in the parallel world with a constant and reliable rhythm. *Sae*'s late husband, a high-ranking nobleman, left her to take on the weighty responsibilities of caring for a large household and for the well-being of their yet unmarried son. The task *Sae* has to undertake is demanding as the family provides the very foundation for the nation, which is patterned in turn upon the model of a great family. *Sae* skillfully runs a large household in which social stratification and order are observed and maintained as a matter of course in the relations among family members and between *nai* (master)

[5] The demonstrations may not have been so much in support of Thaksin as in protest against a government lacking in democratic legitimacy and acting against the interests of the protesters, who had voted, with a majority of the electorate, for a different administration.

and *kha* (serfs). Her position as head of her household requires and at the same time bestows "male" qualities associated with strong leadership. This aspect of her role reconciles traditional views of gender relations with the aspirations of modern middle-class women in Thailand. *Sae*'s leadership derives from acting in lieu of her late husband; therefore, it does not challenge the conservative vision of the role of women. At the same time, the skills with which *Sae* discharges her duties demonstrate that women can take over and succeed in roles of leadership; therefore, her character also holds appeal for the ambitious middle-class women who make up much of the readership and audience of *Thawiphop* and adaptations.[6]

Furthermore, *Sae* serves as a source of knowledge on Thainess, which covers social skills and etiquette as well as "Thai ways" of living, exemplified in the novel by clothing, foodways, and fragrance making. *Sae*'s expertise helps to maintain the identity of Siamese/Thai national society. Unlike other adaptations of *Thawiphop, The Siam Renaissance* omits *Sae*, the mother figure, from the parallel world. *Sae*, in this version, is substituted for by the monarch, who represents the essence of Thai identity. Significantly, the launch of this adaptation coincided with the celebrations of King Bhumibol's diamond jubilee in 2006.

4.2 Nostalgia and the Interpretation of Political Conflicts

Thawiphop and its adaptations also evoke nostalgia for the fight against colonialism, which is represented by Siam's confrontation with France in the crisis of 1893. Initially, *Manee* does not find the prospect of living her life in the parallel world appealing. She comes to realize, however, that in the late nineteenth-century Siam, she will be able to help save the country from French aggression. By comparison, her life in Bangkok in the 1980s seems useless. The *Thawiphop* phenomenon, then, can be seen as the process in which the new Thai middle class have appropriated the heritage of anticolonialism. The memory of the struggle against France has long been enshrined as a defining moment in the master narrative of Thai national history. Through the figure of *Manee*, the middle class seize the episode of 1893 and use it to highlight their role in the fight to preserve national pride, integrity, and independence. This is not merely a matter of historical interpretation or imagination. Nationalistic propaganda portrays the nation as ever threatened, be it from an offer of election monitors by the European Union (Meyer 2007) or from disagreements on border demarcations with Cambodia. As defenders of the nation, the ruling elites claim to be entitled to political power. By highlighting their part in the defense, the middle class therefore assert equality with the ruling elites and their share of power in Thai domestic politics.

The crisis of 1893 took place in the heyday of French and British colonial expansion in Southeast Asia. In order to consolidate its territories in the region, France claimed Siam's tributary states on the eastern side of the *Mae Khong* River.

---

[6] *Sae*'s role as head of household may be understood in analogy to that of queens in the early modern European tradition; see Schulte (2006) and Kantorowicz (1997).

To realize this claim, France sent cannon boats to the mouth of the *Chao Phraya* River and threatened Siam with blockading its access to the open sea. As the Siamese government failed to secure British support and lacked the means to defy French naval power, it was left with no choice but to comply with the French demands (Wyatt 2003).

Historical writing and knowledge is a representation of the past. It does not reveal the truth of what has actually happened in the past but reflects power relations in creating and conjuring up certain memories. The Franco-Siamese episode of 1893 has become a key theme of the master narrative of Thai national history (Winichakul 1994; Kasetsiri 2012). Following the 1932 democratic revolution, the questions of constructing a national society and of legitimacy assumed new urgency. Phibun, the leader of Thailand during World War II, responded to these challenges by introducing a nationalist project which featured modernity, the cult of constitutionalism, and an agenda for regaining the territories Thailand had presumably lost in consequence of imperialist aggressions. This latter theme was likely inspired by the French reaction to the loss of Alsace-Lorraine to Germany in 1871 and especially by the rhetoric and policies of George Clémenceau. It has also become inseparable from the increasing role of militarism in Thai society and from what Chaloemtiarana (2007) calls the "politics of despotic paternalism," which began during the premiership of Marshal Sarit Thanarat (1959–1963).

Why did the crisis of 1893 capture the imagination of the middle class in the late 1980s and in the 1990s? The new interest in the episode forms part of a more general infatuation with Thai history, which marked the 1980s as a decade of nostalgia. Against the backdrop of the period's unprecedented economic boom and soaring foreign investments, the Rattanakosin Bicentennial in 1982 and royal celebrations, especially King Bhumibol's 60th birthday, helped foster a sense of unity and created a nostalgic atmosphere in the country. Yearning for the past, argues Peleggi (2002), gave rise to heritage and nostalgia business, tourism, and state activities. The dynamics of nostalgia that emerged in the 1980s have remained an important part of Thai politics ever since and continue to play a role in the promotion of national unity.

From its very beginnings in the 1980s, the politics of nostalgia has been dominated by royal and official versions of the past that gave prominence, e.g., to the glory of the Kingdom of Ayutthaya and its struggle with Burma. Images of kings and even of a queen fighting on elephant back epitomize this kind of historical memory (Wyatt 2006). Elephant wars were the prerogative of monarchs and thus put a limit on the historical imagination – especially in Thailand, where the educational system promotes the ideology of "nation, religion, and monarchy,"[7] and free speech is encouraged only as long as it remains within this framework. In this

[7] By the turn of the twentieth century, international and domestic developments had led to the adoption of the Siamese national ideology that is still promoted today. The collapse of authoritarian monarchies in Europe at the end of World War I served as a warning to King Vajiravudh against similar threats to his own rule in Siam. Furthermore, the political and financial support the Thai-Chinese community gave to the Chinese overseas movements cast doubts on their loyalty to the crown and the Kingdom of Siam. Their activities appeared all the more threatening to Siam as they played prominent roles in the country's economy. Against this background, the king promoted the ideology of "nation, religion, and monarchy" in an effort to protect his power.

context, the middle class not only sought to participate in the politics of nostalgia but laid claim to nationalism, seeking a gap in the master narrative to insert their presence into the past. *Thawiphop* (2008, Vol. 2: 372) makes clear that

> Siamese-Burmese warfare is a royal diversion, but granting [the French] rights of extraterritoriality under coercion means maiming the country.

The ambitions of the middle class are reflected by Cherd's 1990 silver-screen adaptation of *Thawiphop*, which features the following conversation between *Manee*, her mother, and *Dhep*:

Manee's mother:	My dear, can't you just stay here [in the present]?
Dhep:	Siam is undergoing a time of *seuk* [hostility], and thus needs *karn prabprung prathet* [modernization or reform]. Living there [in the parallel world], we can work better for the benefit of the nation than here. [...]
Manee:	I am happy there, mom. And there...I am recognized as somebody important.

[After *Manee*'s mother has listened to her daughter, her face brightens with happiness.]

The parallel world, as understood by *Dhep* and *Manee*, is a place where commoners can join the old elite in advancing the nation and thus find opportunities for a meaningful life. This view can be easily integrated with the narrative of the crisis of 1893 in official history and popular memory, which do not feature any hero. King Chulalongkorn is conspicuously absent from the standard account of the crisis due to an illness that is commonly explained as the result of the country's helplessness in the face of the French threat.

Manee questions the failures of the Siamese ruling class in dealing with the French, wondering in her thoughts whether or not the old generation had really done their best. Her conclusions, however, do not challenge the official version of the past. She determines Siam succumbed to the military technology and power of France in spite of the best efforts of the country's leaders. In the absence of prestigious hero, *Thawiphop* and its adaptations promote an upper middle-class heroine who uses her proficiency in French and English to help save the nation. *Manee*'s efforts can thus be construed as part of the attempts of the middle class to assert their equality with the ruling elites, especially in saving the nation.

In 1994, a new TV series of *Thawiphop* vividly portrayed the power of the middle class and its heroic role in a narrative that challenges official versions of Thai history with their focus on the monarchs as leaders of the nation. In spite of this somewhat subversive slant, the series swept six of the 1994 domestic Mekalha Awards for outstanding TV productions. Ten years later, by contrast, *The Siam Renaissance* failed to win recognition for its attempt to defend the role of Chulalongkorn and the ruling elites in the crisis of 1893.

By the turn of the twenty-first century, the new middle class seemed overwhelmed by the invisible hand of the global financial markets. In this context, *The Siam Renaissance* articulates another version of the parallel world. *The Siam Renaissance* creates a solemn-looking *Manee* who is not at all an active participant in the parallel world but a lost and exotic oracle, whose knowledge on the future independence of

Siam helps to allay the fears Western encroachments caused among the Siamese elites. Unlike the *Manee* of the 1990s, the protagonist of *The Siam Renaissance* does not stand for the progressive female element of the middle class. Instead, the film promotes the power of masculinity through *Manee*'s relations with ruling-class men. Interestingly, the *Manee* of the 1990s falls for a *Dhep* who is gentle and diplomatic by nature. By contrast, it is a tactless and combative *Dhep* who wins over *Manee*'s heart in *The Siam Renaissance*, sidelining another suitor who bears resemblance to the *Dhep* of the 1990s. More importantly, the powerless middle class cease to declare their talent and ability in their fantasy of the past. Instead, they search emotional stability and assurance in the myth of erudite and visionary monarchs.

The new adaptations of *Thawiphop* and the middle class's claim to nationalism coincided with a flourish of official and royal nationalism, which also manifested itself in well-funded movie projects. The first production of this kind was *The Legend of Suriyothai*, released in 2001. The film is directed by Prince Chatichalerm Yukol, a veteran of his trade, who had already announced his plans to take up the subject in 1997. The film tells the story of Queen Suriyothai of the Ayutthaya Kingdom who died in a sixteenth-century battle with Burma as she tried on elephant back to rescue her husband. Suriyothai has long been recognized as a national heroine in Thai school textbooks and official history (Winichakul 2001). But, it was only in the wake of the 1997 financial crisis that the entertainment industry began to promote the legend of the heroic queen. In 2006, the celebrations of the diamond jubilee of King Bhumibol gave a further boost to the official version of Thai history with its characteristic blend of royalism and nationalism. Prince Chatichalerm contributed once more to this discourse, this time through memorializing King Naresuan whom the master narrative of Thai history enshrines as the greatest ruler of Ayutthaya because he liberated his kingdom from Burmese domination. Prince Chatichalerm has produced a well-funded series of films entitled *The Legend of King Naresuan*, which as of this writing comprises four parts. Emphasizing the significance of the monarchy to the country, the films contribute to the promotion of the monarchy as a source of national unity, which has intensified since the 2006 coup.

In 2011, Thailand witnessed a revival of *Thawiphop* both on stage and on screen, which was linked with the political upheaval in the country since the overthrow of Thaksin. In 2006, ultraroyalists, businessmen, the army, and the Democrat Party sought to suppress the political forces that had rallied around Thaksin (see Chaps. 10, 11, 12, and 13). This mission proved impossible. As a result, supporters of the 2006 coup promoted a new wave of hyper-nationalism to distract from the domestic conflicts of interest. This hyper-nationalism manifested itself in daily life, in political movements in parliament and in the streets of Bangkok and other cities, and in Thailand's relations with its neighbors, in particular, in its policies toward Cambodia (Rungswasdisab 2011; Chachavalpongpun 2012).Thus, the postcoup government escalated a long-standing dispute with Cambodia over the ruins of Preah Vihear Temple on the border between the two countries. The International Court of Justice and UNESCO, which have become involved in the conflict, were accused of being hostile to Thailand. Supporters of the coup skillfully conjured up the ancient specter of a threat to Thai territory. Defending the integrity of the kingdom became once more an implicit justification for authoritarian rule.[8]

Against this backdrop, *Manee* embarks yet another time on her journey to the parallel world. A musical play put on stage by Scenario has *Manee* make it clear that she wants to take part in the nationalist enterprise. Her wish comes true in a spectacular scene in which she fearlessly confronts French soldiers, trying to stop them from arresting and torturing a Siamese nobleman. Scenario's interpretation of *Thawiphop* evokes the love of the nation held by Bangkok's middle class. By highlighting *Manee*'s active contribution to the defense of Siam, the musical tries to ease the anxieties that the conflicts at home and at the borders caused among its audience. At the same time, the play uses *Manee*'s journey to the parallel world to celebrate the monarch as the light of hope and the solution to the country's problems. The song *Golden Land* evokes a utopian Thailand where the monarchs are given from heaven and bring happiness to their people. The land of the Thai will always remain free as long as "we" remain committed to "our" monarchy, united in purpose, and ready for sacrifice.

The second adaptation of *Thawiphop* in 2011, a TV production by Dara Video, adopts a different brand of nationalist imagination. The script has *Manee* criticize Bangkok's new yuppies for their useless lifestyle and their ignorance of social and national problems. At the same time, it offers an alternative construction of self to young members of the urban elites, showing them how they can participate in the patriotic enterprise. The *Manee* of the TV screen is as witty and lively as her character on stage but more playful. Her feminine qualities illustrate conservative ideas of how women can exercise their charms in times of love and war. This interpretation of *Manee* is possibly inspired by Diao Chan, a character in the novel *Samkok*, the Thai translation of the Chinese *Romance of the Three Kingdoms* (Pra Klang [Hon] 1973). Interestingly, the producer of this version lets the audience deal with the "territorial losses" in lighthearted and moderate ways. Furthermore, the series suggests that faced with the challenge of colonialism, the Siamese proudly held up their traditional culture and civilization and successfully used their diplomatic talents to secure the kingdom's independence as a buffer state between the French and British colonies.

The *Manee* of the Dara Video's 2011 TV series was criticized for not being "a good Thai lady" because she shows her affection for *Dhep* too often and too openly. The production nevertheless won the year's Mekalha Award for promoting Thai culture. This award illustrates the significance of *Thawiphop* as a site where modern Thai nationalism has been repeatedly reimagined and renegotiated.

[8]In 1959, Cambodia attempted to settle its dispute with Thailand over Preah Vihear Temple by turning to the International Court of Justice. Marshal Sarit Thanarat exploited the case in an effort to legitimize his dictatorial rule.

5 Conclusion

Thawiphop tells an entertaining story of two young lovers eventually united in spite of all obstacles. But, the novel is much more than a simple romance. It takes the readers to a parallel world created by Thai nationalism. Combined with Tamayanti's talents as a storyteller, this is the key to the success of *Thawiphop*. Since its first publication in 1987, the novel has appeared in more than 15 editions and been adapted several times for television, the silver screen, and the stage. *Thawiphop* has thus become one of the most popular works of Thai literature as well as a social and cultural phenomenon.

Thawiphop demonstrates the discontent of the middle class with the country's present condition, which leads to nostalgia for the Siamese past. The various versions of *Thawiphop* depict a society straining under the high speed of modern urban life and suffering from the erosion of traditional family life, which is a mainstay of official ideas of the nation and of motherhood. By contrast, the Siam of 1893 is fantasized as a land where "Thai" traditions are vigorous and the natural environment pleasant. At the same time, this fantasized land also offers significant opportunities for women to take an active role in shaping and saving the nation.

The *Thawiphop* phenomenon reflects the attempts of the middle class to participate in the politics of nostalgia that have emerged in Thailand since the 1980s. In *Thawiphop*, this participation is achieved through the refashioning of gender roles and the reimagination of colonialism. The nationalism the middle class seek to claim reflects their aspirations in the country's political life. At the same time, the success of *Thawiphop* shows the conservatism of the Thai middle class. At first glance, their brand of nationalism seems novel as *Thawiphop* features a modern and Western educated woman, *Manee*, who tries to save the nation. However, *Thawiphop* gives the story a conservative twist by turning *Manee* into a well-behaved lady of the nineteenth-century Siam, which may be interpreted as an attempt at taming modernity and the modern lifestyle of Thai women.

Acknowledgment I wish to thank Claus K. Meyer for his comments and our discussions on this essay.

References

Aeusrivongse, N. (1993). *The cult of King Rama V* [Lathi sadet pho ro 5]. Bangkok: Matichon.

Baker, C. J., & Phongpaichit, P. (2002). *Thailand, economy and politics*. New York: Oxford University Press.

Bhabha, H. K. (Ed.). (1990). *Nation and narration*. London/New York: Routledge.

Brown, S. (1999). Retro-marketing: Yesterday's tomorrows, today! *Marketing Intelligence & Planning, 17*(7), 363–376.

Carroll, L. (2006). *Alice's adventures in wonderland and through the looking glass*. New York: Grosset & Dunlap.

Chachavalpongpun, P. (2012). Embedding embittered history: Unending conflicts in Thai-Cambodian relations. *Asian Affairs, 43*(1), 81–102.

Chaloemtiarana, T. (2007). *Thailand: The politics of despotic paternalism*. Chiang Mai: Silkworm Books.
Chaochuti, T. (2009). Thawiphop and the narcissism of Maneejan [Thawiphop kap khwam long tua eng khong maneejan]. *Aan, 2*(2), 152–158.
Chaochuti, T. (2012). In the name of the mother(land): Nationalism, psychoanalysis, Thawiphop. [Nainam khong phandin Mae: Chatiyom, Jitwikraw, Thawiphop]. *Rattasatsan, 33*(1), 109–137.
Harrison, R. (2010). Mind the gap: [En]countering the west and the making of Thai identities on film. In R. Harrison & P. A. Jackson (Eds.), *The ambiguous allure of the West: Traces of the colonial in Thailand* (pp. 93–118). Hong Kong: Hong Kong University Press, Cornell University Southeast Asia Program Publications.
Holdsworth, N. (2010). *Theatre & nation*. Basingstoke/England: Palgrave Macmillan.
Inglis, D. (2005). *Culture and everyday life*. London/New York: Routledge.
Jiratikorn, A. (2003). Suriyothai: Hybridizing Thai national identity through film. *Inter-Asia Cultural Studies, 4*(2), 296–308.
Kantorowicz, E. H. (1997). *The king's two bodies: A study in mediaeval political theology*. Princeton: Princeton University Press.
Kasetsiri, C. (2012). Imagined Thai historiography and historical maps from 1930s to the present [Jintakam Prawatisat thai kap phanthee "sia dindan" jak tossawat 2470 thueng 2554]. In C. Kasetsiri (Ed.), *Collected maps: History-geography-politics and colonialism in Southeast Asia* [pramuan phanthee: prawatisat-phumisat-garnmuang kap lhathi aananikhom nai asean-usakhane] (pp. 333–373). Bangkok: Foundation for Promotion of Social Sciences and Humanities Textbook Project.
Lam, M. B. (2012). The postcolonial condition of "Indochinese" cinema from Vietnam, Cambodia and Laos. In S. Ponzanesi & M. Waller (Eds.), *Postcolonial cinema studies* (pp. 107–142). London: Routledge.
López Ricardo, A., & Weinstein, B. (Eds.). (2012). *The making of the middle class: Toward a transnational history*. Durham: Duke University Press.
Matichon. August 13, 1985, p. 1.
Matichon. February 2, 1986, p. 7.
Matichon. October 19, 1986, p. 7.
Meyer, M. J. (2007). The rejected EU's proposal of an election observation mission: A critique of Thai propaganda and policy. *Journal of History* (1), Article 8. Retrieved March 3, 2012, from: http://ejournals.swu.ac.th/index.php/JOH/article/view/1257/1265
Praklang (Hon). (1973). *Samkok*. Bangkok: Bannakan.
Pramoj, K. (2007). *Four reigns* (Tulachandra, Trans.). Chiangmai: Silkworm Books.
Peleggi, M. (2002). *The politics of ruins and the business of nostalgia*. Bangkok: White Lotus.
Rungswasdisab, P. (2011). *Thailand's response to the Cambodian genocide*. Cambodian Genocide Program, Yale University. Retrieved April 10, 2012, from: http://www.yale.edu/cgp/thailand_response.html
Schlesinger, P. (2000). The sociological scope of national cinema. In M. Hjort & S. Mackenzie (Eds.), *Cinema & nation* (pp. 19–31). London/New York: Routledge.
Schulte, R. (Ed.). (2006). *The body of the queen: Gender and rule in the courtly world, 1500–2000*. New York: Berghahn Books.
Siriphaiboon, W. (2008). *Thawiphop* (13th ed., 2 Vol.). Bangkok: Na Banwannakam.
Siriyuvasak, U. (1998). *The economic and political structures of Thai radio and TV system & their consequences for right and freedom* [Krong sang thang sethakitkarnmunag khong rabob wittayu lae thorathat thai lae phon kratob to sithi lae seri phap]. Bangkok: Faculty of Communication Arts, Chulalongkorn University.
Smith, A. D. (2000). Images of the nation: Cinema, art and national identity. In M. Hjort & S. Mackenzie (Eds.), *Cinema & nation* (pp. 45–59). London/New York: Routledge.
Story, J. (2010). *Culture and power in cultural studies: The politics of significance*. Edinburg: Edinburg University Press.
Thompson, E. P. (1968). *The making of English working class*. Harmondsworth: Penguin Books.

Winichakul, T. (1994). *Siam mapped: History of the geo-body of a nation*. Honolulu: University of Hawaii Press.
Winichakul, T. (2001). Suriyothai: A national history of an ideal woman [Suriyothai prawatsart heang chat chabab nang keaw]. *Silpawattanatham, 22*(12), 55–57.
Winichakul, T. (2011). Siam colonial conditions and the birth of Thai history. In V. Grabowsky (Ed.), *Southeast Asian historiography unravelling the myth: Essays in honour of Barend Jan Terwiel* (pp. 20–41). Bangkok: River Books.
Wyatt, D. K. (2003). *Thailand a short history* (2nd ed.). Bangkok/Chiang Mai: Silkworm Books.
Wyatt, D. K. (Ed.). (2006). *The royal chronicles of Ayutthaya* (R. Cushman, Trans.). Bangkok: The Siam Society under the Royal Patronage.

Adaptations of *Thawiphop*

Thawiphop. (1990). Dir. Cherd Songsri. Cherdchai Films.
Thawiphop. (1994). Dir. Charoon Thammasin. Dara Video.
The Siam Renaissance. (2004). Dir. Surapong Pinijkhar. Film Bangkok.
Thawiphop the musical. (2005). Dir. Takolkiet Weerawan. Scenario.
Thawiphop the musical. (2011). Dir. Takolkiet Weerawan. Scenario.
Thawiphop. (2011). Dir. Mawin Deangnoi and Penlak Udomsin. Dara Video.

Filmography

The legend of Suriyothai. (2001). Dir. Prince Chatichalerm Yukol. Prommitr Production Co., Ltd.
The legend of King Naresuan: Hostage of Hongsawadi. (2007). Dir. Prince Chatichalerm Yukol. Prommitr Production Co., Ltd.
The legend of King Naresuan: *Proclaiming independence*. (2007). Dir. Prince Chatichalerm Yukol. Prommitr Production Co., Ltd.
The Legend of King Naresuan: *The naval battle*. (2011). Dir. Prince Chatichalerm Yukol. Prommitr Production Co., Ltd.
The Legend of King Naresuan: *The battle against Nanda Bayin*. (2011). Dir. Prince Chatichalerm Yukol. Prommitr Production Co., Ltd.

Chapter 9
Relatedness: Capitalism and the Sufficiency Economy in Rural Northeastern Thailand

Ratana Tosakul

1 Introduction

During my field visit to Bamrung Kayotha's organic farming in the Northeast (locally known as *Isan*) of Thailand in August 2007, I was struck with his idea and practice of combining the organic farming with the market economy. Bamrung is one of the most famous farmer leaders from Northeastern Thailand and a consultant to the Assembly of the Poor at the national level. Bamrung is a middle-income farmer from Kalasin province in *Isan* who has practiced organic farming according to the philosophy of sufficiency economy over the past 20 years.

My research team and I visited Bamrung at his farm residence several times in 2007. His organic farm was surrounded by various kinds of trees in a rather peaceful, shady, and cool environmental setting. His house was built by a big pond where there were lots of fish. On his farm, there were a range of varieties of plants, trees, and home-grown vegetables, as well as pigs and poultry.

Bamrung and his wife produce chiefly for home consumption and for sale in the local market. They rarely buy any food for their daily consumption, ritual ceremonies, and social contribution. They also warrant that their family will never encounter a problem of food shortage for at least a few continuous years. They believe they have enough food supplies. Bamrung further reiterates his belief that his organic farm is a vivid exemplar of a farm family in *Isan* putting the philosophy of Thailand's sufficiency economy into practice over the past few decades (see also Chaps. 31 and 32 for discussions on sufficiency economy in Thailand).

Similar to many farmers elsewhere in *Isan* who have adopted sufficiency economy, about 30 years ago, Bamrung went bankruptcy because he had depended substantially on mono cash crop production, such as of cassava for his family's income

R. Tosakul (✉)
Faculty of Sociology and Anthropology, Thammasat University,
Tha Phra Chan, Bangkok 10200, Thailand
e-mail: ratanaboon@gmail.com

P. Liamputtong (ed.), *Contemporary Socio-Cultural and Political Perspectives in Thailand*, DOI 10.1007/978-94-007-7244-1_9, © Springer Science+Business Media Dordrecht 2014

generation. Nonetheless, his family had no debt, because they had non-farm production to support. Receiving a fellowship in Japan to study about organic farming, Bamrung returned home in *Isan* and began to put it into practice, mainly for home consumption and for local sale. Still, the family retains some plots of farmland for rice cultivation for export and home consumption.

Likewise, in 2010, during my revisits to Ban Phra and Ban Koke[1] of Khon Kaen province in Northeastern Thailand, I was also struck with the coexistence of sufficiency economy (which I consider as a part of traditional village economies) and the market economy of global capitalism albeit different intensity.

In this chapter, I argue that similar to many villagers in *Isan* and elsewhere in Thailand, villagers of Ban Phra and Ban Koke have combined various modes of economic production to pursue their families' economic interests. In other words, there is a coexistence and relatedness of capitalism and sufficiency economy in the pursuit of their families' economic interests albeit structural political and economic constraints at the national and international levels.

2 Embracing an Opportunity to Participate in the Expanding Market Economy

Since the 1960s, Thailand has supported development ideology that favors modernizing and industrializing the country through capitalist expansion of the economy. Since then, the country has grown substantially,[2] but the rural growth rate has declined relative to Bangkok. The penetration of global capitalism into the rural countryside has been widespread through the commercialization of agriculture (Tosakul 2013).

[1] I first did my ethnographic field research for my doctoral dissertation entitled "Contested Concepts of Development in Rural Northeastern Thailand" in these two communities where I resided for 18 months between 1994 and 1995. The names of Ban Phra and Ban Koke are pseudonyms as to protect their identities. This is because they were very pointed in their political criticisms toward the state development policies and practices.

[2] An economic crisis began in mid-1997, however, delayed attaining the goal of Thailand's becoming the newly industrialized country of Asia. According to the Office of the National Economic and Social Development Board of Thailand, NESDB (2011), and the World Bank Report (2011), Thailand gross domestic product (GDP) has been growing substantially over the last few decades. Between 1960 and the Asian crisis of 1997, GDP annual growth oscillated between 5 and around 10 % per year. From 1988 to 1990, there was growth substantially higher than 10 %. The Asian economic crisis of 1997 caused the first and extensive drop into negative zone. Afterward, growth overall seems to drift around 5 % per year. A second plunge into negative zone occurred with the global crisis of 2008–2009 with negative growth of 2.3 % in Thailand in 2009. Growth in 2010 was measured at 7.8 %, this despite significant political chaos. At the end of 2011, it appeared that the economic growth was quite low about 0.1 % much lower than the expected growth rate of 3.5 % due to the severe damage from the historic flooding in September and October. This made progressive downgrades unavoidable. In 2012, the Thai economy is expected to grow by 5.5–6.0 %, a slight recovery from the last year's flooding. GDP per capita (current US$) in 2010 was 4,613 US$ (source: www.Thaiwebsites.com/, accessed October 1, 2012).

Keyes (2008) traces the changes in Thailand over the past 40 years. He suggests that Thai villagers had left behind what has been called "the sufficiency economy" to undeniably embrace the global capitalist system, but their economic decisions, aspirations, and life choices remain significantly tempered by Buddhist teachings based on moderation and self-reliance. Keyes' (1991, 2008) reminder of the economic world of rural villagers in Thailand provides a good framework for the ways I develop my arguments in this chapter.

I argue that the "sufficiency economy" is not completely abandoned by villagers in *Isan* and elsewhere in Thailand. The sufficiency mode of production, albeit very small in farming production scale and movement, exists within the framework of the market economy. Although villagers of Ban Phra and Ban Koke can no longer be considered as subsistence farmers, they do combine the sufficiency economy (primarily in the sphere of food crop production) with the market economy for their economic security reasons. In my view, the sufficiency economy does not replace or is in conflict with the market economy but does exist within the framework of the market economy.

3 Village Profiles

The villagers of Ban Phra and Ban Koke do share some similarities. They live in the same administrative province of Khon Kaen and share a similar pattern of Thai-Lao culture, village size,[3] access to local economic markets, and other infrastructural facilities, such as being located next to provincial highways. When comparing with these two communities with other villages in the remote areas of the Northeast, these two are relatively better off pertinent to rural economic infrastructure development, as both are located in the core development zone of Khon Kaen, the center of the Northeast for regional development, bureaucratic administration, and higher education. Yet, when considering these two villages within the wider society, they share a similar socioeconomic location within the Northeast, a region situated at the peripheries of the national culture and polity and subject to profound transformations as a result of the modernization and industrialization of the country.

Villagers of these two communities are of Lao origins who share similar linguistic and cultural traits with those living in lowland Laos rather than central Thailand. Since the turn of the nineteenth century, people in the Northeast have been integrated into the political and administrative domain of Siam or Thailand today. Similar to most people of the Northeast, villagers of these two communities often consider themselves citizens of Thailand. They often refer to themselves as *khon Isan*, literally means people or persons of the Northeast, when talking about Thais in other regions of the country. They also refer to themselves as *khon Lao* when talking about other ethnic groups. They use Lao language among themselves but use Thai in public discourse.

---

[3] In 2010, there were 296 and 200 families in total in Ban Phra and in Ban Koke, respectively. Ban Phra was about 200 years old and Ban Koke was approximately 165 years old.

Like the majority of the Thai population, villagers of these two communities follow Theravada Buddhism. Their primary religious beliefs and their ways of life have been largely influenced by a combination of the beliefs in Theravada Buddhism and spirit cults. Similar to most Thai-Lao villagers in other communities, villagers of Ban Phra and Ban Koke practice a custom of uxorilocal residence after they marry. Land is customarily inherited through the female line. However, with the scarcity of available land at present, there is a tendency for many new couples to inherit land from both matrilineal and patrilineal lines. Usually, the youngest daughter marries and lives with the parents and will inherit the parental house and land. In Ban Phra and Ban Koke, kinship relations have laid a very important foundation for village cooperation. I agree with Tambiah (1970) that the basic relationship between kins is organized around economic, political, and ritual matters. Marriage of a couple combines the descent groups of the two families together. All of them will turn to be kinsmen of one another. When problems in life occur, an individual will turn to his/her family and household, then go to the circle of kinsmen, then distant kinsmen, and neighbors and friends. Thus, a Thai-Lao village is characterized by mutual reciprocity and cooperation among kinsmen and neighbors. In Ban Phra, there are four core family names and most people are somehow connected to one another through these four family names. Similarly, most people in Ban Koke are linked through kinsmen.

Pertinent to regional economic disparity, rural villagers in the Northeast have been perceived by the general Thai public as living in poverty, since the Northeast is the poorest region when compared to others, as shown in the following.

Region	GDP per capita (Thai baht)
Bangkok and vicinity	327,321
Central region	241,297
Eastern region	332,798
Northern region	69,773
Northeastern region	42,968
Southern region	98,743
Western region	105,851
All of Thailand	136,511

Source: Office of the National Economic and Social Development Board (NESDB) (2008)

There is no question that the average household and per capita income of Northeastern people have progressed over the past four decades of development. Nonetheless, the regional disparity between the Northeast and other regions, particularly to the Bangkok and city core, still persists.[4]

[4] The statistical data for 2008, as provided by the NESDB, show that there are great differences in gross domestic product (GDP) per capita between the different regions and provinces. The gross provincial product in the Northeast and to a lesser extent in the North is considerably lower than in Bangkok, the Central region, and the Eastern region. The gross provincial product of the Southern and Western regions is placed in between GDPs in Bangkok, and its surrounding provinces are almost eight times bigger than in the poorest (and most populated), the Northeast region of

Economically, most villagers in both communities perceive that the majority of them just have enough for living and eating. The majority of villagers in both communities are small farmers and landless peasants. There is a tendency for the number of small farmers and landless peasants in both communities to rise due to the scarcity of land available and to the breakup of land into smaller pieces through land inheritance. Farmland through tenancy and share-cropping arrangements has existed in the two communities since the 1980s. There are no large landlords in these two communities, but absentee landlords who are wealthy people from Khon Kaen and Bangkok do exist.

Villagers of Ban Phra and Ban Koke have engaged in both on-farm and off-farm production. Ban Phra is characterized as a low flood paddy area. Its topography comprises a gentle land slope down to the east and south of the community where it forms part of the floodplain of the Chi river and where the soil is more suitable for rice and vegetable growing than in the northern and western areas. Rice production in Ban Phra has been under irrigation since 1967. Villagers also produce fresh vegetables for the Khon Kaen city market the whole year through because they have access to irrigation water. Women play a key role in producing and selling vegetables in Khon Kaen city. Actually, women in both communities, like many other villages in the Northeast, have played a prominent role in petty trading in and outside their communities (Kirsch 1982). Small shops with food and grocery items in both communities are run and supervised by village women.

In contrast to Ban Phra, Ban Koke is an undulating area. Its topography is characterized by rolling hills and a gentle land scope down from the northeast to southwest of the community. The community is bounded on the south by the Kok Hin Khao area and the Nam Phong river. Aside from growing rice, farmers of Ban Koke have engaged in cassava and sugar cane production, which have provided the major income for village families since the 1960s.

Rice is the most important cash crop grown in both communities, especially the glutinous rice is the staple food diet of Thai-Lao villagers. Rice is produced for home consumption, although some surplus rice is sold when a family needs cash. Rice production is one factor to determine how wealthy a family farm is, that is, a family farm that cannot produce rice enough for annual consumption and has to purchase rice to eat at a certain period of the year. Many villagers considered this

Thailand. Note that the data provided here are expressed in Thai baht and indicate real GDP. In short, real GDP has reached about 4,000 US$ per year for the whole country, while gross domestic product by purchasing power parity method is equivalent to about 8,000 US$. GDP growth in Bangkok is rather modest. The two regions with the fastest GDP growth are the Central and Eastern regions. Also the Northeast and the North are growing more than 1.5 to 2 times faster than Bangkok. Instinctively, we had thought that Bangkok would be ever getting richer when compared with the countryside, but clearly this is not the case. While the Northeast and the North of the country still have an enormous way to go, the development is promising. The rural development policies of the government between 2001 and 2006 including the universal health care, a farm debt moratorium, village micro-credit programs, entrepreneurial programs, and rice price-pledging schemes likely have been beneficial (source: www.Thaiwebsites.com/, accessed October 1, 2012).

type of family as *kon thuk kon yak* which means people who do not have enough resources to make their ends meet.

Similar to others villagers elsewhere in the Northeast, villagers of Ban Phra and Ban Koke see off-farm production as an important means to earn money for family expenses. As a result of rapid economic growth in Thailand and the Northeast during the past 40 years of development, villagers have embraced an opportunity to participate in the expanding market economy. Khon Kaen city has prospered with land estates and housing development projects during the last 15 years, and the demand for construction has increased. Many people from Ban Phra and Ban Koke commute daily to work in Khon Kaen city and mostly work as construction workers. Many village men are skillful workers and craftsmen. In addition, service-related businesses such as restaurants, hotels, karaoke pubs, pubs, shopping malls, discotheques, and massage parlors have expanded in the city.

In addition, some medium-scale agricultural-based industries, such as fishnet making, fish canning, ice cube making, noodle, sugar, cassava pellet, liquor, garment, and paper factories, have expanded. Similar to what Mills (1999) has found in her work with women from Northeastern Thailand, a number of young women and men in both communities and in other villages of Khon Kaen are motivated to come to work and stay in the city where they come to feel that their lifestyles and identities are different from their parents. Some few young women and men in Ban Phra have migrated to work in industrial factories in Bangkok, whereas in Ban Koke, more have worked in Bangkok. Although Thai-Lao villagers have migrated to work abroad, a small number of villagers in Ban Phra and Ban Koke have done so, for this requires large investment. Based on my village survey in 1995, about 14.5 % of the total families in Ban Phra and 7.5 % in Ban Koke migrated to work abroad. In 2010, the number of international migrants remained more or less the same as in 1995, about 15 %, whereas it was increased to 12 % in Ban Koke. Many have migrated to Japan, Taiwan, and Singapore. Many of those who went abroad mortgaged their farm land for loans. Some were fortunate to make a fortune out of it, and some could pay off their loans and make their ends meet; however, others did not and lost their land.

Like many other rural *Isan* villagers, villagers of Ban Phra and Ban Koke do not live in isolation. They are profoundly involved with international and national markets through the sphere of production (in terms of both farm production and the sale of their labor as a commodity), distribution, and consumption. They have undergone rapid change from being subsistence farmers to becoming commercial farmers through the expansion of the market economy, the development of rural-urban communication and infrastructure, and changes in ecological conditions. People no longer produce only for their families but also for local, national, and global markets. They also rely on the markets for necessary farm inputs such as fertilizers, seeds, pesticides, fuel, tractors, and new machinery and the necessary consumption items such as medicines, clothing, processed food, toothpaste, soap, and shampoo. Fluctuating farm prices in the global market have resulted in the poverty of small rural agricultural producers in *Isan*. Most villagers have complained about insufficient money for home expenses, farm investments, and debts. In 1995, many poor and middle-income family farms had debts charged by merchants in Khon Kaen city or districts with exorbitant rates of interest varying from 5 to 15 % per month. Even debts to kin and neighbors could carry high interest rates, from 2.5 to 5 % per month. Today, this problem still persists. Loans from the Bank for Agriculture and Agricultural Cooperatives (BAAC), which charge varying interest rates from 9 to 12 % per annum (whereas about 12–15 % per annum is charged by a commercial bank), are possible only for certain crops or projects that the government promotes. Most families in both communities have debts to either the BAAC, private users, or both.

Ban Phra and Ban Koke are perceived by local authorities as homogenously poor but relatively better off when compared to remote *Isan* villages. The transformation of the two communities through improvements of rural infrastructure by the state has promoted local production for the market. The communities have access to district and city markets, nearby public hospitals, provincial highways, electricity, and public wells. In addition, the people in Ban Phra have access to irrigation for farming despite their complaints of irregular water supplies and the conflict between water users at the head and tail of the irrigation canals. In addition, a water pipeline system for home use has been installed in Ban Phra since the beginning of 1994. During my field work in 1995, the first private home telephone was installed in Ban Phra, whereas in Ban Koke, people have access to two private radio telephone units. In 2010, all families in both communities already had access to mobile hand phones. Villagers have regarded these infrastructural improvements as signs of progress and modernity.

4 Village-Based Sufficiency Economy Approach

By the 1980s, a call for sustainable development through "sufficiency" farming techniques as a development alternative to modernizing rural agriculture in Thai society emerged, the initiative primarily of some NGOs and village leaders, many of them from Northeastern Thailand. The sufficiency economy approach has, however, been subsequently modified and developed by Thai elites for political and economic reasons. The self-sufficiency approach patronized by His Majesty, the King, has been nationally and internationally known. King Bhumibol has also been credited with a socioeconomic theory of self-sufficiency (see also Chaps. 31 and 32 in this volume).

Local and international NGOs working primarily in the field of integrated rural development to promote the well-being of rural communities in *Isan* and elsewhere in Thailand began to play a significant role in providing a critical view of the state-led capitalist development approach. They perceived that such a heavily market-driven approach could undermine the well-being of rural communities at large. They argued that commercialization of farm production for export was not a feasible strategy for poor farmers, especially for small farmers in Thailand. This was due to unfavorable market price mechanisms, which were not in favor of the rural agricultural farming sector. Small farmers were victims of the exploitative capitalist relations of production and consumption via market price mechanisms. Also, commercialized farming depended heavily on the use of chemical substances which were harmful to humans and the natural environment. These NGOs and some village leaders initiated the idea of sufficiency farm production for rural poor farm households as a development alternative to improve their disadvantaged position in the wider market economy.

The idea of village self-sufficiency economy was initially influenced by European international NGOs, which were major financial donors to several local Thai NGOs between the 1980s and 1990s. These local NGOs were later also exposed to ideas and practices of some Japanese NGOs and farmer movements focused on organic farming, alternative markets, and sustainable development.

The essence of sufficiency economic farming, as practiced by villagers in Ban Phra and Ban Koke and elsewhere in *Isan*, is that it gives priority to integrated organic farming, growing diversified food crops in combination with animal husbandry instead of growing mono-crop agriculture, such as cassava and sugarcane plantations as usually emphasized in capitalist farming in Thailand. The selection of diverse crops to be grown and animals to be raised with sufficient integrated organic farming depends first on the farm family's consumption needs, not driven by market motivations as in capitalism. Whatever is left over from home consumption could then be sold in the market. Additionally, the use of decomposed fertilizer and herbs for agricultural production has been strongly promoted.

It was in the late 1980s that a network for alternative agriculture was formally established among local NGOs and farmer's organizations in Thailand, and later in 1998, the Sustainable Agriculture Foundation (Thailand) was set up to act as a coordinating body for promoting sustainable agriculture in rural development as an alternative to capitalist farming production.[5] The local movement for sustainable development in Thailand also originated in the broad "anti-neoliberalism" feelings of some local NGOs and farmer leaders, particularly from *Isan*. Nonetheless, individuals and groups in the larger overall movement cannot be seen as homogeneous. They each manage their own economic activities relating to sufficiency farming independently. Some are quite different from others in their approach when it comes to definitions, ideas, and practices. Generally, all do share a common orientation of antiglobalization (Bell cited in Walker et al. 2008) and a common belief system, based on Buddhist principles, emphasizing moderation, self-reliance, hard work, patience, and self-restraint in the face of material temptations and desire (Keyes 1983).

According to a database for groups involved in sufficiency economy activities in Thailand, organized by Pipat Yodphruttikan in 2006, there were 626 groups involving in activities relating to sufficiency economy throughout Thailand, primarily at the grassroots level. Of these, 448 were classified as having minimal involvement, 126 as actively engaged in both philosophy and action, and 12 considered as model farmers (Yodphruttikan 2006: 7). The distribution of the total 626 groups by regions is as follows: Central Plains, 140; West, 9; East, 11; North, 51; Northeast, 259; and South, 156 (Yodphruttikan 2006: 5). Economic activities

---

[5] Source: www.sathai.org/, accessed on May 9, 2008.

relating to sufficiency economy can be classified as follows: 25 groups in royal development projects, 64 groups as farmer models, 117 groups as community models, 4 groups as private businesses, 339 groups as community enterprises, 43 groups as saving groups, and 34 groups classified as "others" (e.g., local knowledge masters) (Yodphruttikan 2006: 6). Albeit small in number, the movement indicates a significant historical moment in Thailand where grassroots movement began to emerge, calling for sustainable development in agriculture and providing a development alternative to Thai modernity.

In line with the sufficiency economy philosophy and practice, Bamrung, the prominent farmer leader of the Northeast, is a good role model. He is obviously in favor of the sufficiency farm approach, which his family has practiced over the past 20 years. He believes that this idea can help address the four basic human needs: for food, clothes, shelter, and medicine. If farmers could produce at least 80 % of what they need to consume and use in their everyday lives, this would be the best guarantee of basic security. Nonetheless, Bamrung feels that farm production based on the concept of sufficiency economy alone is not sufficient to help farmers survive. There should be alternative markets for producers and consumers of organic products. This would redress the problem of unfavorable market prices that are biased against the agricultural sector. The state should step in to help organize this. Organic farming production does not aim at profit maximization as in capitalistic farm production. For him, organic farming aspires to enhance peaceful coexistence between humans and nature. Building environmental awareness in the public to help protect our natural environment is a must. Also, this type of farming production stresses the farmers' sufficiency economy. It aims to provide security for both farmers and consumers by promoting a system where producers receive a fair share of the economic distribution and consumers pay a reasonable market price. Thus, direct sale from producers to consumers is a major component of the alternative market. He also believes that the alternative market has to be combined with an alternative way of living, which should correspond to the philosophy of sufficiency economy, highlighting moderation, self-reliance, simplicity, perseverance, moral values, and knowledge, as well as health and environmental concerns.

In addition, Bamrung has mentioned that the philosophy of sufficiency economy would benefit farmers best if it was accompanied by policy support and advocacy to make farmers' problems known to the state and to the public. Farmers in *Isan* and elsewhere need to catch up with the current political-economic issues and be informed on implications of policy and how it impacts local communities. Organizing farmers to defend their political and economic interests is necessary to establish a proper platform for farmers (especially small farmers) to negotiate with other concerned parties, such as state policy-makers and businessmen.

Finally, Bamrung believes that in pursuing their economic interests based on the philosophy of sufficiency economy, farmers need to have allies from different organizations to support their work and to exchange knowledge, skills, and information for updating their organic farming movements, as well as other related activities.

At this point, I agree with Bamrung that the approach may work to guarantee food security of farmers, at least at a certain level. In the case of Bamrung's family, after 20 years of applying the approach, they are not wealthy. They live moderately. I wonder how his family would support the higher education of their only child and what they would do if a family member got ill and needed special medical care in a hospital. As to maximize the contribution of the sufficiency economic approach, the government and other concerned parties need to draft and implement a holistic program to support the initiatives and efforts of farmers at the village level.

The critiques of sufficiency economy approach by Walker et al. (2008) are worth considering. Visiting Bamrung's farm convinced me that the approach places all responsibility for poverty eradication on the farmers themselves. This has made it possible for the government to avoid or play a low profile in addressing any redistribution of resources or income to the rural population of Thailand. Also, I feel that it is possible for Bamrung's family to pursue the sufficiency economy approach because his family currently has no debt. They love what they have been doing on the farm. They do not have many dependents. They are hard working and self-reliant and live moderately.

Let us now turn to the villagers in Ban Phra and Ban Koke who are commercial farmers in contemporary village life. Still, most villagers of these two communities object to neither the market economy nor the sufficiency economy. Approximately 10 and 15 % of the total families in Ban Koke and Ban Phra, respectively, have adopted the sufficiency production through the introduction of NGOs, the media, and the Office of Agricultural Extension in Khon Kaen.

As a result of the commercialization of agriculture patronized by the state development policy since the First Plan in the 1960s, farmers in both communities and elsewhere in Thailand are profoundly involved with the market in the sphere of production, distribution, and consumption (see also Chap. 32 in this volume).

Since the early 1960s, farmers in Ban Koke and elsewhere in *Isan* started to grow maize, beans, and kenaf for the market. When the price of kenaf had been low, they switched to the newly introduced cash crops: cassava and sugar cane. By the late 1970s, the good prices of cash crops motivated most farm families in Ban Koke to engage in cassava and sugar production. Adding to this, Muskat (1994) points out that the opening of the international market, especially the European Economic Community in the 1970s, motivated Thai farmers to actively engage in cassava production for the market. Yet, most farmers in Ban Koke complained that subsequent fluctuation of cassava prices and other farm products caused their families poverty. For instance, a poor farm family told me that in 1994 she invested about 3,100 baht (US$124) in cassava production and by the end of harvesting she received a total of 8,000 baht (US$320) (before the investment cost deduction). She and her husband worked on cassava farm for about 1 year until it could be harvested. Migration has been the best alternative for her family since the 1980s. Her two teenagers commute daily to work in a fishnet-making factory in Khon Kaen city.

As a minor supplement, her family has set aside some parts of farm land for food crop production (such as rice, chili, lime, onion, and green vegetables), for fish pond, and for pig and poultry raising. They primarily rely on their family labor and simple tools and techniques for food crop production. Hired labor is mainly for cash crop production such as rice and cassava. The idea of sufficiency production is first and foremost to produce for home consumption and for sale when the family needs cash. Some farm families also collect some wild native leaves and plants from forests and catch fish, paddy crabs, and frogs from paddy fields, rivers, and canals nearby. In my view, occupational diversifications including working on-farm via engaging in both capitalistic market economy and sufficiency production and working off-farm via migrating to work in industrial factories in urban areas locally and internationally are prominent strategies of family farms in *Isan* to guarantee their economic survival and pursue their economic interests within the structural constraints of political-economic policies and practices nationally and globally.

Villagers in both communities told me that the philosophy and practice of the sufficiency economy are not entirely new to them. Since their forefathers' times, people produced mainly for household consumption rather than for sale. In the early periods of village settlements by the nineteenth century, their forebears grew glutinous rice, chili, and various kinds of vegetables mainly for home consumption, and surplus left would be for exchange locally. They also grew cotton to obtain thread for weaving materials. In other words, they produced mainly for household use rather than for sale. Producing glutinous rice has been their main farming activity until today. In the past, they relied on rainfalls for farming production with the use of family labor and simple technology including water buffaloes for plowing, traditional rice varieties, and manure fertilizers.

Today, this paddy farming production in both communities continues with a change to irrigation technology in some areas such as Ban Phra, modern rice varieties, chemical fertilizers, and the use of some machinery for rice harvesting, winnowing, and milling. Also, today they produce rice for both export and consumption. In times of fluctuating prices for cash crop production, many farmers have chosen migration to be their best alternative. Some chose to strengthen their food crop production based on the idea of the sufficiency economy as a supplement for food security reasons.

Similar to the case of Bamrung, many family farms in Ban Phra and Ban Koke use food products from farms to provide them with some economic security so that they are able to participate in the market economy more effectively. Traditional social relations through families, relatives, and friends have provided young female and male migrants from both communities and elsewhere in *Isan* with job employment information and initial settlements when they go to work in Bangkok or in other major cities in Thailand and abroad. Most migrants remit some money to their parental homes. These young migrants told me that occasionally they brought some rice, dried food, fermented fish, and chili paste from home to Bangkok or abroad as to reduce their food expenses while working in industrial factories or in the service-related business in urban areas. They need to live economically to save some money for their future and to support their parental homes. Buddhist principles play a significant role in shaping village social life. Some young migrants in both communities have mentioned the keys to their success including moderation, self-reliance, and restraint from material temptation and desire.

Food available from their farms helps reducing their food expenses at a certain level, thus being able to partake in the expanding market economy and accepting low wages, especially in an initial stage of industrial development in the 1960s. The market economy has become the most predominant mode of farm production in contemporary village life. Most villagers in *Isan* and elsewhere in Thailand produce rice for both export and consumption. They also produce cash crops for national and global markets. A traditional economy involves in subsistence agricultural production for home consumption primarily with the use of family labor and simple tools and techniques. Traditional village economies may be based on religious beliefs and existing traditional social relations, with economic decisions based on the traditions of community, family, and religion.

5 Conclusion

In this chapter, I discuss the cultural logic of economic action by farmers in the three communities of Northeastern Thailand who have opted to embrace the sufficiency approach in combination with the market economy. Following Meillassoux (1981), I assert that capitalism and a traditional village economy are not in a binary opposition. In pursuing their families' economic interests, most villagers in these two communities are participating and taking advantage of the expanding market economy while making use of their agricultural domestic economies and traditional social relations to enhance the expansion of capitalistic economy. Specifically, I look at economic behaviors of farmers in *Isan* through the case of Bamrung Kayotha, a farmer leader from Kalasin, and villagers from Ban Phra and Ban Koke as expressed in their daily life. I explore how villagers of Ban Phra and Ban Koke regard the sufficiency economy approach and the market economy and what their economic rationality has been in relation to it.

I argue that the sufficiency economy approach as understood and practiced by villagers in *Isan* does not entirely negate capitalism, as the general public in Thailand might have thought. Although the approach proposed by some local NGOs and some farmer leaders, particularly from *Isan*, starting in the 1980s, could be regarded as a critique of Thai state-led capitalist development policies, the sufficiency economy approach, surprisingly, does exist within the framework of capitalism.

References

Keyes, C. F. (1983). Economic action and Buddhist morality in a Thai village. *Journal of Asian Studies, XLII*(4), 851–868.

Keyes, C. F. (1991). Buddhist detachment and worldly gain: The economic ethic of Northeastern Thai villagers. In C. Satha-anand (Ed.), *Collected essays in honor of Professor Saneh Chammarik*. Special issue of *Journal of Political Science Thammasat University*, 16.1–2, 271–298.

Keyes, C. F. (2008, January 9). *The village economy: Capitalist and sufficiency-based: A Northeastern Thai case*. In Keynote speech given at the 10th international conference on Thai Studies, Thammasat University, Bangkok.

Kirsch, T. A. (1982). Buddhism, sex roles and the Thai economy. In P. Van Esterik (Ed.), *Women of Southeast Asia* (Occasional Paper # 9) (pp. 16–41). DeKalb: Center for Southeast Asian Studies, Northern Illinois University.

Meillassoux, C. (1981). *Maidens, meal and money: Capitalism and the domestic community*. Cambridge: Cambridge University Press.

Mills, M. B. (1999). *Thai women in the global labor force: Consuming desires, contested selves*. New Brunswick: Rutgers University Press.

Muskat, R. J. (1994). *The fifth tiger: A study of Thai development policy*. World Institute Development Economics Research (UNU/WIDER). Helsinki: United Nations University Press.

Office of the National Economic and Social Development Board, NESDB. (2008). *Report of the GDP per capita by regions*. Bangkok: Office of the Prime Minister.

Tambiah, S. J. (1970). *Buddhism and spirit cults in North-East Thailand*. Cambridge: Cambridge University Press.

Tosakul, R. (2013). Alterity to modernity: Village-based self-sufficient farm production in Northeastern Thailand (forthcoming).

Walker, A., Unger, D., Glassman, J., & Bell, P. F. (2008, January 9). *Sufficiency economy. A panel discussion*. In 10th international conference on Thai Studies, Thammasat University, Bangkok.

Yodphruttikan, P. (2006). *Database on community groups applying sufficiency economy in their daily lives*. Thai Pat Institute, Rural Reconstruction Foundation under Royal Patronage.

Cited Websites

http://www.ashoka.org.node/3567

http://www.us-asean.org/Thailand/c95.pdf

http://www.Bangkokpundit.blogspot.com/2006/22/differeing interpretations of sufficiency economy.html

http://www.Sagathai.org/

http://www.Thaiwebsites.com/

Part II
Political Aspects in Thailand Today

Chapter 10
Party-Social Movement Coalition in Thailand's Political Conflict (2005–2011)

Aim Sinpeng

1 Social Movement and Party Politics

The literature on social movement and party politics remains largely separated. Social movements are defined as sustained sequences of contentious collective action utilized by those who have new or unaccepted claims and who behave in ways that challenge authorities (McAdam and Tarrow 2010). Social movements are often seen as parallel to parties for they are bounded by different sets of incentives and constraints. Since movements largely come about as a result of lacking regular access to institutions, it stands in sharp contrast to political parties which are bounded by their access to and their roles in formal institutions. In addition, scholars of social movement have long focused more on the disruptive form of contention, thus neglecting other forms such as electoral politics. McAdam and Tarrow (2010) argue in their think piece, *Ballots and Barricades: On the Reciprocal Relationship Between Elections and Social Movements*, which reviewed the development of the field of contentious politics in the past four decades, that scholars ought to make concerted effort to systematically link the studies of elections and movements.

To this end, this chapter seeks to explore the conditions under which political parties and social movements become linked. Thailand provides an excellent case study for a number of reasons. First, there are two social movements that operated parallel to one another but at the same time allowing certain variables, such as socioeconomic and political structure, to be held constant. Second, both movements differ in the extent of their relationship with political parties. Examining the variation between the movements can reveal some valuable insights into the issue of party-movement

A. Sinpeng (✉)
Department of Political Science, University of British Columbia,
C425 – 1866 Main Mall, Vancouver, V5T 1Z1 BC, Canada
e-mail: thaiaim@gmail.com

P. Liamputtong (ed.), *Contemporary Socio-Cultural and Political Perspectives in Thailand*, DOI 10.1007/978-94-007-7244-1_10,

coalition. Third, there is also a variation within each party-movement relationship over time (see also Chaps. 11, 12, and 13 in this volume).

2 Key Assumptions

The main assumption of the research on which this chapter is based is regarding politicians' motives. Politicians are motivated by votes (office-seeking), specific agenda (policy-seeking), or a combination of both. In the office-seeking model, political actors are concerned about rewards, such as "power, prestige, or a place in a lime light" (Budge and Laver 1986: 485). Others are motivated by policy pursuit, which denotes their participation in the policy process in order to further particular policy objectives. Parties, by the same logic, are motivated by office and will take actions that would increase their chance of garnering votes in the next election.

Opposition parties have far less influence on the policy-making process than do their parliamentarians in the government counterparts. As such, oppositional political parties are the candidates most likely to take on extra-parliamentarian strategies to achieve their political end (Almeida 2010). Taking to the streets is, however, a risky business, with many associated high costs. Parties or individual politicians could lose popular support, especially their electoral support base that they would need to maintain (or secure) in order to be reelected. Moreover, they could risk alienating themselves from their fellow party members, who could affect their future party nominations. Since there are many unpredictable variables and uncertainty, they could potentially fail in their objectives.

A key factor that reduces the cost of mobilization is to have a reliable source of popular support. There are two major ways that parties could achieve this: first, establish coalition or alliance with existing anti-government forces (often with various organizations or student groups) and, second, mobilize their existing electoral support base. Key individuals and leaders who participate in both oppositional political parties and social movements act as brokers bringing the movements into closer collaborations with electoral parties (Mische 2008). Such individuals promote the mutual interests of the party and movement in working together on economic policy issues. Membership overlap promotes the coordination of meetings, protest campaigns, strategies, resource exchange (Diani 2004), and shared goals among movements and oppositional political parties. In the absence of such interpersonal ties, there would be much more distance between these two distinct types of organizational arrangements, making alliances costlier in terms of the time needed to build mutual trust.

3 Thailand's Political Conflict: Background

Since 2005, Thailand has been trapped in cycles of mass demonstrations, street violence, marshal laws, and unstable societal conditions. "The most recent clash between the two opposing forces was, by far, the worst ever seen in a 100 years," claims renowned Thai historian Charnvit Kasetsiri (2010, May 20). The battle of colors – between the Red and the Yellow Shirts – in part centers around a highly popular yet polarizing figure, Thaksin Shinawatra, a former prime minister who was ousted in the coup d'état of 2006. The mass demonstrations led by the Yellow Shirts since 2005 sought to expel Thaksin, whom they regard as highly corrupt, manipulative, and authoritarian – a major threat to the country's democracy, monarchy, and national security as a whole. On the other hand, the Reds, the majority of whom were Thaksin's electoral bases, saw the ousting of their much beloved leader as unjust, illegitimate, and a clear regression of democracy.

At the heart of the social movement against Thaksin has been the People's Alliance for Democracy (PAD), or the Yellow Shirts. This is a movement that has brought together a broad range of groups whose interests were adversely affected by the Thaksin regime. This includes some sections of the media, teacher's union, labor, religious groups, nongovernmental organizations, and activists (Songthai 2008: 99). After a rocky start in 2005, the PAD officially formed an alliance in February of 2006 – just months before the September coup. The Yellow Shirts drew mass support from largely the Bangkok middle class,[1] Democrat Party supporters (at various times), and royalists.[2]

The United Front for Democracy against Dictatorship (UDD), or the Red Shirts, was formed in response to the September 2006 coup and the dismantling of the Thai Rak Thai Party. They have become one of the most powerful social movements in recent Thai history. The Red Shirt movement represents what Taylor (2011: 3) describes as "a number of broad interest groups brought together by a desire to see full representative democracy." The class elements within the Red Shirts, while multilayered, are best understood as largely representing "an emerging class of urbanized villagers that straddled both urban and rural society" (Thabchumpon and McCargo 2011: 999). Well-respected public intellectual, Nithi Aeosriwong (2010), has argued that the Red Shirts are largely "lower middle class" – not the poor, but the poorer section of the middle class. As will be detailed below, the Red Shirts were indispensable to the electoral success of Thaksin-backed parties – Palang Prachachon (PPP) and Peau Thai Party (PTP) – and have mastered such broad-based popular support unmatched by any other movements in recent memory (see Chaps. 8, 11, 12, and 13).

4 The Yellow Shirts and the Democrat Party

The Democrat Party and the PAD are loosely related and only coalesce under specific conditions to achieve short-term objectives. The Democrat Party is not a mass-based party and has always been "conservative" when it comes to extra-parliamentarian

[1] Note: On various occasions, PAD leaders and their media call their movement to be urban based and composed of urban dwellers that are middle class. Kraisak Choonhavan, former senator and one of the most vocal members of the anti-Thaksin 40 Senator Group, now Democrat MP, went further: "PAD is the uprising of the middle class" (interview, Bangkok, July 19, 2011).

[2] See Pongsudhirak (2008) and Kitirianglarp and Hewison (2009).

opposition. By nature, the Democrats have a rather elitist approach on politics and would get involved with contentious activities, such as street protests or movements, only when the benefits are obvious. As such, the relationship between the Democrat Party and the Yellow Shirts waxes and wanes over time, depending on expected rewards for mutual support.

4.1 Phase I: Mutual Sympathy, Tacit Support (2005–2006)

The first phase of the PAD-Democrat alliance was marked by mutual sympathy but also ambivalence. There was a recognition of a shared objective, but each pursued different strategies. Before the coup, the Democrats' position toward the PAD was supportive but not overtly so. Frustrated by its inability to check the power of Thaksin, due to institutional constraints, the Democrat members felt they shared similar deep resentment and dissatisfaction toward the Thaksin government as the PAD.

> Parliamentary mechanisms for checking the executive were crippled…We in the opposition couldn't launch the no confidence motion on Thaksin. When his cabinet ministers couldn't respond during questioning period, his MPs did not vote against the motion. In fact so many times parliamentary sessions had to be cancelled because not enough MPs showed up. Thaksin did not respect parliamentary procedures. The Upper House couldn't do anything either. This is a total parliamentary tyranny.[3]

The frustration of the opposition party drove the Democrats to look for allies outside of parliament. The Democrats took some initial steps to mobilize against the Thaksin government, including their planned anti-Thaksin rally and the boycott of the 2006 election, much of which either failed to materialize or proved ineffective. Eventually, some Democrat MPs began to frequent PAD rallies, and some even going on stage to show their support toward the movement.[4] "What the PAD leaders said on stage resonated very much with how we felt in parliament. We saw eye to eye on a number of issues."[5]

The PAD's motivations were clear from the outset: to oust the Thaksin government. Jermsak Pinthong (2008, September 29), one of the earliest and most

---

[3] Dr. Witaya Kaewparadai, Democrat MP and former minister, interview, Democrat Party July 12, 2011.

[4] Democrat MPs that went on PAD stage (various times) include Kasit Piromya, Somkiat Pongpaiboon, Khunying Kalaya Sophonpanich, Anchalee Thepabutr, and Kraisak Choonhavan. Dr. Witaya Kaewparadai, former minister and Democrat MP, confirmed this during an interview: "Democrat Party considered PAD as an ally…indeed some of our members joined PAD and engaged in their activities. Some went on stage, others donated food and money" (interview, Democrat Party, July 12, 2011). This statement is corroborated by the PAD side (interview Somsak Kosaisuk; also Dr. Thamrong Sanegsuriyachan, July 10, 2011; Prapan Koonmee, interview with Khao Sod, reprinted in PAD (2009); Chaipan Prapasawat (Academic, frequent PAD speaker), Interview, June 24, 2011).

[5] Interview with various Democrat MPs, Democrat Party Headquarter, Bangkok, July 2011.

vocal opponents of the Thaksin administration, sums up the anti-Thaksin sentiment: "The Thaksin regime may look like a democracy from the outside, but it is authoritarian because it monopolizes power, interferes with independent institutions, centralizes power in the executive, uses populism to create popular sentiment, makes laws to suit the leader and his cronies, violates human rights and threatens free media."

4.2 Phase II: United (2007–2008)

The second phase of PAD-Democrat alliance is marked by a growing recognition of mutual benefits and expected rewards. The astounding victory of the PPP, a proxy of Thai Rak Thai, pushed both the Democrats and the PAD to the brink of destruction. The PAD changed their strategy. In what their leaders termed "the last war" (Limthongkul 2008), the movement engaged in the longest, most violent anti-government rally to date. The 193-day protest began soon after then Prime Minister Samak Sundaravej of the PPP announced he would seek to amend the 2007 constitution, which the PAD saw as a "national crisis" and that the Thaksin regime was very much alive and remains a threat to Thailand's constitutional monarchy (Katasila 2008). While not engaging directly with the Red Shirts' class-based *Prai* versus *Ammat* discourse,[6] the PAD believes democracy in Thailand will not work like in Western countries because politicians are corrupt, while many citizens sell their votes. For the PAD, elections are essentially steeped in "money politics" (PAD 2008). After a long drawn-out rally that included raiding the Government House, occupying the country's main airport, among others, the PAD declared its "victory" in December 2008 when the PPP was dissolved by the court, paving the way for the Democrat Party to cobble together a coalition and ascend to power.

This period saw the PAD and the Democrats on the united front. As Somsak Kosaisuk, PAD's former core leader, argued "we turned our eyes blind to the differences among us, and focused on our common goal: to rid of the Thaksin regime."[7] The PAD-Democrat alliance ran from top to bottom. At the leadership level, we saw

[6] The term "*Ammat*" was adopted by the UDD leaders, following Thaksin's reference to "extraconstitutional power" (*poo meebaraminokrabob*) who was responsible for his overthrow. The UDD leaders often use the term "*Ammat*" loosely to refer to powerful individuals who supported the coup. In a Red Shirt publication, Thailand in the Hands of *Ammat*, *Ammat* instigated the coup by utilizing the military-bureaucratic mechanisms within the policy, supported by intellectuals, NGOs, and the media who "created conditions for a coup." While *Ammat* is often used broadly, some key individuals have been targeted by the UDD as the core *Ammat*: Prem Tinsulanonda, the army chiefs (Sonthi Boonyaratglin, Anupong Paochinda, Prayuth Chan-ocha), Abhisit (and the entire Democrat Party), Sondhi Limthongkul, PAD, etc. For more discussion on this, see Pongsawat (2011). Kwanchai Praipanna, leader of the We love Udon People Club, explained in an interview that Thaksin is not an *Ammat* because even if he was corrupt, he gave money back to people. That makes people happy (interview, Udon Thani, July 11, 2011). For more discussion on this, see Pongsawat (2011) and Aeosriwong (2010).

[7] Somsak Kosaisuk, interview, New Politics Party Headquarter, Bangkok, July 11, 2011.

a number of Democrat MPs frequented the PAD protest site; many were regular speakers on the PAD stage. Prapan Koonmee, the party's executive member at the time, became part of the PAD's leadership structure. It is an open secret that he is a close friend of the Democrats' MP and one of its largest financiers – Khunying Kalaya Sophonpanich – indicating the coalition approval at the highest level. Indeed, some PAD frequent protesters revealed they have seen Abhisit, the leader of the Democrat Party, visiting the rally site, offering "support" to the PAD leaders backstage.[8] The biggest contribution the Democrat Party could make to the PAD movement has actually been to provide mass support. In fact, Democrat Party leaders admitted mobilizing their mass to PAD rallies – most notably the infamous 193-day protest. While figures vary, according to party estimates, the Democrat Party forces accounted for at least 50 % of total PAD mass.[9] "Democrat Party members, mostly southerners, mobilized the mass to join PAD rallies."[10] Democrat southern MPs, particularly Suthep Thaugsuban, have been instrumental in bringing in the masses from party supporters from its stronghold.

What is clear, however, is that their memberships overlap, which means that the extent to which they support each other's objective has an impact on their popularity. "Officially the [Democrat] Party does not have a specific policy to endorse the PAD. Abhisit told us not to go on PAD stage and let the mass movement take its own course. Unofficially, however, if you [Democrat MPs] want to attend PAD rallies you do it on your own terms," argues Dr. Pusadee Thamtai, Democrat MP and former party executive.[11] The end result of this strong PAD-Democrat alliance is not only sheer mass, but it contributed significantly in bringing down both Samak and Somchai governments and allowing the Democrats to form a government coalition. "It's a victory for the PAD…we are rid of the Somchai government…Abhisit can bring us the new kind of politics with policy innovations and good people to govern the country," proclaimed Limthongkul (2008).

4.3 Phase III: Breakup (2009–2011)

The honeymoon period between the PAD and the Democrats was over soon after Abhisit came to power. The Democrat Party was, in PAD's view, reneging on their promises they made when they fought together against the Thaksin regime. Resentment began to build up as the PAD felt they were not getting their share of

[8] Based on interviews with various PAD demonstrators during the 193-day rally and the 2011 round.

[9] Dr. Witaya Kaewparadai, Democrat MP and former minister. Interview. Democrat Party Headquarter, Bangkok, July 12, 2011.

[10] Thawil Paison, Democrat MP and former minister and a longtime party member (30 years). Interview. Democrat Headquarter, Bangkok, July 12, 2011.

[11] Dr. Pusadee Thamtai, Democrat MP and former party executive. Interview. Democrat Party. July 12, 2011.

what they wanted even though they were responsible for Abhisit coming to power. The straw that broke the camel's back, which became the key issue of the third wave of the PAD protest, was the one involving the Thai-Cambodia territorial dispute. The more radical wing of the PAD included the ultranationalist and ultraroyalist groups.[12] The PAD began to hold anti-government rallies during the Abhisit administration, and the mass of PAD dwindled significantly. One by one, Democrat MPs, who used to vocally and proactively support the PAD, began to distance themselves from the movement.[13]

In the 2011 elections, the PAD's most notable action was the "Vote No" campaign, in which the PAD called on voters to check "none of the above." Although the "Vote No" campaign was a resounding failure, with less than 3 % of the constituency vote, it created a massive rift between the Democrats and the PAD, as well as the latter's breakaway from the party, New Politics Party. The fallout between the PAD and the Democrat Party did make a difference in some constituencies as the "Vote No" campaign took away votes that could have gone to the Democrats and could have meant a victory for the Democrat Party in a tight race.[14] The PAD suffered additional setbacks internally, including dwindling financial support, leadership breakup,[15] poor coordination, and fatigue; losing the Democrat Party support was severely detrimental to PAD mass appeal (Nelson 2011).

5 The Red Shirts and Peau Thai

The UDD came together as a more organized movement in 2007 comprised largely of two groups: the pro-Thaksin supporters (whose electoral base is in the North and Northeast) mobilized by former Thai Rak Thai politicians and the anti-coup civic groups/NGOs. The latter was the first to mobilize immediately following the September 2006 coup – protesting what they believed was the country's unacceptable democratic reversal.[16] This section of the Red Shirts includes NGOs, activists,

[12] For example, the Thai Patriot Network and Santi Asoke.

[13] Kasit Piromya, foreign minister during Abhisit Administration, took part in the PAD's occupation of Suvarnabhumi Airport. He gave an interview to the Telegraph on December 21, 2008, saying that the airport protests were "fun with good food."

[14] A Democrat incumbent from Bangkok reveals, "Before the coup I was attending PAD rallies everyday because the majority of people in my constituency went…I went to garner votes…now the Vote No campaign really hurt the Democrat Party…I was even kicked out from some houses." Interview, District Office, Bangkok, July 14, 2011.

[15] Somsak Kosaisuk, one of PAD core leaders, left PAD in early 2011. He is now the head of the New Politics Party (NPP), a new party formed after the PAD general meeting in 2009. Today the NPP and the PAD are no longer officially affiliated.

[16] Notable groups to protest against the coup in the aftermath of Thaksin's overthrow were the 19 September Anti-Coup Network, Saturday People Say No to Tyranny, Red Sunday Group, White Pigeon Group, 24 June Group, Temujin Network (Chanapat Na Nakorn), and various academics. For a good chronology of protest events since the September Coup, refer to Crisis 19 (Wad Rawi).

intellectuals, students, and some sections of the "idealistic" middle class.[17] The former group, the grass roots supporters of Thaksin, was initially mobilized by the Veera-Nattawut-Jatuporn trio[18] through People's Television (PTV) talk shows and subsequently through a series of Truth Today rallies between 2008 and 2009. While the three leaders were first and foremost former Thai Rak Thai politicians, it was clear that the plight of Thaksin played center stage in the struggle of the Red Shirts.

The UDD solidified their movement between 2008 and 2010 through "socialization in a common struggle," as they quickly found themselves in opposition once again.[19] Immediately following the dissolution of Thaksin-aligned PPP following a controversial court ruling that the party had engaged in corrupt activities, the UDD leaders set up the "Red Land Network" (*Dang Tang Peandin*) and declared "war" on the "*Ammat*." By 2009, in what later would be termed "Bloody Songkran," initially peaceful anti-government protests in Bangkok began to spread to several provinces nationwide. The UDD leaders set April 8 as the "D-Day" when more than 150,000 Red Shirts turned up in Bangkok (Raksaseri 2009). As protesters clashed with state authorities leading to two deaths and hundreds injured, Abhisit declared a state of emergency with scores of Red Shirt leaders arrested. After the April 2009 crackdown, the UDD turned to a less confrontational means to channel their grievances. They collected over five million signatures to petition for a royal pardon for Thaksin. Subsequently, the UDD collected 100,000 more signatures to petition for the return to the 1997 constitution, while pressing ahead with nearly weekly anti-government rallies.

The trigger for arguably the largest mass protest ever in contemporary Thai history came as the Supreme Court seized $1.4 billion of Thaksin's assets. The UDD leaders quickly finalized what they termed "the last battle" – a mass anti-government demonstration where over a million Red Shirts were expected to turn up (*Bangkok Post* 2010, February 23). What was planned as a 7-day rally[20] turned into 64 days of drawn-out protest[21] that ended with a violent crackdown and the deaths of 91 people and more than 2,000 injured. This was the worst episode of

---

[17] Sombat Boon Ngam-anong, founder of the Red Sunday Group. Interview. Red Sunday Group Office, Bangkok, June 2011. The Red Sunday Group was founded in 2010 after the Ratchaprasong crackdown. The group collaborates closely with the main UDD but is not directly under UDD supervision. The Red Sunday Group's main activities are civil disobedience, campaigns, and workshops that focus on raising awareness about democracy, injustice, and human rights.

[18] Veera Musikapong, Jatuporn Prompan, and Nattawut Saikua (the "Trio") emerged as Red Shirt leaders through their talk/comedy show, "Truth Today" (*Sam-Kleu*), in 2008. The show was a meant to mobilize Thaksin supporters to oppose the military-installed government and to continue their fight for justice. The show was initially broadcasted on PTV via satellite, then subsequently via DTV. Truth Today was hugely popular and had a mass following, helping to raise the profile of the Trio.

[19] Jatuporn Prompan. Interview. Klong Prem Remand Prison, Bangkok, July 8, 2011.

[20] "We thought we would succeed in pressuring Abhisit to dissolve parliament and we would all go home after a week," reckoned Kamol, head of Red Shirt newspapers, People Channel online. Interview, People Channel headquarter, Bangkok, July 9, 2011.

[21] The Bloody May lasted from March 14 to May 19, 2010.

mass violence that Thailand has experienced. The incidents of Bloody May 2010, however, were instrumental in pushing the Democrat government to call for house dissolution about a year after the protests. Following Abhisit's announcement in early May, the Red Shirts switched gears and retreated from the street and work to campaign for Peau Thai. Nattawut Saikua (2011), one of the UDD's core leaders and also a party-list MP candidate of Peau Thai, said "because of this Peau Thai would win a landslide in *Isan* and the North."

The landslide victory of Peau Thai, sweeping 53 % of the seat shares, was without a doubt due to the strength of its Red Shirt supporters. From political rallies to the dissemination of voter knowledge, the Red Shirts served as a powerful wing of Peau Thai and were instrumental in the Thaksin party's resounding victory. Despite the risk of running afoul of rules that may limit the relationship between the Red Shirts and Peau Thai, the Red Shirts were deeply involved in the campaign. Red Shirt leader and Peau Thai candidate, Jatuporn Prompan, noted that "this election [2011] the Red Shirts are fighting for Peau Thai…the Reds don't take orders from the party…they support the party on their own initiatives. Without the Red Shirts there won't be Peau Thai today."[22] Kwanchai Praipanna, leader of one of the largest UDD subgroups, "We Love Udon Club," echoed similar concerns: "Peau Thai campaign trails are full of Red Shirt supporters[23] and without the Reds Peau Thai would have long been crushed" (Krungthep Turakij 2011, April 27).

The direct and most immediate beneficiaries of the Peau Thai-led coalition government are undoubtedly the Red Shirts. Since Yingluck was sworn in as Thailand's 28th prime minister just a little over a month ago, her party has secured the release of 132 Red Shirts from various prisons throughout the country a priority.[24] In addition, scores of Red Shirt leaders, be it at national or local levels, became MPs themselves and were given advisory positions in the government. Most importantly, Yingluck made it clear from the very onset that her government would seek ways to bring her exiled brother, Thaksin, back to Thailand – a prospect of which looks increasingly plausible.

6 Discussion and Conclusion

Political parties and social movements have different sets of incentives and constraints. Parties are far more bounded by institutional frameworks, such as party regulations and electoral laws, than movements that they would only ally with movements under

[22] Jatuporn Prompan. Interview, Klong Prem Remand Prison, Bangkok, July 8, 2011.

[23] Fieldwork observations, Peau Thai campaign trail in Bangkok, May–June 2011. Many Red Shirt supporters attended every function where Peau Thai candidates would attend. Based on our observations, they often came in groups of more than eight people, wore red, and often had hand clappers with Yingluck photos on.

[24] Note that thus far only those on charges of terrorism have been granted bail – not those on charges of lese majesty.

specific conditions. The organizational structure of the movement matters to the likelihood and degree of the movement's coalition with a political party. Both the Democrat Party and PPP/PTP became closer to the Yellow Shirts and the Red Shirts, respectively, when they were in opposition and both increased their degrees of separation from the movements once in government. Nonetheless, the UDD-PPP/PTP alliance has been far closer than that of the PAD-Democrat counterparts for the reasons outlined above.

The Democrat Party remains a completely separate entity from the Yellow Shirts. The Democrats, the longest established party in Thailand, is first and foremost a party and does not have any established relationships with movements before 2005. Indeed, prior to the current conflict, the last time the Democrats supported a movement was during mass demonstration in 1992 against the coup government of General Suchinda. Yet, even in that case the Democrats stance was very guarded and not fully in line with the movement. In this conflict, however, the party's failure to win elections, particularly after Thaksin was ousted and his party dissolved, along with the growing strength and popularity of the PAD drove the Democrats to seek an alliance with the movement. Constrained by a set of factors as a political party, officially the Democrats cannot endorse the movement. It, thus, sought indirect ways to support, most importantly through financial and mass contribution. The fact that some of the high-profile Democrat MPs moonlighted as the Yellow Shirt vocal supporters was indicative of the extent to which the party was willing to go to achieve its short-term gains. However, as soon as they became government, their stance completely changed. The party could no longer engage in oppositional politics (or should they have to) in the same vein as they did previously. Since the PAD-Democrat alliance was loose and temporary, it was easy for either to create a distance and eventually they parted ways.

On the contrary, the overlapping organizational structure and the shared de facto leader meant that the Red Shirts and the PPP/PTP are tightly linked. The Reds, the majority of whom are Thaksin supporters,[25] could be counted on as a loyal electoral support base. During electoral campaigns, the UDD switched gears to a campaign mode by endorsing Thaksin-backed parties. Despite the risk of running afoul of rules that may limit the relationship between the Red Shirts and Thaksin-aligned parties, the Red Shirts were deeply involved in campaigning. In times of opposition, the Reds engaged in a number of sustained contentious activities, at times violently, to tip the balance of power in favor of Thaksin and his allies. Over time, the grassroot support that underpins the Red Shirt movement along with sustained shared experience of repression and common struggle has both deepened and strengthened the movement. Red Shirt-aligned parties reciprocated to the movement continued support through the promotion of its leaders into political positions, securing some of the movement demands, such as victim compensation. However, the relationship between Peau Thai and its Red Shirt supporters is without challenge. The ties that bind the party and its Red Shirt counterparts have moved beyond the electoral realm.

[25] This statement is confirmed by various interviews with Red Shirt protesters conducted between 2009 and 2011 also Red Shirts' own publication, Singthong (2010).

Increasingly, Red Shirt leaders from national, provincial, and local levels are demanding more from the party in return for their votes. The Reds want Peau Thai to see their electoral support as "conditional," not automatic. Subnational Red Shirt groups are beginning to act like special interest groups – lobbying MPs on behalf of their members.

References

Aeosriwong, N. (2010). *Reading Thai politics 3: The politics of the Red Shirts*. Bangkok: Openbooks.

Almeida, P. (2010). Social movement partyism: Collective action and oppositional political parties. In N. Van Dyke & H. McCammon (Eds.), *Strategic alliances: Coalition building and social movements* (pp. 170–296). Minneapolis: University of Minneapolis Press.

Bangkok Post. (2010, February 23). UDD to hold decisive rally next month. Retrieved February 20, 2012, from: http://www.bangkokpost.com/news/politics/169431/udd-to-hold-mass-rally-next-month

Budge, I., & Laver, M. (1986). Office seeking and policy pursuit in coalition theory. *Legislative Studies Quarterly, 11*(4), 485–506.

Diani, M. (2004). Networks and participation. In D. Snow, S. A. Soule, & H. Kriesi (Eds.), *The Blackwell companion to social movements* (pp. 339–359). Oxford: Blackwell Publishing.

Kasetsiri, C. (2010, May 20). Chanvit points Bloody May incident the worst in 100 years – Protest crackdown by Abhisit only pleased the Bangkokians; Thaksin was involved in torching. *Matichon Online*. Retrieved from http://www.matichon.co.th/news_detail.php?newsid=1274329841&grpid=&catid=01

Katasila, S. (2008). *The big demonstrations*. In PAD press conference 9/2551 (9/2008), Bangkok. Retrieved from: http://www.manager.co.th/Politics/ViewNews.aspx?NewsID=9510000059495

Kitirianglarp, K., & Hewison, K. (2009). Social movements and contemporary political opposition in Thailand. *The Pacific Review, 22*(4), 451–477.

Krungthep Thurakij. (2011, April 27). Jatuporn warns don't view the Red Shirts as nuisance, p. 4.

Limthongkul, S. (2008, November 23). *Guarding the motherland* [TV]. ASTV.

McAdam, D., & Tarrow, S. (2010). Ballots and barricades: On the reciprocal relationship between elections and social movements. *Perspectives on Politics, 8*(2), 529–542.

Mische, A. (2008). *Partisan politics: Communication and contention across Brazilian youth activist networks*. Princeton: Princeton University Press.

Nelson, M. H. (2011, September 19). *Vote No! The PAD's decline from powerful movement to political sect?* Paper presented at the conference on "Five Years after the Military Coup: Thailand's Political Developments since Thaksin's Downfall". Singapore: ISEAS.

PAD. (2008, November 8). *New politics [speech rally]*. Retrieved from: http://www.manager.co.th/Politics/ViewNews.aspx?NewsID=9510000106471

Pinthong, J. (2008, September 29). The health of Thailand (1). *Manager Online*. Retrieved March 2, 2012, from: http://www.manager.co.th/Daily/ViewNews.aspx?NewsID=9510000115447

Pongsawat, P. (2011). *The politics of prai*. Bangkok: Openbooks.

Pongsudhirak, T. (2008). Thailand since the coup. *Journal of Democracy, 19*(4), 140–153.

Raksaseri, K. (2009, April 15). Key dates in Red Shirt rally. *The Nation*. Retrieved March 2, 2012, from: http://www.nationmultimedia.com/2009/04/15/politics/politics_30100554.php

Saikua, N. (2011, May 18). *No title [speech at a Peua Thai rally]*, Lumpini Park, Bangkok.

Songthai, T. (2008). *The officials call us traitors... but we are the people's warriors saving the motherland*. Bangkok: GPP Publication.

Taylor, J. (2011). *Larger than life: 'Central World' and its demise and rebirth – Red Shirts and the creation of an urban cultural myth in Thailand* (Asia Research Institute Working Paper 150).

National University of Singapore. Available online: http://www.ari.nus.edu.sg/docs/wps/wps11_150.pdf
Thabchumpon, N., & McCargo, D. (2011). Urbanized villagers in the 2010 Thai Redshirt protests. *Asian Survey, 51*(6), 993–1018.

Chapter 11
"For King and Country"? Thailand's Political Conflicts as Dynamics of Social Closure

Allan Lee

1 Introduction

For a country with a rich history of social movements,[1] the recent People's Alliance for Democracy (PAD) movement appeared to be different from other social movements in Thailand's history in several respects. Firstly, despite the heterogeneity within the PAD (Pye and Schaffar 2008), a large portion of its support base consists largely of the urban middle class. This differed from the middle-class-led movement in May 1992, which has been touted as an epitome of democratization in Thailand (see Hewison 1996; Pathmanand 2008). Secondly, never has any movement in the country's history resulted in such a drastic political polarization of Thai society. Empirically, the question of why the Bangkok middle class supported such a movement spills over to an important theoretical question of the relationship between class, democracy, and social movements. This chapter, then, aims to address these concerns by advocating a theoretical framework that allows for a more dynamic appreciation of both historical and empirical realities.

Following the 2006 coup d'état, much work has been done on this political conflict (see Tejapira 2006; Ungpakorn 2007; Case 2007; Ockey 2008; Connors 2008; Connors and Hewison 2008; Phongpaichit and Baker 2008b; Pye and

[1] Somchai Phatharathananunth (2006) examined the struggle of the Small Scale Farmers' Assembly of *Isan* (SSFAI) in Northeast Thailand from 1993 to 2002. Consider also Suthy Prasartset (1980) who looked at nongovernmental group's (NGOs) movements in Thailand since 1969 with the establishment of the Thailand Rural Reconstruction Movement (TRRM), the first nongovernmental development group in Thailand. Jim Ockey (2002) highlights the protest of 22 January 1956, arguing that the protest that took to the streets has been forgotten despite its influence in shaping much of the political sphere in Thailand for a couple of decades after the event itself. The point is that Thailand has a rich history of social movements that spans over at least half a century, yet none of them involved the taking over of airports.

A. Lee (✉)
Department of Sociology, Faculty of Arts and Social Sciences, National University of Singapore, 11 Arts Link, Singapore 117570, Singapore
e-mail: allan.lee.al@gmail.com

P. Liamputtong (ed.), *Contemporary Socio-Cultural and Political Perspectives in Thailand*, 169
DOI 10.1007/978-94-007-7244-1_11, © Springer Science+Business Media Dordrecht 2014

Schaffar 2008; Winichakul 2008; Pathmanand 2008; Funston 2009; Kitirianglarp and Hewison 2009; McCargo 2009; Montesano 2009a; Nostitz 2009[2]; see also Chap. 12 in this volume). While these were certainly commendable, there are several points that ought to be addressed. Many have attempted to answer the important questions of why and how the movement emerged: these explanations revolve around two broader themes of intra-elite struggle and Thaksin's corruption. Albritton and Bureekul (2007: 23), for instance, suggest that Thaksin was seen as competing with the king, by "insinuating himself into ceremonies honoring the 60th year of the king's accession to the throne." Similarly, Connors (2007: 252) emphasized that the movement was a consequence of Thaksin attempting to replace the "old power group – a network based around the palace, Prem, elements of the Democrat Party, members of prominent establishment families and senior bureaucrats – with his own network of intimates and associates" (see also Ungpakorn 2009). On the other hand, scholars such as Pongsudhirak (2008: 142) highlight the "controversies, contradictions, and corruption allegations" of Thaksin's administration and how these contributed to the displeasure toward the ex-premier (see also Case 2007; Connors and Hewison 2008; Phongpaichit and Baker 2008b; Pye and Schaffar 2008; Pathmanand 2008; McCargo 2009 for more explanations[3]). See also Chaps. 8, 10, 12, and 13 in this volume.

Next, in conceptualizing the movement as one about democracy, or even royalism, from the onset, I contend that it limits the appreciation of the phenomenon on hand. In other words, the explicit focus on democracy (see Pongsudhirak 2008; Kitirianglarp and Hewison 2009) assumes that the movement had little to do with issues deeply embedded in Thai society, such as class interests. Many authors, popular media, and pundits have tended to assume and refer to *a* middle class – usually understood as occupying the "middle" of the socioeconomic spectrum. This premise confuses and conflates more than it clarifies, by representing the PAD movement as consisting of the Thai middle class. This has left those who are less attuned to the developments of the movement with the notion that the Thai middle class, as a whole, supports the PAD movement.

This (mis)representation of the PAD supporters has, in turn, placed serious limitations on seeing the movement as one for democracy or even royalism.

[2] Kevin Hewison (2010) provides a relatively balanced review of Nostitz's book, noting that while this written account is "not scholarly, [but] nor is it meant to be" (Hewison 2010: 523), it is influential enough to become "a book that anyone who has a serious interest in Thailand's politics should have" (Hewison 2010: 525). It is important to note as well that, as Hewison highlights, Nostitz's account is not "an entirely non-partisan account as he shows sympathy for the red-shirted campaigners" (Hewison 2010: 523). Nevertheless, the attempt to capture the developments of events places it as one of the foremost accounts on the movement to date.

[3] In addition to these articles, others have attempted to offer a perspective that focused on Thaksin's mistakes in isolating the Bangkokians and his policy mistakes (see, for instance, Tejapira 2006; Connors 2007; Hewison 2008; Pongsudhirak 2008; Montesano 2009b). Nevertheless, I maintain that these explanations are seldom divorced from the idea of a conflict of interests between the Thai elites, such as military leaders and the ex-prime minister.

I maintain that this is an unintended consequence of considering class as a set of fixed categories – usually economic ones – rather than a dynamic outcome of social and economic processes, and conflicts. A weakness of this perspective is that we are unable to move beyond understanding class as "mere incumbents of positions, or embodiments of systemic forces" (Parkin 1979: 4). This is especially salient when we consider how the presence of cross-class alliances among members of both the Yellow and Red Shirts does not negate it from being a class conflict, as some scholars have argued (see Montesano 2009a; Nostitz 2009; Prasirtsuk 2010; see also Chaps. 8, 10, 12, and 13 in this volume). It is precisely because there are groups of people from similar socioeconomic status contesting for dissimilar interests that it would be more useful to think of several groups – or *classes* – occupying the "middle" stratum of society. Accordingly, a Weberian perspective of class seems particularly appropriate.

In that light, I maintain that a perspective that privileges the Marxian conceptualization of class hinders us from fully appreciating it as a dynamic concept. More importantly, it limits the appreciation of the Yellow Shirts movement to a matter of intra-elite conflict, overlooking the significance of the participation of the masses. Following Parkin's (1979: 13) argument that "the relations between classes are to be understood as 'aspects of the distribution of power,'" this chapter proposes a neo-Weberian perspective be included alongside the predominant Marxian stance in examining political conflict in Thai society. In essence, this chapter suggests two things: first, that a neo-Weberian stance offers us constructive insights to appreciating the concatenation of political conflicts in Thai society, and, second, that the recent PAD movement can be understood as an attempt by particular groups of people to secure their interests in response to the social exclusion experienced. This chapter presents a more nuanced understanding of the dynamics between the military, monarchy, and capitalist groups – key actors in the Thai political sphere – as well as the masses, allowing for the involvement of actors from various social positions in society to be included in this struggle for social, economic, and political inclusion. In doing so, I suggest that the occurrences of social movements and political conflict reflect the process of class formation in Thailand as members from various strata of society attempt to consolidate and solidify their social positions, as we shall see.

In other words, this chapter aims to utilize and apply the concept of "social closure" to making sense of the political conflict throughout Thailand's history as well as the recent movements.

2 The Efficacy of "Social Closure" as Theoretical Framework

A Weberian paradigm sees classes and social groups being connected within the sphere of power and attached to the important notion of the distribution of power. For Weber, multiple overlapping dimensions of wealth, power, and prestige determine social stratification (Gerth and Mills 1958). In fact, "the term 'class' refers to any group of people that is found in the same class situation" (Gerth and Mills 1958: 181). Simply put, people displaying similar lifestyle patterns and occupational class and who enjoy similar prestige and privilege constitute members of the same class.

In addition, Weber (1978) argues that there are three features of class: economic interest, life chances, and markets (see also Gerth and Mills 1958). The concept of *interest* is especially useful for not only does it "create[s] 'class'" (Weber 1978: 928), but it is among the "most fundamental and universal components" of human behavior (Weber 1978: 601). Furthermore,

> the concept of divergent sectional 'interests' cannot be limited to economic interests, but must be extended to other spheres of social life. Thus political parties, for example, have interests which derive from their situation as aspirants to, or as wielders of, power, and such interests do not necessarily rest upon shared class situations. (Giddens 1971: 195)

The concept of status groups – defined by the specific lifestyle shared by members of the group – is especially relevant for it not only makes up the social order but is determined by the distribution of social honor. Rather than rely on economic indicators, such as income, occupation, and assets, in stratifying society, status groups consider noneconomic qualities such as political power too. In short, status groups allow us to integrate social, economic, and political power into determining one's social position. More significantly, Weber says that entry into these status groups is often restricted, what he calls *social closure*.

This concept has been elaborated on by Parkin (1979: 44–45) who conceptualizes this process as an exclusionary relationship in which

> social collectivities seek to maximize rewards by restricting access to resources and opportunities to a limited circle of eligibles…securing for itself a privileged position at the expense of some other group through a process of subordination.

Parkin also notes that any group attribute may be emphasized for

> the monopolization of specific, usually economic opportunities. This monopolization is directed against competitors who share some positive or negative characteristics; its purpose is always the closure of social and economic opportunities to *outsiders*. (emphasis in original)

Just as dominant groups seek to exclude others in order to preserve their advantage, groups who have been dispossessed will also attempt to amass opportunities for themselves (see Tilly 1998). In doing so, Parkin (1979: 74) suggests that groups in such an outsider position will mount "usurpationary actions" with "the aim of biting into the resources and benefits accruing to dominant groups in society." For Parkin, "usurpationary closure tends to rely on the public mobilization of members and supporters, as in the use of strikes, demonstrations, sit-ins, marches…and the like."

This concept is especially useful if we were to reexamine the historico-political antecedents in Thai society where we will find important players attempting to exclude and usurp both power and opportunities in the political arena.

3 Social Closure in Thai Political History

From the onset, the fall of absolute monarchy at the start of the 1930s paved the way for a political sphere that has been characterized by the frequent involvement of the military, coups d'état, and the wrestling of power between the army and the state. Led by a group of Western-educated military officers and civilian bureaucrats (Leow 2002), the absolute monarchy was overthrown in the name of democracy in 1932 (Jumbala and Banpasirichote 2001) and came to bolster the political and economic power of Bangkok (Glassman 2010). The royalists did not remain silent, however, following the fall of the absolute monarchy. In fact, they fought for a monarch[4] with as much power as possible within the framework of democracy, albeit with little success (Winichakul 2008). Yet by 1938, the military was, more or less, in full control and began introducing authoritarian policies, this time under the leadership of Plaek Phibunsongkhram (Hewison 1996). The fall of the monarchy ushered in a new economic and political era for Thailand. By the end of the 1930s, Thailand had a well-established "commercialization, monetization, and commodification of the economy" despite not having a full-fledged capitalist system (Hewison 2006: 83). This paved the way for the eventual emergence of the domestic capitalists.

The fear of a growing Chinese-dominated business class, coupled with the potential threat to sovereignty, led Phibun to adopt a "nationalist clientelism" (Ramsay 2001: 61) approach to address this concern. Apart from closing down Chinese-language schools and the mandatory taking of Thai names by Chinese in Thailand, anti-Chinese economic policies were imposed as well (Ramsay 2001). By the end of World War II, the culminated effects of the world depression which forced many Western businesses to withdraw from the country left the Sino-Thais with even more economic influence (Ramsay 2001) while Thailand's economy fell behind the rest of Southeast Asia. The economic surplus remained in the hands of a small group of economic elites – including the Sino-Thai businessmen as well as the "old nobility, tiny new segment of businessmen, professionals and officials" (Phongpaichit and Baker 2008a). Comprising a small proportion of Thai population, this group of elites came to take firm control of Thai economy, controlling the financial and industrial sectors (Hewison 1993). Due to the prevailing animosity toward the Chinese, this group did not, or could not, as a "class," "effectively or adequately control the state and its apparatuses" as the economic and political condition limited the growth of this group after World War II (Turton 1984: 29). This enmity left them fairly small, limiting their wealth as well as political influence (Anderson 1990). With the military government in charge, little protection was given to domestic capital as business families had to subject themselves to the patronage of political

[4] In Thongchai Winichakul's talk entitled "Thailand's Crisis and the Rise of Asia," delivered on June 7, 2011, he made the distinction between monarchy – which he defined as the "network monarchy" (McCargo 2005) – and monarch, referring to King Bhumibol. In this chapter, I borrow these definitions as well to differentiate the various actors. Specifically, in this chapter "monarch" refers to HM King Bhumibol and "monarchy" refers to the institution.

leaders in order to negotiate individual protection (Phongpaichit and Baker 2008a). The Phibun regime eventually faced challenges in 1956 when thousands took to the streets. This incident was touted as a victory for democracy for it signaled that the people were ready to exercise their views and political power (see Ockey 2002). While he was to remain in power for two more years, General Sarit, with the support of students, the monarchy, and the Democrat Party, carried out a coup that finally removed Phibun from power in 1957[5] (Ockey 2002).

This event was to be, in Chaloemitiarana's (1978) opinion, the most important event in the revitalization of the monarchy as it not only marked the removal of the men behind the 1932 revolution but also meant that Sarit, one of the first leaders since 1932 to consistently and consciously build up the monarchy's prestige, was back in a prominent position. The king, concerned about the threat of communism and anti-royalist opinions, allied himself to the military and demonstrated this visibly – dressing in military uniform and adopting the role of the natural leader of the military for instance. The military reciprocated by incessantly promoting the royal family through the celebration of its deeds and highly publicized events (see also Handley 2006; Hewison 2008). Throughout this period, the Chinese business class, perhaps still struggling with the prevailing hostility against them, remained small and lacked substantial political influence (Anderson 1990).

With the influx of foreigners and accompanying investment due to increasing globalization, Thailand began experiencing economic growth and unprecedented modernization in the 1960s (Maisrikrod 1997). The resultant economic growth drastically changed the sociodemographic conditions of Thai society, posing challenges to the authoritarian regime (Ockey 2004). As the economy developed, the demand for education grew alongside the expansion of the middle class that had emerged as a result of the economic boom (Ockey 2004; see also Hewison 1996; Robison and Goodman 1996). These changes meant that politics could not remain authoritarian for long, as the capitalists rode on the new economic wave and capitalized on the government's policy and developed various industries.

The open economy was also "beneficial to democratization" as it threatened to subvert authoritarian repression of democratic ideals (Laothamatas 1996 cited in Jumbala and Banpasirichote 2001). As the economy opened up, the new Thai middle class, emergent from the growing economy, joined private corporations or became entrepreneurs instead of joining the civil service as they had previously done. This departure from government employment, coupled with the liberalization of Thailand's economy, strengthened both the middle class and bourgeoisie class, paving the way for the alliance between these classes in the 1980s. Overall, the development and growth of the economy furthered the cause of the capitalists through the economic expansion as well as the political influence of the business group, securing further protection from the state.

---

[5] Sarit was seen as having cynically manipulated public opinion through his criticism of "dirty elections" and then installed a regime that did away with most of the political system completely (Chaloemitiarana 1978).

By the turn of the decade, the influence of the capitalists had grown, gaining ground in economic policy-making and becoming politically independent and assertive. The relationship between the state and capital was now forced to find a new balance while taking into account the sociodemographic changes in Thai society (Maisrikrod 1997). At the same time, the military appeared to be testing the king's authority when it killed off the parliament the king had pushed for 3 years earlier in 1968. This incident demonstrated the extent to which the monarch had actually cared about democracy – for "while the king had pushed for constitution in 1968, he 'did little to enhance the legitimacy and status of the elected parliament, participant politics…or the institutions created to implement Thai-style democracy…leaving the parliament exposed and vulnerable to…the military'" (Morell 1974, cited in Hewison 2008: 197).

Up until the end of the 1960s, the military, monarchy, and the business "class" had experienced several forms of exclusion, largely as a consequence and result of socioeconomic developments in the region. Nevertheless, the relationship between these historic actors has only gotten more entwined as each attempts to secure economic and political power through various means. The domination of the military and the monarchy, as well as its supporters, in the political sphere had begun to accommodate the rise of the capitalists who had been in control of the economy, effectively sharing a piece of the pie with them. While this tripartite relationship has achieved a dedicated balance, it was in the early 1970s that the scale was tipped, paving the way for an era of social movements that sought to exclude one or more party, with the other attempting to usurp power and gain access to the exclusive political and economic spheres.

The 1973 student-led movement was an attempt to overthrow the Thanom-led regime that had been in power since 1963 (see Leow 2002; Anderson 1990). This demonstrated how the exclusion of the "new middle class" has come to be seen in the attempts of usurpationary actions, usually undertaken by the marginalized and excluded. The impetus behind the 1973 movement was the demand for an immediate "promulgation of a new democratic constitution" (Neher 1975: 1103). The implications of such a proliferation of democracy meant not only a conceding of power by those in power but also the adoption of liberal-democratic agenda – including an autonomous parliamentary system, safeguarding of human rights, the decentralization of power, media freedom, and unbiased economic policy (Phongpaichit 2004).

Most significant during the Cold War era of the 1970s was the recognition that a military dictatorship would pose more danger, not only to the public but to the economy as well. Members of the capitalist group then orchestrated a democratization project (Phongpaichit 2004). Not only did this mark the division of the military-capitalist alliance that had emerged post-World War II, the breakdown of the alliance also signaled the advent of the economic middle class as a strong political actor (Maisrikrod 1997) and ushered in a period of political instability as elections failed to produce stable governments (Connors and Hewison 2008). Another important development was the growth of the economic middle class and the intellectuals along with the deteriorating strength of the military dictatorship as its legitimacy began to erode. The domestic capitalists thus distanced themselves from the army and aligned themselves to the foreign investors who were adverse to the military's style of governance. This also meant the capitalists adopted a position that placed them on the side of the middle class as this new alliance fought for a democratic regime – one that essentially espoused an anti-military sentiment (Maisrikrod 1997). The military was on the verge of being gradually edged out of the Thai political sphere.

However, the espousal of socialist thoughts among the intelligentsia led to fear among the capitalists, who were quick to re-embrace the capitalist system and maintain the status quo, putting an end to the alliance between the capitalists and intellectuals (Maisrikrod 1997). The resultant consequence of this episode was the ideological polarization of Thai politics between the radicals, allegedly out to demolish the national pillars of "nation, religion, and king" (Maisrikrod 1997; see also Niels 2000), on the one hand, and the conservatives, who mobilized the bureaucrats and other religious groups, on the other. The events of this period demonstrated the shift of Thai politics away from the elites to include the middle class. Furthermore, it illustrates the presence of important social groups acting and interacting in Thai society, contesting and asserting different forms of power in an attempt to exclude other players. Anderson (1990: 23) sums this up by noting that this period bears witness to the emergence of parliamentary democracy whereby "ambitious, prosperous and self-confident bourgeoisies feel most comfortable, precisely because it maximizes their power and minimizes that of their competitors."

After 1977, the military continued to exert strong political influence, albeit within a parliamentary framework as Thailand was led by a constitutional and parliamentary regime under the leadership of former military leaders, the most prominent was General Prem Tinsulanonda who was appointed to the position of prime minister in 1980 (Cohen 1991), and the nation entered an era of "semi-democracy" (Girling 1996), otherwise known as "Premocracy." Given the control the military had, political stability and economic growth were accorded greater priority during this period as well (Girling 1996). Although the inclination toward an authoritarian regime was present, Prem chose a conservative style of leadership, one that was acceptable to most of Thai society, and displayed much loyalty to the king, gaining important royal support.

In April 1981, Prem was involved in the suppression of a coup staged by a section of the Thai military – known as the Young Turks – who commanded a significant segment of the armed forces (Cohen 1991; Leow 2002). This faction consisted of younger, lower-ranking field officers who embraced a more radical belief in the Thai military's role in saving the nation and advocating socioeconomic reform – in particular, a full democratic system – under the leadership of the military, not the civilian government (Sirikrai 1982; Leow 2002). Supposedly, it was the internal politics within the military – specifically the rumored transfer of the Young Turks to less significant posts – that sparked off the coup (see Sirikrai 1982). With the lack of support from higher-ranking officials, students, intellectuals, and workers, the coup failed to gather sufficient momentum and was easily contained. An important repercussion of the failed coup was the resulting schism within the Thai army into two main opposing groups led by General Amnart Damrikarn and Major General Arthit Kamlang-ek, the latter having a crucial role in defeating the coup attempt in 1981. However, Amnart's influence continued to pose a serious threat to Arthit's power until his untimely death. Despite the demise of his main rival, Arthit persisted in his efforts to weed out the Young Turks and securing his own position. In a bid to conciliate the factions within the military, Prem called for an election in April 1983 where he was reappointed as the prime minister. The army again opposed constitutional clauses that would have accorded more power to political parties (Cohen 1991).

Overall, the Prem era ushered in both political stability and economic growth, demonstrating the ability of Prem's "grand alliance" – a "new class formation" consisting of capitalists, state bureaucrats and military officers, intellectuals, professional groups, and technocrats – in affecting the power balance of the state (Surin 1997). The Thai political sphere, for the first time, saw businesspeople running for, and winning, parliamentary seats during this period as vote-buying began to spread widely as a means of mobilizing electoral support (Maisrikrod 1997; see also King and LoGerfo 1996). This period also saw the entry of young, well-educated and politically idealistic middle class into influential roles in Thai politics, some of which had migrated to Bangkok from the rural areas. This was especially significant as their presence meant that they were no longer under a feudalistic-authoritarian state apparatus and more importantly, they say saw democracy as an accessible tool to express their opposition against state power (Maisrikrod 1997).

In short, while Prem and his alliance effectively controlled both the economy and the state, the idealistic new middle class continued to pose political opposition from time to time. This was especially so in the late 1980s and early 1990s where the middle class began to demand their inclusion into the system. Prem's "grand alliance," by virtue of its exclusionary nature, had failed to incorporate the politically volatile middle class during its sovereignty. This led to pressures from the middle class who wanted to be included. It did not help that Prem's view of democracy was merely a show of tokenism, with his perceived contempt for democratic institutions and a lack of commitment to the ideology of democracy (Maisrikrod 1997). It was no surprise, then, that the populist Chart Thai Party, fronted by General Chatichai Choonhavan, was elected into power in the 1988 elections.

It was because Chatichai's party's stance coincided with the prodemocratic middle class' scheme that he was able to ride on that wave to power (Maisrikrod 1997). Furthermore, the rise of Chatichai rested largely upon the prevalent anti-Prem, prodemocracy sentiment of that time, which was so strong that practically anybody in parliament could be accepted as the prime minister. In other words, support for Chatichai was, in part, an effort to usurp power, albeit democratically, away from Prem's "grand alliance."

However, the Chatichai government was inundated with blatant corruption – earning the name of a "buffet cabinet" (Maisrikrod 1997; also in Hewison 1993). The parochialism within the Chatichai government – where *jao poh* (or godfathers) and local influential people were dominant (Maisrikrod 1997: 161) – sought to consolidate public power and wealth among members of the "alliance" and contributed to an overarching atmosphere of disdain among the middle class (Maisrikrod 1997; also in Hewison 1993). What infuriated the people even more was Chatichai's final reorganization of the cabinet, which further promoted the financial interests of the various coalition members while marginalizing those who are not part of the group even more (Hewison 1993; Maisrikrod 1997). This led to the eventual downfall of Chatichai just 2 years and 7 months after he first ascended into premiership as a new political alliance emerged. This coalition consisted mainly of state bureaucrats and "enlightened capitalists," but was legitimated by the middle class (Maisrikrod 1997; see also Jumbala and Banpasirichote 2001). It should be noted here, though, that there were variations among the middle class as up until the mid-1980s; they, on the whole, benefited greatly from the export-oriented growth under the Chatichai government. Nonetheless, the military quickly capitalized on the prevailing discontent and staged a coup in February 1991 (Neher 1992; King and LoGerfo 1996; Leow 2002). Support for the coup, as Hewison (1996) notes, was an attack on the Chatichai government that was seen as threatening the balance constituting the state and the political space. More importantly, the coup represented also the manifestation of "inter-clique rivalry[6]" as well as an attempt to reinforce the military's increasingly archaic position in relation to the advent of the new middle class (Hewison 1996).

Following the coup, the National Peace Keeping Council (NPKC) set up an interim government led by Anand Panyarachun (Leow 2002). However, it was the council that held onto the power while preparation was made for the elections in March (Hewison 1993). During that election, many pro-military parties as well as opposition parties participated, but it was the former that won, putting Narong Wongwan in the prime minister seat (Leow 2002). However, Narong's past returned to haunt him and cost him the support of the military (King 1992). The subsequent nomination of General Suchinda Kraprayoon by the military leaders faced much criticism from the public as it indicated a return to military rule (King 1992). More importantly, it was a direct violation of Suchinda's earlier promise that things would be turned back over to the civilians to resume democracy with new leadership.

While the vocal and aggressive middle-business class alliance that brought Chatichai down earlier played a similarly significant role in opposing the Suchinda regime in May 1992 (Maisrikrod 1997; Jumbala and Banpasirichote 2001), it is important to note that for certain groups within the middle class, economic growth and democracy were the perfect complements and the 1991 coup only interrupted this progression. For them, the coup had direct and undesirable impact on the middle class' economic interests. Thus, the appointing of Suchinda became the tipping point in a long process of the military manipulating its dominance in politics. Consequently, the middle class rode on the prevailing "democratization" wave and

[6] The 1991 coup was widely recognized as, partly, a result of conflict between different cohorts of graduates of the Chulachomklao Royal Military Academy, starting as early as in the 1980 and finally culminating in a major division between the military and the government. In addition, leaders of the National Peace Keeping Council (NPKC), which staged the coup, were known to have concrete political ideas and ambitions and wanted a larger share of the corruption pie (King 1992); Pathmanand 2008).

opposed the military-appointed Suchinda government. In other words, democracy was not the end point. Instead, members of this middle class advocated democracy insofar as it provided the political stability and economic development that they desired. Ultimately, the middle class was fighting to protect the source of its privileges – capitalism and development (Jumbala and Banpasirichote 2001).

It was no surprise, then, that the May 1992 uprising – also known as the "Black May" incident – came to be seen as a revolution of the middle and business classes. Popular images from the protests depicted wealthy demonstrators – some carrying mobile phones and arriving in cars (Jumbala and Banpasirichote 2001) – taking to the streets and challenging armed troops (Hewison 1996). From a political viewpoint, it implied that classes that emerged during the postwar economic growth were driving Thai sociopolitical change. Also, the protest appeared to be a revolt against a "conservative, authoritarian, technocratic, and military-dominated coterie" in order to reinstate legitimate political space and a democratic parliamentary system (Hewison 1996). Indeed, it is easy to overlook the underlying workings behind the rise of the middle class against the government and simply regard it as a movement for democracy.

Following the violent suppression of demonstrations, another election was scheduled in September 1992. This time, Chuan Leekpai emerged victorious. The triumph of a civilian government confirmed the end of military rule in Thailand (Leow 2002). While this meant that the military elites no longer dominated politics directly, they maintain firm influence in the area of national defense and security while the ties between them and their associates in the business sector remained intact (Bunbongkarn 1996). However, soon after the Chuan administration assumed office, they faced accusations of having abused a land distribution scheme in Phuket (King 1996). With increasing pressure from the media – an institution owned by the business class – and the lack of support from its own coalition members, Chuan's government was eventually brought down in May 1995 (Phongpaichit and Baker 1997) after the parliament was dissolved. A subsequent snap election was scheduled for July 1995 (King 1996). That particular election saw extensive vote-buying despite efforts from the Poll Watch Committee to curb such actions (King 1996). Eventually, Banharn Silpa-archa became the new prime minster. However, almost as soon as he and his cabinet took office, criticisms began to surface – again, from the privately owned media – claiming that they lacked the technical expertise and qualifications, claiming "infighting among and within government coalition parties" as well as criticizing Banharn's lack of international stature and sophistication (King 1996: 137). Meanwhile, shuffles were made within the military as the Defense Minister Chavalit Yongchaiyudh balanced out the internally competing factions (King 1996). On the one hand, it demonstrated the extent of civilian control over the military. On the other hand, this was in largely motivated by Chavalit's attempt to build up support for himself among the military officers as he prepared for a shot at the premiership in the future (King 1996). True enough, Chavalit took the premiership in the November 1996 election after increasing pressure and conflict within Banharn's coalition took its toll on the Banharn's government, forcing him to resign (King 1996). Chavalit did not last long, however, due to a combination of the Asian economic crisis in 1997 and his failure to manage the country in the midst of the financial crisis (Punyaratabandhu 1998), and Chuan regained the seat of prime minister. It was toward the end of this decade of political instability that Thaksin's Thai Rak Thai (TRT) Party was formed and eventually rose to power (see also Chaps. 10, 12, and 13).

4 Social Closure Under Thaksin's Regime

Broadly speaking, Thaksin's populist policies that resonated with and benefitted the poor meant that they were no longer marginalized. As witnessed by the power of Thaksin's supporters to reelect him into power in the 2005 elections, the implication of this support was that the middle class' votes no longer carried as much influence as it used to. Thaksin's populist policies which translated into mass support and manifested in election votes (see Pongsudhirak 2008; Phongpaichit and Baker 2009) meant that politically and socially, the rural poor were gaining more recognition and regard by Thaksin's government. Politically, the middle class had suffered a minor setback in exerting its voice; economically, it could neither transform its economic wealth to political or social power, nor could it depend on political support to attain economic success. This loss of social and political power together with the declining economy was indicative of the exclusion the middle class was to be subjected to. It also was evident that Thaksin and his associates were beginning to enforce some social closure on the economic and political power they had access to. But, because access to economic and political opportunities was still available to the masses, support for Thaksin's party remained fairly stable and strong: those in the rural areas appreciated his policies, while the middle class seemed satisfied with the actions taken in the handling of the uprising in the South and against alleged drug dealers at that time (Phongpaichit and Baker 2009).

It was acts of nepotism that signaled Thaksin's increasing monopolization of the political domain. With growing dominance and influence, backed by supporters in the military and the police, Thaksin began attacking his critics and gaining control of sections of the media. The extent of his power became further evident in the way he responded to criticisms, using state power unabashedly and treating his opponents with contempt (Hewison 2008; see also Case 2007). Not only was Thaksin monopolizing political power through his influence in the economy, but he was also hoarding alternative voices to his rule (see Chap. 12).

The support from the middle class began to decline when the low-income group was clearly benefitting more from the various populist policies designed and implemented by Thaksin. These include the famous 30 Baht universal healthcare, the one million village investment development funds, cheap loans, and other policies that were extremely popular with the electorate (McCargo 2002; see also Charoensin-o-larn 2009; Funston 2009). Having found that they gained nothing from these policies but were paying taxes to support them, the middle class became more alienated by these policies (Phongpaichit and Baker 2008b). In short, not only were they beginning to be excluded from the political sphere, opportunities for them to voice their discontent were also dominated by Thaksin.

This control over political and economic policies not only restricted the access of resources and opportunities available to groups not within Thaksin's circle but was, arguably, also the source by which he secured the position of privilege at the expense of everyone else. Thaksin's "policy corruption," for instance, was clearly aimed at benefitting his personal concerns and those closest to him (Phongpaichit and Baker 2009; Montesano 2009c). Perhaps the most appropriate of examples is the sale of Shin Corporation immediately following the raising of the limit on foreign ownership of telecommunications firms from 25 to 49 % (Montesano 2009b). In essence, through his control over the state, media, and economy, Thaksin effectively limited the ability of key groups in Thai society from influencing politics and opposing him. His dominance over the economy, coupled by his power to change economic policies, kept the businessmen in check; his control of public space placed a limit on the extent by which independent media and intellectuals could question him or his policies; his authority in the state allowed him to control bureaucrats through both position and tradition (Phongpaichit and Baker 2008b). This thorough monopoly meant that in order for any groups – be it the capitalists, economic, or affective middle class – to obtain a share of the economic and political pie, usurpationary actions, such as social movements, were the best option available. In sum, Thaksin effectively enforced a social closure, alienating and excluding of groups in this social stratum.

Groups in the middle class were not the only ones to be excluded. Thaksin's tendency to appoint his cronies into seats of power meant that the old power group – "a network based around the palace, Prem, elements of the Democrat Party, members of prominent establishment families and senior bureaucrats" (Connors 2007: 252) – was slowly but surely being pushed to the periphery as well. This increasing monopolization of political and economic spheres by Thaksin and the resulting exclusion of the middle class, as well as other groups in Thai society, demonstrate clearly the conditions for mobilization through dissent.

5 Conclusion

The interplay of power among the key players in Thai politics remains deeply intertwined and demonstrates the dynamics of social closure through exclusion by those in power and social closure through usurpation by those marginalized as a consequence of this exclusion. Given the history of Thai politics, it is easy to view the 2006 coup as yet another instance of struggle within the military and the capitalists. However, in highlighting the heterogeneity within each class – such as the middle class which featured strongly in the late 1980s and throughout the 1990s and the division of the military following Prem's rise to the premiership – this chapter suggests that Thai politics has more to do with struggle by groups in society trying to secure or improve their own advantages. To this end, democracy then becomes an ideological tool to legitimize the advancement of both these interests.

In short, this chapter has demonstrated how social closure is a relevant and useful analytical framework for the study of Thai politics for two reasons: first, its ability to incorporate both historical antecedents of political conflict in Thailand, as shown above. Second, in considering the dynamic struggle between forces of exclusion and monopolization on the one hand, and the forces of usurpation and opportunity hoarding on the other, as in the case of the PAD, the movement itself can be understood as a contemporary manifestation of class conflict and contestation in Thai society. More importantly, it allows for the inclusion of existing arguments of the movement being an intra-elite conflict precisely by showing that such conflicts are a result of groups contesting for power, resources, and opportunities. In other words, it explains contestations within and between social strata in society. With this in mind, studies on Thai politics are best appreciated not with a categorical understanding of class but with employing a paradigm that allows for both nuances and dynamism of class interests.

References

Albritton, R. B., & Thawilwadee, B. (2007). Thailand country report: Public opinion and political power in Thailand. In *Asian Barometer: A comparative survey of democracy, governance and development* (Working Paper Series: No. 34). http://www.asianbarometer.org/newenglish/publications/workingpapers/no.34.pdf

Anderson, B. (1990). Murder and progress in modern Siam. *New Left Review, 181*, 13–30.

Bunbongkarn, S. (1996). *State of the nation: Thailand.* Singapore: Institute of Southeast Asian Studies.

Case, W. (2007). Democracy's quality and breakdown: New lessons from Thailand. *Democratization, 14*(4), 622–642.

Chaloemitiarana, T. (Ed.). (1978). *Thai politics: Extracts and documents 1932–1957*. Bangkok: Social Science Association of Thailand.

Charoensin-o-larn, C. (2009). Military coup and democracy in Thailand. In J. Funston (Ed.), *Divided over Thaksin: Thailand's coup and problematic transition* (pp. 49–79). Singapore: Institute of Southeast Asian Studies.

Cohen, E. (1991). *Thai society in comparative perspective*. Thailand: White Lotus.

Connors, M. K. (2007). *Democracy and national identity in Thailand* (2nd ed.). Copenhagen: Nordic Institute of Asian Studies Press.

Connors, M. K. (2008). Article of faith: The failure of royal liberalism in Thailand. *Journal of Contemporary Asia, 38*(1), 143–165.

Connors, M. K., & Hewison, K. (2008). Introduction: Thailand and the 'good coup'. *Journal of Contemporary Asia, 38*(1), 1–10.

Funston, J. (2009). Introduction. In J. Funston (Ed.), *Divided over Thaksin: Thailand's coup and problematic transition* (pp. xiii–xxi). Singapore: Institute of Southeast Asian Studies.

Gerth, H., & Mills, C. W. (1958). *From Max Weber: Essays in sociology*. New York: Oxford University Press.

Giddens, A. (1971). *Capitalism and modern social theory: An analysis of the writings of Marx, Durkheim and Max Weber*. Cambridge: Cambridge University Press.

Girling, J. L. S. (1996). *Interpreting development: Capitalism, democracy, and the middle class in Thailand.* Ithaca: Cornell Southeast Asia Program.

Glassman, J. (2010). 'Provinces elect Governments, Bangkok overthrows them': Urbanity, class and post-democracy. *Urban Studies, 47*(6), 1301–1323.

Handley, P. (2006). *The King never smiles: A biography of Thailand's Bhumibol Adulyadej*. New Haven: Yale University Press.
Hewison, K. (1993). Of regimes, state and pluralities: Thai politics enters the 1990s. In K. Hewison, R. Robison, & G. Rodan (Eds.), *Southeast Asian in the 1990s* (pp. 161–189). Sydney: Allen & Unwin.
Hewison, K. (1996). Political oppositions and regime change in Thailand. In G. Rodan (Ed.), *Political oppositions in industrializing Asia* (pp. 72–94). London: Routledge.
Hewison, K. (2006). Thailand: Boom, bust, and recovery. In G. Rodan, K. Hewison, & R. Robison (Eds.), *The political economy of South-East Asia: Markets, power and contestation* (pp. 74–108). South Melbourne: Oxford University Press.
Hewison, K. (2008). A book, the King and the 2006 coup. *Journal of Contemporary Asia, 38*(1), 190–211.
Hewison, K. (2010). Book review: Red vs. Yellow. Volume 1: Thailand's crisis of identity. *Journal of Contemporary Asia, 40*(3), 522–525.
Jumbala, P., & Banpasirichote, C. (2001). Thai middle classes: Class ambiguity and democratic propensity. In A. R. Embang (Ed.), *Southeast Asian middle classes: Propensity for social change and democratization* (pp. 262–291). Bandar Baru Bangi: Penerbit Universiti Kebangsaan Malaysia.
King, D. (1992). The Thai Parliamentary elections of 1992: Return to democracy in an atypical year. *Asian Survey, 32*(12), 1109–1123.
King, D. (1996). Thailand in 1995: Open society, dynamic economy, troubled politics. *Asian Survey, 36*(2), 135–141.
King, D., & LoGerfo, J. (1996). Thailand: Toward democratic stability. *Journal of Democracy, 7*(1), 102–117.
Kitirianglarp, K., & Hewison, K. (2009). Social movements and political opposition in contemporary Thailand. *The Pacific Review, 22*(4), 451–477.
Leow, L. Y. S. (2002). *Comparative democratization: Elite, civil society and transition process in Thailand and Philippines*. Academic exercise, Department of Political Science, Faculty of Arts and Social Sciences, National University of Singapore.
Maisrikrod, S. (1997). The making of Thai democracy: A study of political alliances among the state, the capitalists, and the middle class. In A. Laothamatas (Ed.), *Democratization in Southeast and East Asia* (pp. 141–166). Singapore: Institute of Southeast Asian Studies.
McCargo, D. (2002). Thailand's January 2001 general elections: Vindicating reform? In D. McCargo (Ed.), *Reforming Thai politics* (pp. 247–260). Copenhagen: Nordic Institute of Asian Studies.
McCargo, D. (2005). Network monarchy and legitimacy crises in Thailand. *The Pacific Review, 18*(4), 499–519.
McCargo, D. (2009). Thai politics as reality TV. *The Journal of Asian Studies, 68*(1), 7–19.
Montesano, M. (2009a, April). *Defending the monarchy: Why and how?* (Asia Research Institute: Working Paper Series, No. 114). Singapore: Asia Research Institute.
Montesano, M. (2009b). Political contests in the advent of Bangkok's 19 September putsch. In J. Funston (Ed.), *Divided over Thaksin: Thailand's coup and problematic transition* (pp. 1–26). Singapore: Institute of Southeast Asian Studies.
Montesano, M. (2009c). Contextualizing the Pattaya summit debacle: Four April days, four Thai pathologies. *Contemporary Southeast Asia, 31*(2), 217–248.
Neher, C. D. (1975). Stability and instability in contemporary Thailand. *Asian Survey, 15*(12), 1097–1113.
Neher, C. D. (1992). Political development and political participation in Thailand. In M. L. Cohen (Ed.), *Asia: Case studies in the social sciences: A guild for teaching* (pp. 414–426). Armonk: M.E. Sharpe.
Niels, M. (2000). *Inside Thai society: Religion, everyday life. Change*. Chiang Mai: Silkworm Books.
Nostitz, N. (2009). *Red vs. Yellow*. Bangkok: White Lotus Press.
Ockey, J. (2002). Civil society and street politics in historical perspective. In D. McCargo (Ed.), *Reforming Thai politics* (pp. 107–123). Copenhagen: Nordic Institute of Asian Studies.

Ockey, J. (2004). *Making democracy: Leadership, class, gender and political participation in Thailand*. Honolulu: University of Hawaii Press.
Ockey, J. (2008). Thailand in 2007: The struggle to control democracy. *Asian Survey, 48*(1), 20–28.
Parkin, F. (1979). *Marxism and class theory: A bourgeois critique*. London: Tavistock Publications.
Pathmanand, U. (2008). A different coup d'etat? *Journal of Contemporary Asia, 38*(1), 124–142.
Phatharathananunth, S. (2006). *Civil society and democratization: social movements in Northeast Thailand*. Copenhagen: Nias Press.
Phongpaichit, P. (2004). *Thailand under Thaksin: Another Malaysia*? (Asia Research Centre Working Paper, No. 109). Perth: Murdoch University.
Phongpaichit, P., & Baker, C. (1997). *Thailand economy and politics*. New York: Oxford University Press.
Phongpaichit, P., & Baker, C. (Eds.). (2008a). *Thai capital: After the 1997 crisis*. Singapore: Institute of Southeast Asian Studies.
Phongpaichit, P., & Baker, C. (2008b). Thaksin's populism. *Journal of Contemporary Asia, 38*(1), 62–83.
Phongpaichit, P., & Baker, C. (2009). *Thaksin* (2nd ed.). Thailand: Silkworm.
Pongsudhirak, T. (2008). Thailand since the coup. *Journal of Democracy, 19*(4), 140–153.
Prasartset, S. (1980). *Thai business leaders: Men and careers in a developing economy*. Tokyo: Institute of Developing Economies.
Prasirtsuk, K. (2010). Thailand in 2009. *Asian Survey, 50*(1), 203–210.
Punyaratabandhu, S. (1998). Thailand in 1997: Financial crisis and constitutional reform. *Asian Survey, 38*(2), 161–167.
Pye, O., & Schaffar, W. (2008). The 2006 anti-Thaksin movement in Thailand: An analysis. *Journal of Contemporary Asia, 38*(1), 38–61.
Ramsay, A. (2001). The Chinese in Thailand: Ethnicity, power, and cultural opportunity structures. In G. H. Cornwell & E. W. Stoddard (Eds.), *Global multiculturalism: Comparative perspectives on ethnicity, race, and nation* (pp. 51–72). Lanham: Rowman & Littlefield.
Robison, R., & Goodman, D. S. G. (1996). The new rich in Asia: Economic development, social status and political consciousness. In R. Robison & D. S. G. Goodman (Eds.), *The new rich in Asia: Mobile phones, McDonalds and middle-class revolution* (pp. 1–16). London: Routledge.
Sirikrai, S. (1982). General Prem survives on a conservative line. *Asian Survey, 22*(11), 1093–1104.
Surin, M. (1997). The making of Thai democracy: A study of political alliances among the state, the capitalists, and the middle class. In L. Anek (Ed.), *Democratization in Southeast and East Asia* (pp. 141–166). Singapore/Chiang Mai: Institute of Southeast Asian Studies/Silkworm Book.
Tejapira, K. (2006, May/June). Toppling Thaksin. *New Left Review, 39*, 5–37.
Tilly, C. (1998). *Durable inequality*. Berkley: University of California Press.
Turton, A. (1984). Limits of ideological domination and the formation of social consciousness. In A. Turton & S. Tanabe (Eds.), *History and peasant consciousness in South East Asia* (pp. 19–73). Osaka: National Museum of Ethnology.
Ungpakorn, G. J. (2007). *A coup for the rich: Thailand's political crisis*. Bangkok: Workers Democracy Publishing.
Ungpakorn, G. J. (2009). Class struggle between the coloured t-shirts in Thailand. *Journal of Asia Pacific Studies, 1*(1), 76–100.
Weber, M. (1978). Status groups and classes. In G. Roth & C. Wittich (Eds.), *Economy and society* (pp. 302–310). Berkley: University of California Press.
Winichakul, T. (2008). Toppling democracy. *Journal of Contemporary Asia, 38*(1), 11–37.

Chapter 12
The Vulnerability of Thai Democracy: Coups d'état and Political Changes in Modern Thailand

Pei-Hsiu Chen

1 Introduction

Five major Southeast Asian countries underwent crucial political transformation and democratic progress at the beginning of the twenty-first century: Gloria Macapagal-Arroyo was reelected president of the Philippines among controversy in May 2003; the peaceful transfer of the regime from Mahathir Mohamad to Abdullah Badawi in Malaysia also took place in October the same year; the political rein was passed over from Goh Chok Tong to Lee Hsien Loong in Singapore in August 2004; Susilo Bambang Yudhoyono beat Megawati Sukarnoputri in the Indonesian presidential election in September the same year to become the new president. The one that has attracted the most attention has to be the reelection of Thaksin Shinawatra as Prime Minister of Thailand in February 2005, whereby an unprecedented absolute majority was obtained, thus fulfiling a "new political era" in Thailand based on election politics.

The diverse connotations of post-financial crisis democratic transition in Southeast Asia have drawn the attention of researchers as well as being labeled as the "new democracy in Southeast Asia."[1] Although democracy within these countries is fast progressing, it is still highly unstable and its vulnerability is thus exposed. On the contrary, authoritarianism still exists and monopolizes political power, forming an alliance of conservative power with entrepreneurs and middle class against liberalism.

As to the vulnerability of the emerging democracies, Karl Popper (1992) suggests that democracy is the best of all systems but also the most vulnerable. It is as vulnerable

[1] For example, a Conference on Political and Economic Transformation of New Democracies in Southeast Asia was organized by the Academia Sinica of Taiwan on October 14, 2005 to discuss systematically such progress, transformation, and predicament.

P.-H. Chen (✉)
Graduate Institute of Southeast Asian Studies, National Chi Nan University,
1, University Rd., Puli, Nantou County 54561, Taiwan
e-mail: phchen@ncnu.edu.tw

P. Liamputtong (ed.), *Contemporary Socio-Cultural and Political Perspectives in Thailand*, DOI 10.1007/978-94-007-7244-1_12,

as a thin piece of paper. If those within the democratic system cannot stay vigilant at all times, then they will lose democracy even politics in the blink of an eye and return to barbarian (Keuth 2004: 55).

The unique political system and democracy of Thailand cannot be clearly defined by typology. Since its adoption of constitutional monarchy in 1932, the framework of such system has remained the same fundamentally. However, in terms of constitutional practice, the principle of figurehead and cabinet system was never realized, and the King of Thailand becomes the ultimate arbitrator of political struggles (see Chap. 11 in this volume). The Thai government was often far from being made up of the constitutional convention of cabinet system prior to 2000, which clearly illustrates that this is not a typical "Tudor" constitutional monarchy and cabinet system of England (Case 2002; Suwannathat-Pian 2004).

Thai democracy sprouted at the end of the 1920s. Many military regimes faced legitimacy crisis as economies collapsed under the pressure produced by the Great Depression in 1929, and Thailand was not exempted either. A semi-democracy system (*prachathipatai khrung bai*)[2] came into being in Thai politics in the 1980s. This was a phase of adjustment and compromise in the civil-military relations during the transition from military authoritarian to civilian politics.

Frequent coups d'état were key influential power in Thai politics, whereas political systems and party politics seemed rather weak in comparison. The "legitimacy" of the Thai coups d'état was based on two sources: first was the incompetence of the civilian government and the chaotic parliamentary politics; second was the approval by the monarch. The Thai King determined the legitimacy of coups d'état based on changes in political scenes and public opinion.

Thai politics was not a typical military regime. Based on the regime typology proposed by Juan Linz (2000), the fundamental characteristics of a military regime include military leaders or a group of military officers controlling governmental decisions, ruling the society under military restrain, military elite occupying key positions in the government, political power monopoly by the military, and politics based on military violence and compulsion. Most Thai military did not monopolize political power after the coups d'état, but monitored the civilian government instead and pulled out soon after the elections and the establishment of constitution or constitutional reform. It is apparent that the Thai coups d'état did not constitute a military regime defined by Linz (2000).

Southeast Asian political researchers often defined Thai-style democracy as bureaucratic authoritarianism. Guillermo O'Donnell (1988) pioneered the analysis on bureaucratic authoritarianism in Latin America. He compared Thai politics with contemporary Argentina and Brazil in terms of characteristics of political regime and concluded that they were highly similar.

---

[2] William Case states that the elite-led democratization in Southeast Asian countries produced a government under democratic procedure, which could not realize the democratic constitutional practice of *ruling party* vs. *opposition party*. The ruler utilized his authority to suppress the opposition as well as reduce the ground of direct political participation by the people, thus producing a *semi-democracy* type of politics.

The bourgeoisie democratic movement in 1992 consolidated the constitutional democracy of Thailand and opened up the political reform for "new politics." However, the ruling power was still monopolized by the elite, the establishment of governmental policies continued to be biased toward the wealthy, and military and bureaucratic groups continued to dominate Thailand (O'Donnell 1988).

Following the setback of financial crisis in Asia and the new constitution coming into being in 1997, Thai politics has gone through the crucial transition that "achieved survival by fighting from a position of certain death."[3] An overhaul of the Thai politics was brought about by the political reform movement that began during the post-financial crisis period. As the history of politics demonstrates, the split of the elite always happened during a national crisis. The accumulated wealth of Thailand from the past few decades was wiped out in an instant during the Asian financial crisis. The disappearance of economic growth meant the elite could only search for legitimate support from the middle to lower class. For the first time in its history, Thailand saw the emergence of a grassroots political part based on social movement – the Thai Rak Thai Party – fast spreading its political turf in rural area (see Chaps. 8, 10, and 13 in this volume).

Instead of a Constitutional Court as in the West, the sacred throne and military authorities in Thailand took over this role. The political culture and progress of the country have elected the King and military to the position of an arbitrator. The impersonalization of arbitrators within the European and American constitutional systems is exactly what Max Weber (1965) advocated. However, the Confucius culture in the East has the tendency of entrusting an individual, who possesses the characteristics of saintliness to attain exterior benevolent dominance, with great ambitions and high deals.

It is inevitable that individuals or designated groups pursue self-interests. The Thai monarchy and military are always protecting their power and personal interests. Thaksin has reshuffled the benefit structure of the upper class and benefited the people through a series of policies. He manipulated populism and nurtured democratic faith in the public, which is a challenge to the authority of the King and military and touched a nerve in the political society of Thailand (see Chap. 11).

When the struggle between populism and conservative power became apparent, social insecurity in Thailand began to spread. Led by media mogul Sondhi Limthongkul, the bourgeoisie whose interests were compromised by Thaksin formed People's Alliance for Democracy (PAD). They invested an enormous amount of resources and carried out fierce street actions. Eventually, under the endorsement of the Thai King, the military carried out a coup that overthrown the democratically elected government of Thaksin (see Chaps. 8, 10, 11, and 13).

Old and conservative elite attempted to return Thai democracy to its established track through military coup and the abolishment and rewriting of the constitution. However, the Thai Rak Thai Party once again won the election through the newly organized People Power Party.

[3] As mentioned by Chuan Leekpai, the Thai Prime Minister appointed during the financial crisis in 1997, in an interview with the writer at the headquarter of Democrat Party in Bangkok on November 18, 2002: "Thailand has become insolvent."

Evidently, the military coup and rewriting of constitution in 2006 did not meet what they set out to achieve. Thaksin was still leading the election politics in Thailand. The only difference was that a big-scale public demonstration has replaced that of the military in the struggle against democracy. The "Yellow Shirts" street protests organized by the PAD in 2008 did not result in military trusteeship, as the foundation for the legitimacy of a coup has become loose. The military coup in 2006 did not change the course of democratic development in Thailand, but instead resulted in the social unrest in 2008. The state apparatus came to a near halt, and even leaders of street politics were requesting "new politics." But the content of such a request differed greatly from its predecessor whereby party politics was emphasized; this one was a political selection system that rejects elections.

The political changes in Thailand personify three classical theses in relation to democratic transformation and consolidation: the correlation between socioeconomic development and democracy, the influence of political culture on democracy, and the role of elite in democratization.

This chapter will, first of all, review the development of contemporary Thai constitution and demonstrate the characteristics of its democracy through the practice of constitutionalism and political system changes. This will be followed by discussions on the social support foundation and ruling strategies of the Thaksin regime and the significance of the effect of "Thaksinization" on "new politics" democracy in Thailand. Thirdly, the cause and effect of the military coup in 2006 that overthrew the Thaksin regime and ended "new politics" will be analyzed in three perspectives, namely, royal family, armed forces, and urban bourgeoisie. Finally, the cause of vulnerability of the Thai democracy will be examined from the aspect of economic and social development, the origin of political culture, as well as the role of the elite.

2 The Course of Development and Characteristics of Thai Democracy

2.1 *Weak Constitutionalism Foundation*

Since the abolishment of absolute monarchy and the launch of constitutional monarchy in 1932, Thailand has declared 18 constitutions. In other words, the *average life span* of a Thai constitution is around 4 years (Siwaraksa et al. 1997).

According to Samuel Finer and colleagues (1995: 2–3) an influential scholar on constitution, constitutions in Thailand are "constantly and continually torn up to make new ones." It is evident in its constitutional history that such high frequency of abolishment (compare to its infamous number of coups d'état)[4] results in the endless cycle of its abolishment and rewrites during the pursuit of a permanent one.

[4] According to the calculation of the writer, there had been 23 coups d'état (19 military coups and four nonmilitary) in Thailand between 1932 and 1991, an average of 2.56 per year.

It is comparable to the cycle of communist revolution and antirevolution, which is almost like trapped in the myth of permanent revolution proposed by Leon Trotsky (Chen 2001).

In the political system of most countries, constitution possesses the sublime position that represents the ruling authority of a nation. But this is the stage for and objective of daily political struggle in Thailand. Whether it was the product of a military coup or a reflection of increasing civilian influence, each political power changeover in Thailand was marked by the passing of a new constitution.

To most countries, constitutional authority is beyond daily political struggle – it is a shared knowledge between politicians. It is only under extreme circumstances that constitution is amended. But this is exactly the opposite in Thailand. In addition to frequent abolishment of the constitution, its amendment is also a common occurrence. Duncan McCargo (1998: 6) compares constitution to a "political football to be kicked around by the winning team."

Constitutional scholars believe that constitutional change does not have to be depended upon democratic transformation. It can be a collective institutional choice. There exists many moments of choice that can influence the constitutional change of a nation undergoing democratic transformation during such dynamic process (Chen 2004: 112).

Not only does constitution not possess the guiding position in the political system of Thailand, it becomes a phase of compromise in politics. As stated by Chai-Anan Samudavanija (2002: 15–17), in Thailand, a constitution does not regulate participation and competition between political groups, but merely a tool in maintaining the power by the ruler. Since the launch of a constitutional government, Thailand has declared 18 constitutions and undergone 23 coups d'état. The continuous loss of the constitutional ethos is the root cause of a political vicious circle and frequent government changes.

In terms of constitution types, the nature of Thai constitutions can be divided into three groups:

1. Democratic: It allows the operation of political parties, elections, and cabinet systems. The parliament is based on election result and adopts bicameralism. The majority party leader from the assembly is appointed cabinet minister, such as the 1974 and 1997 constitutions.
2. Semi-democratic: This allows the operation of political parties and elections, but the cabinet minister does not necessary qualify as a democratically elected congressman. The parliament adopts bicameralism and legislative power is shared between the appointed Senate and democratically elected assembly, such as the 1968 and 1978 constitutions.
3. Nondemocratic: Political parties are prohibited, no elections, the parliament adopts unicameralism, and the executive department (Prime Minister) appoints all congressmen, for example, the 1959, 1976, and 1977 constitutions.

However, the distinction of constitutional typology mentioned above is based on the unique "semi-democracy" of Thailand. Although this distinction is useful in understanding the characteristics of constitutions in Thailand, I believe that the criteria used to measure democracy here need to be clarified in terms of its concept.

First of all, the constitutional system of Thailand always maintains the basics of cabinet system, irrespective of its changes. But, regardless of the type of constitution mentioned above, nothing was left of the fundamental ethos of the cabinet system. The fundamental principle of the system is based on the linkage between execution and legislation, but whether it was the so-called democratic or semi-democratic constitution in Thailand, it was stipulated clearly that "democratically-elected congressmen may not take on ministerial positions" (these was the case with constitutions set up in 1968, 1974, 1978, and 1991).

In fact, the aforementioned stipulation, which departed from the fundamental principle of cabinet system, and another one that stipulated "democratically elected congressmen cannot be on active military service" in the civilian politics were a set measure. Under the disguise of democracy (the assembly was made up of only civilians), a military Prime Minister could legally appoint a military or pro-military individual as cabinet minister in the name of expanding governmental diversity.

Secondly, both democratic and semi-democratic constitutions adopted "bicameralism." There was no clear distinction in the shared constitutional power (budget, legislation, vote of nonconfidence proposition) between the democratically elected assembly and appointed Senate. After the end of a decade long "provisional constitution era"[5] during the Sarit-Thanom regime (1958–1968), the constitution declared in 1968 stipulated that: "[Non-democratically elected] the head of Senate has the countersignature right to the Prime Minister appointed by the King of Thailand" (Neher 1992: 597–601). In other words, the Prime Minister appointed by the Thai King has to be approved by the head of the Senate but not by the democratically elected assembly. But the appointment of senators was done by the Thai King through the proposal of the Prime Minister. This kind of constitutional totally departs from that of a democratic one (Suwannathat-Pian 2004).

Finally, the 1978 constitution enhanced the power of the Senate and stipulated that "the head of the Senate has the right to nominate cabinet minister and both the Senate and assembly shared the rights of budget review and vote of nonconfidence proposition" (Chen 2004: 117). This totally destroyed the ethos of cabinet system and derailed from the democratic principle of *check and balance*, and the democratically elected assembly was restricted by the appointed Senate. The 1991 constitution bestowed upon the Senate the power of nonconfidence regarding the cabinet, and senators were allowed to participate in the debate on governmental policies (Chen 2004).

"Manipulating the constitution" is key to the political "vicious circle" in Thailand (Dhiravegin 1992: 145). Based on such realization, the political elites of Thailand share the value of constitutionalism. But the ethos of constitutionalism never takes root in the actual political operation. The rush to compete in the rewriting of constitution becomes a chronic disease, and constitutionalism becomes what Thai researchers called a *political syndrome* (Chen 2001).

[5] Sarit became prime minister after the 1958 coup. He abolished the 1952 constitution and declared a *provisional constitution* in 1958. The parliament was appointed by him to establish new constitution, which almost became a *legislative bureau* under the executive departments. But, the "provisional" constitution remained in practice for a decade.

Although the authority of Thai constitution is almost nonexistent, people from the academic and political circles still widely regard the realization of constitutionalism a cure to such deep-rooted illness in Thai politics. Since the launch of political reform in 1992, there was an active participation in the rewriting of the constitution from every circle, and various editions of the constitution were proposed. They considered themselves drafters of the constitution, and all seemed to share the vision of creating a *real* constitution for Thailand. But what they had in mind was an eternal constitution, which Thailand has never had during its constitutional history.

If these diligent constitution rewriters ever manage to give birth to an eternal constitution, they would definitely go down the annals of history and become the creator of the authentic people's constitution in Thailand. But, like Duncan McCargo (1997: 119–121) said, the myth of a *real* constitution in Thailand is just like a chimera for an authentic political party in Thailand. It is just a mirage at best.

Bhumibol Adulyadej, the King of Thailand, who is also known as Rama IX, provided the best annotation for the above argument at the New Constitution Drafting Committee in 1997:

> If the constitution draft is reasonable, even it is inadequate, it should be passed and promulgated as soon as possible, because it could be amended later on.... (King Bhumibol Adulyadej 1992: 12)

2.2 *The Instability of Semi-democracy*

Before defining "semi-democracy," it is necessary to clarify the difference in connotation between "semi-democracy" and "semi-authoritarianism." The two terms should not be rashly regarded as synonyms.

Starting off with "semi-authoritarianism," interest groups and opposition parties are allowed by the government. It is a free political participation without elections. However, political hereditary system and corporatism overshadow opposition parties, and political party change is merely a distant hope. Semi-authoritarian gains political power via closed election. Take the "guided democracy" or "tutelage democracy" in Indonesia under Sukarno in the 1960s, for example, semi-authoritarian is not always stable and can easily return to authoritarianism at any moment that crushes civilian participation and dissidence.

By comparison, "semi-democracy" holds regular elections, and opposition parties and interest groups are given some freedom. But, in order to prevent opposition parties from replacing existing power through the election, the freedom of political participation is hugely restricted. The link between opposition parties and interest groups is disconnected, communication and fundraising channels are limited, and many rights are stripped (Case 1996: 439). Although there exist certain structure and procedure related to a democratic system under semi-democracy, the activity of a principal behavioral agent, the political party, is limited. There is also the repression of direct political participation of people to prevent the opposition from taking over existing power in a democratic election (Samudavanija 1990).

Thai politics in the 1980s is often referred to as the semi-democracy[6] period by the academic circle. Semi-democracy, according to the constitutional principles, refers to the constitutional framework regulated by the 1978 constitution (1978–1991) – the longest-living one in the history of Thai constitution. In reality, it refers to Thai politics under the regime of Prem Tinsulanonda (1980–1988) (Dhiravegin 1992).

The 1978 constitution is a political compromise between the military-bureaucratic elite and extra-bureaucratic elite. It reconciliated the old political elements (bureaucratic polity) and new social power (civilian society): the new social power allows the elite to participate in the politics on behalf of the public through fair and open election. The old bureaucratic elite maintains its leading position in politics under the protection of specifically designed constitutional system.

Such compromise in the design of constitution is the key connotation of semi-democracy in Thailand. The design of the 1978 constitution contained both non-democratic and democratic features. Nondemocratic features include the following: (1) the Prime Minister does not have to be a member of parliament under the cabinet system. In other words, the candidate does not have to be a majority leader from the parliament, provided that the parliament majority is obtained or the candidate is specifically supported by military power; (2) cabinet members do not have to be members of parliament only under the cabinet system. Nondemocratically elected members can be recruited to head the departments; (3) cabinet members and departmental heads are allowed to retain their military and/or literary positions (later constitution amendment has abolished this rule); (4) the parliament is bicameral. Members of the Lower House (the assembly) are entirely democratically elected, whereas members of the Upper House (the Senate) are appointed.

Democratic features include the following: (1) the decentralized check and balance of execution and legislation allows the parliament to exercise the vote and debate of nonconfidence proposition on the cabinet. The cabinet minister can dissolve the parliament and hold new elections; (2) the development of party politics is encouraged, and official party registration and their events are allowed; (3) the electoral system is being improved and constituencies re-planed to allow better representation; (4) constitutional amendment stipulates that high-ranking military officers are not allowed to take on the positions in the assembly.

The main reason behind the unstable "semi-democracy" in Thailand is that it departs from the fundamental principles of constitutional monarchy and cabinet system. The "figurehead" holds an important title yet executes little actual power under typical constitutional monarchy, thus does not interfere with constitutional operation. But the King has actual power to interfere in the constitution within Thai politics. The frequent abolishing and rewriting of constitutions resulted in the absurd phenomenon of nominal constitution.

In terms of the cabinet system, the fundamental principle of government constitution is that the majority party should form the cabinet and its leader the

---

[6] The Thai phrase "*Prachathipatai kung bai*" has several English translations including "semi-democracy," "demi-democracy," and "halfway democracy."

Prime Minister. This was not the reality in Thailand, whereby the constitution of the government and the election result were "unhooked." Prem Tinsulanonda, the three-time Cabinet Minister in the 1980s, had never been a majority leader, and neither did he belong to any political party nor involved in elections.

2.3 *The* New Politics *Myth Under the 1997 Constitution*

In the hope of developing *new politics* that was based on political party competition and parliamentary operation, the democratic design of the 1997 constitution in Thailand focused on consolidating the electoral system and reinforcing party politics, thus completely ridding the old shackles of "semi-democracy."

The Election Committee was given a wide range of power by the 1997 constitution, from the output to the input of the electoral system (Article 10 of the Constitution).[7] What faced the Election Committee was not the characteristics and range of its power, but rather the coordination of power between members. They each have the independent power for performance of function, and this caused the disintegration and decomposition of the committee. Five members were comparable to five organizations and five sets of rules (Election Commission of Thailand 1998).

Although the Election Committee was made up of five members only, the secretariat under its command was responsible for the realization of its function. The Election Committee did not work at the national level. Its political maneuver was to decentralize power and devolve upon regional electoral organizations. Regional organizations served as executive tools of the committee and monitored regional electoral institutions at all levels. The Election Committee set up a permanent Provincial Election Committee in each province. Members of these provincial organizations were carefully selected, and they were important as they determined the regional subjects of debate and forwarded them to the Election Committee for consideration. The number of provincial members was based on local population (King Prajadhipok's Institute 2003).

Furthermore, each local election contained three other ad hoc committees. The District Election Committee was the principal mechanism in electoral operation and was in charge of monitoring in the SMD electoral system. There were many District Election Committees under the new electoral system to meet the needs of all the constituencies. But the committees were never responsible for frontline

---

[7] The limits of authority of the Election Committee included (1) controlling and operating the election process, publishing the creeds for general elections, referendums, and local elections; (2) monitoring if governments met their responsibilities while administering the policies; (3) declaring the operation stipulations for electoral institutions; (4) determining the method of constituency division and the rule for ratio representation; (5) investigating and adjudicating election disputes as well as establishing standards for electoral institutions; (6) providing partial or entire vote recount for elections and referendums; (7) declaring elections and referendums, (8) undertaking democratic education on civilians; (9) reporting back on the activities of the committee and its performance each year; and (10) fulfiling duties entrusted on the committee by other legislations.

electoral work. They worked closely with the Polling Station Committee to monitor the progress of voting.

In terms of voting rights at referendums, the new constitution stipulated that it was more of a duty than a right to Thai citizens (Articles 20–23 of the Constitution). It was a political responsibility that eligible voters must vote. If they were not voting, then they would have to report to the Election Committee with the reason. The committee would look into the case and decide whether or not to permit it. Should the reason be judged as inappropriate or insufficient, then voters would have to fulfill their duty to vote, otherwise their designated political rights would be terminated. The measuring standard was ruled by the Constitutional Court not the Election Committee. It was based on the law not politics.

Under the regulation of the new constitution, the 1998 Electoral Law defined voting as civic responsibility. If voters did not vote, they would be stripped of their civic rights. These include the following: (1) losing the right to be candidates at any constituency levels as well as being chiefs of any village or region, (2) losing the right to oppose elections at any level (including those of the village or regional head), (3) losing the right to propose any bills or regional stipulations, and (4) losing the right to impeach officials at any level (Narakorn 2001: 107). Such loss of political rights would last until the next assembly or Senate election. But by stripping away the political rights of nonvoters would not impact the political attitude of voters. The strip of such political rights was so far removed and abstract and might intensify their nonvoting belief once they lose such rights.

To avoid a division in parliament, the new constitution and Electoral Organization Law supported "the consolidation of political parties" (Articles 30, 35, and 38 of the Constitution). All candidates must compete for candidacy in a constituency and the system of ratio representation in addition to being connected to a political party. They have to be referred to the Election Committee by their party leaders. The number of candidate in a constituency and the system of ratio representation were equal between parties. The candidates on the party list were fairly distributed in each region, so as to protect the conventional quota system in Thai politics. Additionally, as there was no natural party identification in conjunction with binding party discipline, there was a widespread lack of loyalty among Thai politicians. Frequent party switching was normal. Members of parliament became what scholars and mass media called apolitical ideologists (Phongpaichit 2002: 9–11).

3 Thaksin Regime and *New Politics* in Thailand

3.1 Basis of the Thaksin Regime

Thaksin, the founder of the Thai Rak Thai Party, was born on July 26, 1949, in Chiang Mai, Northern Thailand. He is a fourth-generation Chinese. His great-grandfather, Chun Cheng Qui, immigrated to eastern Thailand from southern China, where he settled and went into business. He became a tax officer in 1908 and married a Thai woman. They relocated to Chiang Mai in Northern Thailand after the birth of their eldest son and began to trade in Thai silk. Soon he became a man of great wealth (Pathmanand 1998).

Thaksin joined the Royal Thai Police Department in 1973 and later obtained a doctorate in Criminal Justice. He resigned as a lieutenant colonel in 1987 after reaching the position of Deputy Superintendent of the Policy and Planning Subdivision.[8] The computer company he established with his wife began to pick up in 1982 and became one of the few well-known computer companies in Thailand. He, therefore, resigned from the public position to manage the company, working as the president of Shinawatra Computer and Communication, fully devoted to his personal career.

Although the political career of Thaksin has not been long, he moved between political parties and has an in-depth understanding of their operation. Thaksin first joined the Palang Dharma Party led by Chamlong Srimuang, who led the antimilitary uprising of May 1992, and later became deputy party leader. The Chart Thai Party led by Banharn Silpa-archa formed a cabinet in November 1994, and Thaksin was appointed Minister of Foreign Affairs. He later left the cabinet to go into business before returning to take up the position of Deputy Prime Minister in the coalition government.

The Palang Dharma Party and Chart Thai Party were two ends of a political spectrum (the former insisted on moral principles and traditional values, whereas the latter was the symbol of contemporary plutocracy in Thailand). Chamlong Srimuang and Banharn Silpa-archa were people of *different worlds* (the former was called as the "Puritan" of the Thai political scene, whereas the latter was nicknamed "Mr. ATM").

The political career of Thaksin clearly reflected his practicality and flexibility as well as insight into the deficiencies of traditional political parties in Thailand. Political parties in Thailand were highly volatile because there was not one possessing both principles and actual strength. This is closely related to his thinking during his planning and organization of a new party (Chen 2003). He founded the Thai Rak Thai Party on July 14, 1998 and took on the position of party leader and subsequently led the party to an unprecedented victory in the national election in January 2001. He then became the 34th Prime Minister of Thailand on February 9, 2001.

3.2 *Nature of the Thaksin Regime*

Before discussing the nature of the Thaksin regime, I will review briefly the changes in Thai party politics since Thaksin became Prime Minister in 2001. As mentioned earlier, Thaksin has thorough understanding in Thai political party operation and politics. Since coming to power, he has been actively driving the strategy of

---

[8] Police and military enjoy exalted positions in Thai society. This is why the Thai media often calls Thaksin *Police Lieutenant Colonel*.

"party amalgamation." The Thai Rak Thai Party took over parties other than the main opposition, the Democrat Party. First was the Liberal Justice Party, then New Aspiration Party, and finally Chart Pattana Party. The dominance of the Thai Rak Thai Party in the Thai political system was increasing on a daily basis, producing an unbalanced two-party system of a big party (Thai Rak Thai) vs. a small party (Democrat). The competitiveness of the main opposition party, the Democrat Party, weakened as a result.[9] Such development was a far cry from the competitive two-party system set out by the 1997 constitution.

Unlike the usual inefficient coalition government in Thailand, Thaksin was active and determined in the introduction of new policies and demanded to see results. Soon he incurred the ridicule of being "authoritarian." Many of his policies that sought direct public support were criticized as "populist." The academic circle called the implementation of policies by his government "authoritarian populism." It is evident that there was an inherent inconsistency in participatory democratic governance as expected by the 1997constitution (McCargo 2001: 97–99).

Politics in Thailand in the twenty-first century vacillated between *authoritarian populism* and *participatory democratic governance*. Thaksin's first term of office (2001–2004) was the golden period for inspecting the results of political reform and constitutional democracy in Thailand. The influence of political enterprise of the Thaksin government surpassed that of money politics in the past (Laird 2000; Phongpaichit and Baker 2004).

The continuous expansion of the Thai Rak Thai Party was resulting in a one-party state. The arbitrariness and determination of the Thaksin government in following through its policies had caused researchers calling the political change in late 2000 Thaksinization. The Thaksin government had perfectly exemplified *new politics* in Thailand (McCargo and Pathmanand 2005).

From the perspective of seat changes, the Thai Rak Thai Party won 337 seats out of 500 (400 members of single constituency plus 100 members on the party list) in the parliament in the 2005 election. This was an unprecedented victory in comparison to the 255 seats in the 2001 election and has created a never before one-party dominance in the history of politics in Thailand (Sawasdee 2006).

To have won 377 seats meant the opposition party might not obtain the required 125 seats to launch the vote of nonconfidence proposition against the cabinet and ministers. The proposition and debate of the vote of nonconfidence had always been the principal tool used by opposition party to restrain the ruling party since 1980.

In terms of political party support based on regions, the emerging Thai Rak Thai Party had swept all the seats in greater Bangkok and the remotest and poorest Northeastern region. It was also ahead by wide margin in central and Northern Thailand, except in the south. The Thai Rak Thai Party had become a "national" party. The old-line Democrat Party managed to maintain a lead only in southern Thailand

[9] During my interview with Thai politicians in 2003, whether they were the Democrats, Chart Pattana, or even Thai Rak Thai members, they all agreed that the annexation of political parties was to isolate the Democrat and take away its space.

Table 12.1 Main parties' seats in 2005 general election (by region)

	BKK	Central	North	South	Northeast	Single seats	Party list	Party list
Seats	37	97	76	54	136	400	100	500
TRT	32	80	71	1	126	310	67	377
Democrats	4	7	5	52	2	70	26	96
Chart Thai	1	10	0	1	6	18	7	25
Mahachon	0	0	0	0	2	2	0	2

Source: Sawasdee (2006)

and was completely annihilated in other regions, thus becoming a "regional" party bounded to a corner (Table 12.1).

The Democrat Party had successfully prevented the spread of the Thai Rak Thai Party in southern Thailand by sweeping 52 out of 54 seats in the region. But it only scraped together some odd seats in other regions – a total departure from its performance in the past elections.

The Great People's Party (*Mahachon*), which broke away from the Democrat Party in 2004, only managed to obtain two seats and was not able to pass the 5 % threshold to be allocated seats according to the party list. Although Chart Thai Party performed better than expected, it gained a seat in Bangkok and southern Thailand, respectively. It also managed to pass the 5 % threshold to win seven seats based on party list, but it was gradually being marginalized in the Thai political scene.

From *semi-democracy* to *new politics* in Thailand, the primary context of evolution was to hasten the birth of a better-developed party politics as the basis for a solid infrastructure of democracy. The trend of the *simplification of party system* best represented such context. Following the parliamentary election in 2005, a new political territory was established in Thailand. The Thai Rak Thai Party possessed an absolute position of dominance, and the goal of a *one-party dominance* was achieved as declared by Thaksin. As illustrated by election results after 1998, the number of seats gained by the main party was on the rise, and the structure of parties was simplified.

An unprecedented political situation was created in Thailand by the Thai Rak Thai Party after the parliamentary election in 2005. First of all, never before had there been a party with an absolute majority and a cabinet minister with an absolute advantage in the electoral politics of Thailand. The increasing monopolization of Thaksin and his party has resulted in the fundamental destruction of the conventional negotiation and distribution system in Thailand. His refusal to form an alliance with other parties and political powers has contributed to the coalition of anti-Thaksin powers (Sawasdee 2005).

Second, Thaksin gained national prestige and this was due to the "coronation" of the absolute majority public poll. He was the first "strongman" in electoral politics in the 70-year-long constitutional history of Thailand. This had most certainly threatened the absolute authority of the Thai King and had thus become the target of attack by the conservatives.

Finally, Thaksin tried to annex other parties to monopolize the political scene and become a political power that could not be controlled. The rising of Thaksin and his ruling gave a new populist authoritarianism connotation to the *new politics* in Thailand. But this was in conflict with the conventional political structure of Thailand, thus sewing the seeds of future strike back by the conservatives (see also Chaps. 8, 10, 11, and 13).

4 The Significance of the 919 Military Coup in 2006

4.1 The Tradition of Military Coups in Thailand

Samuel Huntington (1968) states, while discussing the development and decay of politics, that there is a positive correlation between the degree of institutionalization and political stability. The higher the degree of institutionalization, the more stable the politics, and vice versa. Military coup plays the most crucial role in the institutionalization of politics because the impact and changes it brought about the political system is most enormous and evident (Huntington 1968).

Talking about military coup in the political scene of Thailand, Sulak Sivaraksa (1998: 74), a social leader from the country and a prominent political commentator, made a concise yet comprehensive comparison: "In Thailand, an unsuccessful *d'état* is like a re-election, a successful one is like a general election."

Ratapraharn, a Thai word for coup d'état, is different from the general perception of the meaning of the word. Japanese scholar, Somsakdi Xuto (1987: 172), suggests that the goal of a coup d'état in Thailand is not to *execute* the country, but to *adjust* its political structure and "modify" its constitution. When coups d'état took place in Thailand, they were simple and easy to control. The coup leaders did not have to mobilize the public to create an image of popularity, and very often, they were not met with mass resistance. Furthermore, the coups never caused social unrest. As a result, only governmental organizations and the ruling clan were directly impacted.

Successful coup leaders have two ways of arranging the new regime: first, set up a military government and the coup leader becomes the Prime Minister (1951, 1958, 1971); second, after appointing an interim Prime Minister to organize the provisional government, the coup leader would announce his return to the military. Regardless of the methods, coup d'état signifies a *way* to change the Prime Minister and his government (Chen 2004).

A comparison and analysis of the political and military organization can illustrate the reason behind the frequent military coups d'état in Thailand. In terms of political organization, weak constitutionalism foundation, inefficient party system, chaotic electoral politics, and the parliamentary politics paved the way for coups d'état in Thailand. In terms of military organization, military coup tradition and the

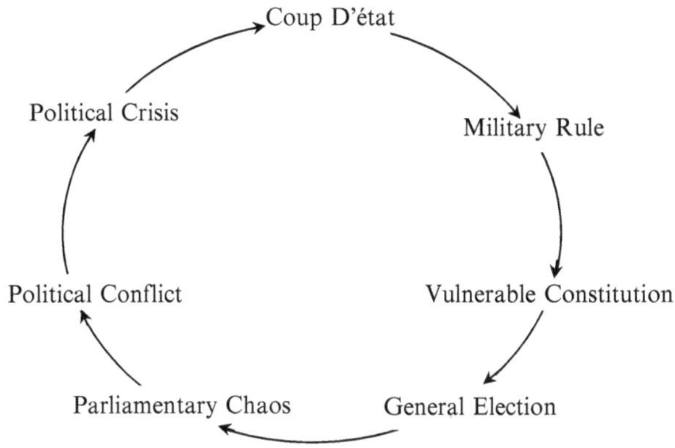

Fig. 12.1 The vicious cycle of Thai politics (Source: Dhiravegin 1992: 145)

practice of military participation in politics were the driving forcing behind military coups (Fig. 12.1).

Behind chronic political dominance of the military in Thailand, decreasing political institutionalization is the key. In regard to this issue, deficiencies in party system and the hollow out of such politics were the two greatest challenges to political institutionalization in Thailand (Chen 2003).

Lucian Pye (1985: 55–57) once mentioned, while discussing political systems in Southeast Asia, that political parties in Southeast Asia were not able to perform their function fully, as there was an existing fundamental problem, as well as that the parties were unable to integrate the ruling class with the general public effectively. Political participation of parties was not enough to set into motion the institutionalization of politics, but was enough to cause fissure among the ruling class. Thailand is a perfect example of this inference.

While on the other hand the chronic dominance of the military in Thailand also matches the theory of Huntington (1968), party system is weak or almost nonexistent in conventional monarchy. In a society lacking colonialism, it is difficult to provoke a mass movement and unfavorable to the development of parties (Huntington 1968). The positions hold by military in the political society of Thailand and the social support that they gain never waned following the economic development and political reform. They are the trusted power behind national development and stability by the people.

According to a nationwide statistical survey conducted by the King Prajadhipok's Institute (KPI) in 2003 on the good governance and development index of the Thai government, the top three social and political institutes in Thailand ranked by the public in terms of trustworthiness were (1) the Constitutional Court, (2) Military, and (3) The National Counter Corruption Commission. The last three were (1) political parties, (2) parliament, and (3) newspapers (Table 12.2).

Table 12.2 Survey of trust in institutions in Thailand

Political institution	Trust	No trust
The Constitutional Court	81.8	18.2
The Military	80.0	20.2
The National Counter Corruption Commission	79.8	20.2
Television	79.5	20.5
The Courts	73.4	26.6
The Election Commission	70.0	30.3
The government system	69.3	30.7
The national government	69.3	30.7
Local government	68.1	31.9
Local MPs	62.5	37.5
Parliament	60.6	39.5
NGOs	59.7	40.2
Police	58.6	41.4
Newspaper	55.7	44.3
Political parties	51.7	48.4

Source: King Prajadhipok's Institute (2003: 34)

Indeed, this is an interesting phenomenon. The three institutions (Constitutional Court, The National Counter Corruption Commission, and Election Committee) set up under the new constitution in 1997 were well trusted by the public, whereas political parties and parliament that the new constitution tried to strengthen were not so well received. Even more thought-provoking was the "newly apolitical" Thai military, which was highly trusted by the public. This clearly demonstrates the contradiction in political consciousness of the Thai people between "political authoritarian" and "participation in democracy."

It is noteworthy that the three constitutional institutions were newly established; hence, the high degree of trust by the Thai public was a reflection of subjective expectation of their future function. The high degree of trust gained by Thai military leading the government was objective proof of the closeness between Thai armed forces and its civil society.

4.2 The Significance and Effect of the 919 Military Coup in 2006

A.D. September 19, 2006 is equivalent to September 19, 2549 in the Buddhist calendar that is widely used in Thailand. Superstitions about numbers are widespread in Thai society and the number 9 above all, the reason being that 9 (*gao*) in Thai sounds similar to *advancement* (*gaao naa*), which implies advancement and achieving both success and fame. See also Chap. 2 for superstitious beliefs in Thai society.

Sonthi Boonyaratglin, Commander in Chief of the army and leader of the coup, met with the Thai King on the 20th and reported on the reason of the coup. He was granted the position of Chief Executive of the constitutional reform group. The King decreed that executive institutions of the country followed Sonthi Boonyaratglin's order, whose position was equivalent to that of a surrogate Prime Minister. The main factor behind the stable politics after Sonthi Boonyaratglin seized power was the support for military coup from the King.

A provisional constitution was declared on October 1, 2006, and an interim military dictatorship was set up. Public figures and intellectuals from all walks of life were called upon to become members of the legislative institute. Surayud Chulanont became Prime Minister. A new constitution was passed in 2007. An election for the Lower House was held in December 2007, and a new democratically elected government was formed and the interim government ended its transitional role. The series of political arrangements were identical to the process in conventional Thai politics.

The 919 military in 2006 revealed a fact about Thai politics. The military obeys the King. The King will support military coups and give up the original constitution and government – even a democratically elected one – based on factors such as to maintain social stability and safeguarding the welfare of the public (Handley 2006).

Since the development of democracy in Thailand, it has had 16 constitutions, and the only constant is the power and symbolic position of the King. A closer look will reveal that political system in Thailand is primarily that of a monarchy. Democracy established by constitution is merely a tool to maintain the orderly operation of politics; the goal was to connect with the global democracy trend. The absoluteness of the royal authority was demonstrated and highlighted in the overt approval by the Thai King regarding the military coup in 2006. However, the King refused to openly execute Article 7 of the Constitution, as he did not want interference to become the constitutional practice. He relied on cultural power and not that endowed by the law, which seemed to keep the royal family from politics (Connors 2008).

Following the oust of Thaksin by military coup on September 19, 2006, political tension between pro- and anti-Thaksin groups has been escalating in Thailand. Continuous political demonstrations by People's Alliance for Democracy (PAD), an anti-Thaksin group, caused the "Yellow Tide" (PAD members dressed in yellow and are known as the Yellow Shirts among international media) (see also Chaps. 10, 11, and 13) and took over the Prime Minister's office. There was almost not a day went by in the Thai political situation without any incidents. The Yellow Shirts took over Bangkok International Airport in November 2008. Political situation in Thailand was reaching boiling point.

People, primarily the bourgeoisie and intellectuals, were calling for military coup to terminate the political chaos. Dozens of university professors even issues an open letter to the Commander in Chief of the Armed Forces, Anupong Paochinda, demanding the military to restore social order via adopting a solid and effective operation (military coup). What is bewildering is: Why is the ultimate wish of the Thai public regarding a political crisis is a military coup?

5 The Weaknesses of Democracy in Thailand

From the political perspective, the "weakness" of an emerging democracy is usually manifested during the political development, as it faces the predicament of two systems: one is the constitutional crisis of the leader, and the other the legitimacy crisis of regime survival. The dilemmas do not necessary happen simultaneously during political changes. However, varying developmental plights frequently bring along more political instabilities and decay to democracies with weak constitutional basis (Ostrom 1997).

Features of political changes in Thailand were embodied by three classical theses in relation to democratic transformation and consolidation: the correlation between socioeconomic development and democracy, the influence of political culture on democracy, and the role of elite in democratization. The democracy weaknesses of Thailand can be analyzed based on these perspectives.

5.1 Observation on the Correlation Between Socioeconomic Development and Democratic Progress

Seymour Lipset (1981) conducted research on the correlation between socio-economic development and democratization in the 1950s and 1960s. Besides, the research undertook by O'Donnell (1988) after the 1970s criticized the simple linear correlation between economic standard and democracy and reconsidered the influence socioeconomic development had on democracy.

The political evolution in Thailand during post-Thaksin era presented a distinct situation of "elite group of pro-negotiation politics" vs. "pro-electoral politics grass-roots." Returning to the research of Lipset, clearly division between rural and city populations eventually led to street political struggle was the result of the difference in living standard between rural areas and cities, and an imbalance in the distribution of economic interests have torn the Thai society apart. The democratic progress in Thailand clearly proved that a country with an apparent caste system, while suffering from chronic imbalance in economic distribution, was susceptible to boycott from the upper-class elite in the transformation and consolidation of its democracy resulting in a division in the social structure.

A vivid caste mobilization is illustrated by the struggle between the anti-Thaksin Yellow Shirts and pro-Thaksin Red Shirts. The former, PAD, received funds and resources from big business and media, and its members were made up primarily of the middle class from the Bangkok metropolis. The latter, United Front for Democracy Against Dictatorship (UDD), was made up of farmers and laborers from far out provinces. It lacked business and media support. The international shocker of the occupation of Bangkok International Airport by the Yellow Shirts in 2008 was clearly the result of police inaction and tacit consent from the military. This was evidently a clash between castes (see Chaps. 10, 11, and 13).

5.2 Observation on the Correlation Between Political Cultural and Democratic Progress

Lucian Pye, in *Asian Power and Politics*: *Cultural Dimensions of Politics* (1985), summarizes and analyzes how Asian cultural bred authoritarianism and proved the reliance of political changes on tradition. Nurtured by Confucianism in East Asia, which is based upon authority and under the influence of religion (mainly Buddhism), the worship of authority in Asian democratic societies is deep-rooted.

Although absolute monarchy was abolished and monarchy constitutionalism was adopted in Thailand in 1932, Thai politics has always been under monarchy control. Its worship for power and individual authority has resulted in its inability to rid the comprehensive control by military, royal family, and bureaucratic groups on the society. In terms of the authority of the royal family, despite the tradition of criticism among academic circle and media in Thailand, the majority of scholars and media do not criticize the royal family, not even some neutral comments. Such phenomenon is likely to derive from fear of lèse majesté prescribed in Thai laws but is also likely to be stemmed from the belief that "the King can do no wrong" (Streckfuss 1996: 13).

Despite the fact that foreign scholars are not likely to be tried for lèse majesté, their comments regarding the Thai King are often reserved. The psychological constraint is evident.[10] A prominent example is that of a politics professor, Ji Giles Ungpakorn, with British-Thai dual citizenship, who wrote the book *A Coup for the Rich* specifically about the military coup in 2006, the content of which involved criticism of the royal family. He was prosecuted for lèse majesté and subsequently exiled to the UK.[11]

As much as the article emphasizes the role of the Thai royal family, there is never the intention to apply indiscriminately the "great man" theory in historical studies or the "strongman" point of view in actual politics. What the article wants to point out is that the Thai royal family is often easily overlooked for the role it plays; it is the key factor that influences and even determines the orientation of democracy in Thailand. This discourse from the observation on the perspectives of political culture is particularly distinct (Hewison 1997: 59).

To quote Karl Marx, the street democratic movement of PAD and its offbeat proposal of new politics, replacing elections with political selections, are typical

[10] According to Kevin Hewison, the four reasons that foreign scholars are not willing to criticize the Thai royal family are as follows: first, they and Thai scholars share the view that the royal family may not be criticized; second, they are concerned about their criticism be misinterpreted as defamation of the royal family, subsequently be prohibited from entering the country by the authority; third, they do not want to hurt their friendship with Thai scholars by criticizing the royal family, and they also worry about implicating people from the academic circle in Thailand; and fourth, it is difficult to find publishers in Thailand who are willing to publish articles or books that criticize the royal family. Furthermore, international publishers are worried about retaliation from the Thai government as well as damage to their business in Thailand.

[11] http://www.bangkokpost.com/breakingnews/136371/lese-majeste-suspect-flees (2009.02.23).

of the counterrevolution of bourgeoisie revolution. Only middle class deep under the influence of East Asian authoritarian culture would propose such an antidemocracy demand.

5.3 Observation on the Correlation Between Elite Politics and Democratic Progress

Proposed by Robert Michels, the "Iron Law of Oligarchy" (Michels 1966) reveals the essence behind the ruling of contemporary political elite, and it is still applicable to this day. Elites can be the creator of social creativity and wealth, advocates of liberty and equality, and guardians of democratic values. However, they can also be looters of public wealth, creators of social caste, and representatives of corruption and decay. Researchers, such as Juan Linz, Philippe Schmitter, and Robert Dahl, generally agree that elite behavior is a crucial variable in the transformation and consolidation of democracy. Such behavior is not constant, and elites make a different choice given different system background, stage of development, and culture and tradition (O'Donnell and Schimitter 1986; Dahl 1991).

For instance, elites from the "semi-democratic" Turkey behave completely different from those in Thailand. During the political crisis in Turkey in 2008, the elite, made up primarily of customary bourgeoisie and military, chose to protect the long-established democracy that has always protected the bourgeoisie since the independence of the country. The upper class and military of Thailand, on the other hand, insisted on the establishment of a parliamentary system based on selection that suppressed the voting rights of the general public (Ungpakorn 2007).

By entrusting the political modernization and democratization of a country upon the strengthening and elevation of position of the elite or bourgeoisie is equivalent to continual consolidation of existing interests of the upper class. To consolidate its collective interests, the upper class, product of authoritarianism, will continue to form an alliance with political elites while participating in the suppression of political demands of the lower class. Buddhism and cultural were employed as ideological tools by elite in Thailand, supplemented by the worship for the King, for tight control of the politics as well as to monopolize the economic benefits. The bourgeoisie in Thai cities was not a firm believer of democracy; some even support authoritarian, as can be gathered from the military coup in 2006 to the social unrest in 2008.

The military coup in 2006 abolished the 1997 constitution, and the military interim government held an unprecedented referendum in 2007 to legalize the constitutional draft proposed by the military. The 2007 constitution is a regression of its constitutional politics. The article 237 that states the court has the right to dissolve political parties is regarded as an "open conspiracy" by the conservative elite to prevent Thaksin from staging a comeback through election and to turn the political situation around and return to negotiation politics.

Both Samak Sundaravej and Somchai Wongsawat were key players in the Thaksin group. The former was well trusted by Thaksin and became Prime Minister after the military coup, whereas the latter was his brother-in-law. Demonstrations by the Yellow Shirts could not force the two out of the office, and eventually the court did so through judiciary adjudication. This was criticized by academic circle in Thailand and the international media as "judicial coup," as the court "collaborates" with political mainstream to determine its adjudication (Ungpakorn 2008: 45–47; Noi 2009: 113–115).

6 Conclusion

Thaksin regime broke down due to military coup is equivalent to the end of electoral politics in Thailand as well as a reverse in its democracy. The political evolution of Thailand in the twenty-first century provided the best annotation for discourse on the vulnerability of an emerging democracy.

The connotation of the "new politics" that Thailand pursued to establish during the democratic progress has always been ambiguous. The "semi-democracy" with decades of practice in Thailand has actually been the best compromise when democratic progress was met with resistance. The authoritarian foundation contained in the political culture of Thailand has given absolute authority to the figurehead in politics, and the civil-military relations in elite politics long dominated the course of democratic development. The intensification and expansion of caste conflict has fuelled the social clash in Thailand after the breakdown of democracy.

Looking from the perspective of the correlation between constitutional changes and the course of democratic transformation, the military coup in 1997 easily torn apart an "authentic constitution" and hastily put together a constitution draft that was put into practice after a referendum. This proved that political elites regarded constitution as a choice of system and highlighted the nonexistence of constitutional authority. As a result, the democratic development of Thailand lacked a solid foundation, thus weakening its democracy.

In terms of the democratic criterion that "democratic politics is party politics," the Thai Rak Thai Party of Thaksin is doubtlessly what Thai researchers call an "authentic party"; "non-Thai Rak Thai" parties, like the Palang Dharma Party and New Aspiration Party before, share the essence of "messiah parties," that is, political leaders with the empty promise of saving the nation and its people but incapable of making that happen (Satori 1984). The breakdown of the Thaksin regime and the disbandment of the Thai Rak Thai Party marked the weak foundation of Thai democracy.

Examining the changes and evolution of constitutions and party politics from perspectives such as economy and democracy, political culture, and elite politics clearly exposed the weakness of Thai democracy. The predicament facing Thai democracy in the twenty-first century is a valuable reference for patterns of change in the emerging democracies in Southeast Asia.

References

Case, W. F. (1996). Can the 'halfway house' stand? Semi-democracy and elite theory in three Southeast Asian countries. *Comparative Politics, 29*(1), 436–461.
Case, W. F. (2002). *Politics in Southeast Asia: Democracy or less*. Richmond: Curzon Press.
Chen, P. H. (2001, May 3–4). *The development of representative democracy in Thailand after May 1992: The 'vicious circle' revived?* Paper presented at the 2001 Taiwan annual conference on Southeast Asian Studies, Nantou, Taiwan.
Chen, P. H. (2003, November 27–30). *Thai Rak Thai and the new politics in Thailand: An authentic party on the march?* Paper presented at the First Asian Political & International Studies Association (APISA) – Asia in the New Millennium: Development, Democracy, and Security, Singapore.
Chen, P. H. (2004). *Thai Rak Thai* and the new politics in Thailand: An authentic party on the March? In Amitav Achaya & Lee Lai To (Eds.), *Asia in the new millennium* (pp. 107–120). Singapore: Marshall Cavendish International.
Connors, M. K. (2008). Article of faith: The failure of royal liberalism in Thailand. *Journal of Contemporary Asia, 38*(1), 143–165.
Dahl, R. A. (1991). *Democracy and its critics*. New Haven: Yale University Press.
Dhiravegin, L. (1992). *Demi-democracy: The evolution of the Thai political system*. Singapore: Times Academic.
Election Commission of Thailand. (1998). *The organic act on the election of members of the house of representatives and senators-B. E. 2541*. Bangkok: Election Committee of Thailand Press.
Finer, S. E., Vernon, B., & Rudden, B. (1995). *Comparing constitutions*. Oxford: Oxford University Press.
Handley, P. (2006). *The King never smiles: A biography of Thailand's Bhumibol Adulyadej*. New Haven: Yale University Press.
Hewison, K. (Ed.). (1997). *Political change in Thailand: Democracy and participation*. London: Routledge.
Huntington, S. P. (1968). *Political order in changing societies*. New Haven: Yale University Press.
Keuth, H. (2004). *The philosophy of Karl Popper*. Cambridge: Cambridge University Press.
King Bhumibol Adulyadej. (1992). *Royal advice by His Majesty the King-20 May 1992/2535*. Bangkok: Office of His Majesty's Principal Private Secretary.
King Prajadhipok's Institute. (2003). *Monitoring the pulse of the nation: Indicators of good governance and development in Thailand*. Bangkok: KPI Press.
Laird, J. (2000). *Money politics, globalization and crisis: The case of Thailand*. Singapore: Graham Brash.
Linz, J. (2000). *Totalitarian and authoritarian regimes*. Boulder: Lynne Rienner Publishers.
Lipset, S. M. (1981). *Political man: The social bases of politics*. Baltimore: The Johns Hopkins University Press.
McCargo, D. (1997). Thailand's political parties: Real, authentic, and actual. In K. Hewison (Ed.), *Political change in Thailand: Democracy and participation* (pp. 114–131). London: Routledge.
McCargo, D. (1998). Alternative meanings of political reform in contemporary Thailand. *The Copenhagen Journal of Asian Studies, 13*(March), 5–30.
McCargo, D. (2001). Populism and reformism in contemporary Thailand. *South East Asia Review, 9*(1), 89–107.
McCargo, D., & Pathmanand, U. (2005). *The Thaksinization of Thailand*. Copenhagen: Nordic Institute of Asian Studies.
Michels, R. (1966). *Political parties: A sociological study of the oligarchical tendencies of modern democracy*. New York: The Free Press.
Narakorn, P. (2001). Reform of the parliamentary electoral system under the new constitution. *Thammasat Review, 6*(1), 105–119.
Neher, C. D. (1992). Political succession in Thailand. *Asian Survey, 32*(7), 585–605.

Noi, C. (2009). *Jungle book: Thailand's politics, moral panic, and plunder, 1996–2008*. Bangkok: Silkworm Books.
O'Donnell, G. (1988). *Bureaucratic authoritarianism: Argentina 1966–1973 in comparative perspective*. Berkeley: University of California Press.
O'Donnell, G., & Schimitter, P. C. (1986). *Transitions from authoritarian rule: Tentative conclusions about uncertain democracies*. Baltimore: The Johns Hopkins University Press.
Ostrom, V. (1997). *The meaning of democracy and the vulnerability of democracies: A response to Tocqueville's challenge*. Ann Arbor: University of Michigan Press.
Pathmanand, U. (1998). The Thaksin Shinawatra group: A study of the relationship between money and politics in Thailand. *The Copenhagen Journal of Asian Studies, 13*, 60–82.
Phongpaichit, P. (2002). Recent popular movements in Thailand in global perspective. *Asian Review, 15*, 1–20.
Phongpaichit, P., & Baker, C. (2004). *Thaksin: The business of politics in Thailand*. Chiang Mai: Silkworm.
Popper, K. (1992). *The lesson of this century*. Cleveland: Ridgemont Press.
Pye, L. W. (1985). *Asian power and politics: The cultural dimensions of authority*. Cambridge, MA: The Belknap Press of Harvard University.
Samudavanija, C. (1990). Thailand: A stable semi-democracy. In L. Diamond, J. J. Linz, & S. M. Lipset (Eds.), *Politics in developing countries* (pp. 266–292). Boulder: Lynne Rienner Publishers.
Samudavanija, C. (2002). *Thailand: State-building, democracy and globalization*. Bangkok: Institute of Policy Studies.
Satori, G. (1984). *Parties and party system: A framework for analysis*. New York: Cambridge University Press.
Sawasdee, S. N. (2005). The 2005 general elections in Thailand: Towards a single-party government. *Philippine Journal of Third World Studies, 20*(1), 48–71.
Sawasdee, S. N. (2006). *Thai political parties in the age of reform*. Bangkok: Institute of Public Policy Studies Press.
Sivaraksa, S. (1998). Loyalty demands dissent. Bangkok: Parallax Press.
Siwaraksa, P., Traimas, C., & Vayagool, R. (1997). *Thai constitutions in brief*. Bangkok: Institute of Public Policy Studies.
Streckfuss, D. (Ed.). (1996). *Modern Thai monarchy and cultural politics: The acquittal of Sulak Sivaraksa on the charge of lèse-majesté in Siam 1995 and its consequences*. Bangkok: Santi Pracha Dhamma Institute.
Suwannathat-Pian, K. (2004). *Kings, country and constitutions: Thailand's political development 1932–2000*. New York: Routledge.
Ungpakorn, G. J. (2007). *A coup for the rich: Thailand's political crisis*. Bangkok: Workers Democracy Publishing.
Ungpakorn, G. J. (2008). *Judicial coups and the settlements of political crisis in Thailand*. Bangkok: Arom Pongpangan Foundation.
Weber, M. (1965). *Politics as a vocation*. Cleveland: Fortress Press.
Xuto, S. (1987). *Government and politics of Thailand*. Singapore: Oxford University Press.

Chapter 13
Politics and the City: Protest, Memory, and Contested Space in Bangkok

Serhat Ünaldi

1 Introduction

On April 3, 2010, when anti-government demonstrators erected a stage right in the middle of Ratchaprasong intersection, downtown Bangkok began to transform (see also Chaps. 10, 11, and 12 in this volume). It slowly turned into a place of memory. About 7 weeks later, the ground of this urban space was soaked with the blood of dozens of demonstrators, of security, and of media personnel. "*Thi ni mi khon tai*," "people died here," became the rallying cry of those who did not want to forget and who regularly returned to Ratchaprasong to commemorate the dead and the injured.

In the years before the gruesome events of April and May 2010, Ratchaprasong was merely a popular urban space centered around two busy intersecting roads, Rama I and Ratchadamri. The sticky air was filled with the noise from Bangkok's notorious traffic jams and saturated with a blend of exhaust fumes from the colorful taxis and incense rising from the sacred Hindu shrines that are grouped here in the shadows of shopping malls, luxurious hotels, and the massive tracks of the elevated sky train. On the face of it, the area appears to be a place of supermodernity, and one is tempted to call Ratchaprasong pre-2010 an empirical non-place, defined by Augé (2008: VIII) as a space "of circulation, consumption and communication" where global flows have triumphed over local "places of identity, of relations and of history" (p. 43). However, even Augé admits that non-places never exist in an absolute sense and some features of Ratchaprasong, such as the places of meeting and of worship, have always qualified it as a real "anthropological space" (p. 43), inscribed with social bonds and history.

Many people who came here before the April and May events of 2010 to do business, to go shopping, to meet friends, and to worship the gods and guardian

S. Ünaldi (✉)
Department of Southeast Asian Studies, Institute of Asian and African Studies, Humboldt-University of Berlin, Unter den Linden 6, 10099 Berlin, Germany
e-mail: serhat.uenaldi@hu-berlin.de

P. Liamputtong (ed.), *Contemporary Socio-Cultural and Political Perspectives in Thailand*, DOI 10.1007/978-94-007-7244-1_13,

spirits did share a *memory of the place*, for example, of New Year's celebrations on the large square in front of one of the shopping malls or of happy get-togethers with friends in hip restaurants. But, Ratchaprasong was not yet a *place of memory* (Truc 2011), not yet a symbolic representation of a particularly dramatic episode of politics in the city.

However, with its transformation during and after the demonstrations of 2010, Ratchaprasong indisputably changed into an anthropological space, defined by Augé (2008: 43) as "places whose analysis has meaning because they have been invested with meaning, [...]. They want to be – people want them to be – places of identity, of relations and of history." When, during the crackdown on the protesters, department stores around Ratchaprasong went up in flames, attention was subsequently drawn to the history of Ratchaprasong before the construction of the shiny shopping malls and hotel complexes (Hon Ayodhya 2010; Lao 2010; Ünaldi 2013a, forthcoming). Local memory, history, and identity had triumphed over global commerce. As Halbwachs (1950: 2) notes: "[E] xtraordinary events [...] occasion in the group a more intense awareness of its past and present, the bonds attaching it to physical locale gaining greater clarity in the very moment of their destruction."

Therefore, this chapter is concerned with the analysis of Ratchaprasong as a place imbued with sociological and political meaning. The main question it aims to answer is why, of all places, did the anti-government demonstrators choose to relocate their protest from Thailand's traditional demonstration site around the Democracy Monument in Bangkok's old city center of Rattanakosin to the modern commercial district around Ratchaprasong intersection? The answer has to do with an extraordinary shift in Thailand's political structure in the wake of the premiership of Prime Minister Thaksin Shinawatra who was ousted in a military coup in 2006 and whose supporters were the drivers of the political protests in April and May 2010. This shift, it will be argued, played out in urban space. An unprecedented demand on the part of Thaksin's followers had to be expressed at an unprecedented point in space, namely, at Ratchaprasong intersection (see also Chaps. 10, 11, and 12).

2 Politics and the City

In 1929, the French litterateur Georges Bataille wrote of architecture's complicity with authority. In a now famous entry in the *dictionnaire critique*, which appeared in the Surrealist art magazine *Documents*, Bataille (cited in Hollier 1992: 47) argued with reference to the French Revolution that monuments "inspire social prudence and often real fear" and that "the taking of the Bastille is symbolic of this state of things: It is hard to explain this crowd movement other than by the animosity of the people against monuments that are their real master."

It is too far-fetched to compare Thailand's May 2010 events with the magnitude of the French Revolution. However, it is true that protests cannot be properly understood without analyzing the places occupied and/or destroyed by the demonstrators. On the one hand, these places function as symbolic representations which can be appropriated and customized by the demonstrators to give a specific shape to their demands. On the other hand, places are productive in themselves in the way they evoke feelings, associations, and memories which may drive or even trigger protests in the first place.

Although Bataille wrote his piece on architecture almost a century ago, its implications for the study of politics and society have long gone unnoticed. It is only recently that space has become an explicit subject of scientific inquiry in the social sciences. Still, in 1989 the geographer Soja (1989: 39) lamented the "despatialization of social theory up to the 1960s" and a "loss of spatial consciousness." In the same breath, he coined the term "spatial turn" to describe the gradual reemergence of that consciousness. Since then, space has indeed staged a comeback, and the study of spaces and places is widely considered as legitimate as the study of the scientifically more established dimension of time, or history, to be more precise. Warf and Arias (2009: 1), who edited the first anthology in English to explicitly address the spatial turn, argue that the approach

> offers a perspective in which space is every bit as important as time in the unfolding of human affairs, a view in which geography is not relegated to an afterthought of social relations, but is intimately involved in their construction. Geography matters, not for the simplistic and overly used reason that everything happens in space, but because *where* things happen is critical to knowing *how* and *why* they happen.

Accordingly, this chapter takes a spatial perspective on the Thai crisis in an attempt to better understand the *how* and *why* of the tragic events that brought the divisive politics of the past years into the heart of the city of Bangkok.

3 From Ratchadamnoen…

On March 13, 2010, thousands of demonstrators gathered at Phan Fa Bridge on Ratchadamnoen Avenue in the heart of Rattanakosin, the historic center of Bangkok. Many of the protesters had traveled a long way from the provinces in support of former Prime Minister Thaksin Shinawatra and to call for the restoration of democracy. Thaksin, a business tycoon-cum-politician, had been the prime minister from 2001 to 2006 when he was constantly reelected due to his extensive support base in the provinces. Thaksin's popularity mainly stemmed from policies introduced by his administration which were responsive to the aspirations of the relativerly poor and the lower middle class, what McCargo and Naruemon (2010) have coined as "urbanized villagers" for pro-Thaksin demonstrators. His critics lambasted schemes such as free healthcare provision and cheap loans as populist handouts, his supporters appreciated Thaksin's ability to tap the hitherto unrealized potential of policies responsive to the needs of the people on the ground.

Although the country swiftly recovered from the aftermaths of the 1997 Asian Financial Crisis under Thaksin's managerial leadership, his popularity in Bangkok was swiftly declining. Business leaders who did not enjoy the prime minister's favor found themselves cut off from government access and felt threatened by the prospect of a political system that was increasingly monopolized and out of their control. Royalists watched anxiously the rising popularity of Thaksin among the poor and the lower middle class which was unprecedented for a national politician. The only political figure who had hitherto enjoyed such veneration among these groups was the King of Thailand. Thaksin was increasingly considered a threat to those who used the conservative royal ideology for their personal gains. Since the interests of royalists and business leaders often overlap – in Thailand royal charisma easily transforms into symbolic and economic capital (Gray 1986: 431–434; Ünaldi 2013b) – the groups opposing Thaksin perceived a common threat around which they united, forcefully supported by influential military figures who had been sidelined under Thaksin and who considered themselves protectors of the monarchy and its associated interest groups. Additionally, sections of the middle class in Bangkok were increasingly frustrated with the electoral system as they voted in vain in light of the massive electoral support for Thaksin in the provinces. The widespread contempt for rural Thais in the capital did not help either. Lastly, Thaksin's disrespect for human rights as exemplified by a bloody war on drugs and the stirring of conflict in Thailand's Muslim-dominated Deep South led to opposition among intellectuals.

These groups came together toward the end of 2005 when Sondhi Limthongkul, a former business ally of Thaksin who eventually turned against him, founded the People's Alliance for Democracy (PAD). The PAD was popularly called *klum khon suea lueang*, or Yellow Shirts, because of the characteristic color of the clothes worn by the group's supporters. Yellow was the color of choice as it is associated with Mondays according to Thai astrological rules which assign a specific color to each day of the week. Monday is the birthday of the Thai King, and it was one of the group's proclaimed aims to protect the monarch from the power of Thaksin (see Chaps. 10 and 11).

The Yellow Shirt movement swiftly gained momentum and prepared the ground for a military coup on September 19, 2006 against Thaksin who has remained in exile ever since. The following years were dominated by continued Yellow Shirt protests against the People's Power Party (PPP), the successor to Thaksin's dissolved Thai Rak Thai party. Yet the PPP remained successful and their executives continued to lead the government in Thaksin's absence until, in December 2008, the governing parties were banned following a controversial decision by the Constitutional Court. The ruling prompted defections and allowed the opposition to form a government under the leadership of Abhisit Vejjajiva, the Oxford-educated head of the Democrat Party. The Democrats had traditionally been favored by the royalist Bangkok establishment and the urban middle class. In late 2008, the Yellow Shirts had achieved their aim of removing Thaksin and his allies from the government (see also Chaps. 8, 10, 11, and 12).

However, after years of military interference and legal meddling on the part of elites in Bangkok, the supporters of Thaksin felt disenfranchised. Even some critics of Thaksin turned against the persistent assault on democratic principles. These intellectuals did usually not deny the wrongdoings of Thaksin but pointed out that Thai politics in general was a messy affair and the punishment of a single party proved that double standards had been applied by a compromised judiciary. Particularly, the failure on the part of the Bangkok establishment to reflect on the reasons for Thaksin's popularity among the lower middle class, especially in the Northeast, came under criticism.

The groups in opposition to the Democrat government and to the events leading up to its formation eventually united under the banner of the United Front for Democracy Against Dictatorship (UDD), or *klum khon suea daeng* (Red Shirts). Coincidentally or not, red is the color of Sunday, the day on which King Taksin was born, the monarch who was dethroned and executed by the first king of the currently reigning Chakri dynasty. The most dedicated followers of Thaksin Shinawatra consider him a reincarnation of King Taksin and the executor of the latter's revenge against the current regime (Krungthon 2010).

With few exceptions – namely, the PAD's brief excursion to Ratchaprasong in March 2006 and the group's controversial occupation of Suvarnabhumi International Airport in November 2008 to exert pressure on the authorities to disband the PPP – most of the protests by Red and Yellow Shirts took place along Ratchadamnoen Avenue. Built during the reign of King Chulalongkorn (r. 1868–1910), Ratchadamnoen ("Royal Progress") connects the Grand Palace and Thailand's most sacred temple, the Temple of the Emerald Buddha, on the banks of the *Chao Phraya* River with the Dusit Palace which had been constructed as the new residence of the Thai kings in the late nineteenth century. After the overthrow of the absolute monarchy in 1932 and the establishment of a military-led government headed by Field Marshal Phibul Songkhram, Ratchadamnoen was chosen as the site for the construction of the Democracy Monument in commemoration of the 1932 revolution. Commissioned in 1939, the *Anusawari Prachathipatai* forms a traffic roundabout where Ratchadamnoen Avenue intersects with Dinso Road. Symbolically, the monument glorifies the three arms of the military and the police as safeguards of the constitution. Four huge fins rise protectively around a round central turret topped by golden-stacked bowls containing an image of the constitution. Koompong (2007: 33) argues that the Democracy Monument was intended to function as "a symbolic device for the state to manifest, legitimize, and maintain power" at the same time as it could be reappropriated and subverted by ordinary citizens. The monument was open to multiple interpretations: first, it functioned as a symbol of the revolution by "disrupting the physical continuity of [...] Rajadamnoen, thus symbolically terminating the monarchical succession [*ratcha damnoen*]" (Koompong 2007: 39); second, it celebrated the military as the protector of the people; third, the golden bowls, which are used in Thailand to present gifts to the king, could be interpreted as the monarchy's acceptance of democracy and its gracious surrendering of absolute power to the people; and fourth, the monument was a modern symbol of secular democracy. As Koompong (2007: 48) summarizes:

> This structure could convey messages both for the constitutional and totalitarian regimes, military and civilian administrations, resistance and violence, liberation and repression, inherited power and meritocracy.

It is ironic that a monument in the heart of the old royal city and a symbol for the might of the coup-addicted Thai military became the physical rallying point around which progressives in the turbulent 1970s united in their call for democracy and social justice. And yet the student-led uprisings of 1973 and 1976 which started at nearby Thammasat University swiftly centered around Democracy Monument, not just for symbolical reasons but because "the conjunction of Modernist open spaces with permeable streets around the Democracy Monument enabled this so-called 'urban insurgency' to persist for some days" (Koompong 2007: 46). The suitability of the site for protests was confirmed again in May 1992 during prodemocracy demonstrations against the military government of then Prime Minister General Suchinda Kraprayoon.

In all these cases the Democracy Monument served as a symbol of the power of the Thai state, a power that was symbolically conquered by mostly middle-class citizens who demanded a say in the running of the country. In most of these protests, portraits of the king and queen were staple items to be hoisted by the demonstrators as a force shield against the power of the military. The protesters found themselves in the middle of the historical royal center and, in many instances, appealed to the power of the king so that the "junta had difficulty arguing that the students were a threat to the throne," as Handley (2006: 210) notes in reference to the student protests of 1973. The use of royal imagery around Democracy Monument surely reached new heights during the PAD demonstrations when Ratchadamnoen Avenue was turned into a sea of royal yellow and calls for royal intervention in the political crisis crossed the line of decency even in the eyes of many royalists.

Owing to the multiplicity of meanings that can be read into the Democracy Monument, it used to serve as a symbol of both secular state power and sacred royal power, whose legitimacy were not questioned per se by most demonstrators of the past (except for the more radical elements among the students who led the uprising of 1976). The institutional setup of the constitutional monarchy was not so much an issue as the way these institutions were run by unaccountable military generals or elected politicians who were close to the members of the royal family and who used these connections for their narrow interests. On the one hand, the Democracy Monument was a symbol of those institutions of which the protesters thought that they should bend to their needs. On the other hand, the monument with its giant image of the constitution evoked the real promise that reform in the interest of the people was possible. As long as this hope remained, Ratchadamnoen was the right place for political protests in Thailand.

Hope for change also drove the first Red Shirt protests in the year 2010. On March 12, 2010, thousands of UDD supporters swarmed into Bangkok in protest against the government of Democrat Prime Minister Abhisit Vejjajiva. Only 2 weeks earlier, the Supreme Court had delivered another controversial verdict against Thaksin by ordering the confiscation of 1.4 billion dollars of the former prime

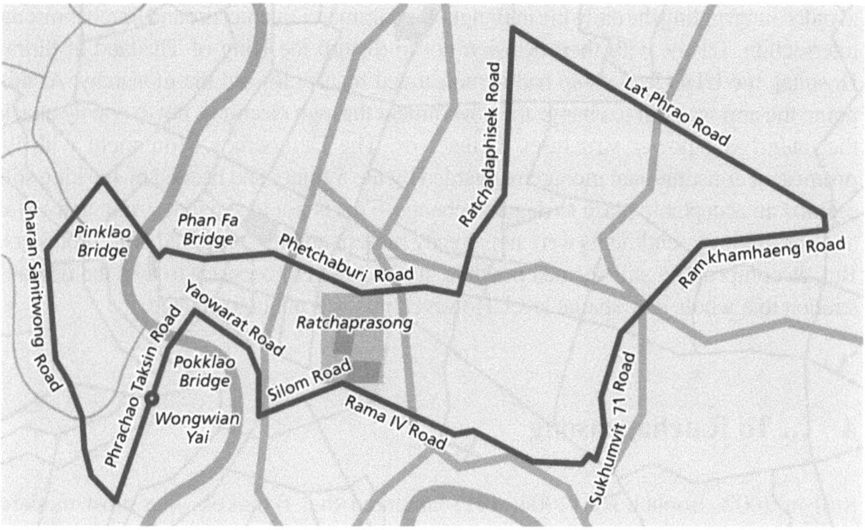

Map 13.1 The route of the UDD convoy on March 20, 2010. The *green ellipse* indicates the location of the protests around Ratchaprasong intersection about 3 weeks later (Source: author) (Color figure online)

minister's assets. In the eyes of the Red Shirts, this was just another proof that no justice could be expected from a vengeful Bangkok establishment. Nevertheless, the first weeks of the protests in Bangkok were relatively peaceful. On March 13, a stage was set up at Phan Fa Bridge just a short walk further up Ratchadamnoen Avenue from the Democracy Monument. The UDD demanded the dissolution of the parliament within 15 days and new elections soon thereafter (see also Chap. 10).

One of the first major demonstrations of force was a convoy of several ten thousands of Red Shirt demonstrators through Bangkok on March 20. Starting at the protest site near the Democracy Monument, the mobile protests covered many of Bangkok's districts (see Map 13.1). However, two features of the protest march stand out. The official route bypassed the Ratchaprasong area in downtown Bangkok, the city's major commercial spot that would a few weeks later become the UDD's main protest site. Secondly, the demonstration crossed the Phra Pok Klao Bridge over to Bangkok's Thonburi side on the west bank of the Chao Phraya River to pass the Wongwian Yai roundabout and its monument to the aforementioned King Taksin. However, the Red Shirt leadership decided at the last minute not to proceed to the nearby Siriraj Hospital where the King of Thailand was hospitalized. The peaceful convoy ended where it started, along Ratchadamnoen Avenue.

An analysis of the route taken by the demonstrators on that day confirms that, at the beginning of the Red Shirt protests in 2010, its character did not yet diverge much from previous protests. The heart of the demonstration was still located in the vicinity of the Democracy Monument. The protest was largely symbolic and nonconfrontational as it avoided interrupting the daily life in Bangkok's commercial center around Ratchaprasong intersection. Lastly, with their decision not to disturb the King of Thailand at Siriraj Hospital, the UDD leadership had demonstrated respect toward the monarchy. At this point, the aim was still to change the government through elections, not to openly attack the underlying power structures themselves. The Democracy Monument with its promise of constitutional monarchy guarded by the military and headed by the king still seemed an acceptable place to demand change. This is not to say that strong anti-royal and anti-military sentiments were not already present among some Red Shirt protesters. But, as compromise still seemed possible, it was not yet necessary to take the demonstration to a whole new spatial level. However, this was about to change.

4 … To Ratchaprasong

Still in 2002, Boonchuen (2002: 401) lamented that Bangkok, like most modern metropolises, was lacking places where citizens could exercise rights of assembly because contemporary cities were increasingly "privatised, commercialized and focused on economic consumption." She noted that temples "as community civic centers have been largely taken over by shopping malls" and that "most people looking for places in which to socialise end up in shopping malls" (p. 405). A lack of opportunities to engage in activities conducive to the development of a strong civil society would lead to social isolation as most commercial places did not provide spaces to congregate "[b]ecause shopping malls are private properties and are privately regulated" (p. 406). In contrast, Boonchuen praised Ratchadamnoen Avenue and the Democracy Monument as "the symbolic epicentre for Thai citizens' fight for democracy: an insurgent space" (p. 413).

The cultural pessimism inherent in such critiques against the modern city, the coining of terms like "non-places" (Augé 2008) to refer to empty places of global flows, and the juxtaposition of civic space and commercial space, of public space and private space, of meaningful space and ordinary space are common among supporters of urban design strategies that are supposedly more responsive to the needs of democratic and historically rooted societies. However, what has been frequently overlooked is that Augé (2008: 91) himself makes an important distinction between non-places as experienced by the individual under supermodernity (places like shopping malls and airports) and political places as envisioned by authoritarian empires, big and small. In that political sense, places are more oppressive than non-places. Augé (2008: 92) contrasts the fluidity of non-places under supermodernity with the oppressive orientation toward places among nationalist regimes:

> Blind to the acceleration of history, […] [Empire]rewrites it; it protects its subjects from the feeling that space is shrinking by limiting freedom of movement and information; similarly (as can be seen from its bad-tempered reactions to initiatives in favour of human rights), it removes the individual reference from its ideology […].

Seen from this angle, Bangkok's monuments in the old royal city of Rattanakosin, such as the Temple of the Emerald Buddha, the City Pillar Shrine, and the Democracy Monument, are serving oppressive ideological purposes. Conversely, and in an admittedly free interpretation of Augé, it may be said that it is non-places, the shopping malls, the spaces of global flows, which offer liberation from those conservative state ideologies.

But, the reason for the Red Shirts to relocate their demonstration from Ratchadamnoen to Ratchaprasong in April 2010 was more complex than that. Indeed, Vorng's (2011: 77) suggestion that "consumer cultures [...] gave rise to new idioms that represent a departure from older modes of status differentiation and articulation of power centralized around the monarchy, bureaucracy, and military" deserves close scrutiny, although it would neatly fit into the place/non-place distinction between old Ratchadamnoen and modern Ratchaprasong. While Vorng (2011: 76) acknowledges that "the business interests of the older political elite are heavily intertwined with property and commercial developments which have modernized Bangkok," she still opens up a binary distinction between two rival city centers, Rattanakosin and Siam-Ratchaprasong, in her view both equally potent. In Vorng's interpretation, both serve a culturally embedded desire for status differentiation, however in different ways – one through the hierarchical belief system that underlies royal power, the other through the symbolic power of material wealth.

But, is Rattanakosin still as powerful as Vorng suggests? Without resolving the apparent contradiction she claims that "Rattanakosin remains a potent, sacred material and symbolic embodiment of the monarchy and Thai democracy" (p. 80) although she admits that "it is no longer significant in the daily lives of most Bangkokians" (p. 73). The architecture historian Chatri Prakitnonthakan, who has extensively written on the symbolism of the buildings and monuments of Rattanakosin (e.g., Prakitnonthakan 2009), points to the increasing monopolization of Ratchadamnoen Avenue by royalists who have deprived the area of the multiplicity of meanings it previously embodied. New museums in celebration of the monarchy are mushrooming in place of secular buildings from the postrevolutionary era and serve as symbols "of the reinforcement of the Monarchic Democracy discourse [...] on Ratchadamnoen" (Prakitnonthakan 2008). A lecturer in architecture at Thammasat University, states that "nobody is interested in Ratchadamnoen anymore because it is in the past" (personal interview, May 13, 2010). Indeed, one might argue against Vorng that the Disneyfication and "museumization" of Thai history and the monarchy along Ratchadamnoen has diminished its potency as a ruling center, an impression that is underlined by the relocation of ministries and other government institutions to the Chaengwattana area on the fringes of Bangkok.

The sanitized version of the Thai state in Rattanakosin thus contrasts markedly with the multiple layers of meaning around Ratchaprasong intersection and the central role it plays in the lives of many people. Far from just being a space of global flows, downtown Bangkok is very Thai – and not just in terms of cultivating a culture of materialistic status display and differentiation. It is, indeed, possible to argue that centers have shifted from the old city to downtown Bangkok around the *skytrain* station Siam and Ratchaprasong intersection. In this reading, Siam-Ratchaprasong becomes an amalgam of the entire scope of sociopolitical and cultural forces in Thailand of whose spatial representation Rattanakosin is increasingly deprived in favor of a stale and one-dimensional display of state ideology. When one chooses to ignore the local roots of Siam-Ratchaprasong, it is easy to underrate the politics of space and that the very existence of the area is unthinkable without the commercial and the dynastic interests of the Thai monarchy (Ünaldi 2012) as well as the connected interests of the military and the business sector. These interests are reflected everywhere, from land ownership patterns over spatial relations to the architecture of the shopping malls and the resulting spatial experience on the part of the *flaneurs* (users of space) (Ünaldi 2013c).

It is important to stress that the area is not just home to these shopping malls and other upscale venues Vorng focuses on, thus leaving the multitude of different places and meanings under theorized, it also houses Chulalongkorn University, Sra Pathum Palace of the reigning Mahidol family, a slum community, a museum for contemporary arts, the National Police Headquarters, Pathumwanaram Temple, and some of the most potent and popular shrines in Bangkok. Academics have written of the Thao Maha Phrom Shrine in front of the Erawan Hotel on the southeastern corner of Ratchaprasong intersection that it has "evolved into […] an unofficial guardian spirit of the city" (Phongpaichit and Baker 2008) and that "it became, in effect, the shrine of Bangkok, overshadowing the *lak müang* shrine in the old royal section of the city" (Keyes 2006: 4).

At the same time, the ownership of the land on which the Erawan Hotel and the shrine were built serves as a good example of the interconnected interests which have shaped this urban space. The land is owned by the Syndicate of Thai Hotels and Tourists Enterprises, a company which was established under the military government of Field Marshal Plaek Phibunsongkhram in the 1950s and continues to be majority owned by the Ministry of Finance (84 %) and CPB Equity (13 %), a subsidiary of the Crown Property Bureau, the monarchy's investment arm. The interests of the monarchy and the state are joined with the interests of two textbook Sino-Thai business families, the Vongkusolkit and Wattanavekin families, who co-own the Erawan Hotel (74 %) together with Thai Hotels and Tourists Enterprises (26 %). Therefore, the Erawan Hotel alone illustrates the manifold and intertwined religious, political, and economic forces that are represented in the physical space that is Ratchaprasong. The bustling area with its global *and* local promises; with its everyday spirituality; with its cultural, educational, and entertainment centers; with its students, slum dwellers, and street hawkers; and with its representations of different layers of royal discourse – Sra Pathum Palace as sacred royal power in built form, hidden from the public gaze, versus various properties as physical manifestations of the monarchy's profane business activities – lays bare Thailand's "antinomy problems" (Gray 1986: 8–10) and thus differs markedly from the increasingly sterile Ratchadamnoen Avenue.

Siam-Ratchaprasong is what Bourdieu (1991: 28) defines as a "space of concentration," "an ensemble of sub-spaces or fields (economic, intellectual, art, university field and so on)." When, after the formal breakdown of the negotiations with the Abhisit government, the Red Shirts first erected their stage at Ratchaprasong intersection on April 3 before permanently relocating there after a bloody military crackdown at their protest site at Phan Fa Bridge on April 10, it seemed the logical outcome of a conflict that had then moved beyond the traditional struggle for democratic change toward more substantial systemic transformations – the transformation of a system whose strands are bundled together at Ratchaprasong intersection. Although some of the business owners in the area had themselves maintained relationships with Thaksin and other Red Shirt leaders (Barnes 2010), the UDD occupation of Ratchaprasong constituted a major attack against business families connected with the Democrat Party and, considering land ownership patterns in the area, the traditional establishment. To communicate their message, it seems the UDD had chosen the appropriate place.

On May 19, 2011, at a commemorative gathering of Red Shirts at Ratchaprasong intersection 1 year after the final crackdown on the Red Shirt protests, Weng Tojirakarn, one of the core UDD leaders, explained the motivations to abandon Ratchadamnoen Avenue for Ratchaprasong in his own words:

> I think last year we came here because we wanted to talk to the Bangkokians, to explain to all the Bangkokians the reason why we had to dissolve the parliament in order to have a new election because Thailand confronted a severe political crisis. [...] That's why we came here, not to disturb people [but] because here is the center of Bangkok and if we speak here we are really sure that the majority of Bangkokians will understand us. We came in order to communicate with the Bangkokians. (personal interview, May 19, 2011)

It seems there was little – and barely a person – left to address at the old site at Ratchadamnoen Avenue. Of course, spreading the message at an appropriate place was not the only reason for the move to downtown Bangkok. During the height of the protests a year earlier, when Siam-Ratchaprasong increasingly resembled a military encampment, another red leader, Wiputhalaeng Pattanaphumthai, explained behind the UDD stage that

> This location is better because it is more pleasant. Strategically, it is more difficult to encircle and to take over this battleground. At Phan Fa Bridge, they could come from all sides and the area was harder to protect. [...] This is a safe island because, due to the height of the buildings, it is also more difficult to attack us by air, for example with tear gas. (personal interview, May 4, 2010, transl.)

Although these strategic considerations did play an important part a third Red leader, Adisorn Piengket, confirmed the point made by Weng a year later when he explained that "we did not have a choice. They forced us to come here. [...] This is the center for the people of Bangkok. We want the world to know and the government to decide quickly" (personal interview, May 4, 2010, transl.).

The occupation of Ratchaprasong was never going to be easy. By blocking the streets in front of the high-end shopping malls and hotels, the Red Shirts, many of them from upcountry, had successfully provoked the most influential forces in Thailand. As Herzfeld (2006: 130) notes: "Those who do not accept the official designation of spatial meaning and use are likely to find themselves defined, quite literally, as beyond the pale and, indeed, as 'matter out of place.'"

Truc (2011: 152) contrasts improvised places to "places of institutional, permanent, and often monumental memory" – of which the Democracy Monument would be an example – and notes that it can be difficult to spontaneously "take over and sanctify [...] a public space, such as a [...] shopping mall" (p. 153) as these must remain open for the free flow of goods and people. Yet Marc Askew (1994: 155) draws attention to "the capacities of Thai people to impose and impart meanings to urban spaces, and through this to create enduring symbols the significance of which go beyond the merely urban." It is impossible to discuss within the scope of this chapter the creative mechanisms with which the Red Shirt demonstrators confirmed Askew's observation and turned Ratchaprasong into their place. In any case, the ultimate violent act that changed Ratchaprasong into a place of memory was beyond the control of ordinary Red Shirts. And when the final military push to clear Ratchaprasong on May 19 claimed the last victims and the retreating Red Shirts torched shopping malls, banks, and other properties of their adversaries, they confirmed "the animosity of the people against monuments that are their real master" (Bataille, cited in Hollier 1992: 47). Crispin (2012:) already notes that "some analysts warn that future street fights could become more personalized than past mobilizations, with rival protest groups openly targeting business groups and interests perceived as red or yellow leaning." In that case, Ratchaprasong will surely see another episode of politics in the city.

5 Conclusion

Ratchadamnoen Avenue with the Democracy Monument at its heart was a place of memory long before the Red Shirts set up their stage at Phan Fa Bridge to make their demands. Here, they were just another group of protesters who seized a place which had previously been imbued with meaning but has now become increasingly depoliticized and sanitized by royalists through "spatial cleansing" (Herzfeld 2006). In contrast, Ratchaprasong was still a relatively blank space in terms of collective memory that – as a center of elite networks, spiritual forces, and Thai modes of capitalism – could be turned into a place relevant to the specific demands of the UDD. Whereas Ratchadamnoen could only be appropriated by the Red Shirts, Ratchaprasong could be made into a place which gave form to their specific aims.

As I have shown, to understand where the UDD protests happened at which point in time helps us to understand why things happened. In the beginning, when the Red Shirts still harbored the hope to successfully push through their demands, the Democracy Monument still seemed an acceptable demonstration site. At that time, the protest was just another example of several political struggles that had taken place in the same area over the previous decades, although this time notably lacking positive references to the monarchy such as portraits or the color yellow. After the breakdown of the negotiations with the government, however, the UDD saw the need to take their protest to the next level and to express their criticism of the system. The appropriate place was Ratchaprasong as the physical embodiment of that system.

By turning downtown Bangkok into their battleground, the Red Shirts had given their movement a new meaning which, because unprecedented in Thai history not just in spatial terms but also in terms of the disrespect shown toward the powers that be, threatened the status quo and thus almost inevitably led to the demise of the protesters who had nevertheless turned Ratchaprasong into a powerful place of memory.

References

Askew, M. (1994). *Interpreting Bangkok: The urban question in Thai studies*. Bangkok: Chulalongkorn University Press.

Augé, M. (2008). *Non-places: An introduction to supermodernity*. London: Verso.

Barnes, W. (2010, June 17). Smoke (and mirrors) behind Bangkok fires. *Asia Times Online*. Retrieved June 20, 2012, from http://www.atimes.com/atimes/Southeast_Asia/LF17Ae01.html

Boonchuen, P. (2002). Globalization and urban design: Transformations of civic space in Bangkok. *International Development Planning Review, 24*(4), 401–417.

Bourdieu, P. (1991). Physischer, sozialer und angeeigneter physischer Raum. In M. Wentz (Ed.), *Stadt-Räume* [City-spaces] (pp. 25–34). Frankfurt: Campus.

Crispin, S. (2012, March 30). Daring double game in Thailand. *Asia Times Online*. Retrieved May 15, 2012, from: http://www.atimes.com/atimes/Southeast_Asia/NC30Ae01.html

Gray, C (1986). *Thailand: The Soteriological State in the 1970s*. Unpublished Ph.D. thesis, Department of Anthropology, The University of Chicago, Chicago, IL.

Halbwachs, M. (1950). Space and the collective memory. In M. Halbwachs (Ed.), *From the collective memory*, Chapter 4. Retrieved April 26, 2010, from http://web.mit.edu/allanmc/www/hawlbachsspace.pdf

Handley, P. M. (2006). *The King never smiles: A biography of Thailand's King Bhumibol Adulyadej*. New Haven: Yale University Press.

Herzfeld, M. (2006). Spatial cleansing: Monumental vacuity and the idea of the West. *Journal of Material Culture, 11*(1/2), 127–149.

Hollier, D. (1992). *Against architecture: The writings of Georges Bataille*. Boston: MIT Press.

Hon Ayodhya (2010). *Athan Wang Phetchabun. Ratchaprasong tong kham sap* [The mystery of Wang Phetchabun: Ratchaprasong must be cursed]. Bangkok: Bangkok Books.

Keyes, C. (2006). *The destruction of a shrine to brahma in Bangkok and the fall of Thaksin Shinawatra: The occult and the Thai coup in Thailand of September 2006* (Asia Research Institute Working Paper Series, No. 80). Singapore: National University of Singapore.

Koompong, N. (2007). The democracy monument: Ideology, identity, and power manifested in built forms. *Journal of Architectural/Planning Research and Studies, 5*(3), 29–49.

Krungthon, T. (2010). Kong kam prawatsat: Taksin returns [The cycle of karma history: Taksin Returns]. *The Voice of Taksin 1*(12), 5–10.

Lao, S. (2010). *Athan: Wang tong ham* [Mystery: The forbidden palace]. Bangkok: Siam Banthuek.

McCargo, D., & Naruemon, T. (2010). Urbanized villagers in the 2010 Thai Redshirt protests: Not just poor farmers? *Asian Survey, 51*(6), 993–1018.

Phongpaichit, P., & Baker, C. (2008, December 2). *The spirits, the stars, and Thai politics*. Lecture, Siam Society, Bangkok.

Prakitnonthakan, C. (2008, January 15). Memory and power on Ratchadamnoen avenue. *Prachatai*. Retrieved May 14, 2012, from: http://prachatai.com/english/node/484

Prakitnonthakan, C. (2009). *Sinlapa-sathapattayakam khana ratsadon: Sanyalak thang kanmueang nai choeng udomkan* [The art and architecture of the People's Party: The principal political symbols]. Bangkok: Matichon.

Soja, A. (1989). *Postmodern geographies: The reassertion of space in critical social theory*. London: Verso.
Truc, G. (2011). Memory of places and places of memory: For a Halbwachsiansocio-ethnography of collective memory. *International Social Science Journal, 62*(203–204), 147–159.
Ünaldi, S. (2013a). Ratchaprasong kon cha mi CentralWorld: Wang Phetchabun kheha sathan thi thuk luem [Ratchaprasong before CentralWorld: The Forgotten Palace Wang Phetchabun]. *Warasan Aan [Read Journal], 4*(3), 170–186.
Ünaldi, S. (2013b). Working towards the monarchy and its discontents: Anti-royal graffiti in downtown Bangkok. *Journal of Contemporary Asia*. Doi: 10.1080/00472336.2013.842260
Ünaldi, S. (2013c). On His Majesty's service: Bangkok's architects between autonomy and heteronomy. *The Journal of Architecture, 18*(3), 425–448.
Ünaldi, S. (forthcoming). Ratchaprasong before CentralWorld: The disappearance of Phetchabun Palace as a reflection of Thai power. *Asian Studies Review*.
Vorng, S. (2011). Bangkok's two centers: Status, space, and consumption in a millennial Southeast Asian City. *City & Society, 23*(S1), 66–85.
Warf, B., & Arias, S. (2009). *The spatial turn: Interdisciplinary perspectives*. London: Routledge.

Chapter 14
The Politics of Change in Thai Cities: The Urban Poor as Development Catalysts

Diane Archer

1 Introduction

In 2003, Thailand introduced the Baan Mankong (secure housing) slum upgrading programme, taking a participatory approach to slum upgrading, by putting the communities at the core of the process, from starting savings groups to negotiating secure tenure, and planning and building new homes. A key organization in the implementation of Baan Mankong is the Community Organisations Development Institute (CODI), a public organization with a strong belief in the ability of community people to take charge of their own development.[1] Since the programme's inception, over 90,000 households across Thailand have benefited from gaining security of tenure and improved living conditions.

At the core of the Baan Mankong process are urban low-income communities (Boonyabancha 2009). Often, the threat of eviction or an associated shelter problem will galvanise one or more communities to organise themselves as a network and carry out a survey of the housing situation in their area, including mapping land ownership and available land for resettlement. A survey is then done of all the communities to build up a database regarding community problems, type of tenure, existing savings, and collective activities. From this database, a plan of action is drawn up, prioritising communities to upgrade on the basis of need and willingness to embark on the project – these communities can then serve as learning opportunities for others in the city, through information exchange and study visits. As communities upgrade, networks can be built up. Throughout this process, the communities may

[1] Originally the Urban Community Development Organisation (UCDO), CODI, emerged in 2000 when UCDO was merged with the Rural Development Fund to work on supporting community-driven development across Thailand. CODI operates under the Ministry of Social Development and Human Security.

D. Archer (✉)
International Institute for Environment and Development (IIED),
80–86 Gray's Inn Road, London WC1X 8NH, UK
e-mail: diane.archer@cantab.net

P. Liamputtong (ed.), *Contemporary Socio-Cultural and Political Perspectives in Thailand*, DOI 10.1007/978-94-007-7244-1_14,

work with and be assisted by other stakeholders such as municipal officials, NGOs, and academics to draw up a city-level plan to improve housing and integrate communities into the city.

At the community level, the process of upgrading requires the formation of a committee in charge of managing the Baan Mankong process and setting up collective savings activities. Communities are entitled to government loans and subsidies for upgrading, administered by CODI, but to qualify for the housing and land loans – totalling a maximum of 300,000 baht per household, to be repaid over 15 years – each community needs to save a 10 % deposit of the total loan amount. The loan is to be administered by a cooperative established at the community level. Community residents must either negotiate for secure tenure in their current site or purchase or lease land elsewhere for relocation. As well as the land and housing loan, the community is entitled to an infrastructure subsidy. Additional subsidies are available, such as for temporary housing during the construction process or to install sewage treatment systems.

Communities should decide collectively what type of upgrading to undergo and how to carry out the upgrading process: whether to hire contractors or do the construction themselves. Decisions will depend on the financial burden each household is willing to accept. For this reason, a survey is carried out by the community residents of each household's income and expenditure, to ensure that the loan taken out can be repaid.

The participatory upgrading process leads to social change, in that the urban poor gain new skills and confidence in various areas, from finance to project management to construction. Another key outcome of the programme has been the creation of the National Union of Low Income Community Organisations (NULICO), a network of community members who are actively involved in the scaling up of Baan Mankong upgrading in communities across Thailand, through the process of community exchanges and learning by doing. NULICO has emerged as a new actor in the community sector and, by working closely with CODI, has become a key actor in changing the role and position of the urban poor in the development of Thailand cities.

Beyond this, Baan Mankong has given rise to further innovative and community-driven solutions to the needs of urban poor communities. A key need for the urban poor, that is, for a flexible financial tool which is accessible to those living and working in the informal sector, is now being addressed by the formation of community development funds (CDFs) at the city and national level, which allows the urban low-income groups to manage funds to carry out their own projects, beyond Baan Mankong (Archer 2012). By pooling together their resources at the city level, for example, by contributing a portion of monthly savings, the communities gain financial empowerment and freedom, as well as a negotiating tool which can draw in other actors, from city authorities to businesses and philanthropists. From the CDFs, or through them, communities can also establish welfare funds, as well as other funds to meet their needs, such as healthcare, education, housing, and disaster relief, funds which can allow revolving loans or grants to address needs. A "Decent Poor" Fund has also been created on a national scale, providing grants for especially vulnerable households, as identified by fellow community members, who may not otherwise be able to participate in community upgrading activities, whilst a community insurance scheme has been established. This chapter examines how Baan Mankong, as a participatory housing project, has catalysed social and structural transformations with regard to the role of the urban poor in Thai cities and filled a number of gaps in the provision of both housing and other services.

2 Participatory Processes for Change

As Baan Mankong is a participatory project, the social relations of those involved in the process are necessarily of relevance, at all stages of the process: before, during, and after upgrading. Somsook Boonyabancha, the former director of CODI, herself said that: "What we need to be stronger … is the sense of power: the sense of politics that how things have been changing. … We can understand why the people's process is important only if we understand this power issue" (ACHR 2008: 9). Participation is seen as part of wider institutional changes, and it is increasingly being related to the rights of citizenship and democratic governance. Community participation should not only serve immediate physical goals but also fulfil broader social development ideals, by strengthening community bonds and demonstrating to the participants what they can achieve themselves, creating opportunities for partnership with the state. Community-managed financial tools, from savings groups to CDFs, allow this to happen on a larger scale and under the control of the people.

The inclusion of state institutions is desirable in participatory approaches, to ensure the more efficient delivery of development and empowerment. Participation itself, through community-driven projects, can be seen as part of a shift towards a "broad-based participatory and decentralized system of governance" (Mansuri and Rao 2004: 25), and therefore part of wider institutional change. The problem is how to do this without the state viewing the communities as a threat to local political interests. The solution is to draw in government authorities as a partner or collaborator, by involving them in all steps of the process and giving them the opportunity to contribute, whether material resources or technical assistance or through an advisory role.

Concurrently, local participants need to be made aware of their importance to the project, as the motivation of the participants and intended beneficiaries is vital for the success of projects. As Appadurai explains, "to break structural inequities in social relations and achieve equitable development it is important to build the 'capacity [of the poor]' to aspire" (quoted in Mansuri and Rao 2004: 27). This necessitates the building of "equality of agency", to create environments to equalise the relational and group-based structures that influence individual aspirations, capabilities, and agency (Mansuri and Rao 2004). This is less likely to occur with a rapid scaling-up process. Community-based development can serve as a rebellion against traditional systems of social organization, which have evolved to manage resources in a manner serving the purposes of entrenched elites (Mansuri and Rao 2004). With regard to housing, it means that they are locked out of access to formal means of finance and hence from secure housing – so community-managed financial tools like community development funds allow a scaling up of the process that remains controlled by the grass roots.

Mitlin (2008: 339) defines co-production as a "strategy used by citizens and the state to extend access to basic services", through the joint production of these services. Co-production can be used to achieve public goods and services and hence higher levels of welfare, when public organizations and citizens share one or more stages of production. Because co-production presents entry-level opportunities for citizens to engage with and influence the state, it is relevant to discussions of community participation. Mitlin believes that co-production is increasingly being used explicitly by grass-roots organizations as a way to strengthen their political position and increase their negotiating power. Baan Mankong can be regarded as an example of co-production in the provision of housing and infrastructure services, and the formation of networks of Baan Mankong communities presents potential for these networks to strengthen the position of the urban poor with the state. Where CDFs successfully lead to the leverage of resources from the state or other actors, they can also be regarded as a tool allowing co-production.

Community participation and collective action for a common goal are more likely where social capital is high (Krishna 2002). Community-driven development, with its emphasis on community participation in decision-making and project implementation, is inextricably linked with social capital. The definition adopted here follows Putnam's (1993, 1998) conception, as used by the World Bank, that social capital is composed of the norms and networks that enable people to act collectively (Woolcock and Narayan 2000; see also Chaps. 4 and 17 in this volume). Specifically, the concept of social capital can be divided into three parts, representing the three levels of analysis: bonding, bridging, and linking social capital (Woolcock 2001). Participation cannot occur without ties between people, whether these ties are horizontal, such as bonding and bridging ties, or vertical, in the form of linking ties. Community finance, in the form of savings groups to CDFs, is a way of strengthening bonding social capital, by gathering people and building trust through the savings process.

Social capital is perhaps the most accessible asset for the poor, as it arises out of social relations, and being part of a social network can be vital to ensuring a better quality of life. Those on low incomes have limited endowments and assets, and therefore sharing assets between neighbours or a community can create community-level assets, and it also makes self-help possible. This mutual aid and cooperation creates bonding social capital within a community, which can be an essential lubricant for self-help. Bridging social capital extends beyond a community, through horizontal ties to like persons, whilst linking social capital can provide vertical ties to persons with power and resources. Thus, whilst bonding social capital may be sufficient to survive, bridging and linking social capital provide opportunities to improve one's situation both economically and socially.

Although community participation at the local level may deal with physical improvements, it ultimately links up to wider institutional change in governance and in how ordinary citizens are perceived and treated by government institutions. The citywide approach to networking and upgrading adopted by Baan Mankong addresses this, by recognising that the city level is the strategic level at which governance issues can be addressed and citizens can play an active role. Citywide networks of communities can actively negotiate with city authorities, all the more so when they have the financial freedom afforded by a community development fund as a bargaining tool.

3 Networks of the Urban Poor as Key Development Actors

The multitude of community networks arising out of the Baan Mankong process were formalised as the National Union of Low Income Community Organisations (NULICO) in September 2006, with CODI's backing. The network is active at multiple levels – city, province, region, and nation – and has two core aims:

1. To solve the problems of community organizations of the poor in cities
2. To collectively push forward policy changes with the state

NULICO works through specialised "teams" who can advise communities: management, information exchange, social welfare, construction, infrastructure, inspection, and finance. NULICO puts into practice the Baan Mankong ideals of information exchange and learning by doing. As community residents who have already completed upgrading and know best what the experience entails, they are better placed to inform their counterparts than government bureaucrats who view things from afar. NULICO also runs meetings, in conjunction with CODI, providing training for communities in how to prepare funding applications and their component parts, such as new community layout plans.

For those who actively volunteer in NULICO, it can be a full-time role, undertaken for a number of reasons. One of these is a desire to help fellow urban poor to develop strong communities and by extension to change government policies. The key role played by NULICO reflects the gap in service provision by other actors in resolving housing problems and empowers them to take an active role in improving not only their own communities but also the wider network of communities within their city and province. NULICO is the agency through which co-production with state agencies can be facilitated.

Forming NULICO has helped to institutionalize the role and position of the urban poor in the Thai social fabric, and its formation was timely, coming when the country's political situation was unstable, and the policies introduced during the Thaksin Thai Rak Thai government were not guaranteed continuation (see Chaps. 10 and 12 in this volume). This instability means that it is the poor themselves who have to ensure they stay on the government's agenda and continue to be allocated funding for the Baan Mankong scheme, by lobbying and negotiating at various levels, from local to national government. Most importantly, NULICO plays a vital role in forming bridges between communities and putting into practice the Baan

Mankong requirement of learning exchange. Networks enable communities to support each other, and they promote access to information, which is vital to achieving empowerment through local organizations (Harriss 2007). NULICO embodies norms which make up social capital, by creating an identity for the urban poor, through a sense of solidarity between communities. This network can do much to bring the urban poor into the wider democratic processes, by encouraging grassroots groups to make their voices heard, not only through demonstrations where necessary, but by showing to society what they are capable of achieving by themselves. Social movements such as these can cement the legitimacy of the Baan Mankong project and the position of the urban poor in the city. The networks also have a policing role, in ensuring that the government delivers on its promises. Community networks increasingly have the capacity to take over from NGOs as the link between the state and communities, and because they are internal to the communities, unlike NGOs, they know exactly what their needs are and what they are capable of achieving. The interaction between the communities and state agencies presents a chance to rectify the imbalances in power which exist in the vertical relationship between these two parties, creating linking social capital in the process. Thus, Baan Mankong, through NULICO, represents an opportunity to bridge the public-private divide.

4 Flexible Finance for Community-Driven Projects

A key problem faced by the low-income communities is access to formal sources of finance, such as loans and mortgages, arising from the informal nature of the assets owned and jobs worked by this sector. The Baan Mankong programme was a response to this, by allowing state-sponsored housing and land purchase loans to low-income communities by making the loans collective. The collective systems of trust arising from social capital within communities serve as the loan guarantee in lieu of title deeds of wage slips, thus addressing the issue of housing finance. However, Baan Mankong loans are only for land and housing-related activities, are limited by the CODI revolving fund for the programme, and require the whole community to be ready to undertake upgrading on a collective basis. It is for this reason that it is preferable, wherever possible, to establish community-managed systems of finance which extend beyond the level of individual community savings groups and are accessible to all communities within a city.

In 2009, an innovative approach to community-based finance was developed, known as city community development funds (CDFs). Whilst CODI can be regarded as a national fund for development, city CDFs are formed by the pooling together of community savings groups on a citywide basis. Each community can retain one portion of savings at the community level, whilst putting another portion into a city fund, creating a city-level revolving loan fund under the control of the communities. The CDFs are managed by a CDF committee which usually comprises representatives from the communities and the local authority and possibly NGOs or other stakeholder organizations. CDFs can be an ideal way to draw in local authorities into community activities, by demonstrating the ability of community groups to manage finance for their own projects, and hence open up opportunities for leveraging contributions to the fund, allowing co-production. Even where local authorities may not have the capacity or the willingness to contribute financially, they may support activities by providing facilities and equipment or by playing an advisory role.

The first two CDFs were established in 2009 with a seed fund from the Asian Coalition for Housing Rights (ACHR), in the town of Chum Pae in Northeast Thailand, as well as in the Bang Khen district of Bangkok (Archer 2012). Since the inception of these two funds, Thailand now has 62 CDFs across the country in operation, whilst 243 are being established, as the value of these funds to local communities is increasingly being demonstrated. Each city uses its CDF in a different way and prioritises different activities, depending on the particular needs of that city, as would have been identified by a citywide survey carried out by the city's communities.

Chum Pae town is the first in Thailand to have achieved the goal of citywide upgrading and hence a city without slums. With a population of approximately 30,000 persons, 5,380 were identified as urban poor. A survey carried out in 2004 by community members and municipal officials revealed 18 slum communities, of which 8 have been upgraded through Baan Mankong and 4 are in process, representing 995 households in total. The communities within the Chum Pae network considered how they could continue to address their housing problems without being entirely reliant on receiving CODI funding for Baan Mankong and agreed to establish a CDF. The CDF would initially focus on resolving housing issues and also assist those outside the Baan Mankong target group, such as families that own land but live in poor-quality housing, as the CDF, being community managed, has the flexibility to address needs as identified by the communities. All 995 households are members of the CDF and have contributed over 52,000 USD to the fund, complemented by a 30,000 USD seed fund from ACHR. As of November 2011, the Chum Pae CDF had provided loans for land purchase to two communities totalling 51,735 USD, benefiting a total of 293 households, at a rate of 4 % over 15 years, allowing households to take a CODI loan for housing only. Of the money earned from interest, 35 % goes directly back into the fund, 25 % into the town's network welfare fund, 35 % supports network activities, and 5 % goes back to members as dividends. The CDF also provided grants to three poorest households in one community so that they could also participate in housing improvement projects – this is part of the Decent Poor programme for assisting vulnerable members of the community as identified by their neighbours, so that they are not left out of projects. One characteristic of loans given by the CDF (as well as CODI loans) is that they are not given to individuals, but to a collective, which functions as a group guarantor.

In addition to addressing housing issues, the Chum Pae CDF also addresses other priorities – one of which is food security. As a result, the CDF purchased a rice paddy field which is a collective resource for all CDF members. The CDF also has its own welfare fund at the city level (in addition to the welfare funds which most communities will run within their communities) arising from a yearly 30 baht (1 USD) contribution per member, which functions as a community-based social security system. A proportion of the CDF also goes towards an education fund and a livelihood fund. As the CDF resources are used by the communities who manage the fund, they have the freedom to adjust the priorities as necessary.

The fund is managed by a joint board, with nine members including community network leaders, municipal officials, representatives from CODI, and professionals such as architects. The joint committee meets monthly to approve loan applications and manage the fund. The CDF is viewed as a tool for facilitating Chum Pae's communities' development, not just with regard to housing but also wider social issues. The Chum Pae communities also benefit from a close relationship with the city administration, being able to use municipal facilities for network meetings, as well as borrowing equipment such as machinery for construction and getting the municipality's backing for their projects.

The case of Chum Pae, as one of the first two Thai CDFs, demonstrates how the fund operates as a flexible tool to meet the communities' needs in various areas, beyond simply land and housing, whilst also reducing the reliance of urban poor communities on CODI loans. Other examples of city funds being tailored to local needs include those of Rangsit, which is focussing on supporting the most vulnerable households within the city, whilst in Udon Ratchatani, the CDF provides loans to stateless households where the government fails to acknowledge them. As the urban poor within the city see the outcomes of using the CDF funds (for housing, land purchase, welfare purposes, or other uses), they will be drawn into also joining the fund, hence increasing its capital base and thus its ability to provide more loans and grants, in a virtuous circle. In addition to this, the larger the size of the fund, the more likely it is to leverage capital from other potential financial donors, either local government, NGOs, or even from the finance sector, as these actors witness the community capacity to manage a large fund for their own development purposes.

Another community financial service which has emerged as a result of the Baan Mankong project is community land and housing insurance, which was launched in October 2010. An annual contribution of 200 baht (6.5 USD) per household will provide insurance to protect housing and land loans, as well as in the case of disasters, from fires to floods. For example, should a person get sick or become injured and lose his or her job and hence the ability to repay the monthly Baan Mankong loan, the insurance scheme will provide a proportion of loan coverage for a certain number of months, depending on the particular situation of the affected family. In the case of disasters, the insurance will cover both borrowers and non-borrowers. The flexibility of this insurance system derives from the fact that it has been developed by community groups for their own use in order to meet their specific needs. Whilst the insurance fund is currently centrally managed and backed up by a CODI guarantee fund, it is planned to decentralise the insurance fund to city CDFs, in order to allow more localised management. The insurance fund is also beneficial to CODI in that it reduces the risk of nonperforming loans (NPLs) and thus helps to maintain a revolving fund for further land and housing loans to other communities wishing to upgrade.

5 Discussion and Conclusion

Baan Mankong, by promoting ties between communities and state agencies, is helping to change relations at the city level, and the growing culture of collective action is reinforced by the financial empowerment of community groups. Baan Mankong connects citizens and public officials across the public-private divide, which is essential for mutual benefit. Upgrading has given residents legal status as tenants of the state or collective owners of a plot of land, and this legality is important for positioning them as members of the city, with a say in its governance and the right to demand services. Additionally, as the residents do the bulk of the upgrading work, they can regard themselves as partners of the implicated government agencies, ensuring that the land is well maintained and facilitating the municipalities' roles with regard to providing sanitation and other services.

The government has provided an enabling environment with incentives for the poor to mobilise, and harnessing citizen action is beneficial for both the state and the people themselves. Participation is most effective if it is regarded as a form of social exchange by both sides, with reciprocity and balance of power (Bowen 2008), and government agencies are realising that it is advantageous for them to allow communities to provide their own solutions to problems, with the agencies providing a degree of support, such as contributing to CDFs.

The implementation of Baan Mankong still faces barriers, such as building regulations which are not suited to communities with very limited space. According to Fox (2005: 6), as well as the state's role in reforming policy, organizations of the poor need to continue scaling up, horizontally and vertically, in order gain the bargaining power necessary to outweigh the "anti-poor elements embedded within the institutions". The two processes can interlock to form a virtuous circle of "mutual empowerment between institutional reformers and social actors in the public interest" (Fox 2005: 6). The most obvious "institutional reformer" in the Baan Mankong case is CODI, which has always pushed the cause of poor communities with the government. It has been the catalyst for Baan Mankong, because of its belief in the power of the poor to help themselves. Increasingly, NULICO is able to take on this role, due to its large, broad-based membership of urban poor communities across the country.

NULICO, by giving the urban poor a chance to play a key role in the urban development of their cities, makes them aware of their importance to the success of Baan Mankong and gives them a forum through which to build upon their experiences, fostering bridging social capital. NULICO is also facilitating the creation of "equality of agency" (Mansuri and Rao 2004) by interacting with government agencies on behalf of urban poor communities, to build linking social capital, facilitated through tools such as CDFs which open up avenues for state participation.

Baan Mankong's ideals of self-help, whilst promoting linkages and offering solutions to the way in which the poor have been marginalized, came at a timely moment in Thailand's political development. The country is reflecting on the meaning of democratic politics and taking note of the social inequalities which have been exposed by the recent political turmoil. This is the right moment for the urban poor to use their capacity for collective action to push for policies which are beneficial to them. The political events in Thailand of the last decade can be regarded as a critical juncture for the country's institutional structures, especially political ones, and the urban poor may have gained enough momentum through participatory projects to ensure that what Murphy (2009) terms mass-based democracy prevails over elite-dominated democracy where the poor have no power.

As Gaventa (2004: 27) states, "when participatory approaches are scaled up from projects to policies, they inevitably enter the arena of government, and find that participation can become effective only as it engages with issues of institutional change". There has been a move away from communities being highly engaged with the state because they are marginalized, hence facing battles against eviction and to gain access to services, towards engagement because they enjoy complementary relations with the state (Woolcock 2001). These complementary relations arise through the cooperation fostered by Baan Mankong, and are especially evident between communities and CODI, and increasingly with municipal officials, through the joint operation of CDFs via joint management committees.

A project like Baan Mankong helps to create political capital, an asset linking individuals or groups to the power structure (Mosse 2005), facilitated by the creation of CDFs as institutions which provide opportunities for government actors to opt in. Thus, it seems that a participatory project can create long-term political value for the poor (Williams 2004), as actions which are not political in themselves have political consequences: self-help in upgrading is a signal from the poor that they do not want to wait for government assistance. The Baan Mankong programme and its associated outcomes (CDFs, community insurance, welfare schemes amongst others) demonstrate the capacity of urban poor groups to manage complex projects to fill the gaps in state and market provision, facilitated by the national NULICO network, which ensures that the interests of urban poor groups remain constantly visible at all levels, from the community, city, to province and nation.

Acknowledgements My thanks go to the Asian Coalition for Housing Rights (ACHR) for developing my understanding of CDFs in Asia. Any mistakes in this text are my own.

References

ACHR. (2008). *E-news: April – May – June 2008*. Retrieved February 1, 2012, from: http://www.achr.net/Download%20Library/Download%20Enews/ACHR%20E-news%20April-May-June%202008.pdf

Archer, D. (2012). Finance as the key to unlocking community potential savings, funds and the ACCA programme. *Environment + Urbanization, 24*(2), 423–440.

Boonyabancha, S. (2009). Land for housing the poor by the poor: Experiences from the Baan Mankong national de Slum upgrading programme in Thailand. *Environment + Urbanization, 21*(2), 309–330.
Bowen, G. A. (2008). An analysis of citizen participation in anti-poverty programmes. *Community Development Journal, 43*(1), 65–78.
Fox, J. (2005). *Empowerment and institutional change: Mapping "virtuous circles" of state-society interaction.* Revised version of paper presented at the Working meeting on Power, Rights and Poverty Reduction, March 23–24, 2004, Washington, DC. Retrieved January 23, 2012, from: http://www.uia.mx/campus/publicaciones/IIDSES/2Empowerment.pdf
Gaventa, J. (2004). Towards participatory governance: Assessing the transformative possibilities. In S. Hickey & G. Mohan (Eds.), *Participation: From tyranny to transformation? Exploring new approaches to participation in development* (pp. 25–41). London: Zed Books.
Harriss, J. (2007, June 30). Antinomies of empowerment, observations on civil society, politics and urban governance in India. *Economic and Political Weekly*, 2716–2724.
Krishna, A. (2002). *Active social capital: Tracing the roots of development and democracy*. New York: Columbia University Press.
Mansuri, G., & Rao, V. (2004). Community-based and -driven development: A critical review. *The World Bank Research Observer, 19*(1), 1–39.
Mitlin, D. (2008). With and beyond the state – Co-production as a route to political influence, power and transformation for grassroots organizations. *Environment and Urbanization, 20*(2), 339–360.
Mosse, D. (2005). Power relations and poverty reduction. In R. Alsop (Ed.), *Power, rights and poverty: Concepts and connections* (pp. 51–67). Washington, DC: World Bank.
Murphy, C. (2009, June 5). Populism erodes Thailand's old order. *Far Eastern Economic Review, 172*, 7–12. Retrieved January 18, 2013, from: http://facthai.wordpress.com/2009/06/12/populism-vs-thailands-old-guard-feer/
Putnam, R. (1998). Foreword. *Housing Policy Debate, 9*(1), v–vii.
Putnam, R. D., with Leonardi, R., & Nanetti, R. Y. (1993). *Making democracy work: Civic traditions in modern Italy*. Princeton: Princeton University Press.
Williams, G. (2004). Evaluating participatory development: Tyranny, power and (re)politicization. *Third World Quarterly, 25*(3), 558–578.
Woolcock, M. (2001). *The place of social capital in understanding social and economic outcomes*. Retrieved January 24, 2012, from: http://www.oecd.org/dataoecd/5/13/1824913.pdf
Woolcock, M., & Narayan, D. (2000). Social capital: Implications for development theory, research, and policy. *The World Bank Research Observer, 15*(2), 225–249.

Part III
Ethnic Issues in Contemporary Thailand

Chapter 15
Language and Cultural Rights in the Ethnic Revival Movement of the Black Tai in Khaoyoi, Petchaburi

Sumittra Suraratdecha

1 Introduction

> In a world of around 250 nations, there are over 6,000 languages. This means that there are very few languages with a country of their own. A language that is not a language of government, nor a language of education, nor a language of commerce or of wider communication, is a language whose very existence is threatened in the modern world. (Hinton 2001: 3)

As the reification and repository of culture, language is a very important part of cultural heritage. Crystal (2000: 34) contends that "if the development of multiple cultures is so important, then the role of languages becomes critical, for cultures are chiefly transmitted through spoken and written languages. Accordingly, when language transmission breaks down, through language death, there is a serious loss of inherited knowledge." The problem of language endangerment is a contemporary issue of interest not only to linguists and anthropologists but one that also affects the public at large. When languages become extinct, there are adverse effects on linguistic and cultural diversity, resulting in irreplaceable losses for the whole of mankind. Krauss (1992) estimates that over half of the world's languages will be extinct within a 100 years. See also Chap. 1 in this volume.

The continuity and vitality of languages and cultures are affected by many social factors, both sociopolitical and socioeconomic. Different languages have different statuses in a community. It is common that a more dominant language will have a better chance of survival than marginalized ones. Thailand is no exception. The survival of many languages in the country is at stake. Previous research has shown that different factors are at play when it comes to saving a language in different contexts. In the case of the Black Tai community in Khaoyoi district, state policies

S. Suraratdecha (✉)
Research Institute for Languages and Cultures of Asia, Mahidol University, Salaya, Nakhon Pathom 73170, Thailand
e-mail: sumittra.sur@mahidol.ac.th

P. Liamputtong (ed.), *Contemporary Socio-Cultural and Political Perspectives in Thailand*, DOI 10.1007/978-94-007-7244-1_15,

and community participation emerge as important factors facilitating, supporting, and nourishing the prosperity of the ethnic group's language in the community.

The study on which this chapter is based is a sociolinguistic study of local community involvement in the initiation and implementation of an ethnic revival movement, with an emphasis on local school curricula in a Black Tai community in Khaoyoi district, Petchaburi province. It looks at how the Black Tai use governmental policies, especially the Basic Education Institutions Curriculum, as a legitimatizing tool to accelerate their ethnic revitalization movement, thus reflecting the importance of legal instruments for cultural revival processes. The study also examines the ethnic revival movement of the Black Tai in terms of a social group's rights-claiming behavior, presupposing groups as "rights-bearers" (Munger 2006/2007). The revival movement is viewed as a collective process of a group that shares similar interests in expressing language rights and cultural rights.

In the following sections, I provide background information on ethnic languages and cultures in Petchaburi province, ethnic minority rights and language rights in Thailand, and state policy on basic education. Then, I discuss the historical stigmatization of the Black Tai in Khaoyoi and how they have gained recognition, which in turn has spurred upward social mobility, by casting off the historical stigma against them as second-class citizens in a collective process of ethnic revival. This is followed by a discussion on language and cultural rights in the Black Tai ethnic revival process and concluding remarks.

2 Ethnic Languages and Cultures in Petchaburi Province

Grimes (2000) and Kosonen (2005) identify 75 languages in Thailand. Beside the "true Thai" and "regional Thai" (Keyes 2008), there are five ethnic groups identified in Petchaburi province. These five groups include Karen, Mon, Black Tai, Lao Phuan, and Lao Wiang (Burusphat et al. 2011a). The Black Tai people are scattered throughout the province in every district, in which Khaoyoi has the highest density of Black Tai population.

According to Burusphat and colleagues (2011a), all five ethnic groups have some kind of ethnic revitalization activities in the communities. Every group has made an attempt to revitalize and preserve their languages and cultures, including ethnic costumes, houses, rituals, and performances like ethnic dances. The most pioneering efforts and outstanding outcomes among all have been witnessed in the Black Tai community in Khaoyoi district. Scholars have characterized the Black Tai as a resilient ethnic group whose ethnic identity and cultural traditions appear to be stronger and more resilient than other ethnic groups in central Thailand.

Recently, the Black Tai community in Khaoyoi district has begun to successfully incorporate the teaching of local history and Black Tai language and culture into local school curricula. Being a Black Tai is now something to be proud of. As a matter of fact, all of the community leaders of every ethnic group revealed their feeling of embarrassment for being a member of their ethnic group in the past; it was an identity they wanted to hide. Now, all of them are proud of their ethnic identity and are trying to promote the pride felt among members of the community. Such process of change is worth examining, from an identity that once embarrassed them to an identity they are now proud to present in public.

3 Ethnic Minority Rights and Language Rights in Thailand

According to the National Human Rights Commission of Thailand (hereinafter NHRC), "human rights" is defined as "human dignity, right, liberty and equality of people which are guaranteed or protected under the Constitution of the Kingdom of Thailand or under Thai laws or under treaties which Thailand has obligations to comply" (National Human Rights Commission, National Human Rights Commission Act, 2542 [1999], section 3, http://www.nhrc.or.th/index.php). Considering the NHRC's definition, the exercise of "human rights" in Thailand is framed and defined according to the Thai Constitution and various other relevant laws or treaties. The Thai Constitution states:

> All persons are equal before the law and shall enjoy equal protection under the law.... Unjust discrimination against a person on the grounds of difference in origin, race, language, sex, age, disability, physical or health condition, personal status, economic or social standing, religious belief, education or constitutionally political view, shall not be permitted.[1]

The Thai Constitution focuses on the equality of individuals regardless of their background, including the language they speak. Despite the inclusion of language, the notion of language rights is not clearly defined in the Constitution or elsewhere. Additionally, to date, Thailand does not have an official language policy. The development of the notion of language rights in Thailand is still in its infancy.

As far as international declarations and treaties are concerned, there are two declarations by the Office of the High Commissioner for Human Rights (OHCHR) and by UNESCO ("Declaration on the Rights of Persons Belonging to National or Ethnic, Religious and Linguistic Minorities" and "Universal Declaration of Linguistic Rights," respectively) that are directly related to the rights of ethnic minorities. However, to date Thailand has acceded to five human rights treaties,[2] none of which specifically addresses language rights or the rights of ethnic minority peoples. The ICERD states that:

> In this Convention, the term 'racial discrimination' shall mean any distinction, exclusion, restriction or preference based on race, colour, descent, or national or ethnic origin which

[1] The Constitution of the Kingdom of Thailand (2007), Part 2, Equality, Section 30, http://www.nhrc.or.th/constitution2007_en.pdf, emphasis added.

[2] International Covenant on Economic, Social and Cultural Rights (ICESCR), International Covenant on Civil and Political Rights (ICCPR), International Convention on the Elimination of All Forms of Racial Discrimination (ICERD), Convention on the Elimination of All Forms of Discrimination Against Women (CEDAW), and Convention on the Rights of the Child (CRC).

> has the purpose or effect of nullifying or impairing the recognition, enjoyment or exercise, on an equal footing, of human rights and fundamental freedoms in the political, economic, social, cultural or any other field of public life (UN Office of the High Commissioner for Human Rights 1965: 2).

While the Thai Constitution and some international treaties the country has signed put an emphasis on the equality of peoples and elimination of discrimination against different groups, the issues of language rights and ethnic minority rights are not directly and specifically addressed in national policy.

In addition, despite the ratification by Thailand of ICERD in 2003, and despite the protection of community rights guaranteed in the 2007 Constitution,[3] instances of stigmatization and discrimination against minority cultural elements, such as ethnicity and language, and the consequences of that stigmatization and discrimination, can still be observed. To give a few examples, inferiority of different ethnic groups in Thailand was outlined in Chiengthong (2003). Keyes (2008: 30) also discusses the discrimination of ethnic peoples, particularly the tribal groups whose cultural uniqueness is commodified for tourism purposes in the country but whose citizenship is still in vain.

4 State Policy on Basic Education

> Unlike majority members, cultural minority members are usually under constant pressure to compromise their cultural identity and assimilate in the majority culture to succeed in other spheres of their lives, like education and career. (Pinto 2009: ii)

Research on language choice and symbolic domination in schooling has shown that while schooling is supposed to provide equal access to all knowledge, it is, as a matter of fact, another site where linguistic and cultural reproduction of existing social hierarchies based on ethnicity, class, religion, and gender, takes place. The kind of knowledge that successfully makes its way into school curricula is usually "the privileged property of the dominant classes" (Heller 2008: 201).

In Thailand, the language of instruction at all levels of education is standard Thai. It started back in the era of King Vajiravudh (1910–1924) who established principles for a compulsory education plan, discouraging other languages. Thai language was set up as the language of instruction to ameliorate threats by nationalistic immigrants of Chinese descent in Thailand, as well as to reinforce the hegemonic nationalist ideology of the Thai state at that time. Being Thai, therefore, required

[3] "Persons so assembling as to be a community, a local community or a traditional community shall have the right to conserve or restore their customs, local knowledge, good arts and culture of their community and of the nation and participate in the management, maintenance, preservation and exploitation of natural resources, the environment and the biological diversity in a balanced and sustainable fashion" (Constitution of the Kingdom of Thailand 2007, http://www.nhrc.or.th/constitution2007_en.pdf).

being educated in the Thai language (cf. Keyes 2008). The use of other languages in class was prohibited altogether in the late 1930s.

Today, such prohibition can be seen as an act of discrimination and a violation of rights. According to Chen (1998: 49), "many aspects of language rights may be regarded as special cases of the general theory of human rights, and the general philosophical justifications of human rights are applicable to language rights.... Violations of language rights can easily be recognized as an injustice and as a failure to give due respect and concern to the dignity of that individual." Examples of violations of language rights include the unavailability of information in a language intelligible to an accused person in court procedures and the subjection of ethnic children to monolingual education in a language other than their mother tongue, resulting in feelings of inferiority and low self-esteem about their own linguistic and cultural background.

Nevertheless, the recently revised "Basic Education Core Curriculum B.E. 2551 [2008]" and the "Basic Education Institutions Curriculum" provide anywhere from 80 h per year for primary students and 240–1,560 h for secondary students in individual schools to create or incorporate their own local curriculum into the core curriculum. Schools have the liberty to incorporate any subjects the local community deem appropriate, unique, useful, and valuable. In some areas, local schools together with nongovernmental organizations have worked together to teach ethnic languages, such as Bisu, Mon, Lahu Shi, Chong, Kui, Northern Khmer, and Pwo Karen, as a subject in school or outside school. Government agencies are not involved in the use of local language in education in Thailand. Such tuition is organized by the nongovernmental sectors only. Overall, only about 50 % of the Thai population has access to education in their mother tongue (Kosonen 2005).

Although the recently revised Basic Education Core Curriculum of 2008 and the Basic Education Institutions Curriculum allow teaching of local content, such as ethnic minority languages, in allocating up to 30 % of the curriculum for local content, not all schools choose to incorporate ethnic languages and cultures into their curriculum. The Basic Education Institutions Curriculum has provided some discretion in its application in local schools. Not all ethnic languages are to be revitalized or will enjoy the same experience of improvement as the Black Tai. The willingness and participation of community members in saving their language and culture is a very important key to the success of ethnic language revitalization. As Romaine (2002: 1) points out, "weak linkages between policy and planning render many policies ineffective. Conventions and treaties adopted by international organizations and agencies recommending the use of minority languages in education usually lack power to reinforce them." One of the key factors is the community's participation and willingness to revive their language and culture. Without supportive governmental policies, sustainable language and culture revitalization movements may arise and succeed through the force of community goodwill and participation. But, without community participation and willingness, revitalization of community's language and culture is basically impossible.

5 Historical Stigma: What's in a Name?

The Black Tai people in Thailand are referred to by different names: Tai/Thai Song Dam, Lao Song, Tai/Thai Song, Tai/Thai Dam, Phu Lao, and Phu Thai Dam. The Black Tai are referred to as "Lao" due to the similar migration history, similar ways of life they share with ethnic Lao, and close linguistic relationship. Both Black Tai and Lao belong to the Southwestern branch of the Tai-Kadai language family. Based on tonal splits and mergers, the Black Tai language is classified into the Tai group (Brown 1965; Burusphat et al. 2011b). With regard to alternate names and different spellings, there are two explanations found in the literature. One explanation is that "Thai" is used to refer to Thai people in general, while the word "Tai" is specifically used to refer to those who speak the languages of the Tai-Kadai language family (Pitiphat and colleagues 1997). Another explanation by Burusphat (1997) suggests that "Thai" is used for those residing in Thailand who speak a Tai-Kadai language, while "Tai" is used for Tai-Kadai speakers outside Thailand. Some linguists still use the term "Tai" to refer to the Tai people in Thailand, such as Tai Phuan and Tai Song Dam.

The place of origin of the Black Tai is believed to have been Muang Thaeng; the location of Dien Bu Phu in Northwest Vietnam today (Sribusara 1979). The Black Tai people in Petchaburi province are descendants of former captives of wars from Muang Thaeng during the reign of King Thonburi, in the Rattanakosin period, circa 1779 (cf. Pitiphat et al. 1978; Pitiphat and Phoonsuwan 1997; Chakshuraksha 2003). Banchun (2009: 48) points out that the Black Tai like to call themselves "Lao Song"; however, they prefer others to call them "Tai songdam" due to the negative connotations of the word "Lao" in the Thai context: "Even though they prefer to call themselves 'Lao Song,' they do not like other out-groups to call them that, as it has the connotation of suppression, insult, and disdain, just as they have been treated since their first arrival as captives of wars until now" [translation supplied]. Klamklomchit (2008) also notes incidents of discrimination, abuse, and rape in the history of the Black Tai during the reign of King Rama V.

In addition, in terms of sociolinguistic study on language hierarchy, the Black Tai language in Thailand belongs to the lower tier in Smalley's dominant hierarchy. According to Smalley (1994), Thailand is a hierarchical society and the ethnic minority peoples are placed at the lower end of the social hierarchy. Belonging to the lower end of the hierarchy means stigma and discrimination that the ethnic minority community has to face, socially, ideologically, and linguistically. Such hierarchy causes discomfort in the contrasting relationship between two groups—"normal" and "stigmatized" individuals (Goffman 1963). Even among the stigmatized themselves, there is a hierarchy. For an internal perspective, an interview with the Black Tai curriculum committee at Khaoyoiwittaya helps illustrate the stigma attached to being called "Lao" in their community.

Excerpt 1: *"...we're the dirty Lao then..."*

Researcher: ... what you said earlier that you said you were embarrassed of being Lao, what happened? Were you teased by others or what was it? Were you teased by your friends?

Interviewee: Not only by people, not only verbally but even written. You "*Lao-gao*" in the story of *Khun Chang Khun Phaen*; they scolded those whose wives were Laotian. Lao was cursed, was suppressed. We tell ourselves that we didn't do right, we made ourselves not clean. We have three kinds of Lao here (...singing "*Chom Khaoyoi*" song), Lao Song, Lao Wiang, and Lao Phuan. One teacher she said she's Lao Wiang she's clean Lao. [person's name] and I thought **we're the dirty Lao then**. I didn't say it out loud but actually, genuinely, we Black Tai are dirty. Like, I went to visit Black Tai in Vietnam. I went up to their houses; they didn't clean their houses. Cats and dogs were all up there. If there're visitors they would use the mat and chairs. It's that we're not clean so we were looked down on by the Thai people. The oil that we used for our hair, we used lard, it stinks, so they despised us.

This is one of several examples of how Black Tai people themselves expressed embarrassment about their own ethnic identity. They related stories of how they were teased and criticized in the wider community in Petchaburi province. In Excerpt 1, the interviewee, who is the community leader, explained that the criticism was conveyed not only orally but also in written form. She gave an example of "*lao gao*," curse words used in a Thai fiction, *Khun Chang Khun Phaen*. Additionally, even among the three Lao-related ethnic groups in Petchaburi—Lao Phuan, Lao Wiang, and Lao Song—the Black Tai are referred to as "dirty Lao." The Black Tai people were looked down on, not only by the Thai people but also other Lao-related ethnic groups in the community. Not only Black Tai adults but children in the community also felt the effects of stigmatization of Black Tai identity.

Excerpt 2: *"...You Lao Song kids! You Lao evil! Get lost! ..."*

Student 1: ...during our scout camp, they teased us saying, **You Lao song kids! You Lao evil! Get lost!**

Student 2: But they are also Lao.

Researcher: Aren't you upset being teased?

Student 1: Not at all. It's better than being teased about something else.

Researcher: Like?

Student 1: Like if you were Karen. They can't pronounce Thai correctly. But actually, if we were born as Karen, we would love to be Karen. Now we were born as Lao, so we love to be Lao. Karen people get teased more. We share their inferiority complex too.

The student in this excerpt reported an incident where her friends and herself were teased by other Lao ethnic kids during her scout camp in the province. She said it was better being teased as "Lao Song" than "Karen." Her story reflects the stigmatization and inferiority the Karen group has to face as well. It is something that they share, being a member of an inferior ethnic group (see also Chaps. 16 and 17 in this volume). The student also said that if she had been born Karen, she would have been proud of her own roots, just as she was proud of being Black Tai now. Her story and comments project the contradiction between feeling inferior and, at the same time, feeling proud of one's own roots.

6 Local Curricula at Watnongprong School and Khaoyoiwittaya School

In linguistically diverse societies, educational institutions could offer monolingual, bilingual, or even multilingual programs depending on the educational policy at the national or institutional level. However, in most countries, the languages included in the formal education policy are typically national languages or a small number of majority languages. When it comes to linguistic minorities, a few viable plans can be considered. The languages and cultures of ethnic minorities could be incorporated into the school curricula in the form of minority-language bilingual education programs or grounded in the so-called multicultural education programs, "a specific policy response to the claims of minority groups for greater recognition within education of ethnic, cultural, religious and linguistic diversity" (May 2001: 173).

According to Banks and Banks (1995: xi), "multicultural education" is "a field of study and an emerging discipline whose major aim is to create equal educational opportunities for students from diverse racial, ethnic, social-class, and cultural groups. One of its important goals is to help all students to acquire knowledge, attitudes, and skills needed to function effectively in a pluralistic democratic society and to interact, negotiate, and communicate with peoples from diverse groups in order to create a civic and moral community that works for the common good." It involves the restructuring of school curricula so that public education can address the ethnolinguistic as well as ethnocultural diversity of the society. A multicultural school curriculum can help fully capture the linguistic and cultural diversity of the society as a whole. In Thailand, research on multicultural education has been conducted since 1998, mostly concerned with the design and development of multicultural programs or multicultural learning units (cf. Yothakun 1998; Suwanruangsri 1999; Jaikliang 2007; Assapaporn 2009; Sungtong 2006, 2009; Farrungsang 2008; Wongtani 2010).

The local school curricula used in Watnongprong and Khaoyoiwittaya schools are more similar to a multicultural curriculum than a bilingual curriculum. Subjects like Black Tai language and tales, traditional songs and games, traditional *khaen* dancing, and Black Tai handicrafts are included in the curricula. Still, they are not real forms of multicultural education, as they do not fully capture the diversity of ethnolinguistic and ethnocultural aspects of the whole community. Rather, they project a number of selected linguistic and cultural aspects of a chosen group, at least at the present time. This tendency seems to confirm Heller's (2008: 201) statement that the kind of knowledge that successfully makes its way into school curricula is usually "the privileged property of the dominant classes."

The Black Tai is now seen as the strongest as well as the most vibrant ethnic group in the province (Burusphat et al. 2011a). The Khaoyoi community is densely populated by Black Tai descendants. The "privileged property" included in the present school curricula mainly focus on Black Tai performances and handicrafts. There is still a lot of work to be done to promote language-related matters or language rights. Attempts to include ethnic languages in Thai schools have so far been in vain.

Kosonen (2005) is of the view that there is no true bilingual education program in Thailand. Nevertheless, it is hoped that, whether true or "in name only," bilingual and multicultural programs will result in positive psychological outcomes, such as better attitudes and higher self-esteem among the students. As Crystal (2000: 31) writes, "local languages are seen to be valuable because they promote community cohesion and vitality, foster pride in a culture, and give a community (and thus a workforce) self-confidence." The local curricula not only make the students proud of their own roots as members of the community but also teach the students to be proud of their roots, whatever they are (see excerpt 2). The positive attitude toward their self-identity is not only held by the Black Tai students but also students of other ethnic groups, as shown below.

Excerpt 3: *"...I want to be Black Tai..."*

Researcher: What are the benefits of the Black Tai curriculum?

Student 1: We get to learn about our roots, our way of life, our origins. We know more and it's fun.

Researcher: What if you had a chance to choose between a regular curriculum and a Black Tai curriculum?

Student 1: Black Tai, we want to learn more about our origins. It makes us love being Lao Song.

Researcher: What about you, what do you think? (talking to a Thai student in the group)

Student 2: The curriculum is good. I live in the community. I can't speak Black Tai, but I kinda absorb it. I want to be able to speak Black Tai. I want to be Black Tai.

Excerpt 4 reveals the students' impressions of the Black Tai curriculum and the teacher. These reactions are positive, not only among the Black Tai students but also among the ethnic Thai students and students of other ethnicities. In this excerpt, Student 2 is an ethnic Thai student who lives in Nongprong subdistrict. The student said she liked the curriculum and wanted to be able to speak Black Tai. Another Karen student from Nongyaaplong made a similar remark elsewhere. In addition, the excerpts from group interviews I carried out show that the local Black Tai students in both Watnongprong and Khaoyoiwittaya schools take pride in being Black Tai and have a good sense of self-esteem. When asked who the "coolest students" in school were—Thai, Black Tai, mixed, or other ethnicity—all the students from both schools said being Black Tai was "the coolest thing."

7 Language and Cultural Rights in the Black Tai Ethnic Revival Process

The revival of Black Tai culture in Khaoyoi, Petchaburi started from the group's interest in ethnic music and performance among people in their own Black Tai network residing in different provinces around the country in the 1970s. It started simply with people from this village traveling to other villages in the same province or other provinces to participate in cultural activities, networking, and enjoying cultural activities. Besides networking, they also wanted to learn more about their own roots. Because of stigma attached to them since the days when they first migrated to Thailand, they have cooperated and networked with one another. This cooperation and networking has made the Black Tai a very closely knit ethnic group. The strong language vitality and cultural preservation have united Lao Song Dam communities. The Black Tai may not have been aware of their rights—like many other groups in Thailand, where the concept of rights is insufficiently acknowledged and promoted—but their ethnic revival movement, their networking, the identification of their roots, and the revitalization of their cultural activities can all be seen as forms of rights-claiming behavior. They have been claiming their rights as Black Tai, to use their own language and to publicly carry out their own cultural activities from the early 1970s.

The Black Tai community leader and schoolteacher in Khaoyoi district described the prejudice and injustice the Black Tai people have had to face. The situation was worse in the past and the group is now stronger than other ethnic minority groups in Petchaburi province. However, some are still embarrassed to be referred to as "Lao" by the majority ethnic Thai. The community leader said that, although the overall situation for Black Tai people today seems to be better than that of some other ethnic groups, Black Tai people have had to face prejudice and injustice from the past up to now. Some Black Tai communities have already assimilated, to a great extent, into the majority Thai society to avoid stigmatization. Furthermore, the community leader's attempts to teach the Black Tai language and culture at school were rejected many times before finally being accepted. At present, more schools are interested in the school classes due to government policies promoting local wisdom, community sustainability, and the recently revised Basic Education Institutions Curriculum. In their recent work, Burusphat and colleagues (2011b: 39) suggest that all Lao ethnic groups in the western region of Thailand take pride in their ethnic languages. These languages are the languages of their ancestors as well as the language used in rituals. Being competent in Lao is an advantage as the language functions as a "secret" language among Lao speakers in all Lao communities.

Through the process of nation building, some ethnic groups may adopt the culture of the dominant group while others opt to maintain and reconstruct their ethnic identity and reinforce group solidarity so as to negotiate and regain social dignity. Instead of assimilating fully into the dominant Thai society, the Black Tai have opted to reconstruct and maintain their ethnic identity to better negotiate rightful access to resources. It could be plausibly argued that their ethnic revival movement and certain improvements, such as increasing acceptance by the wider community and upward mobility, are due to government policies promoting community sustainability and local wisdom. Nevertheless, it is arguable that the Black Tai people would not have been where they are today without the strong will of the community. The ethnic revival movement of the Black Tai elucidates the process of struggle and negotiation with the dominant nation-state and other power sources within the wider community and, at the same time, exhibits the construction and maintenance of ethnic community and ethnic identity in modernity.

From the 1930s to the 1980s, the Thai government was conservative and authoritarian (Hewison 1999). In the process of nation building, homogeneity was emphasized; there was an intense nationalistic movement in Thailand (Chiengthong 2003). Unity of the country was promoted through assimilationist approach and differences otherwise were deemed threats to the unity of the nation (Hayami 2006; Keyes 2008). To this day, of all mainland Southeast Asian states, Thailand is the only country yet to officially recognize its cultural and ethnic diversity numerically (Hayami 2006).

Diversity and difference were repressed in the homogeneously conceived society of Thailand until the emergence of "localism." The localism trend emerged in the Thai state after the economic recession of 1997 in response to efforts to save the country from foreign control over the local economy (Hewison 1999). The collapse of the economy demanded a massive restructuring of the economy; the failure of industrialism has led to the liberalization, "rolling back the state and devolving responsibilities to communities and individuals" (Ryser 2011: 1165). The localism discourse in Thailand is characterized by the following issues: "self-sufficiency; self-reliance; the rejection of consumerism and industrialism; cultural and community; power; rural primacy; and nationalism" (Hewison 1999: 11). Essentially, it emphasizes the strength of local community and self-sufficient economy. It is seen as a source of empowerment for the locals. The promotion of localism brings with it the increasing recognition of diversity and difference, the multicultural aspects of the community. The notion of "Thainess" is thus rearticulated and redefined in Thai society (see Chaps. 1, 8, and 32). The Ministry of Culture, founded in 2002, sets its plans to advocate for ethnic and cultural diversity. Culture is now considered capital for economic and social development. Accordingly, "difference has itself come to mean something else" (Hayami 2006: 287). It has now become a resource.

When the localism trend—promoting the local wisdom, knowledge, and roots of local peoples—began to affect national policies at the end of the twentieth century, the Black Tai became even better known to the public, thus further enhancing pride in their ethnicity. After the Cold War (1945–1991), increasing multicultural awareness and the promotion of ethnic and cultural diversity and local wisdom helped to facilitate the revitalization of Black Tai culture. Indeed, the Black Tai people and their culture became better known through their cultural performances after the rise of multiculturalism in Thailand. Black Tai people whom I interviewed reported having been invited to hundreds of events to perform their traditional *khaen* dancing and to show off their traditional costumes. They were initially embarrassed, but after receiving attention from the public and media, they became proud of what they were doing. After they had an opportunity to perform in front of His Majesty the King, the Black Tai became even more famous. Everybody wanted to see their performances. As a result, community leaders and schoolteachers created several pieces beyond the traditional *khaen* dancing to make their performances more vibrant and varied. They also composed new lyrics to traditional tunes, such as *Chom Khaoyoi* and *Keplep Maeo*. The former is a song about the natural beauty of Khaoyoi that urges people to visit this place where the three Lao groups, the Phuan, Wiang, and Song, live; the latter is about a nutritive local plant, reflecting a Black Tai tradition and way of life. In addition, they also standardized their traditional *khaen* dances, categorized the repertory of *khaen* songs, and added new movements and dance steps to various songs. This body of Black Tai performances represents a newly created cultural identity for the Black Tai in Khaoyoi, Petchaburi; such performances can only be seen here and not in other provinces.

The rise of multiculturalism not only nourished and revitalized the Black Tai's cultural activities but also helped to reduce the historical prejudice against them. Social recognition brings about upward social mobility, and now the other two Lao-related ethnic groups look up to the Black Tai who were once denigrated as "dirty Lao." The trend of multiculturalism triggered a big change for ethnic minority communities. It became something positive to be different.

Excerpt 4: *"...they accept us more because of the media, I think..."*
A schoolteacher at Khaoyoiwittaya school:

> "in terms of acceptance of the wider community, some of the older students were embarrassed by their own ethnicity. Others called them "Lao," and they were embarrassed at the beginning. But after they went to perform and the media liked them, they became proud to be different. In the past, there was not much social acceptance of us being Lao, **but now they accept us more because of the media, I think."**

The role of the media in promoting positive impact was also echoed in another excerpt, a conversation with the Black Tai community leader.

Excerpt 5: *"...TV programs academics and researchers started to come in. Theystarted to take an interest in our ethnic group and we have started to take pride ..."*

Researcher: What causes the change? What brings about the pride that the Black Tai have now?

Interviewee 1: We had opportunities to perform. We were embarrassed then because in the past it was only in the community and the IT was not this accessible. Like, if we went to perform somewhere, say we performed in a hotel, only the hotel people knew about us. The villagers didn't know the kids. The kids who were the pioneer, the first generation of performers, they were proud only among themselves. **But later on TV programs academics and researchers started to come in. They started to take an interest in our ethnic group and we have started to take pride** when we saw

> this and that broadcasted. TV program was broadcasting the Black Tai. We were proud. This was what we did. The villagers started to take pride and those whose children were on TV would ask their neighbors to join them...

Excerpts 4 and 5 reveal the important role played by the media as well as academics and researchers in encouraging acceptance by the wider community and making the ethnic people proud of their own roots.

Additionally, multiculturalism and the recognition of local wisdom and knowledge play an important role in current educational trends. The revised Basic Education Core Curriculum of 2008 and the Basic Education Institutions Curriculum provide approximately 80–1,560 h per year for individual educational institutions to create or incorporate their own local subjects into the core syllabus. The Watnongprong and Khaoyoiwittaya schools have incorporated local history, including Black Tai language and culture, into their local curricula. At the beginning, schoolteachers received academic promotion for writing books or compiling teaching materials on topics related to local history and local wisdom. The Department of Provincial Culture approached schools for cultural performances and everything followed from that; schools and schoolteachers received budgets and awards for incorporating local culture into school activities. The schools become famous in the community. There was a big increase in student enrolment numbers in Khaoyoiwittaya school. Schools also received special supplementary budgets and funds for promoting local culture in their curricula. To promote multiculturalism, the Department of Provincial Culture in Petchaburi province has embarked on a campaign for *rongrian-withi-watthanatham* (culture-based schools). The best culture-based schools are selected and awarded prizes by the Department of Provincial Culture.

Although the national language and its speakers have been advantaged since the National Education Act (1999), the rise of multiculturalism and respect for local wisdom has provided room for ethnic languages and cultures in Thailand. Although there is still no official policy on the languages and cultures of the ethnic minorities or linguistic rights for all citizens, multiculturalism and policies to encourage it are steps in this direction.

8 Conclusion

This chapter has examined how an ethnic revival movement and changes in local school curricula have affected the members of a Black Tai community, including local students. By examining how the Black Tai curriculum has been implemented in local schools, and its impact on local students, I conclude that the Basic Education Institutions Curriculum can be a means of promoting better understanding among different ethnic groups in a community. It helps students to learn more about themselves and others and instills a respect for difference. It also helps to develop pride and fosters self-confidence resulting in higher self-esteem among ethnic minority students. The revival movement has strengthened awareness of ethnic heritages as well as brought them to the surface for broader appreciation.

Looking at the process of revitalization of the Black Tai people in Khaoyoi which started as a stigmatized ethnic group, dubbed the "dirty Lao" among the three Lao-related ethnic groups residing in Petchaburi province, but progressed to a situation where one of the non-Black Tai, Thai-majority students, and an ethnic Karen student said "*I want to be Black Tai.*" Examination of the process allows us to reflect on how the attitude change takes place and how the concept of rights is spelled out in a local context. The Black Tai people may not have been aware of the concept of rights, be it human rights, ethnic minority rights, linguistic rights, or cultural rights, but their ethnic revival movement can be considered as a form of rights-claiming behavior. Instead of assimilating into the majority Thai culture, the Black Tai people try to network and maintain their ethnic identity, reinforcing group solidarity to negotiate and regain social dignity.

The revival movement of the Black Tai people in this study is seen as a collective process carried out by a group that shares common interests, thereby expressing their rights to language and culture. In the context of international covenants and national laws and policies, liberal views tend to ignore the existence of, or even undermine, the importance of group rights. I argue that community strong-will, together with state support, are key factors in the maintenance and prosperity of an ethnic minority community. The state can be important in helping groups exercise their rights to culture. Recognition by the state can provide the spaces in which linguistic and cultural activities are reproduced. These are essential to the linguistic and cultural survival of ethnic minorities.

The Black Tai became known to others before other ethnic groups in Petchaburi did through their cultural performances, through the media, and from the interest of various academics. Other ethnic groups in the province are also trying to keep their ethnic languages and cultures alive, but various factors, i.e., state recognition and support, local power and politics, and the relative social hierarchy of different ethnic groups, may contribute to different degrees of success. In the case of the Black Tai in Khaoyoi, the links and networks they have built within the community and with other Black Tai all over Thailand, the high density of population in the district, the state's support, and the presence of a strong community leader have all played a role in the revitalized identity of the Black Tai today.

Last but not least, the ethnic revival movement of the Black Tai in my study can be seen as "the need to create or continually reproduce dignity and pride" rather than "a wish to return to the past" (Chiengthong 2003: 166). Only certain selective elements are revived to reinforce their uniqueness, namely, costumes and handicrafts, the most vivid elements differentiating the Black Tai from others. The community has to take caution not to fall into "another path to assimilation" or "the institutionalization of culture" (Hayami 2006: 290) whereby culture is mistaken as an object for performance and display only.

Acknowledgments This research was supported under the Culture and Rights Research Project funding scheme, Princess Maha Chakri Sirindhorn Anthropolgy Centre, Thailand.

References

Assapaporn, N. (2009). *The development of housework learning units using inquiry learning activities to promote multicultural understanding and life quality skills of Grade Level 3 students*. Unpublished Ph.D. thesis, Chiangmai University, ChiangMai.

Banchun, O. (2009). Khru thanom khongyimlamai chaoban nongprong [Lecturer Thanom Khongyimlamai Nongprong Villager]. *Warasaan samoson sinlapa watthanatham [Journal of Art and Culture], 30*(3), 48–54.

Banks, J., & Banks, C. A. M. (1995). *Handbook of research on multicultural education*. New York: Macmillan.

Brown, M. (1965). *From ancient Thai to modern dialects*. Bangkok: White Lotus Co. Ltd.

Burusphat, S. (1997). *Encyclopedia: The Black Tai*. Bangkok: Sahadharmmik.

Burusphat, S., Deepadung, S., Suraratdecha, S., Ardsamiti, N., Patpong, P., & Setaphong, P. (2011a). *Kaan chai phaasaa lae thassanakhati to phaasaa lae Kaanthongthiew choeng chattiphan khong klum chattiphan nai phumiphak tawantok khong prathatethai* [Language use and attitudes towards ethnic language and ethnic tourism among ethnic groups in the western region of Thailand]. Bangkok: Saangsue Press.

Burusphat, S., Deepadung, S., Suraratdecha, S., Ardsamiti, N., Patpong, P., & Setaphong, P. (2011b). Language vitality and the ethnic tourism development of the Lao ethnic groups in the western region of Thailand. *Journal of Lao Studies, 2*(2), 23–46.

Chakshuraksha, N. (2003). *Language maintenance and shift in a displaced Tai language: A case study of Black Tai at Nongkhe village, Thailand*. Unpublished Ph.D. thesis, Mahidol University, Nakhon-Pathom.

Chen, A. (1998). The philosophy of language rights. *Language Sciences, 20*(1), 45–54.

Chiengthong, J. (2003). Politics of ethnicity, indigenous culture and knowledge. In K. Mingsarn & J. Dore (Eds.), *Social challenges for the Mekong region* (2nd ed., pp. 147–172). Bangkok: White Lotus.

Constitution of the Kingdom of Thailand. 2007. Retrieved August 12, 2010, from http://www.nhrc.or.th/constitution2007_en.pdf

Crystal, D. (2000). *Language death*. Cambridge: Cambridge University Press.

Farrungsang, B. (2008). The multicultural education knowledge in 3 southern border provinces: Trend for the educational reformation. *Journal of Education, 19*(1), 1–14.

Goffman, E. (1963). *Stigma: Notes on the management of spoiled identity*. Englewood Cliffs: Prentice Hall.

Grimes, B. (2000). *Ethnologue: Languages of the world* (14th ed.). Dallas: SIL International.

Hayami, Y. (2006). Redefining "otherness" from Northern Thailand. Introduction: Notes towards debating multiculturalism in Thailand and beyond. *Southeast Asian Studies, 44*(3), 283–294.

Heller, M. (2008). Language choice and symbolic domination. In M. Marilyn, A. M. de Majia, & N. Hornberger (Eds.), *Encyclopedia of language and education. Vol. 3: Discourse and education* (2nd ed., pp. 201–209). New York: Springer.

Hewison, K. (1999). *Localism in Thailand: A study of globalisation and its discontents* (CSGR Working Paper No. 39/99, pp. 1–27). University of Warwick, Coventry, UK.

Hinton, L. (2001). Language revitalization: An overview. In L. Hinton & K. Hale (Eds.), *The green book of language revitalization in practice* (pp. 3–18). San Diego: Academic.

Jaikliang, W. (2007). *The effects of teaching by using the historical method on learning achievement on the topic of Sukhothai histrorical development, in SOC 32101: social studies, religion and culture, of Mathayom Suksa II students at Banhinlad School in Phangnga Province*. Unpublished Master's thesis. Sukhothai Thammathirat University, Nonthaburi.

Keyes, C. (2008). Ethnicity and the nation-states of Thailand and Vietnam. In P. Leepreecha, D. Mccaskill, & K. Buadaeng (Eds.), *Challenging the limits: Indigenous peoples of the Mekong region* (pp. 13–54). Chiangmai: Mekong Press.

Klamklomchit, T. (2008). *Khunnaang song* [The song elites]. Petchaburi: Petchphumkaanphim.

Kosonen, K. (2005). Education in local languages: Policy and practice in Southeast Asia. In *First language first: Community-based literacy programmes for minority language context in Asia.* Bangkok: UNESCO.
Krauss, M. (1992). The world's languages in crisis. *Language, 68*, 4–10.
May, S. (2001). *Language and minority rights: Ethnicity, nationalism, and the politics of language*. Harlow: Longman.
Munger, F. (2006/2007). Culture, power, and law: Thinking about the anthropology of rights in Thailand in an era of globalization. *New York Law School Law Review, 51*, 818–838.
National Human Rights Commission. *National Human Rights Commission Act, 2542 [1999], Section 3*. Retrieved August 12, 2010, from http://www.nhrc.or.th/index.php
Pinto, M. (2009). *Equality of cultural identity*. Published PhD dissertation, University of Toronto, Toronto.
Pitiphat, S., & Phoonsuwan, S. (1997). *Laosong*: *phonlawat khong rabop watthanatham nai rop song sattawat* [Lao Song: Cultural dynamics in the last two centuries] Research report. Manuscript.
Pitiphat, S., On-dam, B., & Thammaphimuk, P. (1978). *Lao song: Raingan kanwichai* [Lao Song: Research report]. Bangkok: Thammasat University Press.
Romaine, S. (2002). The impact of language policy on endangered languages. *International Journal on Multicultural Societies, 4*(2), 2–28.
Ryser, J. (2011, May 18–20). Whose quality of life? In what kind of city? In *Proceedings REAL CORP 2011* (pp. 1163–1168). Tagungsband.
Smalley, W. (1994). *Linguistic diversity and national unity: Language ecology in Thailand.* Chicago: University of Chicago Press.
Sribusara, M. (1979). *Thai Dam ramphan* [The lamentation of Thai Dam]. Bangkok: Bannakich Press.
Sungtong, E. (2006). *Pramuan khwam ru nai phahu watthanatham: Sueksa changwat chai daen phaktai* [Compilation of multicultural education knowledge in Southern Border Provinces]. Unpublished manuscript.
Sungtong, E. (2009). Strategic leadership in multilingual society: Rethinking concepts, theories and practices. *Journal of Education, 23*(1), 1–16.
Suwanruangsri, K. (1999). *A development of multicultural school and community partnership program for the improvement of preschool teaching in southern Muslim community*. Unpublished master's thesis. Chulalongkorn University, Bangkok.
UN Office of the High Commission for Human Rights. (1965). *International convention on the elimination of all forms of racial discrimination (ICERD)*. Retrieved August 12, 2010, from http://www2.ohchr.org/english/
Wongtani, C. (2010). *Educational travel project for learning about harmonious ways of living in plural community: 'When Muslims visit the temple and Buddhists meet the mosque*. Unpublished manuscript.
Yothakhun, S. (1998). *A development of a multicultural education program to promote self-understanding and preschool children in the Northeastern region*. Unpublished master's thesis, Chulalongkorn University, Bangkok.

Chapter 16
Lahu Students in Thai Schools: The Cases of Som and Noi

Matthew R. Juelsgaard

1 Background

Northern Thailand is home to a variety of diverse ethnic groups and their unique cultures. Included are the Lahu people, who reside throughout most of the countries of mainland Southeast Asia and Southwestern China. Currently, many Lahu children in Thailand attend primary schools[1] located in their home village-communities. After finishing primary school, Lahu students frequently move away from their home village-communities in order to attend secondary school in larger Thai towns or cities. Teaching in a primary school, I observed that many students who left the village-community to study returned within a year or two. Without more than a primary school education, Lahu individuals, who generally occupy the lowest economic class in Thai society, are further disadvantaged. In order to help schools and educators create learning environments that consider the specific schooling experiences of Lahu students and help them to succeed in school, this qualitative study inquired into the formal educational experiences of two Lahu sisters: one who discontinued her schooling after lower secondary school and one who graduated from a well-known university in Northern Thailand.

[1]According to the Thai Ministry of Education, the Thai education system consists of twelve years of schooling: six years of "*Prathom*," or primary school, and six years of "*Mathayom*," or secondary education. Secondary education is further divided into lower secondary, *Mathayom* 1–3, and upper secondary, *Mathayom* 4–6. Eight core subjects make up most of the curriculum: Thai language, mathematics, science, social studies, religion and culture, health and physical education, arts, careers and technology, and foreign languages.

M.R. Juelsgaard (✉)
Department of Educational Foundations, University of Hawai'i at Mānoa,
Honolulu, HI, USA
e-mail: juelsgaa@hawaii.edu

P. Liamputtong (ed.), *Contemporary Socio-Cultural and Political Perspectives in Thailand*,
DOI 10.1007/978-94-007-7244-1_16,

2 The Lahu and Formal Education in Thailand

The vast majority of Lahu, who speak a Tibeto-Burman language, live throughout the mountains of China's Yunnan province, Myanmar, Thailand, Laos, and Vietnam. The Lahu have never controlled a territory of their own and have always lived in the peripheries of more politically dominant peoples (Walker 2003). Walker (2003) claims that there are around 700,000 Lahu worldwide – 59 % in China, 29 % in Myanmar/Burma, 9 % in Thailand, 2.3 % in Laos, 0.9 % in Vietnam, and several hundred refugees from Laos living in the United States.

In Thailand, the Lahu live primarily in the Northern provinces of Chiang Rai, Mae Hong Son, Chiang Mai, Lampang, and Tak. It is uncertain exactly when the Lahu began to settle in parts of the area that today comprises Thailand, although there are written reports of well-established communities by the 1880s and 1890s (McGilvery 1912; Walker 2003). Despite living in Thailand for over 130 years, the Lahu, along with other ethnic minority peoples in the area, are commonly perceived to be outsiders and recent (illegal) immigrants.

The beginnings of formal education, or schooling, by the Thai government among the Lahu began primarily after World War II. The military government of the late 1940s, eager to ally with the United States, developed strong anti-Communist policies. Although there was little government interest previously, the mountainous borderlands inhabited by ethnic minorities gained strategic military importance as communist insurgency became a real threat (Pine 2002; Toyota 2005). The integration, or assimilation, of ethnic minorities into the Thai nation was seen by state authorities as the best way to ensure the Lahu and other ethnic groups accepted the important role of helping to maintain the security of the national frontiers. For many government officials, formal education was seen as the primary tool for integrating ethnic minorities into the Thai nation (Kammerer 1988), and it also served as a means to advance a particular conception of Thai national identity. Regarding this, Keyes (1991: 112) writes: "The primary objective of the national system of education in Thailand has been, and continues to be, to prepare children throughout the country to enter into a 'Thai' national world, a world structured with reference to the Thai state."

With two of the principal objectives of Thai schools being national integration and the promotion of Thai national identity, Lahu students, as ethnic minority students, have a unique perspective on the experience of schooling in Thailand. While researchers have noted the general trend of national integration in Thai schools,[2] little research has been conducted on the day-to-day schooling experiences of individual members of ethnic minority groups, such as the Lahu, who have been recipients of integrationist educational policies.[3] Thus, one of the primary purposes of this study

[2] See Keyes (1991) for a detailed account of how schools serve the purposes of national integration and the promotion of a Thai national identity.

[3] See Johnson (2007) for one of the few insightful accounts of the daily schooling experiences of ethnic minority students in Thailand.

was to inquire into and begin to describe the meaningful schooling experiences of two Lahu students in the Thai schools they attended.

Three research questions were central to this study: (a) What are some characteristics of Lahu students' experiences in Thai schools? (b) What influences a Lahu student to discontinue formal education before completing secondary school? (c) What contributes to a Lahu student successfully completing university study? In attempting to respond to questions (b) and (c), I was specifically interested in the influence of family, peer groups, and schools on the participants' schooling experiences.

3 Theoretical Framework

In their Students' Multiple Worlds Study, Phelan and colleagues (1991, 1998) describe the "worlds," or cultural knowledge and expectations, of family, peer groups, and schools that students' encounter as they move through school. These three worlds interact in the day-to-day lives of adolescents, and students must learn to the navigate borders that arise as a result of knowledge, norms, values, beliefs, and skills in one world being more highly valued than those in another.

Borders can take a variety of forms: (a) sociocultural, (b) socioeconomic, (c) psychosocial, (d) linguistic, (e) gender, (f) heterosexist, and (g) structural. Sociocultural borders can arise when communication, cognitive, interactional, learning, literacy, motivational, or writing styles in one world (family, peer, or school) are seen as inferior to, and not simply different from, those existing in another world. When a student's economic circumstances create significant limitations, socioeconomic borders may exist. Experiences of anxiety, depression, apprehension, or fear that disrupt student's ability to focus, learn, and be in healthy relationships with others have the potential to create psychosocial borders. Linguistic borders may arise when the communication style or language in one world is regarded as inferior to that used in another world (see also Chaps. 1 and 15 in this volume). When roles, aspirations, or estimates of worth differ between boys and girls, gender borders can emerge. Students who find themselves confronted by a world where heterosexuality is superior to other forms of sexuality encounter heterosexist borders. Lastly, structural borders can be defined as characteristics of school environments that prevent student learning (Phelan et al. 1998).

Phelan and colleagues (1998) found in their study that some students encountered few borders while others confronted many. For those who did encounter borders, some transitioned between differing social contexts with ease while others found it difficult. Those who embraced their different worlds and were able to transition smoothly between varied social contexts were often criticized for breaking particular social rules or expectations within each world. And those who perceived the borders as insurmountable were often disengaged from school. Understanding the worlds that students encounter daily, the borders students perceive and the ways in which those borders may or may not be navigated is helpful in creating learning environment in which students can thrive.

4 The Study

In this section, I describe the methods of data collection and analysis used in this study. I also discuss my role as the researcher.

Two Lahu sisters, Som and Noi, participated in this study. Both are from Chiang Rai Province in Northern Thailand, which is also the location of the five schools in my study. Som, who discontinued her schooling after lower secondary school, is 25 years old and lives in Mooban Village in Chiang Rai Province in Northern Thailand. In addition to agricultural work, her family owns and runs a small shop and gas station. Som's sister, Noi, a graduate from a well-known university in Northern Thailand, is 27 years old. After university, Noi worked as a counselor and teacher at a dormitory for ethnic minority students attending the local secondary school. She is interested in the education of Lahu adolescents and the preservation of Lahu culture and identity in Thailand.[4]

Three interviews were conducted in Thai with both Som and Noi. They were asked to participate because of their similar backgrounds, differing educational attainment levels, and previous relationships with me. Participation was voluntary.

The interviews were conducted using a semi-structured format. Each interview was approximately 30–45 min long and focused on the participant's experience of school, what they enjoyed, what they found challenging, and the reasons for discontinuing school, as in Som's case, or continuing school, as in Noi's case. All interviews were audio recorded, translated into English, and transcribed.

I analyzed the interview data by first "asking questions" in order to probe the data for initial concepts and better understand the experiences from the participants' perspectives (Corbin and Strauss 2008). These questions, as well as initial codes that were developed from the data, were recorded in a series of detailed memos. The initial codes were (a) friends/peers, (b) barriers, (c) parents/family, (d) motivations, and (e) responsibility. After reviewing what was coded under "barriers," three sub-codes were generated: (a) feelings of "inferiority," (b) language, and (c) "not knowing." The text coded under "motivations" was also divided into sub-codes: (a) parents expectations, (b) injustice, and (c) future aspirations. The codes were partially influenced by Phelan and colleagues' (1998) "worlds" of family, peers, and schools as I was interested in understanding some of the differing social contexts that Som and Noi encountered as they moved through school and the borders that they navigated.

For a total of 24 months from 2005 to 2009, I was able to live in a Lahu community. Initially, an acquaintance helped to connect in as a volunteer at the community's school. After completing a semester at the school, I became involved with the community in other ways. Having lived in the community, I was able to be more aware of some of the challenges many people faced in trying to go to school. In fact, it was my own experience of observing some of the students I had taught in the classroom discontinuing their schooling that fostered much of my interest in this topic.

---

[4] The names of people and places in this study have been changed to protect the anonymity of the participants.

I am not Lahu, nor do I speak or understand anything beyond the elementary aspects of the Lahu language. I am thus an outsider (Liamputtong 2010) to Lahu worldviews. In order to guard against misinterpretation, I worked with a Lahu research assistant who was more capable of moving between Lahu, Thai, and English contexts than myself. I also attempted to ask more questions to participants than might be necessary in order to clarify what I was interpreting.

5 The Stories of Som and Noi

In the following section, I present the results of the analysis of interviews with Som and Noi. Som speaks of her transitions between different schools and social contexts, the influence of friends and family on her experiences, and the reasons for discontinuing school. Then, Noi describes her initial experiences of school that instilled in her a desire to graduate from university, her encounters with prejudice, and the role of her parents in her schooling.

5.1 Som

Som was a member of the first generation of Lahu students from her village-community to attend Thai public school. At the age of 6, she attended a school founded for Lahu children by the Thai government in her home village-community, Mooban Village. During this time, she lived with her family and she described herself as a "good" student, better than most of her friends. When she was 8 years old and entering the second semester of her third year of primary school, she changed schools. The motivation behind the change was that her parents perceived the schools outside of the village-community to be of better quality. The new school, Baan Primary School, was mostly made up of Thai students, although a few students were from different ethnic minority groups in the region. Importantly, Som's move was not simply a change in schools. As she moved out of the village context and into a Thai town and school, she found herself in a situation that few young Lahu people in her area had encountered before; namely, she was interacting daily with Thai people in a Thai community and Thai school. Her new school, unlike the one in Mooban, was not created for Lahu children, but for local Thais. Under these circumstances, Som needed to learn how to live and act in her new sociocultural context.

Being in this new context brought with it new challenges. In general, she felt "inferior" and unable to keep up with other students. Without the ability to speak Thai fluently, language became a barrier to completing her schoolwork. Commenting on this, she said:

> I was new to the school and I couldn't really speak. Some words I just didn't know and, well, I just couldn't keep up. I couldn't keep up with my classmates. I thought they were Thai, they were *Khon Muang*. I felt inferior. At that time, I just wasn't good in school.

In the face of these challenges, she "just continued to study" primarily because she "had friends to study with." Recognizing that she could get by even if she was not one of the top students, she gave no thought to ending her studies after primary school.

While Baan Primary School was located 8 miles from Som's home community in a Thai town, the secondary school that she attended was located in the small city of Chiang Rai, approximately 30 miles away. Like most families in the community, Som's family had no personal means of motorized transportation. While she could walk home on weekends during her time at Baan Primary School, such a feat was not possible from Chiang Rai. Her physical separation between her family and home community allowed for new experiences but also created misunderstandings between her and her parents.

Som mentioned her new experiences when asked about the differences in the two school settings. She said:

> When I was studying in Baan Primary, I had some friends, not a lot, but some. But when I went to Chiang Rai I made a lot of friends. And then there were a lot of new things, things I never knew and had never encountered. A lot! The school was big, bigger than Baan Primary. It was probably two, three or four times the size. And then there were a lot of people as well, more than 1000. There were several ethnic groups. There were Akha, Lisu, Yao, Hmong, Karen, Thai Yai, Khon Muang and Chinese. I had to change so that I could live together with others because there were a lot of ethnic groups. I had to speak Thai if I was going to understand anything. And then, at that time, I made a lot of friends. When I was in Baan [Primary] and Mooban [Primary] I had about 10 friends. But when I went to live [in Chiang Rai], I had 20 or 30 friends.

Som conveyed her transition with a sense of excitement about the variety of new experiences she was able to have at her new school. Her focus was on new friends, most of who were ethnic minority students.

About twice a semester, Som was able to return home from Chiang Rai in order to visit her family. During these visits, her parents expected her to help farm and to assist with chores around the house. She rarely helped, causing her parents to refuse to give her spending money for school. Without money to spend on items such as new backpacks and cosmetics, which many of her peers possessed, Som felt embarrassed around her friends and questioned her reasons for going to school:

> Sometimes I only had 200 baht when I returned to school. After I paid the bus fare and some other expenses, I didn't have any money to use. So, I thought, why am I studying? I didn't have money to use. I was embarrassed with my friends as well because at that time I was a teenager. They would go to eat together, they had makeup, they had perfume, but I didn't have any money to use. So, I was sad and felt inferior. I asked myself, "Why don't I have the same things that they have? Why do they have these things?" I felt inferior at the time. They had new backpacks and clothes. I didn't have and I felt inferior about it.

Although she was upset that her parents refused to give her spending money, Som eventually came to understand that her parents had little money to give to her. She perceived their support in other ways, especially in the form of spoken affirmations encouraging her to continue her studies. Such affirmation, though, was not enough.

When asked specifically about why she did not continue her schooling, Som, interestingly, speaks about a lack of knowledge:

> I didn't know what the world was like outside of lower secondary school. I didn't know what school to go to for upper secondary school. I didn't know how to get a vocational certificate or anything, because I had never experienced the world outside of school, outside of lower secondary. And so, I couldn't think about what would happen if I didn't study. I could not know at that time. I thought, well, I have mom and dad, and I can go back and live with them. And then well, I didn't know what the future would be like. If I was going to study more, who would take care of me? What will it be like? I would have to make new friends. My friends had to go to several places; and I didn't know what to do. Nowadays, children go on to another dormitory or they rent a place to stay. I didn't know when I left the school what I was going to do. I thought, am I able to take care of myself? I didn't think so at the time. So, I concluded, well, I am not going to study anymore. I can work at home and help my parents. That was all I was able to think to myself.

After finishing lower secondary school, the dormitory where she boarded was no longer able to allow her to board. If she wanted to continue her schooling, she would have needed to find an upper secondary school to attend and a place to stay, perhaps another dormitory. From Som's perspective, a lack of knowledge served to prevent her from transitioning from lower secondary school to upper secondary school. She claims that she was only partially aware of or knowledgeable about the educational opportunities that were available for her. She thought about continuing on to upper secondary school or perhaps pursuing a vocational certificate; however, she did not know in detail what these options entailed or which one might be appropriate for her. While she knew about some of the opportunities available, there was little knowledge about how to go about pursuing these particular educational opportunities. In other words, there was a lack of knowledge with regard to the means to pursue the educational opportunities with which she was vaguely familiar.

In making her decision, Som recognized that she could return home to her parents and help them with farm work. The confusion surrounding what she needed to do in order to continue her schooling made returning home an attractive alternative because there was a familiarity with what life would be like.

From my perspective as a researcher, Som's explanation is important to consider and yet it also seems incomplete if we take into account that her older sister was enrolled in upper secondary school at the time. Although Som did not directly talk about her choice to get married after lower secondary school, I suspect that another reason she discontinued her schooling was to get married and begin a family in her home community. From what I observed during my time in Mooban Village, her choice was similar to other adolescents who frequently chose to discontinue school in order to marry, pursue family life, and work.

5.2 Noi

Noi, like Som, was a member of the first generation of Lahu students in her community to attend Thai public school. Noi started attending school 2 years prior to Som in the village-community of Mooban. She recalls being introduced to the

Thai alphabet and language; but with only one teacher for six grade levels, she says she did not learn much. Having heard that the school in the village-community of Nai Pa Yai offered a higher quality of education, Noi's father decided to send her there along with her two older brothers. The new school was 2 h away on a rugged dirt road, preventing her from seeing her parents more than twice a semester. The school was made up of students from at least four different ethnic minority groups in the area. Noi recalls the initial transition as challenging:

> Every night other students teased me. We all slept together in a dormitory at the school. There were Lisu, Akha, Karen and Lahu. Since we did not come from the same village-community, the other girls I slept with pulled my hair, pinched me and made fun of me. I just could not take it anymore. One night about seven or eight girls came and tried to fight with me. I fought, and I won, probably because I had five older brothers. After that, the other girls never tried to fight me anymore and actually, we became friends.

While the transition from her home community to Nai Pa Yai was challenging at first, Noi eventually began to enjoy her schooling experience. In general, she recalls her time there as instrumental in laying the foundation for her future experiences of school. In particular, two experiences she remembers instilled in her a desire to graduate from university. First, every year they had to introduce themselves to their teachers and the other students. They would have to say their name, where they were from, their age, how many siblings they had, and *what type of work they wanted to have in the future*. Noi claims, in general at that time, many Lahu parents did not talk to their children about future occupations or aspirations. Thus, a teacher asking her about her future educational and economic aspirations was both novel and encouraging for Noi. From my perspective, this orientation toward future "success" is an important aspect of Noi's educational experience to which I will return in more detail in the discussion.

The second experience at Nai Pa Yai school that implanted in Noi a desire to graduate from university occurred while watching a black and white television. Recalling the experience she said:

> I saw a girl on the TV wearing a university uniform and I thought to myself, "I want to wear a uniform." At that time, we did not wear uniforms everyday. We only got to wear uniforms about twice a week. On the TV I saw that they were wearing nice clothes, they looked neat and organized. I thought that would be good if I could study, make it to higher education and wear a university uniform.

Seeing a girl wearing a university uniform instilled in Noi a desire to continue her schooling through university. During her time at Nai Pa Yai school, these two experiences, teachers asking her to think about her future work and an encounter through the television with a women wearing a university uniform, were fundamental in forming Noi's disposition or orientation toward schooling. She began to see school as a pathway toward a fulfilling future.

In her sixth year of primary school, Noi left Nai Pa Yai school and started school at Baan Primary School, where Som had been studying for 1 year at that point. The primary reason for her move was that Baan was closer to home and she could see her parents more frequently. As with her transition from Mooban to Nai Pa Yai, the move to Baan was initially challenging:

> It was the first time studying in a Thai town, in Baan. I wanted to be closer to my family so that I could go home on the weekends. I lived at a dormitory with my siblings. When I went to school there were several other Lahu students at the school. In my classes though I was the only Lahu student. Many of the students would tease me. They would say, "You can't speak Thai." Or "Why can't you read Thai?" Or sometimes they would take rubber bands and shoot me with them and I would not know who shot the rubber band. Some of the other classes had more Lahu students but not in my class. I got angry when they would tease me. They saw me as inferior, as uncivilized, as an alien. They did not see me as a person they saw me as like an alien from some other place.

At Baan Primary School, Noi encountered prejudice for the first time and was the target of stereotypes. Being a member of the first generation of Lahu students to attend Thai schools in the area, she sensed injustice in the way she and other Lahu students were treated. Interestingly, this sense of injustice, of being the target of prejudice, motivated Noi to continue her schooling:

> All of the teasing made me angry, very angry. And it made me want to compete as well, to win. I wanted to show them that I was good, that I was capable, that I could be successful. I wanted people to accept me as a person. I felt that nobody accepted me. At that time, most people thought that the minority people were not capable of studying. They thought that after a little bit of school they would go back to farming. And people used to say that, "Go back to the forest!" So I thought, I need to do this, I need to go to school. This was my motivation. I wanted to fight, to fight for a better life and to be better than others thought I was.

The mistreatment that Noi suffered by being an ethnic minority student served to enkindle in her a strong desire to continue her schooling through university. There was a sense of needing to prove to others, primary Thai others, that she, as a Lahu woman, was capable of academic success and a "better life."

Another important aspect of Noi's educational experience that served as a source of motivation was her parents. Being farmers among the lowest economic class in Thailand, they made observable sacrifices that fostered in Noi a desire to live up to their expectations and not disappoint them. Speaking about her parent's expectations as a motivating force, Noi explains: "I did not want to disappoint my parents. I saw that my father sold his land and sold his fruit orchard in order to send me to school. He sold all the water buffalo and cows … I thought that I did not want to disappoint my parents." Her parent's sacrifice was not for Noi alone but for three of her siblings as well, all of who discontinued their schooling before completing secondary school. Noi offered an explanation as to the significant differences between herself and her siblings:

> He wanted all four of us to graduate but in the end it was just me. My father tried to get us all but it just didn't work … I saw that my siblings upset my parents when they went out with their friends and did not study. My parents told us not to do this but they did. I saw my dad was very sad. He tried his best and he did a great job, but half of the responsibility is on the child as well. Both the child and parents need to commit to going to school.

A sense of responsibility for herself and her future contributed to Noi's desire to continue her schooling. Observing that her parents made sacrifices, she also recognized the need to make sacrifices and made a personal commitment to education. Interestingly, in addition to a sense of personal responsibility for her studies, there was a sense of responsibility to her Lahu community as well. The sense of communal responsibility involved being of service to ethnic minority peoples in the mountains as well as educating non-Lahu people about Lahu society and culture:

> I thought that if I studied I would also be able to help the people who lived in the mountains, the Lahu people. I wanted others to not see us as inferior. I thought about this ever since I was little. Ever since I heard people teasing me, I wanted to bring justice to all the minority groups. I did not want to hear that this minority group is like this and that minority group is like that. I thought about this ever since that time.

Desiring to be of service to her Lahu community, Noi recognized that she would need to attend school to fulfill her hopes. She also recognized that it was not only her Lahu community that was in need; other, primarily Thai, people were in need of learning how to treat the ethnic minority groups justly and with equality. Noi began to envision herself as someone capable of fulfilling this transcultural role.

6 Discussion

This study examined the formal educational experiences of two Lahu students in Thai schools. One of the students, Som, discontinued her schooling before completing secondary school while her sister, Noi, graduated from university. The findings suggest that Som's relationship with her parents, especially with regard to money, and a lack of knowledge as to how to pursue available educational opportunities contributed to her discontinuance of school. Noi's internalization of schooling as a pathway to future fulfillment, the use of discrimination as a source of motivation, her parent's visible sacrifices, and a sense of both personal and communal responsibility were instrumental in graduating from university. In this section, I highlight the implications of my findings for those involved in the education of Lahu students in Thailand, as well as those involved with the education of ethnic minority students elsewhere whose experiences may resonate with that of Som and Noi. In particular, I discuss issues related to (a) encountering borders and building bridges connecting students to available resources and opportunities, (b) motivating students who encounter prejudice, and (c) internalizing the idea that academic achievement is directly related to future opportunities.

6.1 Encountering Borders and Building Bridges

Phelan and colleagues (1998) suggest that students might encounter socioeconomic, linguistic, and structural borders that make it difficult for them to navigate their way through school. Socioeconomic borders arise when economic circumstances create limitations. Both Som and Noi were economically constrained. For Som, this constraint prevented her from involvement with some peers whose economic circumstances were better. Noi, on the other hand, regarded the socioeconomic borders as a source of motivation, and they enkindled in her a desire to continue schooling as a member of a group that generally occupies the lowest economic class in Thailand. The sisters also encountered linguistic borders, a result of the devaluation of languages other than Thai in schools. For Som, the linguistic borders made it difficult to achieve academically; and Noi discussed being teased by her peers for not speaking proper Thai. Lastly, structural borders are aspects of a school environment that prevent, impede, or discourage student learning and continuance in school. Results from this study suggest that Som's inability to access beneficial educational resources contributed to her discontinuance of school. Services and opportunities for furthering her formal education existed and Som was partially aware of these; however, there were no bridges connecting her with available resources.

6.2 *"Challenge Models"*

Cooper (2003) and Cooper and associates (2002) point out that challenges, such as poverty and prejudice, can, under some conditions, motivate students to achieve academically on behalf of their families and communities and prove gatekeepers wrong. The results from my study support a similar conclusion, as we see in Noi's case. In the face of prejudice and other challenges related to being one of the first Lahu students from her community in a Thai public school, Noi felt motivated to achieve academically in order to prove to others that she, as a Lahu woman, was capable of graduating from university. Interestingly, Noi did not only want to prove gatekeepers, other Thai students in this case, wrong, but she also wanted to educate them with regard to Lahu culture and identity.

6.3 *School and Future Opportunities*

Spindler and colleagues (1990) along with Phelan and others (1998) suggest that many metropolitan, upper-middle-class students internalize the idea that academic achievement is tied directly to future opportunities. This orientation toward the future is, in part, characterized by planning for the future, thinking about the future, and worrying about the future. While such an orientation can cause anxiety in many cases, the results from my study indicate that such anxiety may not always be present. Noi, coming from a rural, lower-income background, seems to have internalized the idea that academic achievement is directly related to future opportunities. However, it does not seem to be the case that Noi's orientation toward the future was characterized by anxiety. Rather, Noi's orientation toward the future could be characterized as one filled with hope – a hope to be of service to her community and Thai society in general. A key distinction might be that those students with anxiety internalized expectations related to socioeconomic status or the need to remain at or improve upon one's parent's socioeconomic class. Noi does not seem to embody such expectations; rather, her expectations have to do with being of service to others.

6.4 Implications for Educators

This study has implications for educators of Lahu students in Thai schools and others who are involved in the education of ethnic minority students. First, I recommend that teachers and counselors deliberately work with students in identifying the borders they may encounter. With the help of teachers, students can analyze and deconstruct many of the borders they confront as they move through school. Second, it is important to connect students with available resources. Educators should serve as bridges for students whose parents are not knowledgeable about educational resources. Clubs or organizations for ethnic minority students can provide a place and community within which students can learn about these resources as they move through school. These clubs and organizations can also be places where ethnic minority students feel a sense of solidarity that may help them in using their particular challenges as motivation for academic achievement. Lastly, it seems possible for students to internalize without much anxiety the idea that academic achievement is directly related to future opportunities if students envision themselves as achieving academically for the sake of being of service to others in the future. This is a disposition that can be embraced by educators and passed on to students.

Acknowledgments I thank Gay Garland Reed for her advice in pursuing this project, Lois Yamauchi for her help with conducting the research and feedback on initial drafts, and Natcharat Juelsgaard for her assistance throughout the entirety of the project.

References

Cooper, C. R. (2003). Bridging multiple worlds: Immigrant youth identity and pathways to college. *International Society for the Study of Behavioral Development Newsletter*, No. 2, Serial No. 38, 1–4.

Cooper, C. R., Cooper, R. G., Azmitia, M., Chavira, G., & Gullat, Y. (2002). Bridging multiple worlds: How African American and Latino youth in academic outreach programs navigate math pathways to college. *Applied Development Science, 6*, 73–87.

Corbin, J., & Strauss, A. (2008). *Basics of qualitative research: Techniques and procedures for developing grounded theory* (3rd ed.). London: Sage.

Johnson, T. (2007). Enclothing identity: A Hmong girl's journey into the politics of identification in Thailand. *Teachers College Record, 109*(7), 1637–1662.

Kammerer, C. A. (1988). Territorial imperatives: Akha ethnic identity and Thailand's national integration. In R. Guidieri, F. Pellizi, & S. Tambiah (Eds.), *Ethnicities and nations, processes of interethnic relations in Latin America, Southeast Asia, and the Pacific* (pp. 259–292). Austin: University of Texas Press.

Keyes, C. F. (1991). The proposed world of the school: Thai villagers' entry into a bureaucratic state system. In C. F. Keyes, E. J. Keyes, & N. Donnelly (Eds.), *Reshaping local worlds: Formal educational and cultural change in rural Southeast Asia* (pp. 89–130). New Haven: Yale Center for International and Area Studies.

Liamputtong, P. (2010). *Performing qualitative cross-cultural research*. Cambridge: Cambridge University Press.

McGilvery, D. (1912). *A half century among the Siamese and the Lao*. New York: Revell.

Phelan, P., Davidson, A. L., & Yu, H. C. (1991). Negotiating the boundaries of family, peer and school cultures. *Anthropology & Education Quarterly, 22*(3), 224–250.

Phelan, P., Davidson, A. L., & Yu, H. C. (1998). *Adolescents' worlds: Negotiating family, peers, and school*. New York: Teachers College Press.

Pine, J. M. S. (2002). *Lahu writing and writing Lahu: An inquiry into the value of literacy*. Retrieved from Dissertation and theses database (AAT 3063000), University of Washington, Seattle.

Spindler, G. D., Spindler, L., Trueba, H., & Williams, M. (1990). *The American cultural dialogue and its transmission*. New York: Falmer.

Toyota, M. (2005). Subjects of the national without citizenship: The case of the 'hill tribes' in Thailand. In W. Kymlicka (Ed.), *Multiculturalism in Asia* (pp. 110–135). Oxford: Oxford University Press.

Walker, A. (2003). *Merit and the millennium: Routine and crisis in the ritual lives of the Lahu people*. New Delhi: Hindustan Publishing Corporation.

Chapter 17
Rural-Urban Migration and Ethnic Minority Enterprise

Alexander Trupp

1 Introduction

Throughout the last decades, rural-urban migration of the "hilltribes"[1] of Thailand has become significant. Lack of land rights and low perspectives for education or job opportunities in their home regions as well as a variety of other factors have been facilitating migratory movements to Thailand's urban areas (Toyota 1998; Buadeng et al. 2002). This development resulted in an increasing percentage of highland minorities living in the capital Bangkok as well as in medium-sized cities and tourist centers in the North or in the South of the country. This chapter focuses on the ethnic minority of Akha, and specifically on Akha women, who have migrated into Thailand's urban and tourist areas in order to sell handicrafts and souvenirs. They have become entrepreneurs or self-employed street vendors. In confining the term "entrepreneurship" I use a nonelitist approach similar to that of Valenzuela (2001), where ethnic entrepreneurs are defined as self-employed members of ethnic minority groups, regardless of whether or not they employ other people and regardless of whether they own small business on the margins of economy or large multi-million enterprises (Basu 2007). In addition, they are mainly both owners and managers (or operators) of their own businesses and their group membership is tied to a cultural heritage or origin (Zhou 2004: 1040), whereas ethnic and social embeddedness (Portes and Sensenbrenner 1993) as well as economic transactions play a crucial role. Perspectives of migrant entrepreneurship either highlight the benefits of ethnic business, especially in terms of economic development, urban diversity,

[1] The term "hilltribes" refers to the ethnic minority groups residing in the highlands of Southeast Asia. For a discussion on ethnicity and the politics of ethnic classification in Thailand, see Winichakul (1994) and Laungaramsri (2003). In this article, I use the term ethnic minorities, hilltribes, and highlanders alternately.

A. Trupp (✉)
Department of Geography and Regional Research, University of Vienna,
Universitätsstraße 7/5/C517 (NIG), A-1010 Vienna, Austria
e-mail: alexander.trupp@univie.ac.at

P. Liamputtong (ed.), *Contemporary Socio-Cultural and Political Perspectives in Thailand*,
DOI 10.1007/978-94-007-7244-1_17,

and integration, or warn about precarious working conditions or the formation of enclave economies. By outlining rural-urban migrations of ethnic minorities and exploring their mixed embeddedness and their social practice of economic behavior, this chapter contributes to the neglected phenomenon of ethnic minority studies in Thailand's urban contexts.

While most urban-based hilltribes remain invisible for visitors and other outsiders, one part of a migrant group visually stands out and is about becoming an integral feature of Thailand's urban and beachside tourist centers. Eye-catching female Akha handicraft and souvenir sellers, often wearing colorful and richly decorated hats, became part of an informal sector that is linked to the global tourism economy. The areas of sale of these rural-urban migrants, such as the famous "Kaosan Road" in Bangkok or the notorious "Walking Street" in Patong on Phuket Island, have become interfaces between ethnic minority entrepreneurs and a wider economy consisting of national and international travelers, expatriates, other business owners and workers, officials, and various members of the Thai mainstream society. Although the Akha people in Thailand have a marginalized status and are regarded as a homogenous group, one can find considerable differences within the single Akha category, especially in terms of gender, class, and age. Moreover, the group of Akha entrepreneurs itself is segmented: Some Akha lease booths at markets, others put their goods along footpaths next to the markets, and others again carry their stuff in baskets and roam through the streets of Bangkok or along the beachside streets on Phuket Island as mobile vendors. On the other hand, there are also Akha entrepreneurs who own shops and some are able to export their goods abroad. This chapter provides an overview of the evolvement of urban Akha souvenir businesses over time and space; analyzes the embeddedness of mobile Akha vendors and entrepreneurs in social, political, and economic structures; and explores the strategies and daily routines they employ in order to meet chances and challenges related to their work.

2 Conceptual Frameworks: Agency and Mixed Embeddedness

Since the 1980s, one can observe a growing interest in the studies of ethnic minority entrepreneurship, especially in the United States and in Europe (Aldrich et al. 1990; Kloosterman and Rath 2003; Dabringer and Trupp 2012). Most of the recent labor and entrepreneurial migration studies, however, are concerned with international or transnational migration (Aldrich et al. 1990; Oliveira and Rath 2008) and neglect the fundamental fact that the vast majority of people who migrate do so within the borders of their country of birth (Skeldon 2006: 17). Furthermore, despite the widely acknowledged fact that women as entrepreneurs make a valuable contribution to local and national economies around the world in terms of job creation and wealth generation, they are still the largest underrepresented group in studies of entrepreneurship.

2.1 Networks and Mixed Embeddedness

One popular tool in explaining the success and achievements of various kinds of immigrants and entrepreneurs is the concept of social and ethnic relations (Portes and Sensenbrenner 1993) which refers to the concrete embeddedness of an actor in social and ethnic networks. Social networks consist of more or less homogenous sets of ties between three or more actors (Faist 1997: 193). These actors can be individuals in kinship groups, friendship cycles, households, neighborhoods, or organizations. Social capital, in contrast, is the *ability* to secure resources through networks (see Chaps. 4 and 14 in this volume on social capital). In the context of immigrant studies, scholars point to the importance of reciprocity (Faist 1997) and solidarity among co-ethnics. It is important, however, to note that ethnic social networks transcend geographical boundaries. Portes and Sensenbrenner (1993) were among the first ones who also highlighted the less desirable effects, the so-called negative social capital, such as exclusion of outsiders as a result of community solidarity as well as constraints on individual freedoms and outside contacts due to community norms. Criticizing the one-sided focus on the social dimension, Kloosterman and Rath (2001) propose a more comprehensive concept of (mixed) embeddedness that acknowledges the economic and politico-institutional environment of the actors in question. Thus, it is necessary to analyze market conditions (resource endowment, costs of production, demand side, competition among Akha vendors) and the institutional framework on national and regional/urban level in which they are embedded.

2.2 (Other) Forms of Capital and Habitus

Findings of this study, however, have shown that the concepts of embeddedness do not reveal the complexity of the entrepreneur's situation. It emphasized too strongly the constraints and structural forces while the individual's ideas, motivations, and strategies remain invisible. In order to overcome the dichotomy of structure and agency, Bourdieu's concepts of forms of capitals and habitus have been integrated into the theoretical framework.

Bourdieu (1986) distinguishes four kinds of capital (economic, social,[2] cultural, and symbolic) which enter into power relations and human agency. Economic capital can immediately be converted into money as a ready form of exchange. Cultural capital can exist in three forms: in the embodied/incorporated state, i.e., in the form of long-lasting dispositions of the mind and body (e.g., language skills, production techniques); in the objective state in the form of cultural goods (e.g., books, jewelry); and in the institutionalized state as educational qualifica-

[2] See explanations in Chaps. 4 and 14 on networks and social capital.

tions and certificates. The accumulation of embodied cultural capital requires a process of embodiment/incorporation as it implies labor and time, which must be invested personally by the investor. Symbolic capital is defined as a resource based on prestige, honor recognition, or misrecognition. Bourdieu, talking about conversions and transformations of capital, highlights that one form of capital is translatable into others.

Along with theorizing the forms of capitals, Bourdieu offers "a more nuanced understanding" of agency, via the concept of habitus (Holt 2008: 232). Habitus refers to cognitive structures and is the "universalizing mediation which causes an individual agent's practices" (Bourdieu 1977: 79). It is expressed via embodied dispositions which are durable and acquired through social experience, especially during one's early years of life (Jenkins 2002: 79). It is emphasized that the habitus is influenced as much, if not more, by experience than by explicit teaching: "The power of the habitus derives from the thoughtlessness of habit and habituation, rather than consciously learned rules and practices" (Jenkins 2002: 76). Each individual has a different habitus which is affected by parameters such as age, wealth, sex, physical appearance, and occupation (Ryan 2004). In this understanding, agency is not limited to conscious or deliberate social action and decision making as proposed by rational choice theories. Bourdieu's theory, however, also implies that due to the existence of the habitus, actors are not (unconstrained) free-will actors nor are they entirely controlled by some outside force. But, Bourdieu's concepts of capitals and habitus do not integrate the category gender. In order to understand the economic practices of female entrepreneurs, it is important to study the traditional role and perception of women in Akha society (see Sect. 4.1). Gender is considered as a fluid and relational human construct that is always mediated and negotiated by diverse contexts (Castellanos and Boehm 2008). Therefore, "gender distinguishes between male and female domains in activities, tasks, spaces, time, dress and so on" (Pessar and Mahler 2001: 2).

Consequently, the theoretical framework on which this chapter is based focuses on the interplay of human agency of self-employed female rural-urban migrants and the structural forces they are confronted with and is thus situated within a broader context of political economy. This question of self-determination versus external determination or agency versus structure is still unclear and is one of the pivotal issues in the entire debate about ethnic minority enterprise (Jones and Ram 2007: 60) and is especially interesting in the case of the underrepresented group of female entrepreneurs (Henry 2007).

2.3 *Research on Urban-Based Hilltribes*

My study also contributes to the neglected research on the phenomenon of urban-based hilltribes in Thailand. Many village-based research studies, even concerning the Akha people (e.g., Bernatzik 1947; Alting von Geusau 1983; Tooker 2004) have been carried out, but only a few studies (Toyota 1998; Boonyasaranai 2001; Ishii 2012) have examined the hilltribes in urban contexts. According to Toyota (1999: 2), anthropologists have been inclined to see their task to gather information from the "less spoiled" villages and to record it while it lasts. Research on urban hilltribes, she states further, exists in the area of development studies and has generally been viewed as a part of the "hilltribe problems" or as a result of uneven development (p. 2). Existing studies are limited to Chiang Mai: One of the earliest works by Vatikiotis (1984) focused on the complex issue of what roles minority groups play in urban society and to what extent their assimilation with the Thai mainstream society has taken place. Mika Toyota (1998) explored Akha identity in urban and transnational contexts finding that Akha migrants maintain several identities that enable them to link simultaneously to more than one locality and social setting. Buadeng et al. (2002) developed a quantitative and qualitative profile of hilltribe migrants in Chiang Mai and Chiang Rai providing an overview on migration motives and fields of occupation. And the research of Fuengfusakul (2008) explores the networks and economic strategies of vendors and small entrepreneurs in the Chiang Mai Night Bazaar. This chapter aims to enrich existing literature by integrating data from empirical research carried out in further urban and tourist areas in Bangkok and Koh Samui between 2008 and 2011.

3 Rural-Urban Migration and the Evolvement of Ethnic Minority Enterprises Over Time and Space

3.1 Rural-Urban Migrations of Ethnic Minorities

Internal rural-urban migration, mainly from the Northeastern and Northern region to Bangkok, the Central region, and the mass tourist destinations in the South, has supported the economic development of the country by providing labor for manufactures, constructions, or services (IOM 2011). The movements to urban or tourist areas can be both permanent and temporary including several forms of seasonal migration. These forms of mobility have been facilitated by rapid urbanization, industrialization, and improved transport and communication structures. It is difficult, however, to quantify these migration streams as most migrants are registered in their home regions and not in Bangkok or other urban areas and are thus registered as rural people. Hence, we can only draw on the available census and survey data of the National Statistical Office (NSO): A comparison of the population census from 1960 to 2000 shows that the percentage of lifetime migrants increased from 10.8 % in 1960 to 16.8 % in 2000 and the percentage of 5-year migrants (having moved in the past 5 years) from 3.6 to 6.3 % over the same period (IOM 2011: 14). Data of the annually conducted migration survey reveals a percentage of 2.7 of population who live in a different location than they did 1 year ago (IOM 2011: 14). These numbers do not include individuals who migrated for a period shorter than 12 months and therefore miss many temporary migrants who move during agricultural or tourist high season. Moreover, they can only provide a very general perspective which does not consider the specifics of migration of ethnic minorities.

The settlement areas of Thailand's highland minority groups have always been accompanied by frequent migratory processes. It is thought that some of the mountain peoples, such as the H'tin or the Lua, migrated to what is now Thailand by the beginning of the second millennium, well before the arrival of a Thai-speaking population. The presence of Karen settlements for at least the last 300 years has been verified. The Hmong and Yao have been living in this region since the mid-nineteenth century, and the Tibeto-Burmese ethnicities including the Lisu, Lahu, and Akha immigrated to what is now Northern Thailand in the early twentieth century (Kunstadter 1983: 28). Before the foundation of the Thai nation-state, these different ethnic groups had various types of interaction with the neighboring majority of the population. Contact ranged from almost total autonomy to trading and neighborly exchanges to tribute and allegiance affiliations (Keyes 1995). It is inaccurate to speak of the total isolation of the hilltribes, since there have always been shared influences and contact with the Thai, Burmese, or Chinese ethnicities predominant in Thailand, Burma, or Yunnan. Initially, the Thai government showed no great interest in hilltribe affairs, but this changed drastically in the 1950s and 1960s when they gained attention due to their strategically and politically important position in the context of the East-West conflict and alleged communist insurgency. Two decades later, they became under scrutiny because of their slash-and-burn farming practices (shifting cultivation) which in some cases was linked to the opium cultivation in the Golden Triangle. Even the logging industry as well as lowland farmers, who have moved into the mountains in search for land, are mainly responsible for the deforestation; the problem has been blamed on the minority groups. So, in 1989, the logging ban was enacted by the Thai government. This law enacted a general ban on felling timber for the commercial timber industry as well as for the "simple" farmers of the hilltribes. Theoretically, turning their primary agricultural method of slash and burn into a punishable crime, the law wrenched away an integral part of the hilltribes' livelihood (McKinnon 1997:131). Furthermore, the state largely expanded protected forest areas since the early 1990s which impeded many minority people in maintaining their livelihoods which depend on natural resources (Buadeng et al. 2002: 1). Lack of land use rights and the ban on shifting cultivation are among the most important factors contributing to the increased migration of hilltribe people to urban areas. It is also important to note that due to these developments, the highland ethnic minorities were labeled as troublemakers and forest-destroying drug dealers by the Thai government and in public opinion, especially in lowland urban areas where residents have not frequently interacted with minority people.

Although no official statistical data on Akha migration is available, we can compare different studies which examined the number of hilltribe people in the Northern city of Chiang Mai. In the early 1980s, Vatikiotis (1984: 119) argued that Chiang Mai is not likely to be visited by many highlanders as the city is too distant from the major hilltribe settlements; a statement that soon was to be falsified as the increasing number of urban Akha in Chiang Mai has shown in the decades to come: In the 1970s, their number was estimated to be lower than 50 (Toyota 1998: 210); a survey from 1982 counted 76 (Vatikiotis 1984: 200), but more recent studies assume 1,700 (Boonyasaranai and Chermue 2004) to 2,000 (Toyota 1998: 197) Akha living in the city of Chiang Mai. The reasons for this significant increase of urban migrations of ethnic minority people are manifold. In addition to the mentioned lack of land (rights), Buadeng and colleagues (2002) mention the following migration factors: First, the non-confirmation to village regulations regarding drug addiction or sociocultural rules; second, the quest for higher education and the search for nonagricultural jobs which are rarely available in rural areas; third, the temptation of an urban and more modern lifestyle; and fourth, the opening of trade routes between Thailand and its neighboring countries. These migratory movements have been facilitated by massive improvement in transport infrastructure as well as communication structures and perpetuated by existing social ethnic networks. Studies on urban-based highland minorities carried out in Chiang Mai (Toyota 1998; Buadeng et al. 2002; Ishii 2012) highlight wage laborers as the most prominent migrant group. They mainly work at construction sites, gas stations, or the tourism industry in the hotel or gastronomy business earning around 3.000 baht or less per month. Due to their acceptance of lower than average income, ethnic minority people are preferred employees (Toyota 1998). Another relevant group are student migrants who are often supported by Christian, Buddhist, or nongovernmental organizations (NGOs). Buadeng and colleagues (2002) further mention sex workers in hidden and open service places, traders mainly dealing with agricultural products and handicrafts, as well as a mixed group of government officials, NGO workers, or tourist entrepreneurs as frequent professions in urban Chiang Mai. In the following, however, this chapter focuses on self-employed Akha souvenir sellers by discussing the evolvement of ethnic minority souvenir businesses over time and space; furthermore, it explores the embeddedness of Akha vendors in social and economic networks and illustrates their economic practices.

3.2 *Evolvement of Urban Akha Souvenir Business Over Time and Space*

Ethnic tourism in Thailand started in the 1960s when individual and later on mass tourists visited the highland regions in search for authenticity and adventure (Cohen 2001; Trupp and Trupp 2009). The city of Chiang Mai developed as the tourist center of the Northern region and launched the first tourist attraction such as the Old Chiang Mai Cultural Center and the Night Bazaar which also became the first base for various ethnic minority communities. The hilltribe souvenir business started in the villages. The commercialization of cultural goods is generally not a spontaneous endogenous process initiated by the villagers, but rather an exogenous process introduced by agencies and private companies (Cohen 1983). When profit-oriented motives and the economic pressure to earn money outweigh aesthetic standards and when it is more important to satisfy the customer (tourist) than the artist, then these artifacts can be called souvenir, tourist, or airport art (Graburn 1976). We can date the beginning of urban Akha souvenir business to the early 1970s when some Akha started selling handicrafts on a small scale at the Old Chiang Mai Cultural Center. In 1975, the first Akha woman opened a handicraft stall at Chiang Mai's famous Night Bazaar that has been attracting numerous domestic and international tourists (Toyota 1998). Since that time, many Akha followed her example and this location has become an important center for their social and economic activities. Some highlanders could use these commercial opportunities that were not specifically available to the urban lowlanders. This resulted in an economic niche which may be described as unique to highland minority migrants (Vatikiotis 1984). Over the years, Chiang Mai became the economic and touristic center of the North and the extended domain of hilltribe villages (Toyota 1998). In the 1980s, the market in Chiang Mai changed from mainly selling traditional clothing and jewelry to selling products primarily adapted toward western tourism demand (Choopah and Ness 1997). Akha souvenir and handicraft entrepreneurs may run their own shop, rent a stall at one of the markets, occupy some space on the footpath and on the staircase of a building, or walk up and down with a buckled basket along the streets as mobile vendors. In 2000, there were already about 100 mobile sellers at Chiang Mai's Night Bazaar (Fuengfasakul 2008), but the number was and is not stable as some only come to sell at the markets during tourist high season and return to their home villages for the harvest season. Meanwhile, Chiang Mai features not only a daily Night Bazaar but also a special Friday, Saturday, and Sunday market that have provided both more business opportunities and competition for Akha sellers. Increasing competition, bad selling conditions in Chiang Mai, as well as the motivation of some Akha to discover new destinations and business opportunities led to a spatial expansion of the Akha souvenir business to other urban and touristic areas such as Bangkok, Pattaya, Hua Hin, Koh Samui, or Phuket. The Akha pioneers in Bangkok were very successful in the 1990s as they could sell their products for a good price within a short time. So, they informed their friends and relatives from the home village who later came to accompany them. At the present time, there is a strong fluctuation between the different selling areas and between home villages and selling areas. Some sellers are seasonal migrants who come to work during tourist high season or – in case of being students – during their holidays, while others live as long-term migrants in Bangkok and others again are characterized by a mobile livelihood as they move between different selling destinations and their home village. Thus, one of their main advantages is their high level of mobility and flexibility.

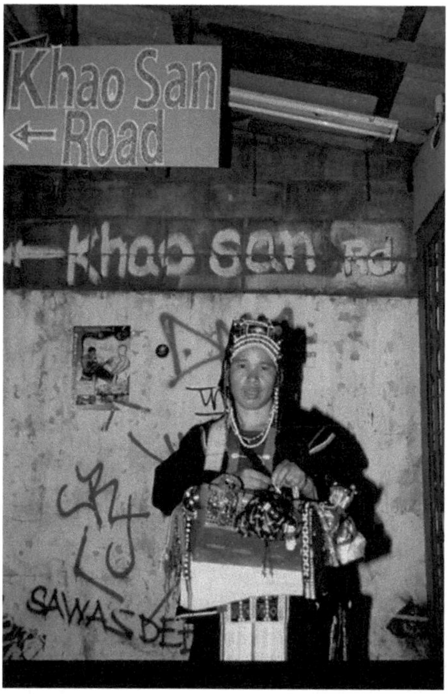

Photo: Mobile souvenir seller on the way to Kaosan Road in Bangkok 2009

4 Agency and Mixed Embeddedness[3]

4.1 Gender and the Division of Labor

Early research carried out by Vatikiotis (1984: 122) notes that females dominated the Akha population in Chiang Mai by 2–1. This trend continues up to the present day (Toyota 1998: 204) and especially holds true in the sector of handicraft and souvenir business where more than 90 % of souvenir sellers and producers are female. Gender as a social construct is part of the habitus and patterns the practice and division of labor. Ethnographic literature about the Akha suggests "that both Akha men and women expressed opinions suggesting that concepts of sexual stratification are important to them" (Kammerer 1988: 34). Traditionally, the Akha have a meticulous gender-based division of labor (Hanks 1988; Kammerer 1988; Yossakrai 2005), whereas household tasks and the production of clothing are seen as women's tasks only. Labor on the fields, however, is done by male and female, although the women's contribution is usually greater (Kammerer 1988). Gender, therefore,

[3] Empirical results of this chapter are based on participant observations and interviews with Akha sellers in Chiang Mai, Bangkok, and Koh Samui between 2008 and 2011.

provides mechanisms of exclusion and inclusion because the centrality of boundaries is crucial to it, but gender is also an essentially hierarchical and inferiorizing discourse and practice (Anthias 2001). Female Akha sellers themselves explain this continuation of gender-based division of labor in the current souvenir business like this: "Men just cannot sell as we do," "men are too shy," and one Akha female mentioned that males are too lazy. Another explanation is linked to the existing images of the exotized and feminized "other" and to the preformed tourist gaze (Urry 1990). Both stereotypes, the one of the pure, real, exotic, or primitive lifestyle of the hill-tribes as well as the one of available Asian women in the context of sex tourism, persist. Ishii (2012: 306) argues that it is difficult for male Akha to find a job in ethnic tourism as this field of occupation mainly requires females and the young in the name exoticism and eroticism. Ongoing analysis, however, shows that men in fact are (although in small numbers) involved in the souvenir business. Some men are learning "typical women work" such as sewing or embroidery, and one might argue that they contest traditional gender roles. But, one has to be careful because the (almost) non-visibility of Akha men does not necessarily indicate that they have no or just a weak function within the Akha souvenir business. Men involved in the souvenir business mainly do not work as mobile sellers as their female counterparts do but sell from a stall or from the footpath. Furthermore, it was observed that an Akha man accumulated a stock of souvenirs in his rented home in Bangkok and became local distributor, in case the women are running out of their own goods. Female Akha vendors refer to oneself as breadwinners of the household, but the question in how far the souvenir sector provided the Akha women an opportunity to be independent from their husbands is still unclear and needs further research.

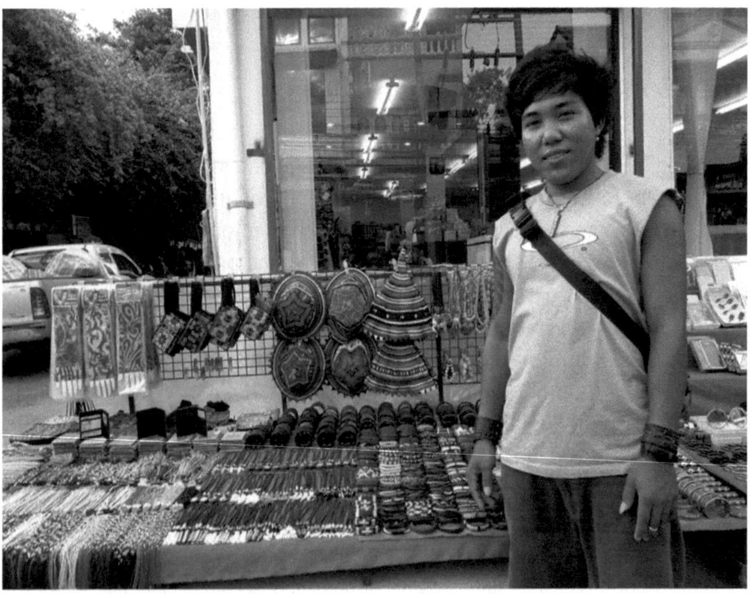

Photo: Male Akha stall vendor on Koh Samui Island 2011

4.2 Bonding Social Capital

Relations "between economic actors are closely related to the socio-cultural context within which such networks are operationalised" (Turner and An Nguyen 2005: 1703). Experienced self-employed Akha sellers have to take care of their family members and close members of the village because they feel a responsibility for them and thus share information and experience. Information concerning selling and living opportunities but also questions about transportation or food in the new destination play a central role, especially for the start-up of a business. Some sellers gained experience at different tourist locations and have a mentoring function for newcomers. Face-to-face exchange but also communication via mobile phone is an important instrument for providing information and support for newcomers or sellers who consider changing their business location. This foundation of social capital can be referred to "value introjections" which emphasizes the moral character of granting resources, learned and introjected during the process of socialization (Portes and Sensenbrenner 1993) and can thus be seen as part of the habitus. Social capital out of a situational reaction of a class of people facing similar challenges is termed "bounded or internal solidarity" (Portes and Sensenbrenner 1993). Many Akha vendors in Thailand's urban tourist areas share the same hard working conditions and similar experiences in terms of discrimination or exploitation: They have migrated to urban areas in search for better work or independence, start selling in the afternoon or early evening, and return home around midnight, and before or after their selling activities, they devote themselves several hours to produce souvenirs. Their hardwork may get appreciated by some western tourists, but they regularly receive complaints from Thai entrepreneurs and municipal policemen who call them annoyers. Such common experiences can create a feeling of togetherness and solidarity within the Akha selling group. In her study about vendors at the Chiang Mai Night Bazaar, Fuengfasakul (2008: 122) made similar observations: She notes that conflicts between mobile sellers occur but they "do not accumulate into antagonism because all of them share the same fate of being the lowest group of vendors and have often been looked down upon by Thai stall holders." Simultaneously, however, forms of negative social capital can be observed. First, while identifying strong relations and solidarity among Akha of low socioeconomic status, social relations and support between "elite Akha" and "ordinary street vendors" are rather weak. A successful Akha shop owner exporting expensive high-qualitative minority products stated that she feels ashamed of the mobile vendors who sell those cheap and simple souvenirs which have nothing to do with Akha culture. Second, several Akha mentioned that over the last years, the number of mobile sellers has increased too fast, especially in Chiang Mai and Bangkok. This is a trend that deteriorates their economic success and can weaken social and ethnic ties.

In addition to these forms of social capital within the Akha communities, ethnic minority sellers and entrepreneurs have built up a set of relations to outsiders such as tourists, expats, and members of the Thai mainstream society. During their long selling hours, the mobile vendors go through negative experiences with customers including conflicts over a negotiated price or sexual harassment. On the other hand, outsider relations can be mobilized and transformed into social, cultural, or economic capital. Many Akha entrepreneurs maintain strong ties to tourists who become steady customers. They can get big orders and export their product to international retailers. Furthermore, especially the younger generation uses the daily contact to international tourists to practice their English and thus accumulate embodied cultural capital.

4.3 Economic and Politico-Institutional Embeddedness

Economic capital is important to start up a business. Compared to other enterprises, the financial entry barriers for the urban street vendors are rather low. To launch as self-employed mobile seller in Bangkok, an amount of 5,000–10,000 baht (about 150–300 US Dollars) which is mainly used for transportation and a small stock of souvenirs and raw materials is necessary. Those sellers, who did not have enough savings for this investment, mainly received financial support from their mother. Interviews and observations indicate an increasing and fierce competition between Akha sellers because the number of mobile vendors grows while the number of tourists in certain areas stagnates. Another reason for more difficult selling conditions lies in the saturation of the consumer's demand as many popular selling areas such as Kaosan Road or Sukhumvit Road in Bangkok receive many returning tourists. An individual economic strategy to counter such developments is to shine out with one's products by diversifying existing souvenirs and creating new products and designs. A prerequisite for being able to design new or products in general is incorporated cultural capital in the form of production skills, thus knowing how to sew and embroider. But, as many vendors are equipped with similar production skills, it does not last long until a successful new product is copied by the other sellers. While some items such as wristbands, handbags, or headgears are (partly) produced by the Akha sellers themselves, other products on display such as necklaces or the wooden frogs are prefabricated and purchased from companies or traders in Chiang Mai, Chiang Rai, or Tachilek (Burma). During their selling activities, the Akha wear to some part their own costume while especially the headgear can be identified as objectified cultural capital that is used for self-marketing in the tourism context. Over the last years, however, I have only met one urban Akha seller who frequently wears her original silver headgear. Most vendors have replaced the heavy original one with a lighter and less expensive piece made of aluminum, and others decided not to wear it at all as it is more comfortable without it.

Another big issue for ethnic minority entrepreneurs is the reproduced negative image among members of the Thai mainstream society. This is also reflected in the fact that Thai tourists hardly buy any products, look down at them, and often call them "*meo*," a negative connoted term. When I presented the topic of this chapter at an international tourism symposium in Bangkok, the president of a Thai university whispered to my colleague that the Akha actually migrated to Bangkok to sell drugs, not souvenirs. This demonstrates that a negative and wrong image of Akha is perpetuated even in academic circles. From a legal perspective, a certain number of Akha is underprivileged by the lack of citizenship (Sakboon 2011). This legal disadvantage, in turn, is limiting their spatial mobility and, therefore, constraining them to start up a business outside of their own district or province. Without citizenship, they are forbidden to leave their district, vote, work, or buy land; they are excluded from the social security and health-care system and have no access to higher education. Moreover, especially on regional and urban level, the practice of law enforcement does not follow a fixed course and varies from time to time and from place to place. There is no official permission for the Akha street vendors yet, but while one and the same woman is accepted at the Night Bazaar in Chiang Mai, she can easily get fined by a municipal policeman for her activity in Bangkok.

5 Conclusion

The development of ethnic minority souvenir business was once initiated by external actors and mainly limited to the Northern region, but over the last years an increasing number of Akha went into business for themselves and migrated southward to Thailand's urban and tourist areas. Despite several constraining structures on economic, political, and socioeconomic levels, Akha vendors highlight the advantages of being self-employed. Being one's own boss is perceived to be better than working as a waitress, housekeeper, or other type of employee; many Akha experienced bad treatments from previous employment. In addition, this autonomy gives them the advantage to visit their home villages and families whenever they want to. Although this occupational independence is highly valued, the preference of working in the city also reflects the limited opportunities in the home villages. Furthermore, life as migrant entrepreneur in the city requires lots of effort as the daily routines of Akha sellers illustrate. They accept long working hours as well as the hassle with police and an urban society that hardly acknowledges their positive impact for the city and tourism. The Akha's entrepreneurship is economically beneficial but brings with it dependence on the market and touristic development. Economic profits from souvenir sales fluctuate strongly and depend on the number of tourist arrivals, the tourist's desire to purchase, and the capital endowment of individuals.

Although the Akha are often attributed with a low social and economic status, they are skillful actors in trade and clearly capable of grasping opportunities. This chapter demonstrates how Akha migrants have carved out their own niches in the tourism industry by entering self-employment and transforming cultural and social resources into economic capital. But, at the same time, these processes are linked with xenophobic stereotypes reproduced by the dominant Thai mainstream society. My findings have shown that ethnic minority entrepreneurs are not entirely controlled by some external structural forces but have shown themselves to be active agents who pursue their own goals and ideas.

Acknowledgments My thanks go to Prasit Leepreecha and Panadda Boonyasaranai from the Center for Ethnic Studies and Development (CESD) of Chiang Mai University for advising and hosting me during the field work period as well as to Kosita Butratana for her field research assistance. I am grateful to the National Research Council of Thailand (NRCT) for granting me research permission. My deepest debt, however, is to the Akha who shared their thoughts and experiences with me.

References

Aldrich, H. E., Waldinger, R., & Ward, R. (Eds.). (1990). *Ethnic entrepreneurs. Immigrant business in industrial societies*. Newbury Park: Sage.

Alting von Geusau, L. (1983). Dialects of Akhazang: The interiorizations of a perennial minority group. In J. McKinnon & W. Bhrukasri (Eds.), *Highlanders of Thailand* (pp. 243–277). Oxford: Oxford University Press.

Anthias, F. (2001). The concept of 'social division' and theorising social stratification: Looking at ethnicity and class. *Sociology, 35*(4), 835–854.

Basu, A. (2007). Ethnic and minority enterprise. In *21st century management: A reference handbook*. Thousand Oaks: Sage. Retrieved September 20, 2009, from http://sage-ereference.com/management/Article_n65.html

Bernatzik, H. A. (1947). *Akha und Meaumeau. Probleme der angewandten Völkerkunde in Hinterindien. Band I+II*. Innsbruck: Kommissionsverlag.

Boonyasaranai, P. (2001). *From the upland forest to the urban city: Akha identity in changing process. Articles on Ethnic Studies*. Chiang Mai: Social Research Institute, Chiang Mai University.

Boonyasaranai, P., & Chermue, M. (2004). *Akha: Lak lai chiwit cak khum khao su muanng [in Thai language] (Akha: From the upland forest to the urban city)*. Chiang Mai: Social Research Institute, Chiang Mai University.

Bourdieu, P. (1977). *Outline of a theory of practice*. Cambridge: Cambridge University Press.

Bourdieu, P. (1986). The forms of capital. In J. G. Richardson (Ed.), *Handbook of theory and research for the sociology of education* (pp. 241–258). New York: Greenwood Press.

Buadeng, K., Boonyasaranai, P., & Leepreecha, P. (2002). *A study of the socio-economic vulnerability of urban-based tribal peoples in Chiang Mai and Chiang Rai, Thailand*. Chiang Mai: Social Research Institute, Chiang Mai University.

Castellanos, B. M., & Boehm, D. A. (2008). Engendering Mexican migration: Articulating gender, regions, circuits. *Latin American Perspectives, 35*(1), 5–15.

Choopah, D., & Naess, M. (1997). Deleu: A life history of an Akha woman. In D. McCaskill & K. Kampe (Eds.), *Development or domestication? Indigenous peoples of Southeast Asia* (pp. 183–204). Chiang Mai: Silkworm Books.

Cohen, E. (1983). The dynamics of commercialized arts: The Meo and Yao of Northern Thailand. *Journal of the National Research Council of Thailand, 15*(1), 69–82.

Cohen, E. (2001). *Thai tourism. Hill tribes, islands and open-ended prostitution*. Bangkok: White Lotus.

Dabringer, M., & Trupp, A. (Eds.). (2012). *Wirtschaften mit Migrationshintergrund. Zur soziokulturellen Bedeutung "ethnischer" Ökonomien in urbanen Räumen*. Vienna: Studienverlag.

Faist, T. (1997). The crucial meso level. In T. Hammar, G. Brochmann, K. Tamas, & T. Faist (Eds.), *International migration, immobility and development* (pp. 187–217). Oxford: Berg.

Fuengfasakul, A. (2008). Making sense of place: A case study of vendors and small entrepreneurs in the Chiang Mai Night Bazaar. In S. Tanabe (Ed.), *Imagining communities in Thailand. Ethnographic approaches* (pp. 107–134). Chiang Mai: Mekong Press.

Graburn, N. H. H. (1976). *Ethnic and tourist arts. Cultural expressions from the Fourth World*. Berkeley: University of California Press.

Hanks, J. R. (1988). The power of Akha women. In N. Eberhardt (Ed.), *Gender, power and the construction of the moral order: Studies from the Thai periphery* (pp. 13–31). Madison: Southeast Asian Studies, University of Wisconsin.

Henry, C. (2007). Women entrepreneurs. In *21st century management: A reference handbook*. Thousand Oaks: Sage. Retrieved September 20, 2009, from http://sage-ereference.com/management/Article_n6.html

Holt, L. (2008). Embodied social capital and geographic perspectives: Performing the habitus. *Progress in Human Geography, 32*(2), 227–246.

IOM (International Organization for Migration). (2011). *Thailand migration report 2011*. Bangkok: IOM Thailand.

Ishii, K. (2012). The impact of ethnic tourism on hill tribes in Thailand. *Annals of Tourism Research, 39*(1), 290–310.

Jenkins, R. (2002). *Pierre Bourdieu*. London: Routledge.

Jones, T., & Ram, M. (2007). Urban boosterism, tourism and ethnic minority enterprise in Birmingham. In J. Rath (Ed.), *Tourism, ethnic diversity and the city* (pp. 50–66). New York: Routledge.

Kammerer, C. A. (1988). Shifting gender asymmetries among Akha of Northern Thailand. In N. Eberhradt (Ed.), *Gender, power, and the construction of the moral order: Studies from the Thai periphery* (pp. 33–51). Madison: Southeast Asian Studies, University of Wisconsin.

Keyes, C. F. (1995). *The golden peninsula: Culture and adaptation in mainland Southeast Asia*. Honolulu: University of Hawaii Press.

Kloosterman, R., & Rath, J. (2001). Immigrant entrepreneurs in advanced economies: Mixed embeddedness further explored. *Journal of Ethnic and Migration Studies, 27*(2), 189–201.

Kloosterman, R., & Rath, J. (Eds.). (2003). *Immigrant entrepreneurs: Venturing abroad in the age of globalisation*. New York/Oxford: New York University Press.

Kunstadter, P. (1983). Highland populations in Northern Thailand. In J. McKinnon & W. Bhrukasri (Eds.), *Highlanders of Thailand* (pp. 15–45). Oxford: Oxford University Press.

Laungaramsri, P. (2003). Ethnicity and the politics of ethnic classification in Thailand. In C. MacKerras (Ed.), *Ethnicity in Asia* (pp. 157–173). London: Routledge.

McKinnon, J. (1997). The forests of Thailand: Strike up the ban? In D. McCaskill & K. Kampe (Eds.), *Development or domestication? Indigenous peoples of Southeast Asia* (pp. 117–131). Chiang Mai: Silkworm Books.

Oliveira, C. R., & Rath, J. (Eds.). (2008, October). Special issue Immigrant Entrepreneurship. *Migracoes. Journal of the Portuguese Immigration Observatory on Immigrant Entrepreneurship* (pp. 1–287).

Pessar, P. R., & Mahler, S. J. (2001, June 30–July 1). *Gender and transnational migration*. Paper presented at the international conference on transnational migration: Comparative perspectives, Princeton University, Princeton.

Portes, A., & Sensenbrenner, J. (1993). Embeddedness and immigration: Notes on the social determinants of economic action. *The American Journal of Sociology, 98*(6), 1320–1350.

Ryan, M. (2004). Agency-structure integration. *Encyclopedia of social theory*. Thousand Oaks: Sage. Retrieved November 18, 2008, from http://www.sage-ereference.com/socialtheory/Article_n3.html

Sakboon, M. (2011). The borders within: The Akha at the frontiers of national integration. In C. Vaddhanaphuti & A. Jirattikorn (Eds.), *Transcending state boundaries: Contesting development, social suffering and negotiation* (pp. 205–244). Chiang Mai: The Regional Center for Social Science and Sustainable Development (RCSD), Chiang Mai University.

Skeldon, R. (2006). Interlinkages between internal and international migration and development in the Asian region. *Population, Space and Place, 12*(1), 15–30.

Tooker, D. E. (2004). Modular modern: Shifting forms of collective identity among the Akha of Northern Thailand. *Anthropological Quarterly, 77*(2), 243–288.

Toyota, M. (1998). Urban migration and cross-border networks: A deconstruction of Akha-identity in Chiang Mai. *Southeast Asian Studies, 35*(4), 197–223.

Toyota, M. (1999, July 4–6). *Cross border mobility and multiple identity choices: The urban Akha in Chiang Mai, Thailand*. Paper presented at the 7th international conference on Thai Studies, Amsterdam.

Trupp, A., & Trupp, C. (Eds.). (2009). *Ethnotourismus. Interkulturelle Begegnung auf Augenhöhe?* Vienna: Mandelbaum Verlag.

Turner, S., & An Nguyen, P. (2005). Young entrepreneurs, social capital and Doi Moi in Hanoi, Vietnam. *Urban Studies, 42*(10), 1693–1710.

Urry, J. (1990). *The tourist gaze. Leisure and travel in contemporary societies*. London: Sage.

Valenzuela, A. (2001). Day labourers as entrepreneurs? *Journal of Ethnic and Migration Studies, 27*(2), 335–352.

Vatikiotis, M. R. J. (1984). *Ethnic pluralism in the Northern city of Chiangmai*. Unpublished PhD thesis, St. Catherine's College, University of Oxford, Oxford.

Winichakul, T. (1994). *Siam mapped: A history of the geo-body of a nation*. Honolulu: University of Hawaii Press.

Yossakrai, K. (2005, April 3–6). *Akha power relations in Northern Thailand: Identity, economics and gender perspectives*. Paper presented at the 9th international conference on Thai Studies, Northern Illinois University, DeKalb.

Zhou, M. (2004). Revisiting ethnic entrepreneurship: Convergencies, controversies, and conceptual advancements. *International Migration Review, 38*(3), 1040–1074.

Part IV
Contemporary Gender and Queer Perspectives

Chapter 18
Learning to Look Good: Thai Women Office Workers and Everyday Consumption Practices at Work

Kosum Omphornuwat

1 Introduction

This chapter problematizes women's lived experiences and everyday consumption practices in relation to their bodies. Particular attention is given to a case study of Thai women office workers and their consumption of makeup and clothes at work. Departing from my keen interest in "the body beautiful" (Gilman 1999), I spent 11 months between 2005 and 2006 carrying out participant observation, photographic research, and in-depth interviews with 32 women employed by two business organizations in Bangkok, Thailand. I initially focused on Thai women's experiences of "beauty practices." However, as the fieldwork began to unfold, the notion of "beauty" appeared to be less relevant. Evidences emerging from my fieldwork pointed to a significance of the notion of "looking good." While dissociating themselves from "beauty," the women repeatedly referred to "looking good" when describing the aspiration that drove their engagement in the consumption practices. Beauty is perceived as an innate quality of the body, while looking good entails the materialization of the body in an attempt to achieve an ideal look.

Elsewhere I introduced a concept of "looking good practices" by examining the ways in which Thai women office workers incorporate looking good practices into their everyday consumption at work (Omphornuwat 2010). This chapter offers another approach to understand looking good practices. By arguing that looking good practices involve learning, this chapter aims to explore how, through their engagement in the consumption of makeup and clothes, Thai women office workers learn to look good.

K. Omphornuwat (✉)
Women, Gender and Sexuality Studies Programme (WGSSP),
College of Interdisciplinary Studies, Thammasat University,
2 Prachan Rd., Pra Nakorn, Bangkok 10200, Thailand
e-mail: kosum@tu.ac.th; kosum_o@hotmail.com

P. Liamputtong (ed.), *Contemporary Socio-Cultural and Political Perspectives in Thailand*, DOI 10.1007/978-94-007-7244-1_18, © Springer Science+Business Media Dordrecht 2014

In understanding how the women learn to look good, firstly, I define a conceptual framework that places learning as central to the analysis. Learning discussed here is different from a conventional approach. Referring to Jean Lave and Etienne Wenger's theory of "situated learning" and the concept of "community of practices" (1991), I conceptualize learning as a process of social participation taking place in the context of everyday life. Secondly, I introduce a debate on "embodied ethnography" (Coffey 1999; Turner 2000; Bain and Nash 2006; Monaghan 2006; Okely 2007) and accentuate the role of the ethnographer's body as an "ethnographic research tool" (Bain and Nash 2006: 99). I argue for the insertion of the ethnographer's visibility and embodied experiences in the conduct of fieldwork, data analysis, and writing of ethnography.

Finally, I draw on my fieldwork at the CEO's office, CAIMEA Banking Corporation [a pseudonym], to demonstrate how the secretaries from the CEO's office learn to look good. While interpreting the women's accounts and experiences, I reflect on my own consumption experiences as a newcomer to the social community. I question how, by participating in the practices of wearing "appropriate" dress, I had learned to become a member of the community of secretaries at the CEO's office.

2 Conceptualizing Learning

As proposed by Lave and Wenger (1991), situated learning theory offers a shift in an analytical viewpoint on learning. The situated learning theory questions a conventional perspective that views learning as an individual process of internalization. That is, a learner as an individual internalizes, absorbs, and assimilates knowledge given and transmitted to her/him. Learning in this sense is an outcome of teaching implemented in a separate environment detached from other everyday activities (Lave and Wenger 1991: 47; Wenger 1998: 3). Lave and Wenger's theory of situated learning is based on an assumption that a learner is a social being who acquires tacit knowledge by actively and continually engaging in a social situation.

In other words, situated learning does not concern a process of internalization, but rather a process of "increasing participation in communities of practices" (Lave and Wenger 1991: 49). A community of practice is a specific kind of community that is defined by "a set of relations among persons, activity and world, over time and in relation with other tangential and overlapping communities of practice" (Lave and Wenger 1991: 98). According to Wenger (2007: 47), "to be able to do their job and have a satisfying experience at work," practitioners as members of the community of practice "develop a shared repertoire of resources: experiences, stories, tools, ways of addressing recurring problems—in short a shared practice." A community of practice is, therefore, constituted by a shared practice among its members.

Lave and Wenger (1991) term a learning process which is situated in a community of practice as "legitimate peripheral participation." Legitimate peripheral participation involves participation as a way of learning. Lave and Wenger (1991: 96–97) argue that a learner becomes a full practitioner in a community of practice not simply through "observation and imitation" but through "participation in ongoing practice as the legitimate source of learning opportunities." It is crucial to note that through this participatory process of learning, a learner engages in not only an acquisition of knowledge which facilitates her/him to master new practices but also a formation of identity which allows her/him to evolve as a full member of the sociocultural community she/he participates in. That is, learners "do not simply learn *about*; they also learn ... *to be*" (Bruner 1996 cited in Brown and Duguid 2001: 200, italics added). From this perspective, Lave and Wenger (1991: 113) argue, "learning and a sense of identity are inseparable."

One of the relevant themes to emerge from my ethnographic fieldwork was that Thai women office workers spoke of their ability or inability to select, acquire, apply, mix, and match their makeup and clothes "appropriately." A notion of "appropriateness" implies the women office workers' longing to belong to and to participate in a social community constructed in the context of their workplace situations. Inevitably, the women are learners who learn to develop their ability to negotiate meanings, to engage in the consumption of makeup and clothes, to share their looking good practices, and to form identities to be accepted as part of the social community they wish to situate in.

By conceptualizing learning as a process of social participation which takes place in the context of everyday lived experiences, I argue that a significant part of looking good practices involves learning.

3 Doing "Embodied Ethnography"

Recent theoretical and methodological literature looking at ethnographic fieldwork has highlighted a significance of the ethnographer's body in conducting participant observation and has called for an intensive investigation to identify the roles and implications of the ethnographer's embodied experiences that potentially contribute to a production of ethnographic knowledge (Coffey 1999; Turner 2000; Bain and Nash 2006; Monaghan 2006; Okely 2007). Amanda Coffey, for example, criticizes the way in which the ethnographer's use of her/his body in experiencing fieldwork has been taken for granted and omitted from the writing and understanding of ethnography. She contests that "all fieldwork can be conceptualized in terms of the body" (Coffey 1999: 68). At the very least ethnographic fieldwork entails the physical presence of the ethnographer in the field.

However, the ethnographer's body is not simply located in the field, but carries with it physical characteristics and appearances that have been documented to have an impact on the conduct of fieldwork (Coffey 1999: 68; Hammersley and Atkinson 1995: 73–75). Martyn Hammersley and Paul Atkinson (1995: 66–67) address the issue of "impression management" that it is necessary for the ethnographer to strategically use her/his "personal appearance" in order to construct identity and negotiate roles during the fieldwork. Impression management through the strategic use of the ethnographer's body is deemed to be important as it offers a greater possibility to the success of the fieldwork. However, it touches only "the surface of the embodied fieldwork perspective." Coffey (1999: 75) comments: "Both the physical body and the symbolic, cultural significance it has are central, rather than peripheral, aspects of ethnographic fieldwork."

An examination of the embodied experiences in the ethnographic fieldwork treats the body as central to the analysis. Nevertheless, it has generally focused on observing, analyzing, and interpreting the uses of "other" bodies rather than the ethnographer's (Coffey 1999: 75; Turner 2000: 53, 55). More recent ethnographic studies argue for recognition of the ethnographer's body in a research process (Turner 2000; Bain and Nash 2006 and Monaghan 2006). Aaron Turner (2000) calls for an insertion of the ethnographer's visibility into research processes and ethnographic representations. Turner questions an epistemological ground that views knowledge as being objective, value-free, preexisting, and discovered. He asserts that the ethnographer "can no longer be seen as an observer recording social facts and processes, but must be seen as an active, situated, participant in the construction of accounts and representations" (2000: 51). That is, the ethnographer has to be considered as an embodied participant whose physical visibility plays a part in the development of a research process (2000: 52).

To illustrate his argument on embodied ethnography, Turner (2000) reflects on the implications of his embodiment during the fieldwork that he conducted with young white men. In his study of doormen's social world, Lee Monaghan (2006) demonstrates how he used his body as a resource for researching "other bodies" in a risky environment. Seeking to understand the entanglement of embodiment and sexuality at a queer bathhouse event, Alison Bain and Catherine Nash (2006) examine how their bodies can be used as an "ethnographic research tool." Paul Stoller (1997) writes about his apprenticeship in Songhay sorcery. In his chapters, The Sorcerer's Body, Stoller (1997: xvi) argues that "one learns about Songhay sorcery not through the assimilation of texts, but through the mastery of the body – through the vicissitudes of pain and illness." The apprentice's body that he used for demonstrating such learning was his own body.

As a methodological approach, embodied ethnography places the ethnographers' bodies as central to the research process. The ethnographers demonstrated how they reflexively examined the implications of their embodied experiences which contributed to an understanding of the experiences and social world of the people they wished to study. Central to my ethnographic work is an attempt to understand Thai women office workers' consumption of makeup and clothes at work. It entails a study of the body in everyday life in which "bodies are most obviously watched, analyzed and noted" (Coffey 1999: 60). I observed and took notes on the clothed bodies of the women office workers. I listened to them talking about their bodies and other women's bodies. I questioned and analyzed their relationships with their bodies.

However, what I wish to emphasize here is that not only were the women office workers' bodies watched, analyzed, and noted but also the ethnographer's body, my own body, needed to be observed, scrutinized, and understood. Working at CAIMEA

Banking Corporation, I endeavored to learn to dress in a similar way to the organization members. I was embraced by the organization's dress culture. I received a guideline of how I should dress for work. I observed my colleagues and learned to dress "appropriately." I interpreted the corporate dress code and appropriated it to be my dress style at work. Retrospectively, I have found that how I dressed myself was beyond the practice of impression management which aimed to facilitate my fieldwork roles and relationships. I shared the practices with the organization members to the extent to which I felt as if I became one of them and began to empathize with why they dressed the way they did in such a particular workplace situation.

I, therefore, accentuate the work of "embodied ethnographers" and argue for the visibility of my body and embodied experiences in the analysis and writing of ethnography.

4 Defining Appropriateness

When asked how they learned about makeup and clothes, most of the women office workers mentioned reading women's magazines, browsing the internet, cruising around shops, taking makeup courses, and talking to friends. In a similar vein, female entrepreneurs participating in Ann Gray's study (2003: 492) of the roles of consumption in the construction of the "enterprising self" attained skills in and knowledge of "self-presentation," "care and maintenance of the body," and "aestheticization of everyday life" through the work of consumption and the use of self-help media. Likewise, women in managerial roles, interviewed by Anat Rafaeli and colleagues (1997: 25–26) in their study of female administrative employees' everyday use of dress at work, reported that they learned what constituted level-appropriate dress by "reading articles on professional women's clothing and fashion in business magazines" and by "transferring notions of appropriate dress from their prior corporate work experience." However, women in clerical roles reported that they learned through "a process of social learning ... by observing what others within their units wore for particular roles and events" (1997: 26).

Although Rafaeli and colleagues (1997) did not focus on a concept of learning, their findings point to a significance of the notion of appropriateness which had been learned and shared by the female administrative employees. To these female administrative employees, wearing appropriate dress was a means to enhance their role execution and performance (1997: 17). "Dress knowledge" shared by the female administrative employees encompasses "a sense of clothing components (e.g., suits, jackets, skirts) that were appropriate to the role of organization member and of the appropriate way of presenting oneself while wearing these components" (1997: 35). In this sense, the notion of appropriateness is a key definition of dress knowledge which informed the female administrative employees' use of dress in facilitating their role execution at one particular workplace. What they needed to learn was not only knowledge about dress in general but also knowledge of how to dress appropriately to their roles in particular situations.

The notion of appropriateness was also significant to the Thai women office workers. Not only did the women office workers talk of their ability or inability to select, acquire, apply, mix, and match their clothes and makeup appropriately, they criticized and commented on other women's ability or inability to comport with the standards of appropriateness they sustained. Mint, for example, recounted her experience when she first joined CAIMEA Banking Corporation:

> I had never worked in an office environment before. … I didn't really know how to dress. At first I just picked and mixed, here and there, looking for a blouse, a sleeveless top or a vest and then covered it up with a jacket. Sometimes, I tried to adapt my own style, mixing casual clothes with work clothes. They didn't match well and looked out of place. I received negative feedback and gradually changed my style. …I just want to know the standard and adopt a style that is right for me. (Mint, 32, secretary)

Working at CAIMEA Banking Corporation, I, myself, witnessed an omnipresence of the notion of appropriateness held firmly by some of the organization members. During my very first meeting with Lux, the PA to the CEO, the expected standard of dressing was prompted in the conversation. "Working here you have to dress appropriately," Lux verbalized her concern. Part of my responsibility at the CEO's office was to answer telephone calls. On a number of occasions, incoming inquiries from the bank's management were to seek advice from the CEO's office regarding appropriate dress codes for forthcoming corporate events. Anticipating how the CEO should look her best in the media and look appropriate in terms of Thai cultural expectations, a few weeks prior to an important corporate event, Lux would prepare a choice of exquisite dresses for her western female CEO to select from. FYI (for your information) emails were circulated in advance among secretarial team members, suggesting an appropriate dress code for a particular meeting.

At CAIMEA's grand ceremonial event where the Ambassador, the CEO, top management, VIP guests, the media, and hundreds of CAIMEA's employees were attended, one of the event coordinators who might have believed she worked behind the scenes was on duty in a white tracksuit while the rest of her team was fully dressed in a black business trouser suit. "Did you see what [her name] was wearing that day?" became an opening line for clandestine conversations for weeks, and the scandalous white tracksuit incident was cited from time to time as an extreme illustration of an inappropriate state of dress that no one should ever repeat.

I argue that appropriateness involves belonging and endeavoring to dress appropriately and explicates longing to belong and to participate in the practices of relevant social community. Mint was not only inexperienced with dressing for an office environment but also strove to learn to dress herself in the way in which she would be accepted. Compared with the lavish attires and black trouser suits donned by event attendees, the white tracksuit was perceived as signifying the coordinator's lack of effort in participating in the bank's most auspicious event and thus was deemed inappropriate.

Unlike Rafaeli's study (1997) which identifies wearing appropriate dress as a means to enhance organizational role execution, the evidence emerging from my fieldwork highlights the wearing of appropriate dress as a means to formulate an identity in order to be accepted as part of a community of practice. This implies that what the women office workers need to learn is not simply an ability to use a combination of clothing and makeup aesthetically but also an ability to tailor themselves appropriately to any social situation in which they participate. Women's magazines, self-help literature, personality development courses, and information from significant persons may be perceived as sources of knowledge about makeup and clothes. However, in developing an ability to dress appropriately and formulate an acceptable identity, learning through an actual engagement in the practices of members of the community is essential. Reflecting on my experiences as a newcomer to a social community, I wish to demonstrate how I learned to become included in a community of practice of the secretaries at the CEO's office, CAIMEA Banking Corporation.

5 Situating the Community of Secretaries

In understanding how Thai women office workers learn to look good at work, I consider working with secretaries from the CEO's office a community of practice. It is not simply because they work together in the same place. I characterize them as a community of practice because "they sustain dense relations of mutual engagement organized around what they are there to do" (Wenger 1998: 74). The secretaries negotiated with one another as to what the meanings of appropriate dress were and how they should present themselves in their workplace.

Mint recounted her experiences as a secretary to the CEO's office where she worked under Lux's supervision for 2 years before relocating to another department:

> The CEO's Office isn't a general office. It's a top executive office. At the CEO's Office, wearing a vest with a knitted cardigan or even with a skirt is not acceptable. She [Lux] said it wasn't appropriate ... At the CEO's Office, we don't really know with whom we are going to come into contact. Some visitors are higher than our CEO. Can you imagine that? ... Our image also reflects our CEO's image. I understand then the necessity of this point. When I worked for the CEO's Office, I had to dress properly all the time...

Lux also associated the meanings of dress with the meanings of workplace. She commented:

> Dress is very important to our corporate image. Dress is also our way to honor the people we come into contact with. If you work in such a high profile organization but dress poorly to welcome customers and visitors, it's wrong. It shows that you don't respect them.

Similar to Lux and Mint, Paan and Kratae, also the secretaries for the CEO's office, emphasized a necessity to dress appropriately. Paan said: "I think the way I dress is appropriate for my workplace because this is a bank. A bank tends to be quite conservative. We aren't dazzling. ..." Kratae talked about being a secretary: "Secretaries meet both internal and external people. We have to look good. We represent our boss. If we look good, the company will look good too." I then asked what Kratae meant by "look good," to which she responded: "We dress appropriately."

Affirming the significance of the notion of appropriateness, the secretaries accounted for their mutual engagement in the practices of wearing appropriate dress. None of them dressed for work in clothing such as t-shirts, jeans, sportswear, sandals, or revealing clothes – clothing officially discouraged by the bank's dress policy and commonly understood as inappropriate dress for a corporate environment. Nevertheless, it should not be assumed that the secretaries all dressed uniformly with conformity to one communal style.

Mint always came to work in a matching dark-colored, suit jacket and skirt. During my visit to her apartment, I was amazed when I saw her wardrobe. It was overflowing with a variety of colorful and fashionable clothes from sexy strappy tops and cute mock-sleeved blouses to trendy knee-length hipsters. She explained: "I don't want to go to work with my own style. It's personal. Some of my clothes shouldn't be worn to work. … When I go to work, I have to respect my workplace, respect the people I'm going to meet." On the other side of her wardrobe, I saw a huge stock of gray, dark gray, and black suit jackets and skirts – Mint's reification of the appropriate dress for work.

Apart from a secretarial qualification from one of the foremost secretarial schools, Lux had a vocational certificate in dressmaking and was very proud of a wedding dress she had made for her younger sister. Lux's best friend ran a fashion house and kept updating her on what the new trends were. Lux said that at home she only dressed in shabby clothes. But most of her work clothes were tailor-made. She would dress in a matching business suit and skirt for important meetings. For ordinary working days, she preferred a color-coordinated blouse and skirt combination. I also noticed that when attending important corporate events, Lux always appeared dressed in exquisite silk garments, mainly in colors that resembled CAIMEA's branding color schemes.

With years of service as a secretary to foreign executives in high-profile banking corporations, Paan accumulated not only work experience and secretarial skills but also a fine collection of tailor-made suits and business outfits. Kratae's mixing and matching of her wardrobe was more diverse. Her favorite dark plum long-sleeved ballerina top was worn with a gray knee-length A-line skirt, a pair of black slacks, or cream linen trousers. Sometimes, Kratae simply wore a pale long-sleeved blouse with dark-colored trousers.

Mutual engagement in the practices of wearing appropriate dress is one of the examples that demonstrate a characteristic of the community of practice of the secretaries from the CEO's office. They negotiated with one another the meanings of appropriateness but reified such meanings differently and formulated distinctive dress styles that suited their individuality.

6 Learning to Look Good

After a few weeks of my placement at CAIMEA Banking Corporation, Kratae, one of the secretaries for the CEO's office with whom I had lunch and went shopping regularly, asked me a very interesting question: "Are you sure you are doing research on this topic?" "This topic" as I had told people around me at the bank including Kratae was concerned with beauty, makeup, and clothes. Upon hearing this question, I went silent for some time pondering the questions that it brought to mind. Why did she ask me such a question? What does she mean? What is she implying? I initially responded with another question: "Why?" She replied: "You look *thammada.*" *Thammada* in this context may be equivalent to normal, ordinary, and, above all, not standing out.

As reported in some journalistic articles, two of the most popular cosmetic surgery procedures sought by Asian women are blepharoplasty for wider eyes and rhinoplasty for a longer nose (Cullen 2002). My small sleepy eyes and tiny flat nose do not seem to fit well with the Thai and Asian ideal of feminine beauty. With regard to my dress, I wore only plain clothes to the bank, generally a white or cream blouse with a pair of dark-colored trousers. My dress may well had complied with the corporate dress code but failed to project my image as a style guru. Sometimes, I showed up to work with the effect of uneven eye makeup, something that I had not even noticed but Kratae had done. I found it difficult to keep my hand steady and draw a flawless symmetrical line on each of my eyelids. Kratae showed me a life-saving tip for a sleepy-eyed woman. The end of each liner should be sharp, slim, and pointing up to give an effect of cheerful wider-looking eyes.

Mint was a secretary from CAIMEA with whom I also became friends. Walking together along the shopping street near the bank, Mint and I enjoyed our lunchtime window-shopping, but it was an extremely hot day. The foundation I had applied earlier did not survive the heat and my face literally started to melt. Mint saw tiny polka dots all over my nose and could not help but diagnose my condition. She prescribed for me a Korean brand of foundation, newly introduced to a Thai market with a sole distributor in Bangkok. I was intrigued by her knowledge and, of course, I followed her suggestion.

Ploy was a secretary whose weight concerns were widely acknowledged among her colleagues. Out of the blue, she looked at me and gave me a compliment. She asked how I managed to stay so slim. Fon, who was a junior trainer, was looking to buy some makeup and asked if I knew any good brands. She cited the name of one particular imported brand and asked to hear my opinion on it.

When I entered the organization, I wished to understand women office workers' experiences. Through participant observation, I thought I was the one who observed the women, looked at them, and looked at their bodies. Apparently, I was not the only one who looked. They too looked at me and looked at my body. The women office workers and I inevitably participated in the practices of reciprocal looking. As I failed to demonstrate my competence in dressing myself flawlessly, some women treated me as a learner and were willing to part with their expertise. Yet, some saw me as an expert who studied makeup and clothes and asked, therefore, for my know-how. Either way, the practices of looking imply an involvement in skills and knowledge that not only inform an ability to select, acquire, and apply makeup and clothes but also constitute our identity as learner, expert or both. These practices of reciprocal looking also affirm a significance of my body in the conducting of ethnographic fieldwork. I was not simply being physically present in the organization but interacting and participating in the practices of looking shared among the women office workers. As such, I agree with Aaron Turner (2000) that the ethnographer has to be considered as an embodied participant whose physical visibility plays a part in the development of the research process. I argue for the insertion of my visibility and embodied experiences in the writing and understanding of the women office workers' looking good practices at work.

When looking at the photographs of me taken with colleagues from CAIMEA Banking Corporation, I began to see why Kratae had said I looked *thammada*. It was my third week with the CEO's office. Lux hosted a dinner party for her team. After the party, we had photographs taken together in front of the restaurant. Paan appeared in a dark-purple tailored jacket and matching skirt. Kratae was in her candy-striped quarter-sleeved blouse and black trousers. Lux looked bright in her light-pink and white floral silk blouse, which matched well with her white knee-length pencil skirt. Standing right behind Lux, I looked peculiarly humble in my neutral-colored, plain, long-sleeved blouse and black trousers. The only accessory I had adorned myself with was a pair of wristbands in support of the bank's good causes and community projects.

A further set of photographs were some snapshots I took with Kratae during a lunch break. At the reception and entrance to the CEO's office, we took turns to pose beside a massive glass wall inscribed with the bank's eye-catching logo and "Welcome" sign. Both Kratae and I appeared in white blouses and dark-colored trousers. A month later, I joined a farewell party for one of the training managers. Again, I was wearing a long-sleeved blouse, this time, pastel pink. Toward the end of my placement, with several dozen CAIMEA working teams involved in the bank's integration project, I was invited to a thank you dinner party hosted by the project director. A professional photographer captured our smiles during this festive event. In one photograph, I was pictured with Paan, Lux, and the project's secretary. Lux was adorned in an elegant, dark-brown, long-sleeved Chinese silk blouse and Paan looked comfortable in her black business suit. The secretary from another department looked more casual in her striped, V-neck, loose long-sleeved top. Unsurprisingly, I dressed in my favorite cream long-sleeved blouse and black trousers. Then, it was my last day at CAIMEA Banking Corporation and I had photographs taken with my colleagues. In one of the photographs, I was standing with Paan by her office compartment. I wore a white short-sleeved blouse and a pair of black trousers.

Reflecting on my experiences of working in the CEO's office, it came as a surprise to me that I reified meanings of "appropriate dress" as a combination of a neutral-colored, plain blouse, and a pair of dark-colored trousers. At the beginning of my fieldwork, I was conscious of making "appropriate" looks through the ways in which I dressed as I simply wished to establish good field relations with gatekeepers and key informants. However, taking a role as one of Lux's assistants, I gradually became engaged in the experience of the world of the secretaries. The making of "appropriate" looks was no longer the intent of fieldwork facilitation, but became part of everyday practices I shared with the secretaries in the CEO's office. I was involved in secretarial work and took responsibility for the tasks I was assigned.

I saw men in suits and women in business dress walking in and out. Back-office operational staff may enjoy the "mix and match" varieties of their momentary "fashion" clothes, yet top management, both male and female, stabilized their styles with "power dressing" and "banker" looks.

Seeing a dark-blue, suit jacket hanging behind the door in a pantry room, I was surprised to learn that it belonged to Noon. Noon's main duty was to prepare and serve refreshments. On top of her spotless uniform, Noon was required to wear a suit jacket when waiting on the Board of Directors and VIP customers.

There had been a long-standing tension between Lux and Kratae regarding a discrepancy between their meanings of appropriate dress. It was not uncommon for her colleagues to witness Kratae's resentment over Lux's strict dress surveillance and unfriendly criticism toward Kratae's work clothes. Although Kratae appeared in well-coordinated non-revealing attire, Lux commented that the ways in which Kratae dressed to work were "too casual." The height of the tension was aggravated when Lux asked Kratae to wear a uniform but Kratae refused. Negotiation between the two resolved that Kratae would wear a suit jacket on top of her "overly casual" work clothes.

The white tracksuit incident truly irritated Lux. However, as her authority was unlikely to be extended beyond the confines of the CEO's office, the only thing Lux could do was to complain to her colleagues. Those who wore jeans, miniskirts, t-shirts, crop trousers, strappy tops, vests, trainers, or sandals would avoid entering or even coming close to the CEO's office. They may leave an inquiry with Kratae at the entrance to the office.

"Dress is an issue here!" I jotted it down in my fieldwork diary in bold and underlined to remind myself of my very first experiences of being in and working at the CEO's office. I took notice of how the secretaries and their colleagues dressed for work. I observed how they received praise and punishment as a consequence of their choice of dress. I shared with them in the advocacy of the notion of appropriateness and felt responsibility in the fostering of orderliness in the CEO's office. I participated in the practices of wearing appropriate dress. To reiterate Mint's account, "I understand then the necessity of this point. When I worked for the CEO's Office, I had to dress properly all the time." Mint negotiated and reified a notion of appropriateness through her practices of wearing a suit jacket and matching somber skirt. To Mint, a suit did not pronounce "power dressing" but rather "safe dressing": "I always wear a suit. It makes me look … umm how do you say, work-ready. … A suit is like a symbol for businesspeople, for executives. But that isn't to say that I wear a suit because I want to look important. I just want to comply with the regulations and look proper for my workplace. I gradually understood this. … A suit is safe. It isn't risky. It covers my shoulders."

In becoming included in a community of the secretaries in the CEO's office, I inevitably participated in the practices of wearing appropriate dress. I negotiated meanings of appropriateness and reified such meanings into my *thammada* look. The ensemble of my pale plain blouse and pair of dark-colored trousers somehow shared a commonality with Mint's matching suit and skirt. It was the safest style as it complied with the bank's dress code and regulations. It was probably the most appropriate style for me to wear during my short-lived experience at the CEO's office. By the time I left the CEO's office and CAIMEA Banking Corporation, I found myself having an "emergency" suit jacket hanging somewhere behind my desk just like Lux, Noon, and Kratae. Had my tenure been an extended period of four or even 10 years, like Mint's and Lux's, rather than 4 months, I would have developed a more comprehensive wardrobe with a fine collection of suits, skirts, and tailored business dress and no longer looked *thammada*.

7 Conclusion

A significant part of looking good practices involves learning. In this chapter, I have explored the way in which Thai women office workers learned to look good through their engagement in the consumption of makeup and clothes. I propose to view learning as a process of social participation taking place in the context of everyday life. Through social participation, not only does a learner acquire tacit knowledge by actively and continually engaging in the practices of social community but also formulates an identity necessary for becoming a member of the community of practices. In understanding learning through a process of social participation, I have argued for an insertion of my visibility and embodied experiences in the analysis and writing of women office workers' looking good practices at work. I have reflected on my experiences as a newcomer to a social community and explored how I had learned to become included in the community of practices of secretaries at the CEO's office through the practices of wearing "appropriate" dress. Looking good entails looking "appropriate." Appropriateness involves belonging and endeavoring to dress oneself appropriately and explicates a desire to belong and to participate in the practices of the social community. I learned to look good, to look appropriate, through my engagement in the process by which I participated in the consumption practices of their local events, negotiated and reified meanings of appropriateness, and produced an identity necessary for becoming a member of the community of practices. Thai women office workers' consumption experiences, as well as my own, demonstrate that the ways in which we learn to look good are informed by our engagement in shared practices and meanings among ourselves in the community of practices.

Acknowledgments This chapter is drawn on the ethnographic work I carried out for my PhD at Loughborough University, UK. I am grateful to my supervisor, Professor Sarah Pink, for her enthusiasm, valuable advices, and insightful comments. She encouraged me to seek creativity in doing ethnographic research, and I could not thank her enough for the learning experience. I am also thankful to my informants who so generously shared with me their experiences, thoughts, feelings, and, of course, beauty tips. Without them, my work would have not been completed.

References

Amit, V. (Ed.). (2000). *Constructing the field: Ethnographic fieldwork in the contemporary world*. London: Routledge.

Bain, A. L., & Nash, C. J. (2006). Undressing the researcher: Feminism, embodiment and sexuality at a queer bathhouse event. *Area, 38*(1), 99–106.

Brown, J. S., & Duguid, P. (2001). Knowledge and organization: A social-practice perspective. *Organization Sciences, 12*(2), 198–213.

Bruner, J. (1996). *The culture of education*. Cambridge, MA: Harvard University Press.

Coffey, A. (1999). *The ethnographic self: Fieldwork and the representation of identity*. London: Sage.

Cullen, L. T. (2002, August 5). Changing faces. *Time Asia*, pp. 48–55.

Davis, J. (1992). Tense in ethnography: Some practical considerations. In J. Okely & H. Callaway (Eds.), *Anthropology and autobiography* (pp. 205–220). London: Routledge.

Gilman, S. (1999). *Making the body beautiful: A cultural history of aesthetic surgery*. Princeton: Princeton University Press.

Gray, A. (2003). Enterprising femininity: New modes of work and subjectivity. *Cultural Studies, 6*(4), 489–506.

Hammersley, M., & Atkinson, P. (1995). *Ethnography principles in practice*. London/New York: Routledge.

Hassard, J., Holliday, R., & Willmott, H. (Eds.). (2000). *Body and organization*. London: Sage.

Jackson, P. A., & Cook, N. M. (Eds.). (1999). *Genders and sexualities in modern Thailand*. Chiang Mai: Silkworms Books.

Lave, J., & Wenger, E. (1991). *Situated learning: Legitimate peripheral participation*. Cambridge: Cambridge University Press.

Monaghan, L. F. (2006). Fieldwork and the body: Reflections on an embodied ethnography. In D. Hobbs & R. Wright (Eds.), *The Sage handbook of fieldwork* (pp. 225–242). London: Sage.

Okely, J. (2007). Fieldwork embodied. In C. Shilling (Ed.), *Embodying sociology: Retrospect, progress and prospects* (pp. 65–79). Oxford: Blackwell Publishing Ltd.

Omphornuwat, K. (2010). *In pursuit of looking good: Thai women office workers and everyday consumption practices at work*. Unpublished PhD thesis, Loughborough University, Loughborough, UK.

O'Reilly, K. (2005). *Ethnographic methods*. London: Routledge.

O'Reilly, K. (2009). *Key concepts in ethnography*. London: Sage.

Pink, S. (2007). *Doing visual ethnography* (2nd ed.). London: Sage.

Rafaeli, A., Dutton, J., Harquail, C. V., & Mackie-Lewis, S. (1997). Navigating by attire: The use of dress by female administrative employees. *Academy of Management Journal, 40*(1), 9–45.

Stoller, P. (1997). *Sensuous scholarship*. Philadelphia: University of Pennsylvania Press.

Turner, A. (2000). Embodied ethnography: Doing culture. *Social Anthropology, 8*(1), 51–60.

Wenger, E. (1998). *Communities of practice: Learning, meaning and identity*. Cambridge: Cambridge University Press.

Wenger, E. (2007). *Community of practice: A brief introduction*. http://www.ewenger.comtheory/index.htm

Chapter 19
Thai Daughters, English Wives: A Critical Ethnography of Transnational Lives

Chantanee Charoensri

1 Introduction

This study on which this chapter is based is about women who found themselves born with limited resources and have been struggling to live up to the social expectations endowed upon them despite this disadvantage. They were born poor women in a poor country and in a part of that country where the opportunity for upward mobility is virtually non-existent, yet they were also situated within networks of position practices that were highly close-knit. The obligations of their roles were so impossibly demanding, given their levels of poverty, that the women felt obliged to get themselves out of this poverty in order to fulfil the demands that were made of them. The study follows the women's life stories in their struggle to be the person their society expects them to be and to perform well in the roles those around them expect them to perform. Finding themselves in a mobile world where 'in order to move up you need to move elsewhere' (Sørensen 2000: 3), some women turned to the path of international migration through sex work and cross-border marriages.

The study aims to break the stereotypes of Thai wives as women who get married only to escape poverty. This will be accomplished by putting their lived experiences within contexts to gain a deeper understanding and reveal their complex relationships with their English husbands. Also, following Garfinkel (1967) and Goffman (1963), I will show that in order to survive in the two cultures and improve their lives, Thai wives need to possess wide arrays of subtle capabilities and sophisticated social skills. To do this, I situate Thai wives' life stories in a meso-level where the existence of the 'ghosts of network others' (Thrift 1996: 54) inhabiting the women's mind-set pressured them to find whatever means they can—within certain limits—to help them conform to internalized role expectations. To achieve this, strong structuration, a refined and more empirically oriented version of structuration

C. Charoensri (✉)
Department of Sociology, Thammasat University, Bangkok 10200 Thailand
e-mail: chantane@tu.ac.th

P. Liamputtong (ed.), *Contemporary Socio-Cultural and Political Perspectives in Thailand*, 299
DOI 10.1007/978-94-007-7244-1_19, © Springer Science+Business Media Dordrecht 2014

theory, will be used as a meta-theoretical framework to capture the analysis of Thai wives' migratory lives.

2 Strong Structuration and Marriage Migration

2.1 Strong Structuration

Strong structuration is a revised version of structuration theory, originally conceived by Anthony Giddens (1984). Giddens develops structuration in response to one of the classic dilemmas in social science: objectivism and subjectivism. In response to this, Giddens places at the heart of structuration the duality of structure. Duality of structure refers to the irreducibility of the relationship between structure and agency which, to Giddens, are two sides of the same coin and not distinct entities. Structures and agency are a duality in the sense that they are both mediums and outcomes of the practices of the agent. In producing practices, agents draw on 'structures' that exist as both 'material levers' and 'memory traces' within them, and in carrying out the practices, agents engage in the reproduction of social structure or contribute to the changing of structures.

Structures in structuration theory are conceptualized differently from the traditional notion of the concept in other sociological theories. Giddens conceptualized structure as 'rules and resources' that agents draw upon in producing actions. It is said to be virtual in the sense it can only be instantiated at the moment when agents draw on it to produce practices. This serves to emphasize the inseparability between structure and agency and to avoid the reification of structure as if it exists completely outside all individuals. Giddens' definition of structures as rules and resources is therefore to emphasize that structure is not an entity in and of itself, divorced from actors, but that it is capable of providing social action with structural elements.

Stones' *strong* version of structuration (2005) attempts to retain the core idea of structuration as duality but with an aim to analyse in situ processes of structuration. To do this, Stones revises structuration and makes two key arguments. Firstly, he points out that the power of structuration as such lies within the meso-level scope of analysis (Stones 2005: 117). Stones asserts that whilst the analysis of structuration process can take into account the macro-historical context of the phenomenon in focus, the latter is not in itself structuration analysis. This relates to Giddens' notion of structure as rules and resources, which is not easily transferable to the macro level. The focus here is thus a focused, micro and meso one.

Secondly, Stones spells out what is implicit in structuration when Giddens talks about agents drawing from internal structures: the temporality embedded in the cycle of structuration. This is Stones' attempt to deal with the much criticised point in structuration theory, most prominently from Margaret Archer (1995) who persistently criticized Giddens for conflating structure and agency. Stones, on the contrary, does not see duality and dualism of structure and agency as incompatible, but argues that both could be true ontologically at the same time. He imposes a temporal dimension into his version of structuration and elaborates it in a model which he terms 'the quadripartite of structuration' (Stones 2005: 75–115). This can be illustrated in a model I reproduce from Stones below:

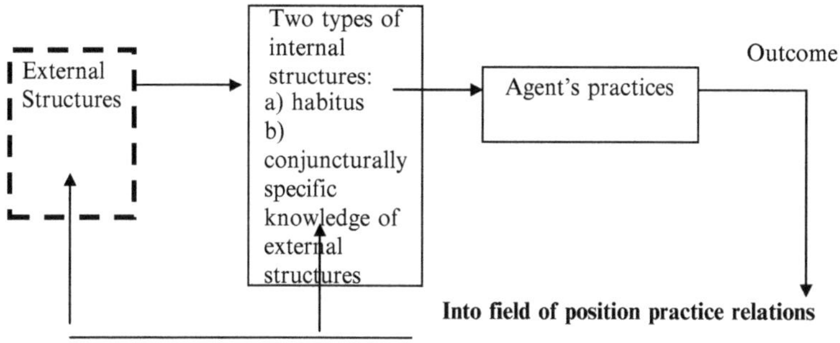

Within this model, Stones defines external structure as the structural context of action, such as networks of position-practice relations, which precede the other three moments of structuration in time and are grander and more extensive in terms of the level of analysis (Stones 2005: 93–94).

There are two types of internal structures or structures *within* the agent: firstly there is the general dispositional, which is similar to Bourdieu's habitus (1977) but less structural prone. It includes internalized cultural discourses, attitudes, dispositions, transposable skills and habits of speech. Secondly, the conjuncturally specific is 'the agent's knowledge of the specific context of action' (Stones 2005: 90) and involves knowledge related to an actor's particular role position and its associated notions of rules and normative expectations. In producing practices, agents must draw on both these two types of structures.

The third moment in the quadripartite of structuration is conduct, which ranges from habitual to highly reflexive, depending on the specific situation and types of actions. These conducts then produce the outcomes that consequentially combine with the outcomes of others' conducts and which reproduce (or change) both external and internal structures in indeterminate ways. For the meso-level of analysis, this outcome then enters the networks of position-practices connected around an agent in focus.

Stones also emphasizes further that this cycle of structuration needs to be viewed as situated continuously within networks of social relations which are taken into account in the actions of individual actors who are situated in their midst. He says that the minds of individual actors are consequently populated by the 'ghosts of networked others' (Stones 2005: 93). The idea of position-practices was coined by Roy Bhaskar (1979) as an alternative conceptualization to an overly passive understanding of roles. In the strong structuration model, position-practice relations have emergent structural properties resulting from agents' conducts, which are the outcomes of both role-taking (agents' slip into structural slots to reproduce structures) and role-making (agents' also engage in more active position taking). These emergent properties of position-practice relations resulting from past practices are then the pre-existing conditions for subsequent actions (Stones 2005: 62).

2.2 *Applying Strong Structuration to the Study of Marriage Migration*

This model provides guidelines of how to look at the career trajectory of Thai women as they have moved spatially and socially from being poor women in rural Thailand to becoming wives of British men. Strong structuration has informed this research by enabling a focus on the interplay between structure and agency in order to arrive at a deep understanding of Thai wives who migrated by means of marriage. In fact, the structure of this chapter will be informed by the theory itself with Sect. 3.1 aiming to portray the women's general dispositions or habitus and how this interacts with conjuncturally specific internal structures at each critical stage in the wives' life trajectories. It will be shown how this interaction conditions the women's conduct at each stage, as they act in specific structural conditions and do so on the basis of their existing personality adapting as best it can to new challenges. Their stocks of habitus, and the character of their habitus, change and develop as time unfolds, with previous experiences leaving their mark. Thus, the chapter will follow through to engage with the women's life stories in successive stages and will attempt to focus on critical conjunctures in order to deepen an understanding both of the structural pressures they have experienced and the active agency they have exerted. It will do this through a hermeneutic engagement with the women's own perceptions (their own durable and evolving phenomenology) of external structural situations at these critical points.

Understanding marriage migrants through the lens of structuration is more specific and more layered than seeing experience simply as the cultural schemas migrants have carried over from their home society as generally been theorized in migration studies. In the case of Thai wives, this means the account of both Thai cultural schemas in general (close family ties and the *katanyoo* values towards one's parents) and also their sedimented and internalized structures resulting from the many specific conjunctural roles enacted during their life trajectories (being poor rural women, being domestic workers and so on, as will be detailed shortly). Thus, whilst the former pulled the women towards transnational familial engagement, the latter led to more mixed feelings. The social injuries of disrespect experienced due to their gendered class status explained the centrality of status in their transnational involvement and also their lack of sentimental attachment to Thailand in general.

Applying strong structuration to marriage migration is distinctive in its ability to focus on two temporal aspects of structuration processes between structure and agency: the temporally extended and the simultaneous. The concept of the general dispositional accounts for the temporally extended dimension in migrants' general dispositional states and allows us to be specific about the different points of sedimentation as experiences are internalized as a result of the agent having occupied particular positions within structures as they proceed in living their lives. Thus, in the case of Thai wives, it would lead us to view the women not only as being Thai but also to their experience as being Thai women of rural origin, something which, as time unfolded, had come into tension, sometimes oppressive, sometimes creative, with the social positions the women came to occupy.

In this current case, I have focused in particular on their primary formation of habitus as Thai daughters with deep and profound attachments to their parents, and subsequently on their habitus as domestic workers and sex workers. The latter has strong associations with disrespect and has resulted in their dispositional tendency to seek betterment and mobility at all costs. These experiences of class injuries contributed to the wives' lack of attachment towards Thai society in general. Social injuries of gender and class were also significant in explaining the centrality of their newly upward status as English wives. This is when the simultaneity dimension became dominant (detailed in Sect. 3.2), in that the focus here is, in a more concerted and immediate manner, on how a particular set of dispositions, inherited from a series of past practices, is seen to engage simultaneously with networked relations in both the UK and Thailand. Transnationalism, understood within the framework of structuration, has been discussed as the encounter between the habitus of the wives and certain forms of reception in the UK. This explains why certain forms of transnationalism have been maintained (familial attachment, transnational investment, frequent visits and the materialization of return) and why their newly upward status as English wives is so central to their transnational practices.

3 From Thai Daughters to English Wives: A Life Story

3.1 From Class Experience to Sex Work: Lives Prior to Migration

Poverty is widely cited as a standard explanation for the growth of sex tourism in Thailand, and it is also extended to international migration of Thai women to Western countries by means of marriage (see also Chap. 20 in this volume). Bishop and Robinson, in their study of commercial sex in Thailand (1998), have rightly pointed out that what makes this explanation standard is the element of truth it possesses. However, although poverty is often a precondition for sex work, it is insufficient to explain the widespread existence of sex work in the country. It also has too little to say about the women's experiences as well as their sufferings and the achievements that they gain from a career in sex work.

To understand how poverty is lived, I will follow the findings/ideas of Beverley Skeggs (1997) who argues that gender needs to be understood in relation to other social positions, most significantly class. I will also resort to the classic work by Simmel (1965) who has shown that it is also crucial to view the poor as a societal creation in order to understand poverty as a stigma. By extending the conceptualization of poverty beyond the identification and quantification of material conditions to the realm of how it is actually lived by the rural women of Thailand, this chapter will illustrate how poverty cross-cuts with other social categories and will also establish an understanding of the women's habitus. This will explain why poor men and poor women in Thailand have quite distinctive dispositions: men are prone to hedonistic retreatism; women are more determined to escape poverty (even by means of prostitution).

This is because most of the women were landless rice farmers who found the economies of their village to be insufficient and thus were forced to migrate to big cities to seek work. It is common for young girls to find employment as domestic workers or live-in nannies. This puts them in a situation where they have to live their daily lives away from people of similar backgrounds and at the same time exposes them to ways of life of those from a higher class. For this specific group, poverty often means living their lives in isolation, experiencing class disrespect and relative deprivation. This is exemplified by what one of my informants, Boonma, told me:

> I was given a healthy sum of money to spend on food every day. I shopped and cooked for them and ate the same menu, but separately in the kitchen. I went on holiday with them and traveled in an s-class Mercedes, but the reason they took me was so that I could take care of their kids so that they could have time to enjoy themselves. I lived my life luxuriously and considered myself lucky, but I was in command of nothing. I knew it did not belong to me and would not last.

Another telling story of how poverty was lived is what Aree told me. It is all about a bowl of *guay tiew* (rice noodle soup).

> It was the day my two kids, then three- and six-years-old, had a craving for *guay tiew* . That was understandable because they had been having sticky rice with *nam prik* [chilli paste] for every meal. I had no money at all, not even a baht. So, I carried the three-year-old on my back with *pah kao ma* [an all-purpose cloth most rural Thai carry around] and went down in a pond to gather morning glory. I then brought all of the vegetables to the *guay tiew* stall in our village and asked if I could exchange it for a bowl of noodle soup. The vendor responded with silence and stiffened her mouth. She did not look at me or my children. I then said 'please, you don't have to give us the meat, just give my kids some rice noodle and soup, they will be very happy'. She was still quiet while my kid's mouths were watering. All the customers were staring at us. The three of us didn't know what to do but stood there, I didn't know for how long until one of the customers broke out: 'Just one bowl of noodle, why don't you give it to them. The vegetable is very good and was a lot'. Eventually, she gave us a bowl of noodles, and with a lot of meat.

The story that Aree chose to tell affected her emotions deeply. My interpretation of the events and why they were chosen to be told is that they significantly changed her perspective on poverty. The event made her seriously consider what way of life, if she remained poor, would be open to her children. It also exposed Aree's poverty in the eyes of the public. In that event, she vividly saw her and her children's position through society's eyes, through the reaction of the noodle stall vendor and all the other customers who were staring at them whilst she begged for a bowl of noodle soup for her children. Both the silence of the *guay tiew* vendor and the helpful customer's reactions had put her in the category of the poor: in one that was lower than the rest—one where they needed help.

This event also points to the role that the social pressure plays in this difficult decision to enter a stigmatized occupation. It was her realisation of the impossibility of complying with the role expectations of a mother and a daughter by conventional means that drove her into sex work. Aree's decision to take the 'deviant' career path seems to confirm Merton's theory of anomie (1957) and also reflects Shilling's point (1997) about 'the mismatching between the bundles of expectation and the resources made available to the incumbent of a position' (Stones 2005: 64). It is this objective, structurally imposed, set of expectations that can lead so easily to feelings of subjective inadequacy and from there to an almost heroic response from active agents that they are not going to put up with this type of situation.

In contrast to the general, commonsense, perception that the decision to enter sex work must typically be made against social pressures, Aree's story has shown that it was actually the structural pressures that pushed her into it. On the other hand, the women, who are generally pushed into sex work by structural pressures, tend also to be torn apart by contradictory moral codes which, at the same time, instruct them to be 'good women'. This structural strain that pulls Aree, for one, into different directions is not easy to cope with, but the women took comfort in the fact that, after all, the job would not be done in front of the eyes of those she deeply cared about but somewhere else. All those who were her significant others would only get what they had always wanted from her without knowing the means she deployed to achieve it—for the women often kept their sex work to themselves.

This gender relation, shaped by class, and coupled with a high position accorded to family within their hierarchy of moral values, and situated within the context of a Thai economy that relies heavily on tourism, all combined to lead the women to perceive that sex work was the best chance they had of complying with the social demands they had been socialised into and which they cared about greatly.

3.2 Compressing and Stretching Community: Lives After Migration

The women's lives after marriage and migration are explored in terms of the relationship between the processes of assimilation and transnationalism. I want to show that the women's retention of transnational ties is necessary for them to counter their limited assimilation. Yet, in the current context of contemporary migration, the limited assimilation has fewer consequences on their migrant lives than it might have had in former times. This is because transnational practices are more effective in sustaining the women's identities, self-esteem and their upwardly mobile status in their home communities. This is due to the fact that, in the contemporary era, transnationalism can extend far beyond the realm of identity and emotional attachment. In the case of Thai wives, many have extended it to mean living in two places. Most couples have properties in the United Kingdom and Thailand, have invested in transnational business, visit regularly and maintain close connections with friends and relatives through daily phone calls. The existing diaspora also lessens the pressure of limited assimilation to a significant level.

Many aspects of Thai women's migratory lives can be captured in two terms: those of the 'compressing' and the 'stretching' of community. The compressing of community refers to the women's relatively closed network of association due primarily to her 'stigma', her limited human capital and the stage in her life course, that of early motherhood, which combined to result in limited assimilation into British society. Mostly, the women confined their social lives within two realms, which are the domestic realm of homemaker and the diasporic community of Thai marriage migrants. Key reason that contributes to why the women lived their migrant lives in such a domestic and diasporically confined way is parallel to Judith Stacey's (1990) explanation as to why lower-class women value the traditional role of homemaker and seem to oppose feminist politics of gender equality. I found that Thai wives also saw the homemaker role as an ideal unrealized (Stacey 1990: 9–12). Thai women grew up within the context of gender ideology that stated that the role of domestic goddess is ideal for women, yet their life conditions had not allowed them to take such a role. Instead, they were forced to seek paid work at a very young age in order to financially support their family. For them, being a homemaker, a caring wife and a mother were thus ideals that remained unrealized. They viewed their good performances in those roles as resourceful in negotiating their spoiled identity. The women felt that they were able to mobilize this resource to negotiate their identity because of the conditions provided by their migration as wives of British men.

Whilst their lives in the UK were compressing in the sense mentioned above, they were also 'stretching' in another sense. Whilst the wives' main role as English wives was that of 'domestic goddess', the main dominant role in transnational community was those of the head of the family back home. This role, as well as their other key role as domestic goddess described above, is vital to the women's identities. Their marginal position within the host society and their personal history, involving the stigmatized occupation as sex workers, were the key reasons why they constructed these reactive identities. Migration has provided the women with resources to acquire the new status as head of the family back home. This came with burdens as stated by Aree:

> My family consults me about everything. My nephew was going to start school, I chose the school. My father was going to be hospitalized, they asked me for the choice of hospital. This is because I can support them now.

The resources, I am referring to in this study, are not only economic resources gained through the marriage with British men but also the cultural competency that Thai wives gained access to through their migration. This included knowledge and information of living in the Western world, which is highly valued by most Thais; language competency; and access to transnational networks. With these resources, many Thai wives had become agents of the widening chain migration by acting as a matchmaker for their friends and relatives back home. This is likely to result in the growth of the Thai diaspora in particular localities where Thais have already migrated in certain numbers (cf. Toskul Boonmathya 2005).

Whilst these resources gained through social and geographical mobilities earned the wives new status at home, it also led to the couples being involved in the complex nexus of dependency. Once the women have married and migrated, the British husbands often join their wives in their transnational practices. By means of marriages, the cross-cultural couples had extended their social capital across borders and this social capital had often been transformed through transnational investment into economic capital and vice versa. This led to the deployment of the wives' relatives by the couple as a cheap labor supply for their transnational investment.

> I suggested to my husband that we should invest in the rubber plantation in Thailand. I let my brother's family take care of it but we take 40 % of the output. It was a good investment and would be a good source of income when we go back to live there. (Boonma)

Yet, at the same time, to sustain the higher transnational status the wives needed in order to encounter limited assimilation, the couples had become exploited themselves. They had to yield incessantly to the demands of their relatives in Thailand which often involved continuous requests for financial support.

> My brother has been so unreasonably demanding. He wanted to invest in a business, he asked me for help. We gave him the money to run a food stall, he did it for, maybe, 2 weeks and just stopped, saying it was no good. Then he told me he had to repay a debt or the loan shark would kill him. I said I didn't care. So, he made my mother call me, knowing I couldn't reject. And I had to ask my husband to help him. (Hansa)

The new status as *farang's*[1] wives allowed the women to gain a higher status within their transnational community (see also Chap. 20 in this volume). This is significant in sustaining the women's migrant lives as it acts as a source of oppositional identity orientation that helps them encounter limited assimilation. However, sustaining transnational status comes with a cost. The wives have to support their extended family financially and this often causes conflicts with their British husbands who see this act as irrational. Yet, that is not the whole story. As many husbands share with their wives the long-term plan to relocate to Thailand, many couples engage in transnational investment that uses the wives' transnational network as laborers. In this way, it would be an oversimplification to suggest that the wives were the only party subjected to being taken advantage of. It would be more accurate to say that the migrated wives, the British husbands and the wives' transnational networks are all involved in this nexus of dependency.

4 Discussion and Conclusion

4.1 Class Injury, Stigma and Lack of Emotional Attachment

Here, I would like to depict how strong structuration as a meta-theoretical framework has helped us arrive at an in-depth understanding of these particular groups of Thai marriage migrants. I will begin by outlining the wives' transnational attachment

[1] *Farang* is a Thai word for westerners. See Chap. 20 in this volume for more information on *farang*.

demonstrating that whilst strong familial attachments, economic transnationalism and returning plans exist, there are hardly any traces of emotional attachment to Thailand in general. This can be explained, and applying strong structuration's terminology, by looking at the relations between the habitus of the women (the early formation of the deep and profound attachments towards their parents, and the latter formation of the betrayal of Thai husbands, experiences of poverty-related disrespect and of sex work) and the conjuncturally specific (segmented assimilation to the Thai diasporic community, yet negative experiences and constraints due to lack of employment opportunity and the perceived stigmas associated with being Thai wives). The relations between the two sometimes creates tension, at other times compounds a sense of injury, and at others provides a sense of gratitude towards the new milieu.

Both the women's compounded sense of injury as migrant wives and the niches in which they felt gratitude and satisfaction need to be viewed in conjunction with their complexly sedimented general dispositions to seek betterment and to overcome their sense of inadequacy as daughters and mothers, and the experiences of disrespect they had encountered as poor rural Thai women. There were clearly a series of tensions or an uneven quality to their experience depending on the specific areas of life we are talking about, and recognition of these can explain the women's particular forms of transnational retention as described in this article.

Many studies on migrants emphasize the centrality of the home-longing sentiment and a closely related nostalgia for the long lost home. This, very often, leads to an idealized romanticizing of 'home' within their imagination, and the preservation of migrants' original culture in a distant place and the mobilization of 'symbolic ethnicity'. But I found hardly any such sentiments among my own informants. The main reason for this, I believe, is the motivation behind the movement of my informants, as migration for them has been more of an escape. Hermeneutically, they understood themselves, albeit not always in these terms, to be escaping from poverty, class injury and the sex worker stigma. For this reason, migration for my informants is a quest for betterment, but it is also much more than this; it is also in many ways a rejection of key aspects of their home society.

Another factor contributes to the missing emotional attachment to their home country among Thai wives is the constant renewal of their knowledge of current conjunctural conditions within Thailand through their regular visits and intense communication with friends and relatives back home, as well as with those from the diasporic community who 'have just been there'. Thus, the negativity engendered by their past experiences limits their nostalgia, whilst the opportunities allowed by their current sets of position-practice relations mean there is no possibility of a chasm opening up between their image of Thailand and the changing reality.

4.2 *Prospect of Return*

The myth of return is commonplace among migrants. Thai wives are no exception. However, the word 'myth' is not quite accurate in their case, for the phrase has been employed to signify migrants' home-longing sentiments that never come true. But, in the case of Thai-English couples, many of them not only plan to return but have materialized the returning plan by building houses, businesses and social connections in Thailand. Two couples in this study did eventually return. One of the two subsequently came back to the UK due to the fact that they found living in Thailand was no longer a means to achieving their preferred lifestyle: which in this case was running a bar by the beach. Part of the explanation of the difference is that the current condition of global connections has rendered moving across borders less consequential. Relocation between two places was seen by many Thai-English couples as an open option to realized the best possible level of well-being and pleasurable lifestyle. It is crucial to note, however, that living in Thailand might have different meanings for the husbands than the wives. Whilst some husbands stated that to live there was personal escapism (one of my informants' husband used exactly these words) and the route to their dream lifestyle, this situation was more complicated for the wives. One reason, among others, for this is that their migration is not only their means *towards* well-being, socially and economically, but also an *escape from* social injuries of class inferiority. Thus, for the women, their return meant more than simply fulfilling a home-longing sentiment. I have already mentioned that they did not have the kind of nostalgia from home possessed by other migrants (see especially Karanfil 2009), and so return for them, if pursued, would have to mean something different. For them, the act of returning was a contingent act in that if they were to return at all, it would have to be a triumphant homecoming. In effect, anything less than a success in terms of status mobility would defer their return.

Certainly, their lack of awareness of required skills and capabilities, the absence of emotional attachment towards Thailand as a country, the excessive value they gave to Western culture, their anger and their migration understood as an escape will all contribute to the contours of their future lives after they return to Thailand, if and when they do return to Thailand. As I insisted throughout the chapter, Thai women see their marriage migration as an achievement and pride themselves for having been able to gain well-being for themselves and for their transnational family. To return to Thailand then is in a way an act of triumph and defiance, especially when we look at this with regard to their past experiences resulting from their position within the lower strata in Thai society. However, this is not a sweeping triumph across all dimensions and certainly they are not upwardly mobile in every aspect.

I have noted throughout this chapter that this is a story of a group of women struggling to move spatially and socially away from economic insufficiency and painful experiences of class misrecognition and disrespect, and I would like to end with some evaluation of the success of their quest. I would also like to make a brief assumption about the prospects for their lives after their relocation back to Thailand with regard to the journey they have made both socially and spatially resulting from their cross-border marriages. In general, one can say they are upwardly mobile in terms of economic status, but that this does not come with social mobility. Although they can go back to Thailand with the pride that they can now support their family and have given the people they care about better lives, encounters with people from higher strata can still induce misrecognition and disrespect. This was clearly the case when Suda went back to Thailand and checked in at a five-star hotel. She was asked by a staff member to show her identity card in order to prove that she really was registered as a guest there. This is an act which Bourdieu would call a 'soft form of domination', resting on a symbolic form of violence, where people are kept within their place in a social structure despite gaining some economic capital. Suda as well as other Thai wives knew too well that they would never gain enough cultural capital to achieve a new status in social circles/networks other than those they originated from.

Maybe these are the reasons why my informants decided to return and settle in their existing networks of relationships or in a coastal town crowded by tourists where they could live their lives somewhat free from being reminded of their backgrounds. In those two settings, their economic capital and some cultural capital gained from living abroad, such as the ability to speak English and their experiences of living in Western society, are more valuable and are easier to transform into social capital. Specifically, for those who chose to resettle in their hometown and among their current networks, they can easily pass to a new respectable status, for they can now well perform the roles expected of them. The hope for well-being and lives lived free from class inferiority may only be possible for the next generation, and maybe that is not too bad an achievement considering their starting points.

References

Archer, M. (1995). *Realist Social theory: The morphogenesis approach*. Cambridge: Cambridge University Press.

Bhaskar, R. (1979). *The possibility of naturalism: A philosophical critique of the contemporary human sciences*. Brighton: Harvester.

Bishop, R., & Robinson, L. (1998). *Night market:Sexual culture and the Thai economic miracle*. New York/London: Routledge.

Bourdieu, P. (1977). *Outline of a theory of practice* (R. Nice, Trans.). Cambridge: Cambridge University Press.

Garfinkel, H. (1967). *Studies in ethnomethodology* (p. 1967). Englewood Cliffs: Prentice Hall.

Giddens, A. (1984). *The constitution of society*. Cambridge: Polity Press.

Goffman, E. (1963). *Behavior in public places: Notes on the social organization of gatherings*. Glencoe: Free Press.

Karanfil, G. (2009). Pseudo-exiles and reluctant transnationals: Disrupted nostalgia on Turkish satellite broadcasts. *Media, Culture and Society, 31*(6), 887–889.

Merton, R. K. (1957). *Social theory and social structure* (Rev. ed.). Glencoe: Free Press.

Shilling, C. (1997). Reconceptualizing structure and agency in the sociology of education: Structuration theory and schooling. In C. Bryant & D. Jarry (Eds.), *Anthony Giddens: Critical assessments* (Vol. IV, pp. 342–364). London: Routledge.

Simmel, G. (1965). The poor (C. Jacobson, Trans.). *Social Problems, 13*(2), 118–140.

Skeggs, B. (1997). *Formations of class and gender*. London: Sage.

Sørensen, N. N. (2000, July 7–9). *Notes on transnationalism*. Paper presented at the workshop on transnational migration: comparative theory and research perspectives, University of Oxford, Oxford.

Stacey, J. (1990). *Brave new families: Stories of domestic upheaval in late twentieth century America*. New York: Basic Books.

Stones, R. (2005). *Structuration theory*. New York: Palgrave Macmillan.

Toskul Boonmathya, R. (2005). Cross-cultural marriages of Thai women to western men in Northeastern Thailand. *Journal of Mekong Society, 1*(2), 1–53.

Thrift, N. (1996). *Spatial formation*. London: Sage.

Chapter 20
The Expat Life with a Thai Wife: Thailand as an Imagined Space of Masculine Transformation

Megan Lafferty and Kristen Hill Maher

1 Introduction

For most of his life in England, Edward[1] considered himself poor. He was 40 and working as a librarian in Sheffield at the time that his parents died and left him a fair sum of money. A friend then invited him to join him on a holiday to Thailand, and Edward decided to take him up on the offer since he had always wanted to visit the landscape of rice fields he had seen in Vietnamese films. However, once he landed in Pattaya, he never made it out to the countryside. He met a 24-year-old bar girl[2] named Nat on his first night while playing pool and ended up spending the rest of his vacation with her. Upon returning to England, Edward started evaluating his life. He did not especially enjoy his job at the library and was sick of playing pool in the pub with "the same old blokes night after night." He thought, "I could come here, and I'll never be rich, but I could come here and just live. I thought, 'Just do it. What do I want to do?' I thought if I didn't go, I'd always ask myself what would it have been like. Would we have had a baby?"

Edward returned during school holidays and eventually took an unpaid leave of absence to stay longer than a month. He and Nat hired a car and drove out to her home village, a small rice-farming community about a 5-h drive northeast. Edward fell in love with the village life and enjoyed the simplicity. When he arrived to see

[1] All names from the field study have been replaced with pseudonyms.

[2] The "bar girl" position and term is most often synonymous with sex work.

M. Lafferty (✉)
Anthropology, School of Social and Political Sciences,
The University of Melbourne, Parkville, VIC 3010, Australia
e-mail: megan.lafferty@gmail.com

K.H. Maher
Department of Political Science, San Diego State University,
5500 Campanile Drive, San Diego, CA 92182-4427, USA
e-mail: kmaher@mail.sdsu.edu

P. Liamputtong (ed.), *Contemporary Socio-Cultural and Political Perspectives in Thailand*, DOI 10.1007/978-94-007-7244-1_20, © Springer Science+Business Media Dordrecht 2014

Nat's parents' place, he explained his excitement, "So we were in this shack, just nailed together, and I'm thinking, 'right on!' I'm in the middle of nowhere, which is great, fantastic. And then Billy [another Englishman] comes along from two doors down saying, 'hello mate.'" It turned out that four other villagers were already married to foreigners, most having moved abroad, but Nat's cousin and Billy had built a house right there in the village, near the place where Nat and Edward eventually built a three-bedroom home and are now raising their daughter.

The story of how Edward came to live in provincial Thailand is more complex than his own narrative reveals, and it represents a larger trend of western men moving to Thailand and settling there at least semipermanently with Thai wives or partners. In some cases, they settle in tourist enclaves, but others move to their partner's home village in more remote provinces where their presence transforms the local landscape, economy, and social relations. A 2003 survey found nearly 20,000 women married to European men in the Northeastern region of *Isan* alone; in the Nakhon Ratchasima Province, these marriages accounted for 21 % of all marriages. In many villages, half of the residents had foreign family members (Limanonda 2007).

Thailand has long attracted western men, after a leisure and sex industry developed in the wake of the Vietnam War. As a result, Thailand has become a top sex tourist destination in the world as well as being a popular source of brides for transnational marriages facilitated by the Internet. Both of these industries have historically generated relationships between Thai women and western men that have often resulted in the women migrating abroad. However, growing numbers of western men in relationships with Thai women are now the ones who undertake an international migration (see also Chap. 19 in this volume). What are the circumstances under which Thai women and western men have begun to marry and settle in Thailand, especially in Northeastern provinces? To what extent are the men's experiences and subjectivities grounded in the same kinds of economics, desires, and subjectivities that underlie the sex tourism industry? How does their position of privilege get constructed and transformed once they settle, and how do the men negotiate these transformations?

To answer these questions, we begin by examining the historical development of sex tourism and marriage migration between Thailand and the West. We then turn to qualitative interviews held with western men living in Thailand to examine how their structural privilege plays out once they settle. We find that these men's social positions are much more complex than those represented in sex tourism literatures, which emphasize the position of domination and control that enables men to enact fantasies of masculine transformation. While western men who settle in Thailand benefit from the same kinds of privilege that comes from whiteness, masculinity, and global position, their structural privilege in this new context can simultaneously generate new insecurities and social alienation. Our analysis illustrates some of the ways men in this position negotiate the shifting landscapes of power and identity through their own self-narratives in relationship to Thai women, Thai men, and other locally settled western men.

2 A Political Economy of Sex, Tourism, and Marriage

The story of how western men have come to live in provincial Thailand relates to the larger story of Thailand's relationship to the West and to global sex tourism markets. There had long been pressure for Thailand to open its economy,[3] but Thailand's economic policies began a major shift in the 1950s when foreign-educated ruling elites consolidated a new power bloc with the Thai business community and military. According to Truong (1990: 159), this bloc had two main objectives: to "open Thailand's economy to foreign investment in local industry" and to invest "in new ventures in the leisure and service sector catering to the needs of the US military." These dual economic strategies began a process of opening Thailand to international lending, transnational capital, and the US military. The World Bank provided loans for Thailand to build up its infrastructure to stimulate investment in a new tourism industry, and the USA established military bases in Thailand as part of its Cold War strategy in the region, placing most of its troops in *Isan*.

Military bases were surrounded by brothels, massage parlors, and go-go bars, where thousands of *Isan* women worked in industries serving American soldiers. Whereas most of the bases were located in *Isan*, the resort and recreation areas sprang up around Bangkok and the nearby beach town Pattaya, catering to US and other foreign servicemen with hotels, restaurants, bars, and sex. Prostitution in Thailand did not begin with US military bases or "Rest and Recreation" (R&R) practices, but American military men changed its public display as they walked openly with "rented wives" down main streets (Van Esterik 2000: 175).

When US troops began withdrawing from the region, the industries that depended on soldiers withered. Thai officials turned to the World Bank and negotiated an agreement to transform the entertainment industry created for R&R into a global tourist industry (Truong 1990; Bishop and Robinson 1998; Van Esterik 2000).[4] Mies (1998) describes this transition as the movement from one foreign occupation to the next, as imperialist industrial capital followed the imperialist military, both working to strengthen the sex industry.

The Thai government then facilitated the industry through its domestic policies, such as the Prostitution Suppression Act of 1960, which defined prostitution as a crime of promiscuity that only applied to the seller and not the buyer (Truong 1990: 155), and the Service Establishments Act of 1966 that made it possible for

---

[3] Jackson (2007) argues that Siam, then Thailand, had "colonial" economic relations with imperial powers in the form of unequal trading relations, even while it was never formally colonized.

[4] Gregory (2003) notes that the World Bank, the World Trade Organization, and the United Nations were all aggressively promoting tourism "as an economic panacea for the Third World" (p. 329), and that such neoliberal development policies rest on the naturalization of gender and other social differences, insofar as export processing zones and tourism all depend upon the participation and exploitation of particular groups of women (p. 328).

"entertainment places" to provide euphemized "special services" at the request of customers who continued to be exempt from penalty when those services included prostitution (Truong 1990: 155–6).[5]

The Tourism Authority of Thailand (TAT) has also played a role in generating sex tourism, beginning with "the '1987 Visit Thailand Year' campaign, which clearly targeted the traveler interested in sexual experience" (Hamilton 1997: 148) and continuing thereafter with promotional images of beautiful young women representing Thailand's character and tourist appeal.[6] Sex tourism gradually expanded into a diverse industry geared toward particular nationalities of men, with different establishments for Middle Eastern, American, German, Japanese, and Malaysian tourists (Hamilton 1997: 148; Van Esterik 2000: 180). The marketing of Thailand's sex tourism industry has been so successful that this image pervades the construction of Thailand that one sees in western media, Internet, and popular culture (Nuttavuthisit 2007).

The sex tourism industry has wide-ranging effects within Thailand, one of which is that it entails a rural-to-urban migration of young women, particularly those from groups already marginalized ethnically and economically. Many of the women who work in the tourist-oriented sex and service industries around Bangkok and Pattaya have migrated from the rural North or Northeast (Lyttleton 1994; Van Esterik 2000; Cohen 2003). After hosting the American military, *Isan* – the Northeastern area with an ethnic Lao majority – developed networks that made it a key source of sex workers that catered to western men. Within Thailand, these women are racialized – considered culturally unsophisticated, indigenous, and darker than ethnic Thais, and therefore, less attractive (Lyttleton 1994; Howard 2008). *Isan* is marginalized culturally in the rural-urban hierarchies of Thai society, and economically, consistently ranking as the least developed region (Mills 2005: 389–90). As Thai development policies have disrupted subsistence farming in *Isan*, it has become a source of internal migrants, especially among unmarried women between the ages of 15 and 25 (Mills 2005: 387),[7] who find work in factories, domestic service, and in services related to tourism.

---

[5] This act was replaced in 1996 with the Prevention and Suppression of Prostitution Act (B.E. 2539), which continued to criminalize prostitutes, but added crimes for those involved in prostitution businesses and those who procure sex. Given the flourishing sex trade that remains, these additions are apparently not enforced. B.E. 2539 particularly raised penalties for those involved with the trafficking and prostitution of minors. (ILO National Laws on Labour, Social Security and Related Human Rights [NATLEX] database: http://www.ilo.org/dyn/natlex/docs/WEBTEXT/46403/65063/E96THA01.htm)

[6] Officially, the state discourages sex tourism and all forms of prostitution. Van Esterik (2000: 159) writes that the TAT has become increasingly careful to avoid images that would promote sex tourism. Yet, Johnson (2007) finds some advertisements aimed at foreigners that included sexualized, orientalized images of Thai women that were omitted from ads aimed at domestic tourists.

[7] Of course, it is not only the young women who are migrating. Mills notes that nearly half of the adult men in the *Isan* village where she conducted her study had served as overseas contract workers in the Middle East or nearby Asian countries (2005: 394).

The earnings from work in sex tourism are much greater than those in other jobs open to these migrant women,[8] and although the sex industry is widely disparaged within Thailand, marriage to a foreigner has gained respectability among the lower classes as a means of long-term financial support for the extended family (Cohen 2003; Howard 2009).[9] Based on ethnographic interviews with workers in sex tourism, Askew (1999: 118–20) argues that immediate life circumstances also play into some women's decision to work in bars for foreigners, such as the impulse to "spite one's life" out of frustration or anger or to seek out "laces of difference or danger" in response to tedium or social constraints.

In the sex tourism locales in developing states, the nature of prostitution can be less circumscribed or apparently commercial than it is in western countries. Cohen (1986, 2003) describes the "open-ended prostitution" in Thailand, which can originate almost anywhere there are tourists and not involve immediate demand for payment, but instead later entreaties for money to pay rent or help family members with a financial crisis. To westerners, the interaction can feel very much like any other affair or romance, blurring the lines between commercial sex, "rent-a-wife" arrangements, and genuine emotional intimacy. In this regard, men who do not identify as sex tourists can enter into ambiguously commercial relationships with women who may not identify as sex workers (O'Connell Davidson and Sanchez-Taylor 1999: 42). Relationships that begin this way can transform into longer-term relationships and marriages that result in westerners – locally known as "*farang*"[10] – settling near their wives' families in Thailand. As *farang* settle in Thailand and more cash flows through rural communities, more families want a *farang* to join them so that they can have access to cash.[11]

The phenomenon of western men touring in Thailand and settling there with Thai partners has certainly been shaped by various policies and practices and the sex tourism industry, as well as the economic and social circumstances of individuals. However, political economy is more than a backdrop for making sense of this

[8] Truong (1983: 541) estimated that prostitution in Bangkok generated $1,875–18,000 per year, compared to $250 for restaurant waitressing or $312–450 for factory work. Askew (1999) later estimated factory wages at 2,000–3,000 baht per month, while sex work among foreigners could earn 10,000–50,000 baht.

[9] A Khon Kaen University study found that when asked what they want for their daughters, 90 % of the respondents in the rural Northeast replied, "I want for them to marry a foreigner" (cited in Bernstein 2007). However, Hamilton (1997: 164) claims that respectable Thai women from the urban middle class would not marry a *farang*, given the reputation of these relationships that would tarnish their social status.

[10] The term *farang* refers to "white-skinned Westerners" (Hamilton 1997, ftnt 4). According to Cook and Jackson (1999: 18), it is "a ubiquitous Thai cultural-ethnic term which conflates 'Caucasian (race)' and 'Western (culture).'"

[11] This pattern strongly resembles the cycle that ensues from remittances flowing into home communities by migrants from developing states. As families with a migrant gain more access to cash and goods, other families feel both relative deprivation and perhaps greater actual poverty when local prices rise. Hence, emigration spurs greater emigration, just as the *farang* influence in rural communities lays the groundwork for further transnational relationships and *farang* migration.

West-to-East migration; it also shapes desire and the most intimate relations between people (Constable 2003: 143). It informs how people think about Thailand or "the West" as places, about their own relative position in a social order, and their expectations in relationships.

3 *Farang* in Thailand

It is hard to know exactly how many westerners live in Thailand, but Howard (2009) reviews the best available information and estimates 100,000, with the largest proportions coming from the UK, Germany, the USA, the Netherlands, France, Canada, and Australia. Of the total respondents from his online survey, virtually all were men, and nearly half were married to a Thai or had a live-in Thai partner.[12] In this way, the population of westerners in Thailand differs somewhat from other contexts in which we see western enclaves of expats and retirees, where it is more common to see western women, couples, and families (Howard 2008). There was a substantial age spread, with the median age at 43. They were generally well educated, and 70 % lived in the tourist locales or Bangkok, with smaller proportions living in more remote provinces. Those still living in Thailand had been there, on average, just 3.5 years (Howard 2009: 205–6) (see also Chap. 19 in this volume).

The narratives we analyze here come from a set of qualitative interviews that Megan conducted in 2007–2008 with 13 western men living in Thailand with Thai partners or wives. She focused especially on the Northeastern region of *Isan* and the Northern region surrounding Chiang Mai. Most interviews took place in participants' houses and were supplemented with informal conversations and participant observations in the surrounding areas.

The majority of the men whom she spoke with had first come to Thailand on a holiday or for short-term work, but several men had made a decision to begin a new life in Thailand before ever visiting. There were also American men who were stationed in Thailand during the Vietnam War, returned to the USA with Thai wives, and retired together in Northern Thailand decades later.[13]

The interviews from this field study were rife with material about how these men were constructing themselves as ideal white masculine subjects in ways that would be less possible back in their home countries, while simultaneously responding to insecurities and the loss of control they experience, as we discuss in the following

[12] The 2005–2006 survey had 1,003 respondents. The survey was posted in various websites for expats, newsgroups, English language newspapers, and the magazine "*Farang,*" and hence relied on self-selection instead of random sample.

[13] The former military men in long-term marriages had much less of an age gap with their spouses (3–4 years) than the others (average of 25 years), and they were more integrated socially in Thailand. However, they occupied a similar social location as the others in terms of structural privilege. One of these men had started seeing a much-younger Thai girlfriend after his spouse died.

two sections. Throughout our analysis, we relate our materials to the very limited existing literature on *farang* men in Thailand[14] as well as to the broader literature on masculinity within sex tourism.

4 To Be a White Man: Thailand as an Imagined Space of Masculine Transformation

The men interviewed for this study have not all been tourists of any sort, and we do not want to conflate their relationships with prostitution; however, their social position in Thailand bears some resemblance to that of white sex tourists, whose power and privilege are constituted in part through their relations with Thai women, Thai men, and other *farang* men. A key theme that runs like a thread throughout the tourism literatures as well as in our interviews is the vision of Thailand as a space of masculine transformation and self-discovery. Thailand is being produced as an imagined geography within which white men can differently invent and position themselves.[15]

Much of the literature on masculine transformation within sex tourism emphasizes the ways in which sex tourists constitute themselves as subjects through relations with local women. Some authors focus on the exercise of power, domination, or control that becomes possible for some men in sex tourism encounters. For instance, O'Connell Davidson and Sanchez Taylor (1999: 52–53) argue that:

> In the Third World, neocolonial relations of power equip Western sex tourists with an extremely high level of control over themselves and others as sexual beings and, as a result, with the power to realize the fantasy of their choosing. They can experience sexual intimacy without risking rejection; they can evade the social meanings that attach to their own age and body type; they can transgress social rules governing sexual life without consequence for their own social standing.

Gregory's (2003) work echoes this theme and adds that sex tourism destinations function as a "theme park" that permits men not just to be entertained but also to constitute themselves as boyish adventurers who thrive on risk and competition. This cultivated masculinity rests on a construction of the destination as an "illicit space" or "an Adventure Zone for adults in which civilized norms of western male behavior could be abandoned and taboos breached" (Broinowski 1992: 39).

---

[14] These include Howard's (2008, 2009) survey, two analyses by Cohen (1986, 2003) of which the latter appears to be based on interviews or participant observation in Thailand and the former on correspondence between partners, Askew's (1999) writing based on participant observation and interviews in Bangkok's sex tourism sector (though he focuses primarily on women), and Hamilton's (1997) analysis of novels written by *farang* authors about *farang* characters in Thailand.

[15] As Berg and Longhurst (2003: 352) note, "masculinity is both temporally and geographically contingent," making the production of new identities possible in different locations.

The transformation in status and potential for remaking oneself as a privileged subject are possible in part because first-world currencies go further in Thailand. As Brennan (2004: 20) notes, "globalization can enrich not only local elites and (already capitalized) foreign investors in the developing world, but also cash-poor foreigners who create expatriate communities of relative privilege." However, the transformation in status among white westerners also rests on their capacity to position themselves as neocolonial expats and capitalize on the status of whiteness.

Edward, one participant, spoke at length about the transformation in status that had happened both to him and to other *farang* men: "You can see the *farangs*, in England or wherever, they would be a no one. Then they come to Pattaya, maybe even myself as well. You're not a big fish, but you come to Pattaya with your money." Despite this, Edward expressed considerable ambivalence about his status in the village, which was gratifying on one hand, but was also uncomfortable in that it felt "wrong" to his democratic instincts:

> These people [villagers] will walk past me and try to be lower than me. They think I'm better than them. I hate it because I think we're all equal, irrelevant of money [...] I like it because it makes me feel more important, but I know it's wrong. You're equal. Everyone's equal.

It is not only his relative wealth but also his whiteness that buys Edward a position of superiority in a context where white complexions and facial features are fetishized and buy status. Whereas Thai-European children, or "*luk khrueng*," used to be largely socially ostracized (being seen as the illegitimate offspring of GIs on R&R), by the mid-1990s, these children had gained status from lighter skin and began to serve as models for advertisements and entertainment images (Persaud 2005: 214–219). In talking about his daughter, Mattie's standing among village children, Edward said: "Everybody in the village loves her. Everybody in the village treats her differently because she is so special."

Most of the interview subjects articulated their sense of privilege and power only obliquely,[16] such as in the ways they described their intimate relationships as if they had been the only one with the agency to choose an appropriate partner. For instance, Paul, who was Edward's 68-year-old American neighbor, positioned himself as a classic "boyish adventurer" in Thailand: "I was staying in the States and finding old fat women and living the life in America, which when you're older it's not as exciting as when you're young, particularly when you're single." He anticipated that the dating landscape in Thailand would work more in his favor. A Thai friend introduced him to his wife of three years: "She was everything I'd been looking for. She was in her mid-30s, I think quite attractive, and extremely nice. I'm extremely happy with my pick and couldn't ask for anything better."

[16] The outlier in this regard was Bill, a 61-year-old American in Thailand, who openly claimed a superior status over Thais and women more generally. He spoke critically about Thais, calling them lazy, unsophisticated and stupid, yet he was engaged to a 28-year-old Thai woman whom he had been seeing for 6 months. In his account of visiting his Thai fiancé's home, he said that all of her family would be seated on the floor socializing, but that he refused to sit on the floor and instead would sit on a chair to tower over them.

A 48-year-old named James from London moved between third and first person pronouns while describing the appeal of a place where an older western man can reclaim his masculinity within a relationship:

> Ok, so a guy's 50, he's overweight, he's losing his hair – it doesn't make him any less of a man. He's had a few failed marriages because he can't adjust to being the 'new man,' modern man, whatever you call it. I think some of them want a traditional marriage. [...] Maybe the women's careers become important. I think a lot of us guys find it hard to adjust to the demands of western women. [...] They come here looking for something different [...] We feel we're in charge of marriage, we're the breadwinner, maybe it's we weren't able in keeping up with western ways.

James did not ever articulate why he imagined his 32-year-old wife had married him (a first marriage in his case), but this question hovered just beneath the surface in many interviews.

As the following section explores further, the role of money in these relationships underlies any number of insecurities, such that few subjects explained their partner's interest in them in these terms. Instead, the more common explanation involved comparing themselves favorably to Thai men in a kind of "White Knight" (Garrick 2005) rescuing discourse. Cheating Thai men are stock characters in this narrative. It constructs his white masculinity as essentially desirable and lays the ground for trust by downplaying the role of financial security. The men we interviewed widely reproduced this narrative: they talked about their own emotional sensitivity and ability to provide a strong home environment, whereas they constructed Thai men as weak, unfaithful, lazy, and unreliable.[17] Part of what is going on in the White Knight discourse is the projection of a national and racial frame onto personal histories. No *farang* narrative attributed a Thai partners' bad relationship with a Thai man to the failings of a particular person; instead, they focused on the failings of Thai masculinity, implying that Thai women need to look not just to a different man but to a different nationality and race in order to secure a happier future. *Farang* narratives about cheating Thai men also ignore the fact that some of their Thai partners have also had bad experiences with *farang* men who lied, cheated, were abusive, or disappeared. While the subjects often criticized other *farang*s' moral behaviors and relationship manners, when comparing themselves to Thai men, they uniformly tended to agree that white men made superior lovers.[18]

---

[17] Another discourse about Thai men by western tourists paints them as effeminate, given a smaller body size and less muscular frame, a de-masculinization that Malam (2008) found challenged by heterosexual Thai bar workers in the tourist setting of Pha-ngan Island in southern Thailand through sexual liaisons with tourist women, harassment of transgendered people, and other performative behaviors.

[18] Another variant of the White Knight discourse prominent in the sex tourism literature is the story about saving women from the systemic poverty that supposedly drove them into the sex industry. They are represented as nice girls who had to engage in prostitution to survive or to support their families (whereas only "bad" women in the West sell themselves). This rescuing discourse frames the money exchanged as a kind of benevolence on the part of the westerner rather than a commercial exchange, part of the way that these relationships are seen as "real" intimate relations (Bishop and Robinson 1999: 195; Davidson and Taylor 1999: 49). See also Garrick 2005; Cook and Jackson 1999: 14. We did see some evidence among our interviews of a discourse about rescuing women from poverty, though not from sex work.

With a western income and whiteness as key resources, a *farang* who settles in Thailand can constitute a masculine identity as a neocolonial expat, as a "real (white) man," in large part via his relations with a Thai woman and her family and through discursive comparisons to Thai men. This identity is not mobile but rather rests on being socially situated in Thailand among other *farang* men who validate the narrative. In these regards, the structural position and narratives of some men settled in provincial Thailand do resemble what has been written about sex tourists to some extent. Alongside the power or privilege that ensues from this position is the desire to believe that it is not money (or whiteness, or western privilege) that is the source of their power, but instead their essential masculinity (Gregory 2003: 350). However, beyond these similarities, the larger picture of what happened after settling was much more complicated, as the transformation in status also introduced new forms of vulnerability.

5 The Consequences of Privilege

Being a *farang* in Thailand clearly permits a shift in status that would not be possible at home; however, those who settle there in longer-term relationships end up in a much more complex position than those who have transient tourist experiences. In many ways, the very bases of their privilege in Thailand tended to undermine their potential for social incorporation into Thai society and the trust and intimacy of their relationships. Even while the space of Thailand made the reinvention of new masculine selves possible, such masculinities were contingent and unstable (Berg and Longhurst 2003: 352), subject to internal contradictions and attrition.

5.1 The Social Position of the Village Farang

As the story about Edward in the introduction illustrates, part of the appeal of rural Thailand for him was its simplicity, its distance from "civilization" as he knew it in Sheffield. While his surroundings in *Isan* bore little resemblance to his former life, the novelty of living in such a radically different context had evolved into a routine in which he played scrabble and golf with other *farang* and drank and played snooker in a nearby pub in the evenings (just as he had before leaving England). He was not socially integrated, as he spoke little Thai, and his wife spoke limited English. This inability to talk with his wife about complex topics also left him feeling a certain social isolation even within his marriage.[19] While not all the men

[19] In his earlier writing on Thai-*farang* marriages, Cohen discusses what he calls their "extreme heterogamy" and how the common differences in educational levels can play out in "misunderstandings, tensions, and conflicts once a newly contracted marriage becomes routinized. … The very traits, which have frequently been the initial source of attraction, become over time the basis of material problems" (Cohen 2003: 68).

were living in a village as remote as Edward's, few had built Thai social networks outside of their family.

This scenario begins to illustrate how the place in which a *farang* settler can gain social status and a radically simplified life[20] can end up leaving him in a world apart. Most of the men interviewed for this study had developed some separation between their social life and their Thai partner's social life. Most had few language skills in Thai[21] and often their Thai partners' English was limited to what they had picked up working in tourist settings. At the same time, these men had to rely on their wives for translating and handling matters such as finances, and even daily shopping, a dependence that entailed a loss of control.

It is not simply the issue of language that can produce alienation, but also the stereotypes and expectations that accompany *farang* status. Whereas this structural identity confers privilege and power, it can also reduce a person socially to a caricature, "just another *farang*" instead of a complex individual with a specific history, tastes, and range of social roles. In his village in *Isan*, Edward did not have anyone who knew him well as an individual, as a former librarian from Sheffield with a past in a commune and a fascination with horticulture. Rather, his *farang* relationships were superficial and transitory, and his relationships with Thais centered on his *farang* status and the financial support he could offer.

Some men dealt with this isolation and loss of control by constructing it as a choice. For example, James explained that he is learning some Thai but had no desire to assimilate because of cultural differences in "the way you deal with problems." However, he also blames Thai society for his alienation: "As long as I'm here they'll never accept me as anything other than a foreigner even though I'm married here, I have a business here, I've got a child here." James raises a key point in his observation: even if *farang* men were to try to assimilate into Thai culture, they would always be marginalized socially as perpetual foreigners, a loss of status compared to the cachet they gain from defining themselves as expats of the West. They occupy a more privileged position as first-world outsiders than they would as

[20] Askew (1999) writes about the desire for "radical simplicity" that draws western men to Thailand and how language differences in a relationship feed that feeling: "The pidgin English of love and flirtation enhances the mystique of involvement in a new and refreshing life space. The differences in education levels add to this male experience of the exotic Asian woman, primal and close to nature" (pp. 118, 129). Hamilton (1997) also speaks to how novels by *farang* authors construct an "essential woman" in Thailand who cannot communicate fully with the *farang* man, and that in some way "adds to her allure and mystery. She is not devoted to the ceaseless round of rational discussion, demand, insistence, requirement, justification, and so on which is taken to characterize relationships with Western women" (pp. 154–5). But, she notes, the lack of communicative intimacy also keeps the *farang* partner from knowing what is going on and underlie the "misrecognition" in Thai-*farang* relationships (155, 164).

[21] The main exceptions were two of the American men who were stationed in Thailand during the Vietnam War and have been married to Thai women for 30 years. One other American who had lived in Thailand for three years had also developed fluent Thai (Charley). Of the respondents in Howard's (2009) survey, 16 % claimed fluency in Thai.

"immigrants" who have come to Thailand to join their wives' families,[22] and this outsider position also likely buys them more freedom from Thai mores and customs.

Many *farang* men instead socialized with each other, often at western-styled bars and restaurants. The relationships that develop between *farang* could be double-sided. On the one hand, they provided familiar social connections and a place of belonging, regardless of particular nationalities. On the other hand, the ways those we interviewed talked about their *farang* friends evidenced some distrust, tension, and competition. Although Paul and Edward both lived near each other, they each spoke critically about the other when apart, and Edward said, "I thought I'd meet a lot more nicer *farangs* to be honest, but I see them at the store and say hello and they look at me like, 'what are you doing?' [...] Because I'm abroad in a foreign country, I feel a connection with a *farang* and just want to say hello."

5.2 "I'm Sure She Loves the Likes of Me"

Men may end up feeling isolated not only among their social networks in the village but also within their most intimate relationships. The masculine identity as a "real (white) man" that can be produced in this space partly via relations with Thai women is something fragile and prone to erosion and doubt. Western men who were positioned as privileged and wealthy in this context could end up uncertain about the bases for their intimate relationships, and while they may have claimed superiority to Thai men as lovers, the role of money in the relationship arose as a source of widespread anxiety.

In part, such insecurities were fed by popular representations of Asian women that have emerged from the conflict between western fantasies and anxieties: on the one hand, they are represented as innocents from the countryside, delicate Lotus Blossoms who make ideal wives; on the other hand, they are constructed as whores and Dragon Ladies, scammers who are just after money (Hamilton 1997; Constable 2003). Cohen (2003: 67) describes various stories appearing in the press of Thai women, depicting them as "professional tricksters, who repeatedly married, or promised to marry, foreign men and abandoned them after relieving them of considerable sums of money."[23]

Farang discourse sometimes projects this money-obsessed image onto all Thais. Howard's (2008, 2009) survey turned up a lot of similar material in the open-ended

---

[22] Constable (2003: 172) notes how western men who move to the Philippines or China "often jokingly refer to themselves as 'mail-order husbands,'" which is only a joke because of the strength of the normative image. The movement of western men into less developed states contradicts the global imagination of migration unless they are positioned as neocolonial expats.

[23] Of course, Thai women are also globally stigmatized by the international reputation of the sex tourism industry, which conflates Thai femininity with prostitution and inhibits Thai women's ability to travel comfortably and safely in the world (Cook and Jackson 1999: 13; Van Esterik 2000: 169).

questions, including talk about how materialistic Thais are as a culture and warnings to others about how Thais are all really just trying to swindle westerners out of their money.[24] As James also affirmed, "a lot of guys end up getting more than they bargained for; they're walking ATMs."

Another reason that insecurities about love and money arose over time was that the first-world currency that enabled middle or working class tourists to live the high life while on holiday did not last forever. Particularly if a marriage was grounded in part on the desire for financial security, there was a danger that a Thai woman who later realized that her husband was not as rich as she thought may leave him for someone who is a more secure provider.

For relationships that began in ambiguously commercial ways in sex tourism districts, this doubt seems especially likely to arise.[25] For example, Edward said he had heard about a lot of men ending up broke after their Thai wife "ran away" with their money. Despite Edward's generally positive assessment of his own marriage, he pondered aloud whether his wife had genuine emotional ties to him:

> Nat always tells me she loves me. Every day, she tells me, 'have I told you I love you today?' And I do hope she does. I know she did it for an economic reason. I know she has a past, but I've got a past. [...] You know, I mean, that's not an issue with me. She instigates sex; it doesn't always come from me. If she didn't love me, would she do that? Probably not. There is an age gap and whatever, and I was worried about that. [...] We have 17 years between us. I think I look young for 43. If I had hair, I'd look even younger.

Aware of economic circumstances and uneasy about the age difference, Edward said he trusts Nat, but he still felt the need to look for evidence that she loved him, something he was unsure of: "She says she loves me, and *I'm sure she loves the likes of me*. Maybe she loves me. I don't know. I hope so" (emphasis added).

Questions about real love were also evident in relationships that developed independent of the tourist scene.[26] Nigel, a 56-year-old Englishman, decided to make a fresh start in Thailand after he went through a divorce back home. Wanting to meet a Thai woman, he used an online dating service, thinking his chances of meeting someone genuine by chance would be difficult. Nigel searched for a well-educated

---

[24] Interestingly, Howard (2008: 161) himself takes all these warnings at face value and passes them on to an imagined potential *farang* readership as a point of analytic advice: "The many swindles directed at foreigners should be avoided, particularly taking a wife who is only concerned with money."

[25] In his analysis of correspondence letters between Thai bar girls and their *farang* boyfriends, Cohen (1986) finds that although a *farang* often feels sexual and personal dominance over an apparently submissive Thai woman in the beginning of the relationship, the power balance and identity politics reverse as soon as a *farang* leaves Thailand but hopes for a continued relationship (p. 121). He finds himself with doubts and anxieties about her sincerity, insecurities, and tensions that are the product of how the relationships begin and the fuzzy or open-ended practices of prostitution in sex tourism.

[26] Cohen (1986: 125) makes more general claims about the ambiguous relationship between the emotional and material in *farang*-Thai relationships: "in the back of their minds they are aware of the unrealistic aspects of their relationships, their enthusiasm mixes with forebodings, their hopes with fears and their trust with doubts."

woman from a middle-class background, and after corresponding with women for about 4 months, he "narrowed it down to Lin," his 30-year-old wife who had a bachelor's degree and worked for an insurance company.

Despite their similar education and class standing, Nigel raised some of the same kinds of poignant questions about whether his wife loved him:

> People hear that Thai girls are targeting western husbands purely for the economic gain. I think for a Thai woman… that the financial security does play a bigger part of the relationship, certainly initially than in the West. […] To be honest, with the age difference, I've thought long and hard. First of all, is it right even to get married, but also now whether or not we have children… Not that I'm bad looking, but I'm quite sure she could do better than me in the looks department. Part of the attraction to her has been that I can provide security to her… But I do see… the genuine parts of the relationship evolve between us. Silly things like she'll wake up the middle of the night and roll over and put her arms around me. And that's almost in her sleep. That's not something you do with someone you don't share deep feelings with. There are lots of instances like that. But I've realized part of the attraction is knowing I can look after her well. But, I also treat her well; that comes into it.

Nigel's story illustrates tensions that arise from the ambiguous relationship between love and material security that left him looking for evidence of authentic emotion.

Of course, financially strategic relationships can deepen and last, and there is no reason to assume that women who enter into such relationships do not also hope for love.[27] Part of the *farang* insecurity in this context surely derives from western notions of love and marriage that consider true love and pragmatic concerns to be incompatible (Constable 2003: 128). While western sexual relationships still often involve gifts and masculine gestures of "providing" (such as paying the bill on dates), such financial transactions are carefully packaged as romance. For this reason, men who accept the western dichotomy of marriages as being grounded either in opportunism or authentic emotion may struggle to reconcile the two if they acknowledge any pragmatic motives on the part of their partners. This struggle is not unique to *farang* men in Thailand, but it is surely heightened by their structural position there, the widespread discourse about scamming Thai women, and the realities of financial expectations by the women and their families. One irony in the discourse about Thai women's opportunism is that it has been produced largely by men who experience a substantial improvement in status in Thailand and who may have begun relationships with Thai women in part based on their physical assets rather than a pure emotional connection. Violations of western notions of romantic love hover like a specter on both sides.

[27] For instance, Brennan (2004) found romantic hopes among women working in the Sosua sex tourism district in the Dominican Republic alongside fantasies of how a first-world passport could open doors to a better life off the island. For this reason, she talks about Sosua as a "sexscape" or a "space of transformation" where *both* locals and tourists engage in fantasies of their own transformation (p. 14). In her study of correspondence marriages between western men and Asian women, Constable also emphasizes the wide diversity of motivations among both partners and how such relationships are not reducible to economics or power relations, even while they are shaped by them (2003: 9, 122).

The above narratives about alienation, insecurity, and loss of control illustrate some of the potential repercussions from occupying the position of a neocolonial expatriate. That is, the status that these *farang* men gained from their relative wealth, whiteness, and "expat" position also tended to leave them socially isolated and uncertain about the bases for their intimate relationships. In response to this vulnerability and loss of control, some of them adopted self-narratives centering on conscious choices and successful masculinity.

6 Conclusion

The settlement of western men in provincial Thailand transforms social geographies at the same time as it leaves global hierarchies unchallenged. These men have been able to frame their move overseas to live near their partners' families in a way that does not make them "immigrants," but rather, "expats" who occupy a privileged position that derives from their western income stream, whiteness, and first-world outsider status. In this regard, their structural location does resemble that of sex tourists.

However, the existing literatures on masculinities in sex tourism enclaves do not capture the complex balance between power and vulnerability that was apparent among men who had settled in Thailand. The very things that permitted them structural privilege in the short run had a series of repercussions for their social and intimate lives. Remaining a western outsider instead of attempting to assimilate within Thai society may have helped buy them freedom from the discipline of social expectations, but it also left them without a place to fit in other than in a superficial role as a *farang*. Their ability to provide financial security to lower-class Thai women and their families bought them status and access to younger women than might have been possible back home; however, the role of money in the relationship sat in awkward and anxiety-producing tension with their own western notions of marriages grounded in romantic love. The interviews from this field study illustrated the heady potential of transforming oneself into an ideal masculine subject in a radically simplified life, as well as the alienation, insecurity, and loss of control that this transformation entailed.

The strategy of western migrants such as these to remain expats in their daily lives in Thailand has repercussions not only for the men themselves but also for social and economic structures in the provinces in which they settled. The foreign income *farang* men bring with them also transforms rural economies, with families with a *farang* connection rising in status, and local businesses catering to the consumption desires of a *farang* clientele. Families without this tie to western income likely experience a sense of downward mobility as local goods become more expensive and as their neighbors can buy things they cannot. Finally, the influx of western marriage partners will surely have implications for the dynamics of race, gender, and kinship in these areas.

The Thai state seems ambivalent about the settlement of westerners on a permanent basis. Short-term visas are no longer renewable,[28] and while marriage to a Thai gives residency, naturalization is difficult, and foreigners are not allowed to own houses or land and so must register them under a Thai citizen's name (Cohen 2003; Howard 2009). These policies suggest that the Thai state welcomes the short-term flow of currency that tourists and investors bring into Thailand and may even have an interest in promoting short-term marriages, but that it holds a nationalist line against the permanent incorporation of *farang* men. It is hard to say how long any particular western settler will remain in provincial Thailand, but the transformations occurring there appear to be self-reinforcing. Of course, *farang* men are only one of the relevant set of actors in this instance of western expatriate communities forming in a developing state; surely, Thai women and men are also renegotiating their own identities and locations in local and global terms as geographies transform, rich topics for further study.

References

Askew, M. (1999). Strangers and lovers: Thai women sex workers and western men in the 'pleasure space' of Bangkok. In J. Forshee, C. Fink, & S. Cate (Eds.), *Converging interests: Traders, travelers and tourists in Southeast Asia* (pp. 109–148). Berkeley: International and Area Studies.

Berg, L., & Longhurst, R. (2003). Placing masculinities and geography. *Gender, Place, and Culture, 10*(4), 351–360.

Bernstein, R. (2007, August 12) Variations on a theme: Thai women and foreign husbands. *The New York Times*. http://www.nytimes.com/2007/08/12/world/asia/12iht-letter.1.7087394.html

Bishop, R., & Robinson, L. S. (1998). *Night market: Sexual cultures and the Thai economic miracle*. New York: Routledge.

Bishop, R., & Robinson, L. S. (1999). Genealogies of exotic desire: The Thai night market in the Western imagination. In N. Cook & P. Jackson (Eds.), *Genders and sexualities in modern Thailand* (pp. 191–205). Chiang Mai: Silkworm Books.

Brennan, D. (2004). *What's love got to do with it?: Transnational desires and sex tourism in the Dominican Republic*. Durham: Duke University Press.

Broinowski, A. (1992). *The yellow lady: Australian impressions of Asia*. Melbourne: Oxford University Press.

Cohen, E. (1986). Lovelorn farangs: The correspondence between foreign men and Thai girls. *Anthropological Quarterly, 59*(3), 115–117.

Cohen, E. (2003). Transnational marriage in Thailand: The dynamics of extreme heterogamy. In T. G. Bauer & B. McKercher (Eds.), *Sex and tourism: Journeys of romance, love, and lust* (pp. 57–81). New York: The Haworth Hospitality Press.

Cook, N. M., & Jackson, P. A. (1999). Desiring constructs: Transforming sex/gender orders in twentieth-century Thailand. In N. Cook & P. Jackson (Eds.), *Genders and sexualities in modern Thailand* (pp. 1–27). Chiang Mai: Silkworm Books.

[28] Whereas many foreigners in Thailand used to have access to endlessly renewable 30-day tourist visas, this loophole was eliminated in 2006, and thousands of westerners are arrested and deported for overstaying their visas (Howard 2009: 200–202). Retirees over 50 who have an income of at least US$23,000 per year can get a one-year renewable visa.

Constable, N. (2003). *Romance on a global stage: Pen pals, virtual ethnography, and 'mail order' marriages*. Berkeley: University of California Press.
Garrick, D. (2005). Excuses, excuses: Rationalisations of Western sex tourists in Thailand. *Current Issues in Tourism, 8*(6), 497–509.
Gregory, S. (2003). Men in paradise: Sex tourism and the political economy of masculinity. In D. S. Moore, J. Kosek, & A. Panadian (Eds.), *Race, nature, and the politics of difference* (pp. 323–355). Durham: Duke University Press.
Hamilton, A. (1997). Primal dream: Masculinism, sin, and salvation in Thailand's sex trade. In L. Manderson & M. Jolly (Eds.), *Sites of desire, economies of pleasure: Sexualities in Asia and the Pacific* (pp. 145–165). Chicago: University of Chicago Press.
Howard, R. W. (2008). Western retirees in Thailand: Motives, experiences, wellbeing, assimilation and future needs. *Aging and Society, 28*, 145–163.
Howard, R. W. (2009). The migration of Westerners to Thailand: An unusual flow from developed to developing world. *International Migration, 47*(2), 193–225.
Jackson, P. A. (2007). Autonomy and subordination in Thai history: The case for semicolonial analysis. *Inter-Asia Cultural Studies, 8*(3), 329–348.
Johnson, A. A. (2007). Authenticity, tourism, and self-discovery in Thailand: Self-creation and the discerning gaze of trekkers and old hands. *SOJOURN: Journal of Social Issues in Southeast Asia, 22*(2), 153–178.
Limanonda, B. (2007) *Motivation and process of marriage migration: A case study of Thailand.* Paper presented at PAK/IPAR conference on international marriage migration in Asia in Seoul, Korea.
Lyttleton, C. (1994). The good people of Isan: Commercial sex in northeast Thailand. *The Australian Journal of Anthropology, 5*(3), 257–280.
Malam, L. (2008). Bodies, beaches and bars: Negotiating heterosexual masculinity in southern Thailand's tourism industry. *Gender, Place, and Culture, 6*, 581–594.
Mies, M. (1998). *Patriarchy and accumulation on a world scale: Women in the international division of labour*. London: Zed Books.
Mills, M. B. (2005). Engendering discourses of displacement: Contesting mobility and marginality in rural Thailand. *Ethnography, 6*(3), 385–419.
Nuttavuthisit, K. (2007). Branding Thailand: Correcting the negative image of sex tourism. *Place Branding and Public Diplomacy, 3*(1), 21–30.
O'Connell Davidson, J., & Sanchez-Taylor, J. (1999). Fantasy islands: Exploring the demand for sex tourism. In K. Kempadoo (Ed.), *Sun, sex, and gold: Tourism and sex work in the Caribbean* (pp. 37–54). Lanham: Rowman and Littlefield Publishing.
Persaud, W. H. (2005). Gender, race, and global modernity: A perspective from Thailand. *Globalizations, 2*(2), 210–227.
Truong, T. D. (1983). The dynamics of sex tourism: The case of Southeast Asia. *Development and Change, 14*, 533–553.
Truong, T. D. (1990). *Sex, money and morality: Prostitution and tourism in Southeast Asia.* London: Zed Books.
Van Esterik, P. (2000). *Materializing Thailand.* Oxford: Berg Publishers.

Chapter 21
Women NGOs' Movement for Fighting Against Domestic Violence

Suangsurang Mitsamphanta

1 Introduction

When a female baby is born, she wishes to be raised in a loving family. When she becomes a girl, she wishes to have a loving boyfriend. Once she marries with her beloved man, she wishes him to be a loving husband. She wishes to have a good marriage and a happy family. In reality, however, women experience domestic violence at least once in their lifetime.

Domestic violence against women is a type of violence performed in families which should be the safest and happiest area for everyone (Kapoor 2000; WHO 2005). The perpetrators of domestic violence normally are intimate partners of the victims (Feminist Majority Foundation 2012). It is an epidemic that cuts across the world, from country to country, developed and developing countries, and cuts across every socioeconomic status (Kapoor 2000; WHO 2005). It directly affects women's rights, security, and health, and its consequences are both economic and social. For example, the cost effect is cost of services used in treating or preventing violence and the indirect influence is the pain and suffering of the victims. Additionally, domestic violence impacts the labor force, general productivity, interpersonal relations, and the general quality of life from both an economic and societal perspective (Kapoor 2000).

In Thailand, as well as other countries, domestic violence is presented as a common problem between intimate partners (Manager News Paper, 12 Nov, 2007). It is identified as a "normal" thing (WHO 2005). Domestic violence is never seen as a women's rights issue or crime (Kemp 1998; Satha-anan 2010). Rather, it is seen merely as a family or private problem (Bubphamas 2007). It is also not perceived as a big problem.

S. Mitsamphanta (✉)
Department of Public Administration, Faculty of Political Science,
Chulalongkorn University, Henri-Dunant Rd. Pathumwan, Bangkok 10330, Thailand
e-mail: lbsms10@gmail.com

P. Liamputtong (ed.), *Contemporary Socio-Cultural and Political Perspectives in Thailand*,
DOI 10.1007/978-94-007-7244-1_21,

Domestic violence became an offense when the Thai Parliament ratified the Act for Protection of Domestic Violence's Victims in November 2007. The Act was drafted with the cooperation of many parts of the society which included women NGOs, government organizations, concerned politicians, academics, and community networks from Bangkok and other provinces (Mitsamphanta 2011; Thai Health Promotion Foundation 2009).

As the Act was initiated by women NGOs, it is interesting to learn about the success of these NGOs in solidifying the issue of domestic violence in a patriarchal society like Thailand. This chapter focuses only on the role of nongovernmental organizations in fighting domestic violence. It first describes the evolution of women NGOs in Thailand, the attitude of women NGO's toward domestic violence, how and when they became involved with the issue, and their concerns and tactics used in combating the issue.

This chapter is based on my qualitative research in Thailand. The data was compiled from interviews, group participation, and literature review. The information was mostly gained from formal and informal interviews with people who could be considered stakeholders in the domestic violence issue. The key informants were women NGO workers, politicians, and government officials. Additional information came from the observation of meetings between women NGOs and their network.

2 Historical Perspective

2.1 The Beginning of Thai Women NGOs

According to Pandey (2003), the evolution of Thai Women NGOs is divided into three phases which are the periods before 1932, 1940–1979, and 1975–1995.

At the first phase, women NGOs in Thailand were established as women's clubs, groups, or associations. All those women's groups were established by elite women with two different ideologies. The women's groups, which were formed based on the idea of conservatism, were set up to provide educational access to women, in order to promote the notion of being a "good wife" and a "good mother." Another type of women's association was created by female reformists aiming to empower disadvantaged women in terms of economic and legal status. They then offered skill training and legal advice for girls and women. Those organizations were the Association of Women Lawyers, Guides Association of Thailand (GGAT), and the Committee for Women's Social Welfare. All these groups worked under the auspices of the National Council of Women of Thailand (NCWT). They were also patronized by the royal family.

The second move of Thai women NGOs was between 1940 and 1970. This was the transformational period of women activists' ideology. In regard to the world political situation, women activists were inspired by left-wing political ideology. Additionally, Western feminism was introduced by elite women who had been educated abroad. These two political ideologies were first launched among university students and middle-class intellectuals in Bangkok. It was then spread out and strengthened solidly across the country. During this period, one of the important Women NGOs emerged. The Promotion of Status of Women Group (now the Association for the Promotion of the Status of Women) was created in 1974 by a former lawyer in the elite class. The guarantee of women's rights and abolishment of discrimination against Thai women were the goals of the association. Subsequently, this group expanded their activity from legal counseling services to shelters and skilled training centers as well as running a research institute (APSW 2012a).

In the third phrase (1975–1995[1]), Thai women NGOs' perspectives and activities were affected by the International Organization, especially the declaration of UN Decade for Women (1975–1985). Also, in regard to the changing of social structure and the increasing of educated middle-class people, the activists were young educated middle-class women. These young women concentrated more on the issue of women's liberation. As a result, their activities were expanded and they began moving into public areas such as the regional protests against Japanese sex tourism. After participating in that movement, the activists regrouped as the first women NGO—Friend of Women Group in 1980—and then they had developed the group to be Friends of Women Foundation (FOW). The roles of FOW mainly focus on women's rights protection and providing assistance to women in crisis (FOW 2012). Soon after that, Women's Information Center which is now known as the Foundation for Women (FFW) was instituted in 1984. This organization has been chiefly supporting activities for the purpose of respecting, protecting, and promoting the rights of individual women and girls based on human rights principles (FFW 2012). Besides, HOTLINE Center Foundation, a phone counseling service for vulnerable women was formed in 1984 (HOTLINE 2008). Some years after that, the EMPOWER foundation, an advocate to sex worker's rights, was founded in 1992. All these women activist groups are the pioneers of women NGOs of Thailand.

2.2 *Women NGOs Who Fight Against Domestic Violence*

Although there are many women NGOs in Thailand (Online Women in Politics 2012), there were few NGOs available for interviews about their movement on domestic violence during the field work. The two organizations that I was able to interview were the Association for the Promotion of the Status of Women (APSW) and Friend of Women Foundation (FOW).

In 1974, Ms. Kanitha Wichiencharoen and women and men who were concerned about women's issues founded the Status of Women Promotion Group. The goals of the group were to encourage women's rights and eliminate discrimination against women in Thailand. Over the years, the activities of the group became more

[1] In regard to Kemp (1998), in the 1970s, the new movement concerning abused women began and expressed at the grassroots level in establishing shelters for battered women.

concrete. In 1981, the first Emergency Home was started with the help of the Women's Lawyers Association of Thailand and the Girl Guides Association of Thailand. It is a shelter for disadvantaged women. The group became a legal charity in 1982 and is called the Association for the Promotion of the Status of Women. The second Emergency Home and the Children's Home were begun in 1986. Three years later, the Jimmy-Rosalynn Carter Women's Clinic and Nursery and the Sasakawa Women's Education and Training Center (We-Train) were opened at Don Muang, Bangkok, the current location of the association. The Women's Clinic provides services to women with unplanned pregnancies. Also telephone services are available for consultation on women's reproductive health problems. In 1990, APSW expanded its reach in the research field by establishing the Gender and Development Research Institute. The research institute conducts action research on policy issues and provides policy advocacy in order to improve the status of women and promote gender equality. Besides, We-Train International House was set up and run as an on-site conference center. It helps in fund-raising for APSW. Additionally, in 1955, APSW founded a Don Muang Youth Center in Don Muang district and Women's Health Clinic in Dusit, Bangkok. In 2003, they opened their latest sanctuary for women in crisis and is called the Kanitnaree Center (Rape Crisis Center). Here, rape victims are provided with sensitive care by professional staff at the center.

APSW (2012b) has been developing and extending their activities and services for decades in order to empower women to be equal, to acknowledge and improve their skills, to support disadvantaged women and children, and to improve their quality of life. The center also works in association with other governmental and nongovernmental organizations inside and outside the countries working in the same area.

FOW (2002) emerged from young women and men who are interested in women's problems grouping together and exchanging their views. FOW was established with the intention to expand the public awareness on women's issues and inequality and coordinate with other organizations to ensure women's equality. FOW has been working for women for decades with the objective to create and to promote new social attitudes that value gender equality. These include social equality as well as fair economic and cultural treatment of women. There has also been extra work to improve the general public's understanding of the issues of rape, forced prostitution, domestic violence, economic discrimination, work dismissal, and sexual discrimination.

Recently, the FOW worked intensely on the issue of sexual crimes and harassment of women. In order to support their work, FOW set up functions such as a women's rights protection center, shelters, legal counseling services, telephone counseling services, a health center, a women's publishing house, a documentary library, gender analysis training, and income-generating projects for women. Furthermore, FOW expanded its network by joining in many activities of other women's organizations.

APSW and FOW have been working with disadvantaged women for decades. Many of them came to these organizations mostly as victims of domestic violence (Mitsamphanta 2011). They provide many kinds of assistance to these women in order to reduce their suffering and protect them from further abuse. From their experiences, it is interesting to know how they understand domestic violence.

3 Women NGOs and Domestic Violence

3.1 Its Perspective on Domestic Violence

3.1.1 Domestic Violence Is Not a Private Problem

Generally, people consider domestic violence merely a family problem. However, APSW and FOW (Mitsamphanta 2011) recognize it as a public problem which directly affects women's rights and dignity. It is the beginning of a series of violence against women. Furthermore, it has many significant consequences on women's lives, health, and economic status—women are also a part of the labor force in the market. It indirectly impacts the national development as well. Additionally, the violence has a direct affect on women's rights. Women should have the right to protection by the law.

3.1.2 Forms of Violence Are Varied

> The injuries that appear on women's bodies are various, like bruises, cuts, burns, etc. Some are injured seriously. Some are splashed with acid and get horrible burns. Some are betrayed by their unfaithful husbands, having mistresses and taking away her money. There are many forms of assaults, physical, psychological, and economic. Forms of violence are various and sometimes you can see the injuries on a woman's body. You cannot guess what happened to her or how it happened? Sometimes it's really horrible. (Director of Women's Rights Protection Center (WRPC), FOW, personal interview, 2007)
>
> Wives cannot refuse when husbands want to have sex. In addition men control sexual desire. Men decide when to have or not have sex, use or not use a condom. (Manager of FOW, personal interview, 2007)

Domestic violence has many forms and degrees. The perpetrators use violent behavior to control their intimate partner. The assault can be physical, sexual, psychological, and/or economic. The attack can be with or without weapons or anything that can harm another person (Chothirat 1994; Wirawatanodom 1997; Navaboonniyom 2001; Karmen 2004). The levels of violence vary. It can start from a minor argument to an accidental physical attack such as pushing. In worse cases, the attack can cause serious injuries, disability, and even death.

3.1.3 Causes of Domestic Violence: Macro and Micro Level

> Domestic violence happens because of many factors. It is not only from poverty but it roots on the imbalance of power, culture and law which help men to perform violence against women. Also unfaithfulness, lack of responsibility of the husband, and male superior idea and patriarchy are the main causes of problem. There are no laws to protect women from domestic violence. (Director of WRPC, FOW, personal interview, 2007)

> Domestic violence occurs because of patriarchal perspective, and gender inequality. It makes men think that their wives are their property. (Manager of FOW, personal interview, 2007)
>
> Domestic violence reflects the gender inequality of the society. (Director of GDRI, APSW, personal interview, 2007)

The factors that contribute to domestic violence are complex (Jewkes 2002). For a clearer understanding, the causes can be separated in two levels—macro and micro. At the macro level, domestic violence is embedded in social norms and structures and includes the concept of patriarchy. This makes women unequal and subordinated to men. Men are the ones who control all the power, economy, and property, including women. The belief in male superiority contributes to the use of violence as a tool for controlling women (Kemp 1998; Kapoor 2000; Jewkes 2002). Furthermore, no one dares to interfere to save the victims. As a result, domestic violence is disregarded by law, legislation, politics, and the economic system.

> Alcohol is the main cause of violence performed in our society. A lot of husbands after getting drunk, use violence against their wives. (Manager of FOW, personal interview, 2007)

Looking down to the micro level, the background of the abusive perpetrators, drug and alcohol addiction, and poverty are all risk factors in evoking violence between intimate partners.

FOW's and APSW's perspective on domestic violence precisely recognizes it as a gender inequality problem caused by patriarchy which is reflected in cultural norms, social attitudes, and social institutions. As a result of the damage of domestic violence on the victims, women NGOs called for social attention in order to raise public awareness about the issue.

3.2 *Support Provided for Domestic Violence Victims*

The women NGOs provide assistance to the victim in two stages which are protection and prevention.

Both APSW and FOW (Mitsamphanta 2011) provide many services as protective measures. All the caring measures aim to save the victim from repetitive assaults and abusive environments and to improve their mentality. The services provided include counseling (telephone, face-to-face, and group), cooperation for prosecution, house visits, shelters, and group therapy programs. All the assistance is run by the social workers of the NGOs, lawyers who have received social skill training, and women who have experienced violence. All services are offered based upon the beneficiary's needs and problems.

In order to solve the problem, only protection is not enough. Consequently, prevention measures are necessitated at every level of the society from the individual to national level. Women NGOs offer many activities so as to prevent domestic violence. Empowerment programs are set up for the individuals. The programs supply the necessary knowledge, education, and skill training such as sewing courses, cookery courses, and hairdresser courses. Education and training skills will decrease the economic dependency of women on men. It can help battered women to leave their abusive husband easier.

Additionally, community cooperation is significant. Thus, women NGOs form a workshop in their network communities. The workshop permits both women and men to participate. The activities will be created on the gender equality concept. NGO staff will be only facilitators acknowledging and stimulating participants to think, realize and figure out the cause and solution of domestic violence in the community by themselves.

3.3 Limitations of Women NGOs Responses to Domestic Violence

For decades, women NGOs have been working with great effort on decreasing domestic violence and ensuring women's rights. Nevertheless, they cannot complete the goal. That is because of the lack of funds, the limited number of women NGO workers, lack of network, and lack of the intervention authority as their limitation.

All the activities of protection and prevention of domestic violence necessitate permanent ongoing funding. The financial support for NGOs mainly is from donors and the government. Nonetheless, all this financial support is not constant. The government financial support is insufficient, while the donations are project-driven and depend on many factors. In addition, sometimes the donor requests something from women NGOs which is not related to their work (Director of WRPC, FOW and Director of GDRI, APSW, personal interview, 2007). The dependency on donations creates difficulty in running the movement. Consequently, women NGOs need persistent funding from the government.

Because its intention is to stop domestic violence across the country, it needs a large staff and many branches. However, the number of employees and network offices in communities are inadequate for this incredibly difficult task (Director of WRPC and Manager, FOW, personal interview, 2007).

Another important factor is the myth that domestic violence is an intimate problem or *reung phua mea*.[2] With this notion, it is difficult to save the beaten wife from continued brutal actions. Therefore, it is very difficult for women NGOs and any witnesses to help the battered women. Thus, to protect the victims of domestic violence, authority for intervention and a new attitude about domestic violence are imperative.

[2] *Reung phua mea* refers to the problem or fight between intimate partners which an outsider should not be involved with. The belief is that the outsider will have problems with that couple when they resolve their problems.

4 Movements for Fighting Domestic Violence

Because of these limitations, women NGOs urged cooperation from society and the government. Many strategies were employed in order to obtain the obligation of the private and public sectors for unraveling domestic violence. In the private sector, women NGOs aim to improve social attitudes and increase awareness of domestic violence, as well as the network of antiviolence against women. Simultaneously, in the public sector, the schemes were designed to influence the government to take responsibility for mandating policies and programs that relate to domestic violence.

4.1 The Movement in the Private Sector

Movement in the private sector was done via networks and alliance building and campaigns. Networking and campaigns were very important in order to expand the idea of antiviolence against women, challenge the myth of domestic violence, and enhance women's rights awareness.

The networks and alliances were built by the cooperation between women NGOs and other NGOs who could understand or at least were not against the idea of gender equality. The cooperation was done via joint projects and joint activities. As gender issues and domestic violence are considered sensitive issues in Thai society, when women NGOs were working with other NGOs, they did not show their strong feminism. Instead, they insinuated gender ideas such as gender equality, antiviolence against women, and women's rights into the activities' content. They had high complexity in working with others. They did not coerce the other to agree with their points. Nonetheless, they gradually and gently acknowledged their gender perspective to their networks via some activities such as group discussions and workshops, until other NGOs understood and accepted the ideology and became a part of their alliance (Manager of FOW, personal interview, 2007). Their partners were NGOs fighting against the HIV/AIDS epidemic, antialcohol drinking clubs or "Don't Drink Clubs," and women's training groups (Director of WRPC & Manager of FOW, Director of GDRI, APSW, and M.P., personal interview, 2007).

Raising social awareness was the second strategy employed in the private sector. Women NGOs and their network campaign on many occasions related to women such as International Women's Day and Antiviolence Against Women Day. The campaigns were created in several areas across the country and published through various kinds of mass media such as television spots, radio spots, posters, and newsletters (Director of WRPC & Manager of FOW, Director of GDRI, APSW, personal interview, 2007). During the campaign, several activities were utilized, for example, marches, dramas, and parades. These activities were aimed to encourage people to understand domestic violence as violence against women. With this comprehensive and continuous effort, the women NGOs believed that people in society would become conscious that any kind of violence should not be tolerated, and no one has the right to use violence against another.

It can be concluded that women NGOs (FOW and APSW) mainly focus on acknowledgment of gender ideals and the idea of antiviolence against women especially domestic violence via many media and activities. The campaigns and activities aim to affect society both in the private and public sectors. They are not only for raising social attention toward domestic violence but also for activities in the private sector that will lead to government attention and response to the problem as well.

4.2 *The Movement in the Public Sector*

With the long-term intention to solve the problem systematically, especially within the legal system, women NGOs and their networks apply many strategies at all levels to urge the government to respond and commit to new domestic violence legislation.

4.2.1 At the Constitutional Level and Its Outcome

The most important and basic factors necessary to solve domestic violence is to ensure women's rights and equality in the constitution of the country. Women NGOs believe that once women's rights are guaranteed by the highest laws, it will lead to other following laws, policies, and regulations responding to women's issues. Accordingly, women NGOs tried to utilize the constitution for improving gender equality and protecting women's rights. The provision of gender equality will transform social stance and empower women (Thomson and Bhongsvej 1996). Additionally, it will lead to laws, policies, and budgetary allocations that will empower women in several important areas including domestic violence.

At this stage, women NGOs applied social forces and lobbying as their means to push women's rights into the constitution. With the leading of Women and Constitution Network, APSW, FOW, and female members of the Constitutional Drafting Assembly (CDA), they started to lobby the constitutional legislators of CDA to identify women's rights in the constitution. Additionally, they referred to international laws especially the Convention on the Elimination of All Forms of Discrimination against Women (CEDAW) as a tool to pressure the government to answer women's issues (Thomson and Bhongsvej 1996). Furthermore, a female MP (personal interview, 2007) mentioned that some of CDA's members who are in the women's network try to convince other committees who seem to have gender sensitivity to pay attention to women's issues. It is known that not everyone will be interested in women's issues or concerned about domestic violence and women's problems. Thus, strong evidence of the problem such as reports and research of women's issues was significantly utilized for reinforcing the lobby and for the committees to accept the point.

Because of this relentless effort, in 1997, women's rights and language against all forms of violence against women were stated in the 1997 Constitution of the Kingdom of Thailand. They were mentioned in Sections 4, 5, 28, and 30. Additionally, domestic violence was addressed separately in Sections 53 and 80. Ten years later, because of a Thai political situation, Thailand passed the 2007 Constitution of Kingdom of Thailand. However, the recognition of women's rights and the prohibition of all violence against women were still provided in Sections 4, 5, and 30, while domestic violence was identified specifically in Sections 52, 80 (1), and 81 (5).

4.2.2 At the Legislative Level

Once women's rights and domestic violence were recognized in the constitution (especially in 1997), women NGOs (specifically, Women and Constitution Network, Friend of Women Foundation, Foundation for Women, Empower Foundation, Association for the Promotion of the Status of Women, Circle of Female Lawyer, Thai Labor Organization, Women Lawyers' Association of Thailand, and Volunteering Muslim Women's Group) moved forward for particular laws on domestic violence (Tamthai 2003). With the same strategy and Female Parliamentarian Group as the alliances, they lobbied high-ranking officials of the Office of the National Commission on Women's Affairs (NCWA) to be a main respondent of the issue. Furthermore, in regard to the professional experience and the movement of women NGOs on women's issues, they were appointed to an ad hoc committee of the Legal Advisory Sub-committee of the NCWA. Then they pushed forward to lobby with other members of the National Assembly (NA) to pass a law directly responding to domestic violence. Once they had a broad network and many alliances, they started to draft a law on domestic violence. With the hope that the law would help in protecting the victim and provide more choices on legal procedures, the drafting process was started. Nonetheless, because of the Thailand Bureaucratic Reform in 2002, the drafting process was paused. This was a good sign. In 2002, the Ministry of Social Development and Human Security was established as an outcome of the reform. Under this ministry, there is the Office of Women and Family Affairs which is the first government office established to directly take care of women's issues. The drafting process on the domestic violence law was continued with the new main respondent, Ministry of Social Development and Human Security. The draft was completed and presented to the Cabinet in 2005. Before that, it was revised several times. After approving the draft, the Cabinet assigned the Ministry to form the ministerial regulations for supporting implementation. In March 2007, the draft was verified by the Ministry and submitted to the cabinet and then the National Assembly in April.

Once the National Assembly accepted the draft of the law, women NGOs and their allies changed to lobby the members of the National Assembly to agree with and pass the law. In the law, sexual assault and rape are counted as forms of domestic violence; accordingly, women NGOs pushed their effort to amend Penal Code Section 276 in order to extend this protection to cases of marital rape.

Furthermore, a female MP (personal interview, 2007) stated that social force or mass movement was another strategy they utilized for pressing politicians or members of the parliament to pass and amend the law. The activities included sending postcards with messages urging lawmakers to ensure women's rights and equality in the constitution. They did this by contacting their representatives in each province via the women's network. Parades were also arranged in order to show their power and stance for the protection of their rights and dignity.

At the conclusion, on August 14, 2007, the "Act for Protection of Domestic Violence's Victims" was promulgated and published in the Thailand Gazette, Volume 124. Subsequently, on November 13, 2007, the law became effective. Also in the same year, the Penal Code section was amended by removing the clause "who is not his wife" (Director of WRPC, FOW, personal interview, 2007). The result of this deletion is that the new law will protect women from marital rape.

As a result, at the legislation level, the outcomes were the Act for Protection of Domestic Violence's Victims which was the first specific law on domestic violence, and the amendment of Penal Code Section 276 which protects women in cases of marital rape.

4.2.3 At the Policy Level

Only ensuring women's rights in the constitution was not enough; precise policy to purposely stop violence against women was still required. Women NGOs attempted to add this provision at every step of the implementation. As a result, the women's network and women NGOs pressed the government to consent to other policies and plans. Lobbying, proposing measures or ideas for resolution, and campaigns were used as their approaches.

Lobbying was performed with the high-ranking administrative officials such as ministers, the permanent undersecretary of ministries, the deputy director of government division, and the provincial governor. This is because they had the authority potency to introduce the policy and plan the budget for the implementation or to carry out the policies. The lobbying was done by the women NGOs and their network by directly contacting high-ranking officials and other related policy-makers. They expressed their ideas and attitudes about the problem. Then they convinced them to understand the problem and agree to take action (Manger and Director of WRPC, FOW; Director of GDRI, APSW, personal interview, 2007). Thus, the women NGOs and their networks, as the lobbyists, lobbied hard against those people.

> In general, we speak to the high-ranking administrators of many related ministries. We try to explain our ideas to them and make them understand the problem. This will lead to budget changes and policy upgrading. (Director of WRPC, FOW, personal interview, 2007)

In addition, women NGOs proposed some policy models or blueprints of the plans for the related government offices to solve the problem. These policy models and plans were drafted with the cooperation of women NGOs, academicians, and representatives of government offices (Director of WRPC, FOW, personal interview, 2007). Examples of the plans that women NGOs proposed to the cabinet via NCWA were the eight measures to solve violence against women, the Policies and Plans to Eradicate Violence Against Children and Women.

Furthermore, campaigning in society was the indirect channel of women NGOs to induce policy-makers to act on domestic violence issues. They believed that the movement in society could increase women's rights awareness for the policy-makers. The campaigns mostly were parades and public speeches on International Women's Day and in the month of elimination of violence against women. The Manager and the Director of WRPC (FOW, personal interview, 2007) further mentioned that all those activities were arranged simultaneously in many places across the country. Sometimes, the advocacy was done via posters with reminiscent messages exhibited in public areas such as governmental organizations (Director of GDRI, APSW, personal interview, 2007).

> Many activities were arranged continuously in these several years, and then the government repeated our paths on creating the same sort of activities. (Director of WRPC, FOW, personal interview, 2007)

Women NGOs applied many strategies at this level with the expectation for particular policies and plans concerning domestic violence to be created. Consequently, on June 22, 1999, the cabinet announced the month of November to be a month of Antiviolence Against Children and Women. Seven days later, the Cabinet also declared the eight measures to solve violence against women. About a year later, the Policies and Plans to Eradicate Violence against Children and Women was approved by the Cabinet on May 16, 2000. In regard to the Policies and Plans to Eradicate Violence against Children and Women, the One Stop Crisis Center (OSCC) was set up in several hospitals as a first contact center for the victims of domestic violence.

4.2.4 At the Implementation Level

Implementation was a very important step for practicing the policies. Also, the persons implementing the policies are the government officials or the bureaucrats. The bureaucrats have to work under the bureaucracy rules and obligations which are somewhat gender blind. However, they are government agencies who will work closely with the issue and the victims of domestic violence. It is very important to acknowledge and encourage them to be gender sensitive. As a result, they will not aggravate and can really help the victims.

Based on this principle, women NGOs offered several training programs such as gender sensitive training programs, and case resolution programs to the officials who work with domestic violence. The training programs were typically set up in the form of workshops and round-table seminars. In the workshops, the facilitators used real cases for the attendees to study and practice. As domestic violence is a sensitive issue and needs several dimensions of support, trainings were always conducted with a multidisciplinary approach. The trainees came from every related government office, for example, police officers, medical staff, government social workers, and legal staff.

> We formed several workshops aiming to expand the assisting network for victims of domestic violence. We also expected that the workshop will provide a network of officials who are involved in the issue. We tried hard to make the connection between agencies. (Director of WRPC, FOW, personal interview, 2007)

With the reputation and experience of women NGOs handling the domestic violence cases, sometimes they were invited to be facilitators in gender-sensitive training by governmental organizations. As facilitators, women NGOs suggest some means to help the victims of domestic violence (Director of WRPC, FOW, personal interview, 2007).

Women NGOs tried to cooperate with several governmental agencies that related to domestic violence. The cooperation was mostly done via the training programs. The cooperation could be begun by either women NGOs or the government agencies. Women NGOs training programs assisted in increasing gender awareness and gender sensitivity to the government officials at the implementation level.

5 Discussion and Conclusion

From the information described above, the movement of women NGOs in the private and public sectors can be represented by the following schemas (Tables 21.1 and 21.2).

From the schema, it shows that the methods of movement were different following the space, level of movement, and target persons. In the private area, women NGOs mostly used activities that were easy for people to access and easy to remember and understand. In the public area, women NGOs preferred the persuasion technique and pressuring the center of state power in order to get a government response. Although the methods of movement were different, the main purposes were the

Table 21.1 The movement in the private sector, methods, and the outcomes

Level of movement	Actors	Type of movement	Target group	Activities	Outcomes
Societal level	Women NGOs	Network and alliance building	Other NGOs	Joint project, joint activities, group discussion, workshop	Expanding network
		Campaign	People in the society	Marching, drama, parade, media spots	Increasing people awareness

Table 21.2 The movement in the public sector, methods, and the outcomes

Level of movement	Actors	Methods of movement	Target group	Outcomes
Constitutional level	Women and Constitution Network, Association for the Promotion of the Status of Women, Friend of Women Foundation, Female members of the CDA	Lobbying	Constitutional Drafting Assembly	1997 Constitution of Kingdom of Thailand; sections relates to women's right 4,5,28, and 30; sections relates to domestic violence 53 and 80
		Social advocacy References to international human rights documents such as CDEAW, Beijing Platform for Action	Constitutional legislators	2007 Constitution of Kingdom of Thailand sections relates to women's right 4,5, and 30; sections relates to domestic violence 52, 80 (1), and 81 (5)
Legislation level	Women and Constitution Network, Friend of Women Foundation, Foundation for Women, Empower Foundation, Association for the Promotion of the Status of Women, Circle of Female Lawyer, Thai Labor Organization, Women Lawyers' Association of Thailand, Volunteering Muslim Women's Group	Lobbying Being ad hoc committee of the Legal Advisory Sub-committee of NCWA Social advocacy	Highrank officials of the Office of the National Commission on Women's Affairs (NCWA)	Act for Protection of Domestic Violence's Victims Penal Code section 276
Policy level	Friend of Women Foundation, Association for the Promotion of the Status of Women	Lobbying Proposing measure or idea	High-rank administrative officers	The Policies and Plans to Eradicate Violence against Children and Women One Stop Crisis Center (OSCC)
Implementation Level	Friend of Women Foundation	Providing training programs	Bureaucrats	Increasing of gender sensitivity and awareness of the bureaucrats

same. They were challenging the domestic violence myth, the increasing of women's rights awareness, and the concrete responsibility of the state toward domestic violence as a social policy issue as well as a criminal one (Ball and Charles 2006). Accordingly, they tried hard to get the state to be responsible for solving all aspects of the problem (Kapoor 2000). Also international women's rights declarations were employed as a reference and a tool to call for the government's real obligation to offer a pragmatic measure (Zhang 2009). From the outcome, it shows that women NGOs can ask the state to be responsible at every level and in every government sector such as criminal justice, health, and social work.

List of Interview

The Director of Women's Rights Protection Center, Friend of Women Foundation, the Office of Friend of Women Foundation, Bangkok, Thailand

The Manager of Friend of Women Foundation, the Office of Friend of Women Foundation, Bangkok, Thailand

The Director of Gender and Development Research Institute, Association for the Promotion of Women Status, the Office of Gender and Development Research Institute, Bangkok, Thailand

A Female Member of the Parliament, the Office of Democrat Party, 7 February, 2008, Bangkok, Thailand

Acknowledgments This paper was first presented at the 11th International Conference on Thai Studies, Bangkok, Thailand, July 2011.

References

APSW. (2012a). *Major activities of APSW*. Retrieved March 14, 2012, from http://www.apsw-thailand.org/Intro.htm

APSW. (2012b). *APSW's objectives*. Retrieved March 14, 2012, from http://www.apsw-thailand.org/About%20APSW2.htm

ASTV Manager News Paper Online. (2007). *Thai tid undab lok chai khwam run reang nai krob krua*. Retrieve November 12, 2007, from http://www.manager.co.th/Lite/ViewNews.aspx?NewsID=9500000134219

Ball, W., & Charles, N. (2006). Feminist social movement and policy change: Devolution, childcare and domestic violence policies in Wales. *Women's Studies International Forum, 29*, 172–183.

Bubphamas, N. (2007). *Sieng sathon thee jak kwham thong jam thee mi arj leum*. Retrieved February 16, 2012, from www4.eduzones.com/haloha123/995

Chothirat, S. (1994). *Kwamrunrangnaikrobkrua: Koranee sami thamrairangkai panraya nai ked phuenthi krungthepmahanakorn lea jangwad klaikeang*. Bangkok: National Institute of Development Administration.

Feminist Majority Foundation. (2012). *Domestic violence facts*. Retrieved February 8, 2012, from http://feminist.org/other/dv/dvfact.html

FFW. (2012). *Foundation for women*: *The foundation for women*. Retrieved March 14, 2012, from http://www.womenthai.org/eng/aboutus.html

FOW. (2002, January–December). *Friend of women foundation newsletter* (Vol. 13). Bangkok: Documentation and Publicity Section Friends of Women Foundation.

FOW. (2012). *Friend of women foundation: About*. Retrieved March 14, 2012, from http://support.iz.vc/go.php?http://www.friendsofwomen.or.th/index.php?key=Y29udGVudD1hcmN0aWNsZSZpZD0xMDM=&PHPSESSID=c52d0546544a6eeb2b78ebffbf6efdbc

Jewkes, R. (2002). Intimate partner violence: Cause and prevention. *The Lancet, 359*(9315), 1423–1429.

Kapoor, S. (2000). *Domestic violence against women and girls*. Innocenti Digest, no. 6. Florence: United Nations children's Fund, Innocenti Research Center.

Kemp, A. R. (1998). *Abuse in the family: An introduction*. Belmont: Brooks/Cole Publishing Company.

Mitsamphanta, S. (2011). *State responsibility in addressing domestic violence: A case study of Thailand*. Saarbrücken: LAP LAMBERT Academic Publishing GmbH & Co. KG.

Navaboonniyom, V. (2001). *Kwamrunrangtorpanraya: Kortedjing jag phuthukkrathamtharun preabtheabkab phukratamtharun lea thadsana jag chumchon (Violence against wives: Fact from abused, abuser and community attitude)*. Nakornpathom: Mahidol University.

Online Women in Politics. (2012). *Women's organization*. Retrieve March 14, 2012, from http://www.onlinewomeninpolitics.org/thai/thaiorgs.htm

Pandey, S. R. (2003). *Roles and challenges of civil society in Thailand: A case study of women NGOs* (WARI Working Paper # 14). Bangkok: WARI.

Satha-anan, S. (2010). Bod bannathikarn: Trung sukaphawa phuying wai rawang wattanatham lea kodmai. In S. Satha-anan (Ed.), *Jud yuen: Warasan Satreeniyom Thai* (*Stance: The Thai Feminist Review*) (Vol. 4, pp. xi–xvi). Chiang Mai: Women's Studies Center, Chiang Mai University.

Tamthai, P. (2003). *Prachasangkom reum sang: Rang por ror bor kajad kwamreunrang nai krob-krua (Civil society and the law on the elimination of domestic violence)*. Bangkok: Friedrich-Eber-Stiftung.

Thai Health Promotion Foundation. (2009). *10 pee kan ron na rong yuti khwam run reang tr phu ying kab parakit yong mai sin sud*. Retrieved February 16, 2012, from http://www.thaihealth.or.th/healthcontent/featured/12433

Thomson, S., & Bhongsvej, M. (1996). *Sitthi satrithai nai ratthammanun*. Bangkok: Gender and Development Institute, Association for the Promotion of the Status of Women.

WHO. (2005). *Summary report WHO multi-country study on women's health and domestic violence against women: Initial results on prevalence, health outcomes and women's responses*. Geneva: WHO Press.

Wirawatanodom, N. (1997). *Kwamrunrangtorsatri: Suksanaiklumphuying ayu 15–44 pee thee marabborikan na panaekphupuainok rongphayaban jangwad Chainat (Violence against women: Study of 15–44 year-old women at Outpatient Department, Chainat Hospital, Chainat province)*. Nakornpathom: Mahidol University.

Zhang, L. (2009). Domestic violence network in China: Translating the transnational concept of violence against women into local action. *Women's Studies International Forum, 32*, 227–239.

Chapter 22
Women's Agency in the Malay Muslim Communities of Southern Thailand

Andrea Katalin Molnar

1 Introduction

Women have been described as "victims" in the literature on women's political participation in Southeast Asia. Moreover, publications tend to focus on the formal political arena of elected officials, often highlighting the obstacles that women face when entering politics. Even such obstacles have been discussed through the lenses of a discourse on women as "victims"—victims of patriarchy or of the "old boys" network or of culture and so on. This discourse obscures women's agency. Literature that addresses women's political engagement through civil society is not very voluminous for the Southeast Asia region, particularly in the sense of highlighting the impact of women's actions on significant human security issues. Yet, women are politically engaged—whether through the formal political arena as politicians or, more commonly, through civil society as leaders and activists in social movements and NGOs. Women are agents of change and their political engagement makes significant impact on various issues of human security issues, including peace-building efforts in various parts of Southeast Asia. This chapter examines Malay Muslim women's agency in the Deep South of Thailand, focusing on civil society engagement.

The chapter is based on field research in 2007, 2008, 2009, and 2010 in the Pattani and Yala regions. This chapter does not address the full extent of the ongoing research project, but is addressing some of the key aspects of the overall project. The project focuses on political engagement among Muslim women of the Malay ethnic minority of Thailand and aims to investigate women's agency and specific historical and cultural processes that empower and enable women's political participation. Political engagement is defined here in an inclusive sense of both informal and formal political participation and leadership roles—whether with reference to

A.K. Molnar (✉)
Department of Anthropology, Northern Illinois University,
DeKalb, IL 60115, USA
e-mail: andreakatalinm@gmail.com

P. Liamputtong (ed.), *Contemporary Socio-Cultural and Political Perspectives in Thailand*,
DOI 10.1007/978-94-007-7244-1_22,

civic organizations, NGOs, common interest groups or civil service, elected government office, and political parties. This chapter emphasizes women's political engagement through civil society and thus what I define (for analytical purposes) as the informal political arena. The formal political arena, in contrast, concerns women's political engagement through running for elected office, engagement in political parties, and serving in government officials and officials in other state institutions (e.g., local district government and in the military). This chapter examines aspects of political engagement among women of the Muslim Malay ethnic minority, particularly in comparison to the results of such studies among Thai ethnic women and to women from other parts of Southeast Asia (including Timor Leste). Since the project focuses on the conflict-torn Deep South of Thailand and thus on women engaged in the informal political arena—such as local women's organizations, networks, grassroots groups, and NGOs—it also endeavored to investigate links between women's political engagement through civil society and local peace-building processes. Historically, Muslim women of the south of Thailand have been always an economic force, given that they do the majority of trading, as well as work in agricultural fields and rubber plantations and in small-scale fishing, and indeed engaged in grassroots activities focused on development issues. This chapter explores the different ways in which Muslim women from Southern Thailand have been increasingly engaged through civil society since 2004, and argues that women are not passive victims but are active agents of change. Furthermore, the chapter utilizes comparative material from Timor Leste. The paper addresses several interrelated questions: Is women's engagement through grassroots groups political engagement? If so, to what degree are local Malay culture, Islamic religion, and especially the ongoing violent conflict encourage or impede such political engagement? And What kinds of potential impacts can Muslim women's political engagement through civil society have on women's empowerment, future political participation—in both formal and informal political arenas—as well as for building lasting peace in the Deep South?

These questions were informed by data from the available literature on women's political participation in the developing world, in Southeast Asia, and specifically in Thailand. Furthermore, these research questions were also influenced by the comparative sources from another Muslim society of Indonesia.

The research employed anthropological qualitative research methods with particular sensitivity and ethical considerations for conflict zone research. Data was collected through participant observation, focus group discussions, and 193 in-depth interviews (both unstructured and structured) with various stakeholders. While the majority of interview subjects were women, interviews were also conducted with men from the Deep South. Participant observation also included participation in NGO meetings, project activities, and training workshops for women.

In this chapter, I focus on women's engagement through the lenses of a discourse that places women into the role of agent. By focusing on women's agency, the chapter tries to shed light on the important contributions of women through civil society that is often obscured by a focus on women's political participation in the formal political arena as elected politicians. Yet, the participation and leadership that women engage in through civil society also have significant political implications with a view to their contributions to human security, and in conflict-torn regions, work toward peace-building efforts. Therefore, a central goal is to shift the tone of discourse on women from victims of sociopolitical systems to agents of change and as active contributors from a political anthropology perspective.

2 Conceptual Considerations

Before considering the Southern Thai case, it might be useful first to clarify how I interpret and use certain analytical concepts and frameworks. For the concept of civil society, I use the multifaceted definitions of Muthiah Alagappa and his contributing authors in *Civil Society and Political Change in Asia: Expanding and Contracting Democratic Space* (2004a; see also 2004b, c). Alagappa (2004c) views civil society as an "arena of power, inequality, struggle, and cooperation that is populated by a wide array of voluntary and nonvoluntary groups" (2004c). Furthermore, he describes civil society as:

> A distinct public sphere of organization, communication and reflective discourse, and governance among individuals and groups that take collective action deploying civil means to influence the state and its policies but not capture state power, and whose activities are not motivated by profit. (Alagappa 2004c)

The analytical concept of "agency" also requires further consideration. Quoting Comoroff and Comoroff (1999), Ahearn (2001:112) points out that social scientists have often neglected to define the way they use the concept of human agency and indeed have often misused this analytical concept. She cautions researchers to not only address what "agency" means to the analyst but also the meaning of agency for the people under study and the ways in which such meaning changes over time. Abu-Lughod (1991:41–55) also highlights the ways in which anthropological discussions of power that have been influenced by Bourdieu and Gramsci tended to focus on resistance. Thus, the agency of the subaltern has been inadvertently equated with resistance instead of resistance being a "diagnostic of power." Ahearn and Abu-Lughold's arguments highlight that any discussion of agency needs to be contextualized in terms of the dynamic processes of power relations in a society that are historically situated (from a diachronic understanding). Ortner (1994:372–411) also discusses the issue of agency in her considerations of the practice-based models in cultural anthropology focusing on the notion of power, power relations, and the dynamic interrelationship between action, motivation, and social-cultural system (ideology, discourse, structural aspects of the system, and so on). Thus, I treat agency in the context of the arguments advanced by these anthropologists given that these arguments go beyond and refine the theoretical positions argued by Bourdieu (an action theorist). I do not view the concept of women's agency in terms of resistance alone, that is, resistance to the Thai state's power or to the dominant Thai ethnic group. Rather, my research investigates participation and engagement in the political process and thus views women's agency as a process which is dynamic in relation to historical and cultural processes that empower and enable women's participation. Therefore, instead of focusing on political structures, my ongoing and long-term research examines process in the framework of processual analysis in political anthropology: "the processes involved in determining and implementing public goals and in the differential achievement and use of power by the members of the group concerned with those goals" (Swartzet et al. 1966:7). Women's political participation, women's empowerment, and the concept of power itself will be viewed with a reference to (1) Foucault's (1977, 1980) discourse as system of knowledge that influences the limits of thinking and acting but is largely unconscious, and (2) dynamics of power relations from the orientation of civil society (cf. Comoroff and Comoroff 1999). My analytical framework derives from political anthropology, and I investigate Thai Malay Muslim women's "voices" and perceptions of political participation. As Susan Gal (2002:215) points out, recent feminist analyses in the anthropology literature "suggested that women's 'voice' often differ significantly in form as well as content from dominant discourse."

By dominant discourse, I mean the national and dominant cultural discourse on women and women's roles (cf. Foucault 1980). The existing literature on Thai women's political participation highlights the factors of women's domestic roles and duties as wife and mother, being subjugated in a patriarchal system, and images of femininity, as barriers to political participation (see, e.g., Ockey 2004 and Raksasataya 1968 among others); yet, these are integral parts of a national and cultural discourse on women and women's roles in Thailand. The theme of women as victims is heavily emphasized. Thus, the dominant discourse has direct implications not just for national policies that affect women's political participation but also for the ways women themselves view political participation and the means by which they choose to participate in the political arena. Such arguments, however, ignore that at the same time, women may "choose" to be empowered by utilizing "women as victims" discourse in their participation; for example, NGOs who focus on "victims" of violence in Southern Thailand or women's organizations with specific social welfare foci (see also Chap. 21 in this volume). Therefore, I reject women as universally dominated by men and as victims, in the spirit of James Scott's (1985) arguments that the subjugated classes do have agency (Bond and Gilliam 1997). It is through an investigation of their voices that we can discover the agency that Thai Malay Muslim women possess. While Tsing (2002:331) also argues against female marginalization, Lewellen (2003:203–206) highlights the fallacy of relegating the marginalized into a subjugated category as passive victims. Thai Muslim women of the Malay ethnic background are anything but passive as this paper tries to demonstrate.

3 Political Engagement of Muslim Women in Southern Thailand

In this section, I want to consider the many different forms that Muslim women's engagement takes in the Deep South of Thailand. My research findings indicate that the ongoing conflict has been an important driving force behind a rapid increase in the engagement of Muslim women through civil society, and thus engagement has taken a more organized, extensive, and less ad hoc form than previous grassroots engagement at local community levels that focused on development issues. The current historical experiences of the ongoing conflict very strongly shape women's lives, perceptions, and motivations for political engagement through civil society. Since the flare-up of violence in 2004, there has been a rapid increase and proliferation of various informal local NGOs, women's networks, and associations, many of them working under the umbrella of larger and formal regional NGO organizations (see also Chap. 21).

While my cultural informants expressed great reluctance to engage in the formal political arena for a multitude of reasons, mirroring the factors reported in a number of studies on political participation among Thai ethnic women (e.g., Iwanaga 2008a, b, c, d), with the current security situation, Muslim women became highly active in the informal political arena through grassroots activism. Initially, this activism took the form of mass female protests and blockades. Thai English language media—The Nation and Bangkok Post—has frequently reported on this phenomenon between 2004 and 2007. These protests were described by interview participants as spontaneous undertakings out of sheer frustration and feelings of helplessness and being made "voiceless," with "nobody listening to their concerns, questions or providing any answers." Women protested at police stations, in front of military installations, and in front of government buildings. The "female blockades" concerned justice issues or, in local interpretations, feelings of miscarriage of justice. Local explanations by Muslim women for these "female blockades" overwhelmingly emphasized that the protestors were "mothers and wives" who want to protect their own families and desire justice, peace, and security. They unanimously and very vehemently denied the state's interpretation that it is the separatist men who are behind these protests figuring that authorities would not dare to harm Muslim women. The lack of satisfying results in the state's dealing with a multitude of justice issues very strongly contributed to the rapid emergence of a great number of grassroots organizations that focus both directly and indirectly on these issues in a more formal and coordinated manner. These local women's networks, associations, and NGOs, aside from justice issues, also focus their attentions on women and children victims of violence. The rapid proliferation of these grassroots organization provided women with a new venue and vehicle through which their voices and concerns might be heard. An interpretation for the virtual disappearance of female protests since 2007 has been attributed to this process of rapid emergence of and coordinated actions by a multitude of local NGOs.

The discussion of the active engagement of Muslim women in the Southern border region highlights the following spheres: the separatist movement, proliferation and nature of engagement of local women's NGOs, engagement in state institutions, and implications for transition to engagement in the formal political arena.

While in Timor Leste women were also active as separatist fighters, commanders, and couriers, I have found absolutely no evidence for such forms of engagement among women in Southern Thailand. Although it has been reported that the Thai military estimates that 1 % of Malay Muslim women are also active in the insurgency (Levett 2007), a couple of interviews instead hypothesized that women who might be either involved with or sympathetic to the goals of separatists have duties that focus on the maintenance of Malay cultural identity. They focus on the teaching of local history, religion, and especially the local language. Bajunid (2005:9) argues that "to be Malay is to be Muslim" and that "Malay is still the definitive Islamic medium and the undisputed marker of Islamic identity among Muslims who live as real minorities in the Malay cultural heartland in Thailand and in the provinces of Yala, Pattani, and Narathiwat."

My research suggests that Southern Thai Muslim women of the Malay ethnic background are instead very heavily engaged with local women's networks, associations, and NGOs, particularly since the proliferation of such grassroots organizations. These grassroots groups tend to be led by highly capable and well-educated middle-class women, many of them lecturers and working with other women with university degrees and student volunteers from local universities. They also train women from the villages through various workshops that often have support from national and/or international NGOs and other organizations. Those local NGOs that are also engaged in peace-building efforts usually collaborate with non-Muslim, Buddhist NGOs of the Deep South and indeed address the needs of victimized Buddhist communities as well. The Muslim women's NGOs are also collaborating with more formal NGOs (i.e., those registered as NGOs with the Thai state) often expanding their own groups' projects under the umbrella and support of these local NGOs. Local Muslim women's networks and NGOs also affiliate with Muslim organizations or specifically Muslim formal NGOs. It is important to point out that the diversity of Islamic traditions present and tolerated in the Deep South does not seem to impact on the local women's NGOs and network's work and indeed such local women's groups and NGOs can affiliate with formal and indeed larger NGOs of a variety of Islamic traditions—e.g., a local women's group that is constituted in membership of Sunni women would work well with a larger former NGO which is mainly Shi'a in leadership and composition. Local women's networks, associations, and NGOs engage in activities that address a multitude of urgent issues that the local populations of Pattani, Yala, and Narathiwat deem not to have been addressed by the state governance apparatus (either not at all addressed or not sufficiently or unjustly addressed).

The recent Muslim local women's grassroots organizations' activities focus on widows and victims of violence. They provide grief counseling and also guidance to the acquisition of resources/compensation that ensure these women have the ability to provide education for the children of the household, mainly through educating victimized women about their rights as citizens of the Thai state. Indeed, the educational function that these local women's NGOs fulfill, given that the focus is on a form of civic education, has the potential to impact socialization of democratic principles. While a tangential outcome of the actual focus of activities by local NGOs, the potential future implication of these civic education endeavors should not be underestimated and indeed could be further fostered and enhanced. Local Muslim women's grassroots organizations also attempt to train grief counselors, albeit with a lack of funding. Another type of active engagement of such women's networks, associations, and NGOs concerns village projects that provide skills training to women and job training for youth—thus focusing on enhancing economic capacities and is a form of local development. Another program focuses on drug use prevention and rehabilitation among the youth—this is a serious problem in the Deep South and local women's grassroots organizations feel that governmental program efforts have been insignificant and inefficient in addressing this crucial problem. Thus, again these women's groups are trying to address the gaps that exist (in local perceptions) in state initiatives. My interviewees argued that drug abuse prevention also contributes toward peace-building efforts, since separatists might not so easily recruit such youth for carrying out terrorist acts. They argue that the youth who are addicts tend to be those who have experienced the effects of violence or are unemployed and with no hope for a future—or in other words, they have nothing to lose. Another focus of local women's NGOs and networks concerns justice issues through collaboration with national-level human rights NGOs by securing legal counsel and support to those accused, detained, or indiscriminately rounded up. In their view, women should also be involved in human rights work since it has direct implications for the welfare of family when men are rounded up indiscriminately and might not get released (often without ever being charged) for two or more years or when men who fear such round up would not go to work—thus women are forced to become the sole providers for their family. All the various programs that local Muslim women's groups are engaged in are culturally sensitive to the Muslim (and Buddhist communities in cases of ministering to the needs of victims in these communities).

More recent initiatives of women's groups build upon these various engagements. A local community radio show provides the population with local cultural content but more importantly gives a "voice" to women who are given an opportunity to tell their experiences of the conflict in the Deep South. This initiative also provides for potential delivery of assistance to those women who might need psychological trauma counseling since the group consults with a medical professional when screening these interviews. The radio program engages local women and the hosts are women as well. Thus, it is women telling women's stories and experiences. Furthermore, the radio hosts get an opportunity to hone their self-confidence in speaking out.

The overall agenda of various local women's NGOs has been described as "human security" which is part of "national security" as some of my NGO informants expressed it. They view their activities as a national security issue since without human security ("security of livelihood and justice"), peace cannot be achieved in the south. Therefore, from their perspective these women's grassroots organizations are working toward peace building. As some of the leaders of these local women's groups expressed it: "Women better understand other women, therefore it is important for women to be actively involved in supporting other women who experienced the effects of violence, and to lobby the government for peace, justice, as well as for compensations and scholarships."

During 2010, there was a further development in the range of issues that local formal NGOs are addressing in the communities of the Deep South that fully engages women. A new initiative of the larger Islamic NGOs of the Deep South began a consultation and discussion with stakeholders concerning their vision for a peaceful Southern border region under a decentralized civilian government as a solution to ending the conflict and violence. In this ongoing dialogue, women's voices, visions, and hopes are given consideration through the representation of women's civil society organizations. Therefore, women's NGOs and networks have an active engagement concerning political matters.

The organization of women's civil society groups is diffuse in the Deep South where many women's groups, networks, and other women's grassroots groups emerged in many different locals. My research suggests that there is competition among Southern Thai women's grassroots organizations, particularly for funding, and thus, they have not yet optimized their ability to network and to "solidify their voices" against injustices. They are not yet at a stage where they can readily "forge network links and political coalitions among themselves to strengthen their voices" (Tantiwiramanond and Pandey 1991:157). My data suggests that instead these women's groups tend to forge political coalitions with the few larger formal Islamic NGOs of the region that are not exclusively women's NGOs.

While women's engagement is most visible through civil society in the Deep South, it should be mentioned that Muslim women have been reported to be engaged through more formal venues, however, in much smaller numbers. There have been reports of female rangers from among the Malay Muslim women; these tend to be of the younger generation who see their role as protecting their communities and contributing to establishment of peace. I am unaware of Muslim women of Malay ethnic background from the south being members of official government forces either in police or military. However, there are indeed women of Thai ethnic background engaged, aside from administrative and secretary positions, in the capacity of community liaison work. At least one Air Force woman of Thai-Buddhist ethnic background who worked as a community liaison person tended to view all Muslim Southerners of the Malay ethnic background, particularly those who had any "justice" issues or complaints, as being "all separatist." This prevalent ideology and mode of thinking among members of the military could be one of many reasons for a lack of interest by Malay Muslim women in joining security forces. However, it should be emphasized that there are both male and female security forces members who are dedicated to peace and to finding solutions to deep-seated problems of the region.

Women's political engagement in Pattani, Yala, and Narathiwat appears to be mainly through NGOs or civil society. Formal female politicians that represent issues of human security from the perspective of women are lacking in the Deep South. During my fieldwork, two women were singled out by my informants as formerly active in the formal political arena. One was viewed by women as largely ineffective, not interested in women's issues or in issues of the Deep South. Her engagement in politics was viewed as no different from male politicians. The other female politician was viewed only in a slightly better light and mainly due to her political family's connections and her activities in the medical profession. In local Muslim women's views, there is low representation of women's issues and women's voices in the formal political arena, and there is not a preference for female candidates since both male and female politicians would behave the same way in addressing (or in this case not addressing) problematic issues of the region. However, informants pointed out and even emphasized that it is not politicians (either male or female) but women who are engaged through civil society who are the ones championing issues of human security for all women and men. The perception is that these women's NGOs and networks work tireless to tackle problems that the politicians either neglect or are highly ineffectual in addressing, lacking political will.

4 Discussion

My research data indicates that Muslim women of the Southern border region are not simply "voiceless" victims but are active agents toward change and address those issues that are of concern not only to themselves but for the entire population of this conflict-torn region—namely, justice and human security issues. In this section, I want to further consider the implications of such active engagement for Muslim women's political participation through civil society. Particularly, I want to consider the following questions:

- Is Muslim women's engagement through civil society a political engagement or simply the continuation of women's work on development issues?
- How might their engagement contribute to change?
- Will their engagement decrease or even cease after the conflict subsides and peace is established?
- Can their engagement become the platform for formal political arena engagement, and if so, what potential factors would contribute to a successful transition from the informal to the formal political arena?

Kittitornkool (2005:217) and other Thai researchers highlight that women's grassroots engagement in development programs focused on three main areas: (1) involving supplementary income-earning skills, (2) involving the fulfillment of housewives' duties, and (3) involving childcare. She, like other researchers, has pointed out that these types of participation "tend to focus on the improvement of the traditional role of women as wives and mothers" (Kittitornkool 2005:218). I would argue that the nature of engagement of the newly emerged Muslim (and Buddhist) women's networks and NGOs in the Deep South has a much more expanded focus and is not simply an extension of "development engagement." Aside from the more recent involvement in consultation concerning forms of civilian governance that the population desires in Pattani, Yala, and Narathiwat, which would seem a more clear-cut case of political engagement, their activities in educating of women about their rights as Thai citizens and thus attempting to empower women goes beyond development initiatives. Whether their motivations are "political" in nature or not, the programs do have political implications and "side effects." Furthermore, "human security," the rhetoric used by women's groups when they talk about their activities, and linking it to achieving political stability, peace, and the end of the violent conflict, also suggests a different mode of thinking than those concerning development issues. Among these women's NGOs, their grassroots activities are described as filling in the gaping holes that the formal political arena has either not addressed or nominally and ineffectually treated. Therefore, based on my findings, I argue that women's networks, grassroots organizations, and NGOs are the spheres of political engagement for Muslim women of the Deep South. Research on Muslim women's political engagement from the Middle East and Africa also suggests that social movements, social networks, voluntary associations, and NGOs, local and transnational, are arenas for women's political engagement (Moghadam 2003; Al-Mughni 2000). As Tantiwiramanond and Pandey (1991:157) point out,

> Women's own political empowerment is necessary and their participation important because political power not only permits the acquisition of resources but includes their continuing acquisition as well. Some women working in NGO groups learn participatory decision making, and acquire leadership and organizational skills.... Group discussions familiarize women with current issues at hand, and develop their consciousness.

These observations also seem to apply to Southern Thai Muslim women's NGOs. However, the intersection of agendas between local and transnational grassroots organizations as well as national government agendas must also be noted, since not all of these organizations will automatically empower women. In the Southern Thai case, current programs that I observed through my research do indeed aim to empower women. Many of these programs of women's grassroots organizations have been supported and aided by national and regional level formal NGO organizations as well as by international organizations such as the USAID, Canadian International Development Agency, The Asia Foundation, the European Union, and even the Asian Development Bank. The programs that received cooperation from the international groups specifically focused on empowering women through civic education and teaching women about their rights as citizens.

Several works on Thai NGOs and associations have pointed out that these organizations are not necessarily independent of the agendas of the nation state, as Coordination Committees exist between the government and development-oriented NGOs and they need the government's support and cooperation (e.g., Tantiwiramanond and Pandey 1991; Pongsapich 1995; Suksawat 1995). The alliance of women NGOs with state bureaucracies to attain their ends has been highlighted in other parts of the world (e.g., Lang 2002:290–304). This is not quite the case for the Southern Thai women's NGOs. My data thus far suggests that instead of aligning themselves with state bureaucracies, these local Muslim women's NGOs are aligning themselves with lager formal Islamic NGOs. Based on my interview data, I suggest that this has less to do with religious affiliation but more to do with these women's groups having emerged relatively recently and, therefore, did not yet have sufficient time for refining their organization and cooperation and coordination. At this stage, they do not yet seem to have the level of solidarity or unity of voice that would allow for any coordinated aligning with state bureaucracies; but from what I have observed and recorded, *some* of the women's groups are on a trajectory to achieve this level.

Pongsapich (1995:43) argues that in Thailand, there are four different types of grassroots organizations and only two of these four may be attributed with "empowerment" since they seek minimal contact with government agencies or have an approach that is critical of government policies and programs, and are interested in activities at the local rather than national levels emphasizing awareness of rights and "consciousness raising." In her critical examination of a Northern Thai NGO whose activities focus on gender and development, Costa (2008:215–238) cogently demonstrates that this grassroots group's work and ideology is shaped by "gendered and sexualized nationalist discourses" with significant implications for Thai women's rights and citizenship (Costa 2008:217). My research findings are in complete agreement with this conclusion concerning the Thai national discourse on women. Costa's arguments also highlight that some of these NGOs do not empower women of a community but might empower the women leadership of the organization. It has been also observed in studies on women NGOs from other parts of the world that the transformation of local social movements, networks, and other grassroots organizations focusing on women's issues and rights as citizens into formal NGOs replicates and reproduces formal institutional hierarchies and bureaucracies, while negotiating and reproducing gendered discourse of the government seems to be counterproductive to the effectiveness of "empowering" women and creates a disjuncture between the members of such women NGOs and the women in the communities they serve (Lang 2002; Sangtin and Nagar 2006).

In the case of women's grassroots organizations in Southern Thailand, I would argue that these observations hold to a certain degree. It is true that the women leaders of the organizations are indeed empowered by the engagements and processes I discussed in this chapter. But the women leadership is also engaged in providing many workshops to train village women in order to empower them, indeed often funding these initiatives from their own pockets. Those villagers that receive the training are obliged to take back the skills and knowledge they acquire to their villages and train women in the villages themselves. Of course, there will be variation as to what degree village women will carry out such obligations.

In Southern Thailand, Muslim women's engagement is impacted by the current political situation. The many women's grassroots groups and initiatives that emerged try to address the devastating consequences of the Southern situation. These groups engage in educating, empowering, and mobilizing women—whether in terms of protests or advocacy activities or the much needed local programs that these Muslim women's groups implement. So, can these women's networks and NGOs in Thailand's Deep South affect or contribute to change? I would argue that aside from the socioeconomic effects in village communities (strictly development-oriented activities) and the justice and human rights advocacy they engage in, these grassroots organizations do have the potential to affect change in terms of *transforming modes of thinking* through civic education, teaching *both* men and women of village communities about their rights as citizens, and indeed being a moderating voice. In most of my discussions and interviews, my cultural informants directly emphasized the need for civic (as well as religious) education of *both* genders in order to bring about lasting change and to achieve peace in the Deep South.

The women leaders of grassroots organizations advance programs and discourse that is unfriendly to "extremism/radialization" and instead promote reconciliatory and cooperative modes of thinking. Furthermore, if women's discourse and visions concerning the types of decentralized civilian governance for the Deep South are taken seriously by the local Islamic NGOs in collaboration with all the stakeholders of the region, there is the potential for affecting political change in the future. For now, at least, women through grassroots organizations have been included in these discussions.

Will women's political engagement through civil society continue post-conflict or will it regress to a strictly welfare focus in the domain of development? With the absence of men due to factors I already mentioned, space opened up for women to engage. The male-dominated Malay Muslim culture in the south emphasizes the wife and mother (home caretaker) gender roles for women—even women's highly visible economic roles as agricultural workers and traders and sellers at markets are viewed in terms of household economy. Thus, village women's interest in the political situation appears to be directly influenced by the ongoing violence and its impact on their livelihood and families' security. Village women's engagement then probably would continue through the development and welfare domain. Although if the civic education and learning about their rights as citizens is thoroughly socialized through the program initiatives of current women's grassroots organizations, there is the potential for village women to remain engaged, at least in their participation and their choices in local elections. However, at this stage it is hard to gauge the real efficacy of the "empowerment" programs of the multitude of women's networks and NGOs in the Deep South, in order to make more convincing predictions. The potential does exist, however, and the extension and deepening of civic education by Southern NGOs among the wider populations could produce a highly positive impact. Masdit (2008:272) argues that educating women and providing them with knowledge of the democratic process of elections and the role of MPs in Parliament is crucial. She forwards an argument for such "transformative politics" (Masdit 2008:274):

> The concept of transformative politics is a spontaneous social movement to push for political reform by empowering women. Through continuous and systematic training, women from all parts of society can broaden their democratic education… Transformative politics is not limited to their roles as potential politicians since the roles of voters, the contributors, the canvassers and the campaigners are equally important.

I would note that a more concentrated effort on a more extensive civic education could also potentially contribute to finding democratic forms of political solutions to the plight of the conflict-torn Deep South. Therefore, the nature of civic education programs carried out by local NGOs can have politically transformative significance. However, it also must be noted that once peace returns, funding potentially is also likely to dry up for such civic education activities for Southern NGOs from governmental and NGO sources both at national and international levels.

There are many worthwhile projects that work on empowering women so that they can be transformed from victims to active participants in their region's future and peace building. Many of those fulfilling leadership roles in local women's networks and NGOs are academics and teachers and often rely on volunteers (many of whom are female university students) and their own wages to undertake their projects. They show commitment to and confidence in their grassroots organizations' agendas and activities to bring about change. These well-educated and middle-class women leaders (and student volunteers) are gaining invaluable experience through their engagement in civil society that would prepare the most capable among them for a transition to participation in the formal political arena. But, before I discuss these latter implications, I would argue that the individual characteristics of women NGO leaders and current female university students in Southern Thailand and their passion to serve the public would most likely keep them actively engaged in civil society even post-conflict. These women would face local cultural obstacles to a much lesser degree than village women to stay engaged through civil society and engage in programs focused on issues that promote justice and social equity in a Muslim cultural context.

The political engagement of women leaders of local NGOs and women's networks has the potential to become the basis for formal political arena engagement. However, there are several potential factors that could contribute to a successful transition from the informal to the formal political arena. These women are acquiring skills and knowledge—whether in terms of advocacy or negotiation—and are learning how to network, how to garner support from politicians, key political stakeholders, and the wider population, and they understood the rules of the "political game" given that their ongoing engagement and experiences occur in an area that is politically charged and indeed at times a minefield due to the separatist conflict that is going on.

The inhibiting cultural factors for women's public engagement, particularly in the formal political arena, were and remain just as acute as those cited for Thai women's political participation. In his comparative study on non-Southeast Asian Muslim societies, Fattah (2008:44–45) found that it is literate (cf. educated) women in all Muslim countries included in his study who were more supportive of democratic institutions than were Muslim men. He also pointed out that educated Muslim women were more aware of their plight and other inequality issues in the society at large. In Fattah's study, educated Muslim women who advocated more democratic forms expressed these ideals in terms of an Islamic context and did not view Islam as a limiting factor, but instead, they viewed men and male-centered cultural norms and ideology as "depriving them of the rights given to them by sharia" and "not give women a fair share even by Islamic standards." In this comparative study, Fattah reported that most educated women "argued for a more active role for women in politics," and he argued for a quota system in political positions as a way to empower Muslim women. My interviews with Southern Thai Muslim women NGO leaders and with university students (women in their early twenties) made similar arguments about women's political participation in the formal arena. The majority did envision sometime in the future a greater participation of women in politics. Vichit-Vadakan (2008a:49; see also 2008b) points out that according to the opinion survey of the UNDP in 2006: "While there was no strong opposition to women attaining high political offices, there were some mixed feelings about women's leadership abilities." Like the Muslim women in Fattah's (2008:45) study, in my research I found that educated middle-class Muslim women of the Deep South do foresee Muslim women politicians in the future, but they all expressed discomfort at considering formal political leadership positions being held by Muslim women (governor, Prime Minister, and so on). The discomfort was expressed in terms of NOT women having less of an ability to have policy vision and implement these but more in terms of dealing with male opponents (whether Buddhist or Muslim) who may have different agendas. Thus, in the conceptions of my cultural informants, "lack of ability" was expressed in terms of dealing with male opponents who would undermine their leadership abilities. Only in a few cases did young university female students suggest that the Islamic religion had anything to do with the discomfort about a Muslim woman leader. I would also note that the female leaders of local women's grassroots organizations also shied away from being labeled as a "leader" and preferred to talk about their work in terms of service and being a "coordinator." Therefore, local conceptualizations of power, politics, and leadership as currently existing in women's cultural worldview have to be taken into account when assessing Southern Thai Muslim women's attitudes, motives, and interpretations of their political engagement in civil society.

Southern Thai Muslim women's transition into the formal political arena would also depend on the further training and support invested in them. There are some Islamic NGO organizations (particularly those linked with Muslim student activism) that showed a much greater enthusiasm and support for Muslim women being engaged in formal politics, including for providing necessary training to capable women for such engagement. Another promising line of argument and initiative I have encountered through my research in this regard concerns plans for establishing a women's studies program at a major local university's Islamic college since the goal of such a program is to prepare educated women to engage with and contribute to the public sphere—using their education to better the lives of the people from the Deep South. In the interviews concerning this particular plan, the male participants argued that the traditional stance of Muslim males for keeping women out of the public sphere tended to focus on women's lack of knowledge and understanding of the world due to a lack of education. However, they argued that this factually does not hold true anymore, and used the demographics of their university's student population as an example where a large portion are Muslim women. Indeed, I have observed this myself on the Pattani campus, even in traditionally male-dominated fields (e.g., political science) where half the students were Muslim women. Therefore, my participants argued that there is a need to prepare and train such educated Muslim women for greater public sphere engagement.

The factors that limit Muslim women's political participation in formal politics are in many ways no different than those that have been identified for Thai women in general (see Vichit-Vadakan 2008a:32–43; see also 2008b): stereotypes of women which is an integral part of Thai national discourse on gender roles, lack of confidence and self-esteem, lack of gender awareness in political parties, lack of money and finances, greater public scrutiny and harshness of media toward women politicians and candidates, the harsher critiques of women politicians by other women, and the need for a family legacy of politics or for patrons. My interview with one former Muslim woman politician in the Deep South raised most of these obstacles. My research findings are in agreement with these obstacles in a qualified sense. In some ways, these obstacles to women's political participation in the formal arena are present globally, whether in the Southern or the Northern Hemispheres. Not all women have the interest or capabilities to be running for office in the formal political arena. It takes connections and a great depth of finances to run for office. And indeed, the media and other women tend to be harsher on female candidates.

The overall Thai national discourse on women's roles indeed does impact on the perceptions of the public on women in politics. However, such a discourse can be mitigated by the individual characteristics, skills, and actions of specific female candidates. Not all highly dedicated and successful female leaders of women's grassroots organizations in the Deep South have an interest in formal politics. Those who do have distinguished themselves through their personal character, skills, actions, advocacy, negotiation, and networking skills do indeed have the potential for garnering support should they transition to formal politics. These are articulate, well-educated women, who do not have self-confidence and self-esteem issues, albeit they might play down their own achievements to fit the mold of gender roles as per the national discourse. I would emphasize that it is the national discourse on women's roles and not specific Malay or Islamic discourse that has the greatest relevance here. With regard to women's self-esteem or lack of confidence issues, I argue that this assessment is based on whether women are outspoken about their views, assessments, and opinions in a public setting. Both my interview and participant observation data indicate that women from women's NGOs, networks, and grassroots organizations are highly articulate and outspoken in those situations where they constitute majority—whether in NGO meetings or activities. In situations where there is a mixed group, Muslim women are less outspoken if the male participants are in majority. Therefore, in my assessment the issue is less women's lack of self-esteem or confidence, but the culturally ascribed behavior expected of them and the public space allowed for their "voices."

Kittitornkool (2005:223) points out that women are skillful in network building, internal communication, and negotiation, due to their experience and that "in conflict resolution processes it is more likely women leaders than men who maintain their integrity and public interest while dealing and negotiating with the powerful." These are all characteristics I have observed myself among the Muslim women leaders of local women's networks and NGOs. Therefore, it is not necessarily an issue of capabilities in the sense of skills, networks, and so on for highly capable NGO women leaders to transition into the formal political arena. Kittitornkool also suggests that "in spite of the greater degree of social acceptance of women's public involvement in different Southern contexts," there is agreement that the extent to which such roles are significantly recognized remains limited due to the persistent cultural ideologies concerning gender roles. Again, I would agree with this assessment in general, but I would also argue based on my research findings that the most capable women leaders in local Southern Thai NGOs belong to the well-educated middle class whose current engagement through the informal political arena already go against the grain of "persistent cultural ideologies" yet their engagement has found acceptance. Furthermore, women in Malay culture have always been engaged in the public sphere and the Malay cultural worldview could potentially provide greater opportunities to well-qualified Muslim women to enter the formal political arena.

5 Conclusion

Muslim women of Pattani, Yala, and Narathiwat are not simply passive victims of the ongoing conflict and violence. They are actively engaged through civil society to do something about women's plight and that of the rest of the population. They are active agents in the ongoing processes of negotiating to find a political solution to the problems of the Deep South and thus build peace in the conflict-torn region through a variety of programs and actions. Their engagement through civil society is political engagement, and if their engagement is supported, developed, and valued, there is the potential for their engagement in formal politics as well. Listening to the voices, aspirations, and wisdom of half the Southern region's population and utilizing the unique skills and viewpoints they bring to the table will have implications for building lasting peace—whether through their continued political engagement through civil society, or as elected representatives to the provincial civilian decentralized governments of Pattani, Yala, Narathiwat, or as those who keep "radicalization" at bay. But NOT all women and not all women leaders of local grassroots organizations will have the abilities and capabilities to become politicians. Those that do have the abilities should be supported by the various stakeholders in Southern Thailand, as this is already recognized by some educational institutions and Islamic NGO organizations in the case of women's participation through civil society. Enhancing civic education of both men and women at all levels of society would not only benefit women's political engagement but could potentially impact democratic processes of the Deep South and indeed the whole Thai nation.

Acknowledgments I would like to thank my "Thai Patrons," my Thai colleagues who have supported the development of the different phases of this research project through academic discussions, linking me into cultural informant networks and stimulating my academic thinking about the various issues under investigation—thank you Dr. Chaiwat Satha-Anand, Dr. Juree Vichit-Vadakan, and Dr. Srisompob Jitpiromsri from Thammasat University, NIDA, and Prince of Songkla University, respectively. I also would like to thank the following instances for small travel grants that allowed me to travel to Thailand over the course of the project: the Center for Southeast Asian Studies at NIU for foreign travel awards and especially for the Royal Thai Fund supporting faculty research travel, and the Lillian Cobb Fellowship (at NIU). I also would like to thank Professors Danny Unger and Judy Ledgerwood, my colleagues, who have read an early draft of this manuscript and provided invaluable feedback. I wish to express my deepest thanks to all individuals and organizations that have participated and continue to support my research engagement in the Deep South.

References

Abu-Lughod, L. (1991). The romance of resistance: Tracing transformations of power through Bedouin Women. *American Ethnologist, 17*(1), 41–55.
Ahearn, L. M. (2001). Language and agency. *Annual Review of Anthropology, 31*, 109–137.
Alagappa, M. (2004a). Civil society and political change: An analytical framework. In M. Alagappa (Ed.), *Civil society and political change in Asia: Expanding and contracting democratic space* (pp. 25–57). Stanford: Stanford University Press.
Alagappa, M. (2004b). *Civil society and political change in Asia: Expanding and contracting democratic space*. Stanford: Stanford University Press.
Alagappa, M. (2004c). Introduction. In M. Alagappa (Ed.), *Civil society and political change in Asia: Expanding and contracting democratic space* (pp. 1–21). Stanford: Stanford University Press.
Al-Mughni, H. (2000). Women's movements and the autonomy of civil society in Kuwait. In R. L. Teske & M. A. Tetreault (Eds.), *Feminist approaches to social movements, community, and power, Vol. 1: Conscious acts and the politics of social change*. Columbia: University of South Carolina Press.
Bajunid, O. F. (2005). Islam, nationalism, and the Thai state. In W. Sugunnasil (Ed.), *Dynamic diversity in Southern Thailand* (pp. 1–19). Chiang Mai: Silkworm Books.
Bond, G., & Gilliam, A. (1997). *The social construction of the past: Representation as power*. New York: Routledge.
Comoroff, J. L., & Comoroff, J. (1999). *Civil society and the political imagination: Critical perspectives*. Chicago: University of Chicago Press.
Costa, L. M. (2008). Gender, sexuality and nationalism in a northern Thai nongovernmental organisation. *Asian Studies Review, 32*(2), 215–238.
Fattah, M. A. (2008). *Democratic values in the Muslim world*. London: Lynne Rienner Publishers.
Foucault, M. (1977). *Discipline and punish: The birth of the prison*. New York: Vintage.
Foucault, M. (1980). *Power/knowledge: Selected interviews and other writings 1972–1977*. New York: Pantheon.
Gal, S. (2002). Between speech and silence. In J. Vincent (Ed.), *The anthropology of politics: A reader in ethnography, theory, and critique* (pp. 213–221). Malden: Blackwell Publishing.
Iwanaga, K. (2008a). Women in Thai politics. In K. Iwanaga (Ed.), *Women's political participation and representation in Asia: Obstacles and challenges* (pp. 173–209). Denmark: NIAS Press.
Iwanaga, K. (2008b). Introduction: Women's political representation from an international perspective. In K. Iwanaga (Ed.), *Women's political participation and representation in Asia: Obstacles and challenges* (pp. 1–26). Denmark: NIAS Press.
Iwanaga, K. (Ed.). (2008c). *Women's political participation and representation in Asia: Obstacles and challenges*. Denmark: NIAS Press.
Iwanaga, K. (2008d). *Women and politics in Thailand: Continuity and change*. Denmark: NIAS Press.
Kittitornkool, J. (2005). Southern Thai women in development: A tale of two villages. In S. Wattana (Ed.), *Dynamic diversity in Southern* (pp. 213–240). Chiang Mai: Silkworm Books.
Lang, S. (2002). The NGO-ization of feminism: Institutionalization and institution building within the German women's movement. In B. Smith (Ed.), *Global feminisms since 1945* (pp. 290–304). New York: Routledge.
Levett, C. (2007). Women join front line in Thailand. *The Age*. Retrieved March 24, 2004, from www.theage.com.au/news/world/women-join-front-linein-thailand/
Lewellen, T. C. (2003). *Political anthropology: An introduction*. Westport/London: Bergin and Garvey.
Masdit, S. (2008). My story as a woman in Thai politics. In I. Kazuki (Ed.), *Women and politics in Thailand: Continuity and change* (pp. 265–278). Denmark: NIAS Press.
Moghadam, V. M. (2003). Engendering citizenship, feminizing civil society: The case of the Middle East and North Africa. *Women and Politics, 25*(1/2), 63–87.
Ockey, J. (2004). *Making democracy: Leadership, class, gender, and political participation in Thailand*. Chiang Mai: Silkworm Books.

Ortner, S. B. (1994). Theory in anthropology since the sixties. In N. B. Dirks, G. Eley, & S. B. Ortner (Eds.), *A reader in contemporary social theory* (pp. 372–411). Princeton: NJ.

Pongsapich, A. (1995). Strengthening the role of NGOs in popular participation. In J. Boonyarattana-soontorn & G. Chutima (Eds.), *Thai NGOs: The continuing struggle for democracy* (pp. 9–50). Bangkok: Thai NGO Support Project.

Raksasataya, A. (1968). The political role of Southeast Asian women. *Annals of the American Academy of Political and Social Science, 375*(1), 86–90.

Sangtin, W., & Nagar, R. (2006). *Playing with fire: Feminist thought and activism through seven lives in India.* Minneapolis: University of Minnesota Press.

Scott, J. C. (1985). *Weapons of the weak.* New Haven: Yale University Press.

Suksawat, R. (1995). Behind the Thai NGOs. In J. Boonyarattanasoontorn & G. Chutima (Eds.), *Thai NGOs: The continuing struggle for* (pp. 51–68). Bangkok: Thai NGO Support Project.

Swartz, M. J., Turner, V. W., & Tuden, A. (Eds.). (1966). *Political anthropology*. Chicago: Aldine.

Tantiwiramanond, D., & Pandey, S. R. (1991). *By women, for women: A study of women's organizations in Thailand.* Singapore: ISEAS.

Tsing, A. L. (2002). Politics on the periphery. In J. Vincent (Ed.), *The anthropology of politics: A reader in ethnography, theory, and critique* (pp. 325–337). Malden: Blackwell Publishing.

Vichit-Vadakan, J. (2008a). Women in politics and women and politics: A socio-cultural analysis of the Thai context. In I. Kazuki (Ed.), *Women and politics in Thailand: Continuity and change* (pp. 27–53). Denmark: NIAS Press.

Vichit-Vadakan, J. (2008b). A glimpse of women leaders in Thai local politics. In I. Kazuki (Ed.), *Women and politics in Thailand: Continuity and change* (pp. 125–167). Denmark: NIAS Press.

Chapter 23
Trafficking and Coerced Prostitution in Thailand: Reconceptualizing International Law in the Age of Globalization

Erin Kamler

1 Introduction

The trafficking of women for the purposes of coerced prostitution is a global problem that has particular relevance in Southeast Asia. The International Organization for Migration estimated that 200,000–225,000 women and children from Southeast Asia migrate to other countries annually for purposes of informal and often coerced labor, making this region the largest source of trafficked women in the world (Farr 2005). Thailand, which the US State Department designated a "Tier 2 Watch List" country in 2011, has been classified as a source, transit, and destination country, due to its relative affluence in the region (U.S. Department of State Office to Monitor and Combat Trafficking in Persons Report, 2011). International human rights law has taken important steps to address the issue of trafficking within the global economy. International law falls short; however, when it comes to defining coerced prostitution as being a transnational issue since, it is not always linked to the crossing of physical borders between sovereign states. In failing to address the transnational nature of coerced prostitution, international law also fails to address the needs of women who are in precarious labor and migration situations. This, in turn, relegates coerced prostitution to the domestic realm where often prostitutes are criminalized rather than supported by strategies that could foster their emancipation. In this chapter, I argue that coerced prostitution, particularly in Thailand, is a **transnational** (my emphasis) issue. I illustrate how the limited view of prostitution in the human rights discourse points to larger issues about the role of international law in the context of globalization, and I use contemporary globalization theory to show how the institution of international law functions in an outmoded paradigm.

E. Kamler (✉)
Annenberg School for Communication & Journalism, University of Southern California, 3520 Watt Way, Los Angeles, CA 90089-0218, USA
e-mail: erin.kamler@gmail.com

P. Liamputtong (ed.), *Contemporary Socio-Cultural and Political Perspectives in Thailand*,
DOI 10.1007/978-94-007-7244-1_23,

2 Conceptual Framework: Coerced Prostitution and Globalization

In examining prostitution in Thailand, I will make two important assumptions. First, prostitution, when it is coerced by virtue of the lack of other viable means of income-generating alternatives for women or when it is imposed on children, is a violation of human rights. The issue of whether prostitution can be considered a "choice" as opposed to a "coerced" activity has been subject to a great deal of scholarly debate between abolitionist and pro-rights feminists (see Barry 1995; Bindman and Doezema 1997; Jeffries 1997; Doezema and Kempadoo 1998; O'Connell Davidson 1998; Doezema 2002; MacKinnon 2007; Segrave et al. 2009; Shobha 2009), but I will not address this debate here. Rather, I will make the assumption that in circumstances when prostitution has **clearly** been coerced—whether by virtue of the fact that the prostitute is underage, is working in a locked brothel, or has no alternative means of viable, sustainable income-generating activity available to her due to social, political, and economic deprivation—it should be viewed as a human rights violation, falling under the auspices of the UN Declaration of Human Right's Article 5, which states that "no one shall be subjected to torture or to cruel, inhuman or degrading treatment or punishment" (The Universal Declaration of Human Rights, retrieved on April 7, 2010). Rather than unpacking the definition of coerced prostitution and showing how it is "cruel," "inhuman," and "degrading," I will assume this to be the case and focus instead on why coerced prostitution should be understood as a transnational issue.

Second, I will use the terms "globalization" and "transnationalism" interchangeably, to evoke the conceptual framework set forth by Castells (2004a, b): that in the context of globalization, networks offer a system of logic that is more relevant to the needs and functions of modern society than the "vertically organized, command and control structures" (Castells 2004a: 5) which make up hierarchically dominating institutions such as sovereign states. Evoking this concept, I assert that both human traffickers as well as consumers of coerced prostitution from various regions of the world participate in a network of exploitation to which international law must respond. The involvement of these global actors constitutes a "network of purveyors" that contributes to coerced prostitution's emergence as a transnational issue in the age of globalization.

3 The Treaties and Their Histories

In recent decades, the UN has developed treaties and conventions intended to suppress human trafficking and coerced prostitution. The 2001 United Nations Protocol put forth a definition as to what constitutes human trafficking and its relationship to prostitution:

> The recruitment, transportation, transfer, harbouring or receipt of persons, by means of the threat or use of force or other forms of coercion, of abduction, of fraud, of deception, of

> the abuse of power or of a position of vulnerability or of the giving or receiving of payments or benefits to achieve the consent of a person having control over another person, for the purpose of exploitation. Exploitation shall include, at a minimum, the exploitation of the prostitution of others or other forms of sexual exploitation, forced labour or services, slavery or practices similar to slavery, servitude or the removal of organs.

Thailand is a party to this convention, which is supplementary to the convention against Organized Crime. Thailand has taken additional measures to address trafficking in persons under international human rights law by adopting the *National Policy and Plan of Action for the Prevention and Eradication of the Commercial Sexual Exploitation of Children* (1996) and the 1997 amendment of the *Act on Prevention of Traffic in Women and Children* to include boys (Derks 2000: 33). In 1992, Thailand ratified the *Convention on the Rights of the Child* (*CRC*) and more recently adopted the *Optional Protocol on the Sale of Children, Child Prostitution and Child Pornography*.

I will now briefly outline the history of anti-trafficking treaties and agreements made under international law in order to illustrate the trajectory of this discourse. In doing so, I will illustrate how the treaties have made important inroads into viewing coerced prostitution as a transnational issue rather than merely a domestic one. Throughout the better part of the past century, anti-trafficking policy has introduced important connections between trafficking and prostitution. The first such connection involved the protection of European women from being sold into slavery in the former European colonies and was named The International Agreement for the Suppression of White Slave Traffic in 1904 (the "1904 Agreement") (Derks 2000: 33). The agreement distinguished between "pure and innocent" women and those who formerly worked as prostitutes, a distinction that supported the dichotomy of victimhood versus consent that is mirrored in many current debates about whether or not the prostituted have "choice." Interestingly, the 1904 Agreement excluded the detention of a woman within a brothel (after she had been trafficked) because of presumed conflicts with domestic jurisdiction and state law—perhaps foreshadowing the notion of "noninterference" that contemporary international law assumes in allowing states to prosecute international trafficking crimes in the domestic arena. In tandem, the International Convention for the Suppression of the Traffic in Women and Children (the "1921 Convention") and the International Convention on the Suppression of the Traffic in Women of Full Age (the "1933 Convention") continued to consider the outcomes of trafficking crimes to be a matter of domestic jurisdiction.

The League of Nations introduced a new urgency to the issues of trafficking and coerced prostitution and, in so doing, began to establish a conceptual link between these issues and the notion of transnationalism. The International Agreement for the Suppression of the White Slave Traffic (Article 23(c)) entrusted the League "with the general super-vision over the execution of agreements with regard to the traffic in women and children" (Castendyck 1944: 231), and in 1927, the League appointed investigators to research the trafficking of persons in the Americas, Europe, Asia, Far East, and the Middle East. For the first time, an international lawmaking body found that trafficking and coerced prostitution were international, transnational problems that must be addressed beyond the domestic realm.

In 1933, the League introduced important amendments extending protections to nonwhite women while eliminating idea of "consent" as a viable defense (Reanda 1991). By 1937, the League of Nations had identified the brothel as the key site at which the trafficking of women in Asia was enacted. This new view of the brothel as being a mechanism for suppressing women was, perhaps, the first identifiable moment when trafficking and prostitution were collapsed and defined as intersecting elements of the same circumstance. Consent, as a concept, was removed from the discourse entirely, and "prostituted" women were viewed as victims of a coerced experience.

The 1949 convention was the "first international instrument to consider forced prostitution a matter of international law, rather than strictly an issue of domestic jurisdiction" (Chuang 1998: 75). Originally proposed in 1946 by the United Nations Economic and Social Council, the Convention was designed to address the League of Nation's initiatives in the social realm. Its goal was to establish a legal framework asserting that procurers of trafficking and prostitution should be punished, regardless of issues relating to victim's age or consent. In so doing, this initiative advanced the notion that prostitution is inherently demeaning to women and communities and a violation of human rights (i.e., the "abolitionist" perspective). These measures, while importantly broadening the issue trafficking to fit within an international framework, simultaneously simplified its definition.

The conditions set forth in the treaties also introduced a level of complexity to the penalization of criminals. For the first time, punishable offenses were considered "extraditable." State parties were made to agree to establish systems of informational exchange, in which states would work domestically to reduce prostitution through initiatives such as education. These factors introduced a challenge within the international legal system; rather than adopting a unified global governance approach to coerced prostitution, the Convention allowed it to be regarded and penalized in ways that varied domestically. The Convention introduced no provision for international supervision and only required states to report "periodically" on their progress—bound by no mandatory timeframe (Reanda 1991: 201–211). These conditions introduced flaws in the international legal realm in allowing states to respond to coerced prostitution ambiguously. The law did not insist that coerced prostitution be viewed as a human rights violation when it came to the treatment of its procurers in the domestic arena.

Another important legal initiative came in the 1975 UN Convention on the Elimination of All Forms of Discrimination (CEDAW), which sought to define and elaborate on general guarantees of women's rights and guidelines against discrimination (Convention on the Elimination of All Forms of Discrimination Against Women, retrieved on August 29, 2009). CEDAW worked to decriminalize prostitution throughout the international arena for the express purpose of ending penalization against women who are trafficked and forced to work as prostitutes. CEDAW's continued assertion that prostitutes are not criminals carries particular significance in countries such as Thailand, where prostitutes often fear criminal persecution if they turn to the law for advocacy and protection. According to the United Nations Association of the USA,

> ...in such situations, these women have no recourse for action, either to seek treatment for sexually-transmitted diseases such as HIV/AIDS or to gain their release, because they are afraid of arrest if they contact the authorities (Convention on the Elimination of All Forms of Discrimination Against Women, retrieved on August 29, 2009).

CEDAW recognized the need for the international community to view coerced prostitution as a human rights violation, rather than a criminal act warranting punishment. This view has been met with resistance in societies who view women's sexual activity as threatening, shameful, and deserving of punishment, as well as from the abolitionist policy agenda of the Bush Administration, which refused to provide services to women who saw their engagement in prostitution as a form of "choice" (Doezema 2000; Global Alliance Against Traffic in Women 2007). Nevertheless, CEDAW's conceptual stance underscores the notion that coerced prostitution is a transnational process and therefore should be supported within the international legal discourse.

Spurred by the achievements of the UN Universal Declaration of Human Rights, other international organizations have brought trafficking and coerced prostitution into the center of the international human rights law discourse. UNESCO and the World Tourism Organization made sex tourism a focal point of their agenda in the 1980s (Segrave 2009: 253). Additionally, the 2000 UN General Assembly Protocol to Prevent, Suppress, and Punish Trafficking in Persons, especially Women and Children (the "Trafficking Protocol"), supports the criminalizing of procurers (Segrave 2009: 253).

Thailand has enacted similar legislation. In 1997, Thailand passed the Measures in Prevention and Suppression of Trafficking in Women and Children Act and has since implemented a strong NGO anti-trafficking presence including organizations such as ECPAT, UNIFEM, GAATW, UNESCO, ILO, local NGOs, as well as 97 government-funded shelters operating throughout the country (Segrave 2009: 254). Despite these measures, to date there is no single trafficking policy operating within Thailand.

3.1 The Problem with the Domestic Arena

As with all conventions adopted under international law, state parties are responsible for upholding the standards and conditions set forth and for enforcing criminalization on the domestic level when laws are broken. The Protocol requires:

> ...state parties to provide, if appropriate and possible in accordance with their national laws, assistance to the trafficked persons and set up mechanism and co-operation to tackle the issue more effectively. However, it was felt that the wording in this section of the Protocol does not oblige state party to seriously provide assistance to trafficked persons because the state can set condition to act in accordance with their own national laws but not according to the international human rights standard (Skrobanek 2003: 1).

This statement illustrates a fundamental flaw in international human rights law as it is presently conceived. The difficulty with allowing international crimes to be prosecuted in the domestic arena raises the problem of interpretation. By leaving prosecution and policing in the hands of states, rather than an international criminal court, states are given the leeway to interpret the details of these crimes subjectively, allowing for the possibility of misinterpreting the intentions of international law. In the case of Thailand, many NGOs have observed that police efforts to prosecute criminals and purveyors of commercial sex often fall short, with crimes notoriously going unnoticed and, in some cases, with the police themselves demonstrating complicity (Personal communication with anonymous NGO employee, July 2009, August 2010, August 2011). These observations point to the need to strengthen the reach of international law.

But, while many anti-trafficking NGOs advocate for punishing traffickers and procurers, these organizations are well aware that on a local level, the mandates of international law are often considered irrelevant. Since the decisions about criminalization rest in the hands of domestic law enforcement, ultimately international law is open to vastly subjective interpretation. The power of such domestic interpretations of international human rights law endangers women whose lives and security are at risk, but whose needs are not being heard. Additionally, the implications of this relativistic approach to human rights point to the potential ineffectiveness of treaties intended to have a transnational reach.

3.2 Weaknesses in the Treaties

The UN treaties on trafficking accurately define human trafficking as being a transnational crime involving the crossing of national boundaries. When a state party ratifies these treaties, it agrees to adhere by the principals of criminalization set forth in the treaty. As I have explained, however, since the world does not employ a single international court to address human rights violations, the process of penalizing traffickers is always tried in the realm of the domestic courts. The danger in giving domestic courts such power involves the potential conflicts of interests some governments have in supporting female migrants and trafficking victims and criminalizing them due to their status as prostitutes or noncitizens. Whereas I argue that no sex worker should be criminalized or condemned for her engagement in prostitution (whether voluntary or by force), many governments continue to treat prostitutes as criminals. As my field research in Thailand has indicated, this discrepancy creates a conflict in the policy measures designed to suppress and prevent trafficking as it is often consenting sex workers who are punished in the state's attempt to locate and assist trafficking victims (Kamler 2009). Additionally, women who migrate informally across sovereign borders and enter into sex work are often subject to discrimination on the basis of their non-citizenship status (Brennan 2005). The limited reach of the treaties allows state agendas of criminalizing prostitution to go unchecked, often with detrimental consequences to women.

In addition, problems occur in domestic courts' relativistic interpretations of crime. Indeed, notions of criminality, justice, and rights are often a matter of cultural interpretation. Such a relativistic interpretation can be seen, for example, in the recent case of the Saudi Arabian "sorcerer" conviction. In April 2010, Ali Hussain Sibat, a Lebanese man, was tried and convicted in Saudi Arabia for offering "predictions and advice to callers on a Lebanese television network" (Jamjoom 2010: 1). Initially slated to be beheaded on the grounds of breaking Sharia law, his sentence has been delayed in what one article described as a "domestic political power play… by conservatives who may be seeking to embarrass reformist leaders such as King Abdullah" (*Los Angeles Times* 2010: 1). Despite the fact that the accused was not a Saudi Arabian national, nor had he committed the alleged "crime" on Saudi Arabian soil, Ali Hussain Sibat was nevertheless tried in a domestic Saudi Arabian court. The fact that international law allows for such loopholes in its system of global governance exemplifies the danger and precariousness of this institution in the context of globalization. Unless Saudi Arabia agreed to ratify and uphold a treaty honoring the human rights of freedom of opinion and expression and freedom from religious persecution (set forth in the UN Declaration on Human Rights in Articles 16 and 18, respectively), the state, as an independent actor, is free to determine to its own satisfaction the parameters of human rights law.

A similar problem exists in regard to the domestic courts' varying interpretation of coerced prostitution. Despite the conceptual linkage between trafficking and coerced prostitution that the international treaties and conventions have established, many domestic courts view prostitution in ways that vary according to local cultural perceptions. In examining different states' views of prostitution, it becomes clear that prostitution is a highly contested act, containing multiple layers of meaning that result in policies that differ vastly according to context. In Sweden, for example, prostitution was legalized in 1999, at which time the act of procuring, rather than prostituting, became criminalized (Women's Justice Center 2010). This is not the case in the USA, a country in which, in many jurisdictions, prostitutes are penalized as criminals, while customers remain unpunished. Similarly, in Thailand prostitution is treated as a crime in itself unless the prostitute can prove that she or he is a victim of human trafficking. The fact that domestic courts employ such vastly different understandings about the nature and definition of prostitution (as well as the problematic collapsing of forced and voluntary prostitution) points to the weakness in international human rights law.

The anti-trafficking treaties also possess a generally weak understanding of women's lives and realities. While the treaties offer a basic framework and definition as to what constitutes human trafficking, they fail to recognize, give voice to, or otherwise acknowledge the circumstances that lead to trafficking and prostitution, particularly in the developing world. Reanda (1991) has argued that mass prostitution always develops in tandem with high levels of military troops, or circumstances in which groups of men want to be "serviced." This may explain how coerced prostitution in Thailand emerged largely as a response to the US war in Vietnam. Despite arguments asserting that it is imperialistic for the West to assume responsibility for sex trafficking in Southeast Asia, the rise of Western sex tourism has had measurably detrimental effects on migrant women and children due to structural inequalities perpetuated under the conditions of globalization. The failure of the treaties to acknowledge the historic occurrences, which set the scene for today's exploitation of women in Southeast Asia by Western tourists, points to the West's complicity in the systemic violation of women's rights in the developing world (see also Chaps. 19, 20, and 25 on sex industry in Thailand).

In tandem, the treaties fail to address political, economic, and social "push factors" that lead to circumstances of vulnerability in migration contexts and subsequent scenarios of human trafficking. Economic disparity, which is seen most sharply in circumstances faced by women, is a primary cause of women's migration through and beyond Southeast Asia for purposes of prostitution (Personal communication with Volunteer Coordinator at D.E.P.D.C., July 2009). Additionally, the new informal migration process occurring under globalization fosters "new forms of cross-border solidarity and identity formation that represents new subjectivities" (Sassen 2000: 261).

According to the United Nations (2011: 1):

> Women represent 70 percent of the world's poor. They are often paid less than men for their work, with the average wage gap in 2008 being 17 percent. Women face persistent discrimination when they apply for credit for business or self-employment and are often concentrated in insecure, unsafe and low-wage work. Eight out of ten women workers are considered to be in vulnerable employment in sub-Saharan Africa and South Asia, with global economic changes taking a huge toll on their livelihoods.

Acknowledging the reality that women generally face harsher, more dire economic circumstances than men is a critical, yet often overlooked part of the discourse on trafficking. Additionally, it is essential to acknowledge that working as a prostitute in a destination city (such as Bangkok) is likely to earn a woman a higher wage than she would otherwise earn working in a rural village in Burma, for example, as Burma is a nation "near the bottom with regard to levels of education, healthcare and protein consumption" (White 2004: 14) and lacking protections against child labor (US Department of State 2002).

Economic disparity as a "push" factor in women's migration processes may be seen as a violation of human rights in itself. My recent research has indicated that prostitution in destination cities in Thailand is preferable to situations of dire economic hardship in countries such as Burma. In forthcoming work, I examine the "push factors" that compel female migrants to enter Thailand in search of viable economic opportunity. Indeed, contrary to many myths that abound about migration and sex work being uniformly "forced" or "coerced" processes (Kempadoo et al. 2005; Parreñas 2011), my research indicates that many women migrate from Burma into Thailand voluntarily, as conditions in Burma are so dire that the precarious labor experiences they face in Thailand are more preferable. Theses disparities point to the way political economy factors in home countries violate women's rights to economic and social security. The UN conventions and treaties should explicitly acknowledge these circumstances, yet they fail to do so.

This weakness speaks to the failure of the treaties to approach human rights frameworks from the needs of women, as opposed to from the needs of the state. Rather than focusing on economic and social rights, which, theoretically are designed to protect victims *from* human rights abuses, the language of the treaties is structured to support civil and politically oriented rights, often thought of as *right to* types of rights. Such rights deal primarily with issues related to the public sphere and political processes, for example, the right to vote, the right to bear arms, or the right to engage in free speech. Female migrants facing economic hardship and material deprivation are seldom as concerned with civil and political rights, as they are caught in the mire of having to first defend their economic and social rights. As Pogge (2007) has noted, world poverty is as much a cause of weakness, vulnerability, and injustice as it is a result. For impoverished people around the world, and particularly for women and girls, civil and political rights that treat people as independent, rational actors yet dismiss systems of engrained economic disadvantage and social discrimination are not the types of rights they need defended most. The anti-trafficking treaties fail to adequately address the systemic issues that lead to these violations.

4 Globalization Theory and International Law

I will now turn to a broader examination of international law as it relates to contemporary processes of globalization. Saskia Sassen (2007) has introduced the issue of the nature of the global versus the local in the context of the changing conception of the modern state. Sassen asserts that in the modern world, globalized processes can be found not just in transnational networks or existing in a "global" sphere, but are actually located within states themselves. That is, processes of globalization have penetrated local environments, changing the nature of various social issues and institutions. This notion serves as a frame for my assertion that prostitution is a transnational process, rather than a local one. Sassen points out that this "localization of the global" (2007: 80) requires that we not only renegotiate the concept of the national but also reexamine the social sciences themselves and reframe our thinking about various political institutions. Building upon the analysis of the treaties that I have presented, I argue that international human rights law is one such institution. While international law provides a framework for responding to transnational criminal activity, this framework is limited conceptually. In essence, it is a step behind the globalization process that Sassen analyzes. Because of this, international law must be reimagined to adequately view coerced prostitution as a global crime that takes place within local spheres.

During the past century, the UN charter has established conceptual parameters of transnational processes through implementing and recognizing state sovereignty. The paradigm of sovereignty, which initially emerged as a result of the Treaties of Westphalia in 1648 was solidified in the 1933 Montevideo Convention on the Rights and Duties of States, which established that state sovereignty would encompass "three main requirements: a permanent population, a defined territory, and a functioning government. An important component of sovereignty has always been an adequate display of the authority of states to act over their territory to the exclusion of other states" (International Development Research Center 2010: 83). This concept of sovereignty plays a significant role in the discourse on human trafficking. State parties are responsible for ratifying and upholding anti-trafficking conventions, and the international-versus-domestic criminal divide is viewed by the law through the lens of sovereignty.

This, in turn, has many implications for women who are trafficked and who work as coerced prostitutes within the boundaries of a sovereign state. In the cases of trafficking and coerced prostitution, unless the crossing of an international border occurs, international law has not been violated. Conversely, international law offers no protections to people who are trafficked and/or engage in coerced prostitution unless they cross physical, politically defined boundaries from one sovereign state into another. Given that domestic laws often fail to punish trafficking crimes, we may logically conclude that many crimes against women who are trafficked domestically—despite the transnational *processes* that may contribute to creating these circumstances—often go unnoticed. I will return to this idea shortly.

Sassen questions the concept of state sovereignty under the ever-evolving conditions of globalization. She points out that as we work to "re-code the national" (2007: 91), our previous notions of state sovereignty and territorial land boundaries must shift. While she does not argue for a return to pre-Westphalia notions of territory, Sassen proposes an important conceptual shift in what should constitute a political boundary. She also asserts that certain institutions that have historically been viewed as "distinct" and "mutually exclusive" (2007: 91) from one another must now be reexamined:

> Key among these are some components of the work of ministries of finance, central banks, and the increasingly specialized technical regulatory agencies, such as those concerned with finance, telecommunications, and competition policy. In this regard, then, my position is not comfortably subsumed under the proposition that nothing much has changed in terms of sovereign state power, nor can it be subsumed under the proposition of the declining significance of the state (Sassen 2007: 91).

I add to Sassen's list the institution of international human rights law. As I have illustrated, treaties do not reach into realms traditionally considered to be "local," functioning under domestic, state jurisdiction. Further, these treaties provide limited definitions of what constitutes transnational criminal activity and, in the case of coerced prostitution, whether purveyors of commercial sex should be held criminally accountable.

International law must be reimagined in the context of globalization, in order to encompass the ambiguities of criminal activities that do not necessarily involve the crossing of land boundaries between sovereign states. To reimagine coerced prostitution as warranting such attention would mean treating this issue with more gravity and importance than it presently receives.

5 Coerced Prostitution Is Transnational

The transnational nature of coerced prostitution is apparent in several processes that occur under the conditions of globalization. The most apparent of these is migration. Migration across sovereign borders, as well as within the borders of a state, is commonly associated with the issue of coerced prostitution. In the example of Burmese women who migrate informally to Thailand, whether migration occurs under threat of violence, deception, or with an understanding on the part of the migrant of what conditions await them in Thailand, the fact remains that upon arrival, many women find themselves in situations of gross labor exploitation. According to the Development and Education Programme for Daughters and Communities, an NGO working to prevent trafficking among stateless minority women and children in Thailand's North, Burmese migrants often possess no legitimate legal or citizenship status in Thailand, subsequently rendering them unable to claim even the most basic protections under Thai law (Personal communication with Volunteer Coordinator at D.E.P.D.C., July 2009). Having no access to health care, education, "legitimate" employment opportunities, or even police protection, many Burmese migrants find themselves in situations of exploitation. Even migrants who enter sex work consensually may face exploitative conditions working in brothels such as quotas, restricted movement, or high fees given to brothel owners (Personal communication with anonymous NGO employee, August 2011). The precarious conditions encountered by many women during their migration processes illustrate the way coerced prostitution may be viewed as a transnational process.

Another process that relates to the transnational nature of coerced prostitution involves the shifting public-private divide under conditions of globalization. Kaupr (2007: 225) argues that global governance should extend its protective reach into newly emerging "informal," previously seeming "private" realms. He discusses the failure of political structures and institutions to support transnational processes that encompass these realms:

> Globalization—particularly the massive growth in the extent, intensity, velocity, and scope of cross-border interactions (Held et al. 1999)—has not been met by a corresponding increase in our capacity to exercise political control over this enmeshed world. We have gaping holes where governance should be.... In the face of dramatic de facto changes in economic and political power, there has been a combined failure to reconstruct political theory and to transform our political institutions—to the dramatic extent commensurate with this new reality (Kaupr 2007: 225).

Kaupr articulates the danger of political institutions lagging behind the present conditions of globalization, as these conditions warrant a shift in the way such institutions are viewed. Indeed, the private has become more political than ever before, in that activities previously rendered as belonging to the domestic sphere are now directly connected to global processes (the "feminization of survival" being one powerful example). The implications on global governance and the ethical responsibility of the world community in addressing these issues are grave. Coerced prostitution, viewed ambiguously across cultures and over time, must no longer be rendered to such vast disparity in interpretation. As the above examples demonstrate, it is a global process that international law must now explicitly address.

6 The Case of the Development Organization for Daughters and Communities (DEPDC)

I will now briefly present a case in which these issues come together to illustrate why domestic-level prostitution is a concern in the international arena, and should not be merely relegated to the domestic criminal realm.

In 2009, I traveled to Mae Sai, a small city in Thailand adjacent to the Burmese border, to conduct research on the trafficking of women and girls into and within Thailand. I worked at an organization called the Development Organization for Daughters and Communities, an NGO dedicated to trafficking prevention among ethnic minorities in the Mekong Subregion. While at DEPDC, I learned that ethnic minorities in Thailand are often more vulnerable to the problem of trafficking than Thai nationals because their citizenship status leaves them lacking many basic rights. Without citizenship rights, many families succumb to the forces of poverty and crime, each in turn becoming driving factors for child trafficking. DEPDC is explicit in its mission to prevent child trafficking among the many ethnic minority communities in Thailand, Burma, Laos, the Yunnan province of China, Cambodia, and Vietnam. Among these groups are the Shan, Kachin, Karen, Tai-Yai, Hmong, Lahu, and Akha peoples of the *Lanna* region of Thailand's North (D.E.P.D.C. 2009a, b).

In addressing the concerns put forth by NGOs such as DEPDC, Thailand has adopted numerous initiatives to comply with the United Nations' efforts to combat human trafficking, demonstrating a willingness to implement policies that treat human trafficking as a crime. Yet, Thailand's reputation abroad is still that of a trafficking hub, and the Thai government has been sluggish to penalize traffickers. Thailand's public diplomacy initiatives remain underdeveloped, and its single campaign to "re-brand" Thailand's image in order to steer public attention away from viewing the country as a sex-tourism hub has been a failure (Nuttavuthisit 2006). In contrast to its neighbor Cambodia, for example, a country that has taken significant steps in its public diplomacy efforts to combat child trafficking, such awareness campaigns in Thailand are rarely effectively geared toward the general public. Despite a 1998 report, in which the International Labor Organization estimated that 100,000–200,000 Thai women and girls worked in the commercial sex industry overseas (Lim 1998: 411), Thailand's measures to combat its image as a destination for sex tourism have been few and far between.

Additionally, while the Convention is designed to protect Thai citizens from trafficking abuses, the Government of the Kingdom of Thailand has maintained two reservations on this initiative: Article 7, regarding birth registration, and Article 22, regarding children seeking refugee status in Thailand (ECPAT International 2006: 21). These reservations reveal that while the government is taking a policy stance against the trafficking of Thai citizens, it is unwilling to extend these efforts toward refugees and stateless ethnic minorities living within Thailand's borders. Thailand's efforts to protect or even recognize the rights of ethnic minority women and girls—the populations most vulnerable to trafficking and other exploitative labor situations—are barely existent.

7 Thailand's Lenient Stance

Several factors explain why the Thai Government has been largely dismissive of trafficking and coerced prostitution within and beyond its national borders. Among these are examples pointing to the globalized, transnational nature of the crimes in question. In this section, I will illustrate how Thailand's lenient attitude toward trafficking and coerced prostitution is connected to the nation's role as a transnational actor.

The first factor is sex tourism. Sex tourism in Thailand is, perhaps, the largest issue exacerbating the spread of coerced prostitution among young girls in Thailand. According to a recent article by a Pulitzer Crisis Center reporter in Bangkok, "North Americans comprise 25 % of sex tourists in the world and are directly complicit in economically supporting this industry" (Guzder 2009: 1). In the late 1990s, Thailand's reputation as a destination for sex tourism increased (see also Chaps. 19, 20, and 25). Due to the 1997 Asian economic crisis, women from the rural Northeast and other economically deprived regions of the country migrated to Bangkok to find work as unskilled laborers, many working in prostitution. The trafficking of children for sexual exploitation also increased. During this time, it was widely thought that police corruption played a large part in the issue. With Western television shows promoting its beaches as easy places to purchase sex and bar girls crowding Bangkok's tourist-district streets, Thailand's image as a destination for sex tourism was on the rise.

In 2003, the Thai government recognized the need to correct its negative image abroad by addressing the problem of coerced prostitution and trafficking in its nation-branding strategy. The government implemented the "Branding Thailand Project" which identified the positive associations tourists made with Thailand, such as "exotic," "friendly," "fun," and "cuisine" as well as negative associations such as "sex/prostitute," "cheap," and "poor" (Nuttavuthisit 2006: 23). Despite these re-branding efforts, however, as of 2006 "no public officials or law enforcement officials were arrested for being complicit in trafficking" (www.humantrafficking.org, 2008), and the Thai government had failed at substantially documenting and tracking the victims of sex trafficking. While Thailand has made attempts to correct its negative image, the fact remains that coerced prostitution is embedded in the tourist-based economy that makes Thailand thrive.

Another factor that plays into Thailand's participation in the global trafficking and prostitution problem involves Thailand's national identity vis-à-vis ethnic differentiation. Thailand, in order to maintain its national identity and thus its differential status within the region and within the world, uses ethnic differentiation to cement its national identity. Bangkok elites go to great lengths to set themselves apart from the many "hill tribe" ethnic groups living along Thailand's Northern borders. Cementing this ethnic differentiation and thus creating a (fictionalized, yet conceptually very real) national identity can be seen as an issue relating to culture, globalization and, identity (see also Chapters in Part III of this volume).

Castells (2004a, b) has introduced a framework for the relationship between globalization and culture, suggesting that at the advent of the twenty-first century, cultures began to trend toward a kind of contraction, a rigid self-definition, in the face of globalization's ever-widening pull. The instinct for cultures to become increasingly nationalistic, Castells suggests, is in fact a reaction against the threats of globalization that they perceive are occurring. Thailand's national identity project relates directly to such a perceived threat. In order to uphold its notion of identity, Thailand has become increasingly permissive of the crimes of sex trafficking and prostitution that occur so widely within its borders. This curious case, in which transnational crime actually *supports* the establishment of national identity, has dangerous implications on the relationship between nationalism and globalization—implications that should not be overlooked in the international human rights law discourse. Additionally, the circumstances occurring within Thailand support Sassen's assertion that global processes have local effects (2007: 79) and are playing out in new ways that existing international institutions must address.

Closely connected to this idea of upholding national identity is Thailand's desire to maintain regional economic hegemony. This national goal also relates to the prevalence of prostitution in Thailand, in that Thailand's participation in the global criminal economy helps uphold its status as a regional economic hegemon. It can be argued that Bangkok's identity as a sex trafficking hub draws money and resources into Thailand much in the way that other countries attract real estate or manufacturing investment. Indeed, as China is known for cheap manufacturing of goods, Thailand's cheap labor is the service of sex. This reality presents another example of how coerced prostitution is, in fact, a transnational issue.

8 Conclusion: Does the West Have Responsibility?

International law is lagging sorely behind the realities of globalization. Problems such as trafficking and coerced prostitution, which pervade the global arena while situating themselves within local realms, are conceptualized and handled in antiquated ways. How should the West respond to these issues? Thomas Pogge's thought-provoking essay (2007: 211) articulates the difficulty in reconciling Western attitudes toward the global poor with issues of inequality:

> World poverty appears as one overwhelming—Herculean or rather Sisyphean—task to which we, as individuals, cannot meaningfully contribute. One makes a disaster relief contribution after a tsunami and finds that, two years later, the damaged areas have been largely rebuilt, with our help. One makes a contribution to poverty relief and finds that, two years later, the number of people living and dying in extreme poverty is still unimaginably large.

> The former contribution seems meaningful because we think of the task as limited to one disaster—rather than including the effects of all natural disasters, say. The latter contribution appears pointless. But such appearances arise from our conventional sorting categories. Seeing the global poor as one vast homogenous mass, we overlook that saving ten children from a painful death by hunger does make a real difference, all the difference for these children and their families, and that this difference is quite significant even when many other children remain desperately hungry.

Pogge suggests that Western neglect of the structural issues that underlie world poverty cannot be justified under the current conditions of globalization. Concurring with this, I argue that globalization processes warrant global responsibility. Transnational processes have now come to the people and are affecting local economies and cultures worldwide. As consumers of global labor, including labor in the sex industry and other informal sectors, Western nations, organizations, institutions, and individuals have an obligation to provide safety measures for women and children who bear the brunt of these structural inequalities. In order to advance the discussion about Western responsibility, however, the international legal discourse must also advance. The first step in this direction involves international law's explicit recognition of coerced prostitution as a transnational issue fostered by structural inequalities and bound to processes of migration. In so doing, treaties must support the decriminalization of prostitution worldwide and instead, work toward the criminalization of those who exploit others' labor in the domestic arena as well as across sovereign borders. Reimagining the international as also encompassing the local will allow us to advance the discourse on international human rights law at this crucial, albeit fragile moment in our history.

Acknowledgments I would like to express my appreciation to the many NGO employees, volunteers, women, and children who continue to open my eyes to the circumstances and realities of human trafficking, prostitution, and labor migration in Thailand. Specifically, staff members at ECPAT International and DEPDC during my field research in 2009 made important contributions to this chapter. I also wish to thank faculty at USC's Annenberg School for Communication and Journalism, particularly Dr. Manuel Castells, Dr. Larry Gross, Dr. Patricia Riley, and Dr. Nicholas Cull for their support. Finally, I wish to acknowledge the female migrant laborers and sex workers in Thailand who, despite their voices often being suppressed in policy initiatives and scholarly research, possess real expertise about the current state of trafficking, labor migration, and prostitution in Thailand.

References

Barry, K. (1995). *The prostitution of sexuality: The global exploitation of women*. New York: New York University Press.

Bindman, J., & Doezema, J. (1997). *Redefining prostitution as sex work on the international Agenda*. Retrieved April 15, 2011 from http://www.walnet.org/csis/papers/redefining.html

Brennan, D. (2005). Methodological challenges in research with trafficked persons: Tales from the field. *Data and research on human trafficking: A global survey.* Geneva: International Organization for Migration.

Castells, M. (2004a). Informationalism, networks, and the network society: A theoretical blueprint. In M. Castells (Ed.), *The network society: A cross-cultural perspective* (pp. 3–48). Northampton: Edward Elgar.
Castells, M. (2004b). *The power of identity*. Oxford: Blackwell Publishing.
Castendyck, E. (1944). Social problems. In H. Eager Davis (Ed.), *Pioneers of world order: An American appraisal of the league of nations* (pp. 229–239). New York: Columbia University Press.
Chuang, J. (1998). Redirecting the debate over trafficking in women: Definitions, paradigms, and contexts. *Harvard Human Rights Journal, 11*, 65–107.
D.E.P.D.C. (2009a). *About us*. Retrieved July 6, 2009, from http://depdc.org/eng/aboutus/target_group.html
D.E.P.D.C. (2009b) *Home*. Retrieved July 6, 2009, from http://depdc.org/index.htm
Derks, A. (2000). *Combating trafficking in South-East Asia: A review of policy and programme responses*. Geneva: The International Organization for Migration.
Doezema, J. (2000). Ouch! Western feminists' 'wounded attachment' to the 'third world prostitute'. *Feminist Review, 67*(Spring), 16–39.
Doezema, J. (2002). Who gets to choose? Coercion, consent, and the UN trafficking protocol. *Gender and Development, 10*(1), 20–27.
Doezema, J., & Kempadoo, K. (Eds.). (1998). *Global sex workers: Rights, resistance and redefinition*. New York: Routledge.
ECPAT International. (2006). *Global monitoring report on the status of action against commercial sexual exploitation of children: Thailand*. Bangkok: ECPAT International.
Farr, K. (2005). *Sex trafficking: The global market in women and children*. New York: Worth Publishers.
Finnerty, C. (2008). *Cross border migration and prostitution in Thailand: Is there a fine line between trafficking and voluntary migration of women and girls?* Unpublished MA Development Studies Dissertation, University of Leeds, UK.
Global Alliance Against Traffic in Women. (2007). *COLLATERAL DAMAGE: The impact of anti-trafficking measures on human rights around the world*. Bangkok: Global Alliance Against Traffic in Women.
Guzder, D. (2009). *Thailand: The world's sex tourism capital*. The Pulitzer Center on Crisis Reporting. Retrieved October 31, 2009, from http://pulitzercenter.typepad.com/untold_stories/2009/08/thailand-flesh-market.html
Held, D., et al. (Eds.). (1999). *Global transformations*. Cambridge: Polity.
Humantrafficking.org. (2008). *Thailand- The situation*. Retrieved October 25, 2008, from http://www.humantrafficking.org/countries/thailand
International Labor Organization. (1998). *Sex as a sector: Economic incentives and hardships fuel growth*. Retrieved October 24, 2008, from http://www.ilo.org/public/english/bureau/inf/magazine/26/sex.htm
Jamjoom, M. (2010, April 2). Condemned 'sorcerer' won't die Friday, lawyer says. *CNN*. Retrieved April 15, 2010, from http://www.cnn.com/2010/WORLD/meast/04/01/saudi.arabia.sorcery/index.html
Jeffries, S. (1997). *The idea of prostitution*. Melbourne: Spinifex Press.
Kamler, E. (2009, October 15–18). *National identity, the Shan and child trafficking in Northern Thailand: The case of D.E.P.D.C.* Working paper presented at the International Conference on Shan Studies, Bangkok, Thailand.
Kempadoo, K., Sahghera, J., & Pattanaik, B. (2005). *Trafficking and prostitution reconsidered: New perspectives on migration, sex work, and human rights*. Boulder: Paradigm Publishers.
Kupur, A. (2007). Reconstructing global governance: Eight innovations. In D. Held & A. McGrew (Eds.), *Globalization theory: Approaches and controversies* (pp. 225–239). Cambridge: Polity Press.
Lim, L. L. (1998). *The sex sector: The economic and social bases of prostitution in Southeast Asia*. Geneva: ILO.

Los Angeles Times. (2010, April 2). *Saudi Arabia: Factional politics may be at heart of legal dispute over psychic's fate*. Retrieved April 15, 2010, from http://latimesblogs.latimes.com/babylonbeyond/2010/04/saudi-arabia-lebanese-tv-psychics-death-sentence-stayed.html

MacKinnon, C. (2007). *Are women human? And other international dialogues*. Cambridge: Harvard University Press.

Nuttavuthisit, K. (2006). Branding Thailand: Correcting the negative image of sex tourism. *Place Branding and Public Diplomacy, 3*(1), 21–30.

O'Connell Davidson, J. (1998). *Prostitution, power and freedom*. Cambridge: Polity Press.

Parreñas, R. (2011). *Illicit flirtations: Labor, migration, and sex trafficking in Tokyo*. Stanford: Stanford University Press.

Pogge, T. (2007). Reframing economic security and justice. In D. Held & A. McGrew (Eds.), *Globalization theory: Approaches and controversies* (pp. 207–224). Cambridge: Polity Press.

Reanda, L. (1991). Prostitution as a human rights question: Problems and prospects of United Nations action. *Human Rights Quarterly, 13*(2), 202–228.

Sassen, S. (2000). Women's burden: Counter-geographies of globalization and the feminization of survival. *Journal of International Affairs, 53*(2), 503–524.

Sassen, S. (2007). The places and spaces of the global: An expanded analytic terrain. In D. Held & A. McGrew (Eds.), *Globalization theory: Approaches and controversies* (pp. 79–105). Cambridge: Polity Press.

Segrave, M. (2009). Order at the border: The repatriation of victims of trafficking. *Womens Studies International Forum, 32*(4), 251–260.

Segrave, M., Pickering, S., & Milivojevic, S. (2009). *Sex trafficking: International context and response*. Portland: Willan Publishing.

Shobha, S. V. (2009). *No woman fights to become a prostitute. Boloji.com*. Retrieved November 1, 2009, from http://www.boloji.com/wfs6/2009/wfs1241.htm

Skrobanek, S. (2003). Human trafficking: From vertical to horizontal journey. *Voices of Thai Women*. Retrieved October 25, 2009, from http://findarticles.com/p/articles/mi_7068/is_20/ai_n28149390/pg_4/?tag=content;col

The International Development Research Center. (2010). *State sovereignty*. Retrieved April 15, 2010, from http://www.idrc.ca/en/ev-28492-201-1-DO_TOPIC.html

U.S. Department of State Office to Monitor and Combat Trafficking in Persons Report. (2002). Retrieved April 26, 2012, from http://www.state.gov/j/tip/rls/tiprpt/2002/

U.S. Department of State Office to Monitor and Combat Trafficking in Persons Report. (2011). Retrieved August 13, 2013, from http://www.state.gov/j/tip/rls/tiprpt/2011/

United Nations Association of the USA. (2009). *The UN convention on the elimination of all forms of discrimination against women (CEDAW)*. Retrieved October 31, 2009, from http://www.unausa.org/Page.aspx?pid=935

United Nations Division for the Advancement of Women Department of Economic and Social Affairs. (2009). *Convention on the elimination of all forms of discrimination against women*. Retrieved August 29, 2009, from http://www.un.org/womenwatch/daw/cedaw/

United Nations Entity for Gender Equality and the Empowerment of Women. (2011). *Women, poverty and economics*. Retrieved April 25, 2012, from http://www.16dana.ba/en/info/women-poverty-and-economics-2/

White, J. A. (2004). Globalisation, divestment and human rights in Burma. *Journal of Corporate Citizenship, 14*, 47–65.

Women's Justice Center. (2010). *Sweden's prostitution solution: Why hasn't anyone tried this before?* Retrieved April 15, 2010, from http://www.justicewomen.com/cj_sweden.html

Chapter 24
Gender and Buddhism in the Wake of the Tsunami

Monica Lindberg Falk

1 Introduction

The December 26, 2004, was a Sunday and the weekly Buddhist holy day in Thailand. The children were free from school, and many people, especially women, were at the temples making religious merit when the Tsunami waves hit the Thai shore. Initially, after the Tsunami, the Buddhist temples became important places for people to seek refuge. Rescue camps were established on temple grounds and in close connection with temples, and temples were significant for keeping thousands of dead bodies. The Thai people turned to the monks for consolation, for explanations about life and death, and the monks were important in conducting rites and ceremonies and for restoring continuity and order.

This chapter explores local adaptation strategies and examines religious and spiritual beliefs as key elements in the recovery. It provides example of ways in which Thai Buddhist monks, nuns, and laypeople employ Buddhism to cope after having lost family members, friends, neighbors, their homes, and means of livelihood. Most of the ethnographic accounts presented in this chapter are based on in-depth interviews and participant observation, together with repeated visits to villages in Phang Nga province. Conventional anthropological fieldwork procedure of participant observation, in-depth interviews, and narratives were used in order to explore how people deal with their situation after the disaster.[1] I have worked together with an assistant, and the informants are Buddhist monks, nuns, laywomen, and men who have survived the Tsunami and family members and relatives of victims of the Tsunami.

[1] Since the study is primarily based on information collected from personal observation and interviews, consideration of ethical questions is important. I have masked the identity of the informants, and all personal names in this article are fictitious.

M.L. Falk, Ph.D. (✉)
Social Anthropology, Centre for East and South-East Asian Studies, Lund University, Lund, Sweden
e-mail: Monica.Lindberg_Falk@ace.lu.se

P. Liamputtong (ed.), *Contemporary Socio-Cultural and Political Perspectives in Thailand*,
DOI 10.1007/978-94-007-7244-1_24,

2 Impact of the Tsunami in Thailand

The Indian Ocean Tsunami on December 26, 2004, hit the shores of 13 countries. Almost 280 thousand people lost their lives. According to the Thai government's official statistics, there were 8,327 dead or missing in Thailand. About 8,500 people were injured in Thailand. These figures do not include the many migrant workers who died in the Tsunami. Many of them lived and worked in Thailand without proper documents, and their relatives in Burma (Myanmar) have not reported them missing. Oxfam reported that more women than men died in the Tsunami. Among the Thai who died were 54.8 % female and 45.2 % male (Isalapakdee 2006).

Six provinces in the south of Thailand were struck by the Tsunami. The population in the coastal areas is multiethnic. Many of those who were hit by the Tsunami were fishing families and migrant workers, and the Tsunami had devastating consequences for them, first through loss of lives and second through damage and losses of houses and fishing boats. Small fishing households live under economically strained circumstances and have few assets apart from a small boat and some fishing gear. Their houses are modest, and alternative sources of income are irregular (Lebel et al. 2006).

The provinces of Phang Nga and Phuket had a booming tourist industry that attracted Thai people from other parts of Thailand to work. Immigrants from the neighboring country Burma/Myanmar also worked as unskilled laborers in the area. Many of the affected people came from other provinces in the south, central, northern, and northeastern parts of Thailand, and most of them worked as construction workers or in the service business (Isalapakdee 2006).

3 Phang Nga Province

The most seriously hit province in Thailand was Phang Nga, and some villages were almost wiped out by the Tsunami. After the Tsunami, rescue camps were established on temple grounds and at areas belonging to the local governments' administration. The situation for the inhabitants in the coastal areas is, many years after the catastrophe, still troublesome, especially concerning livelihood.

In Phang Nga, 29 subdistricts and 69 villages were affected by the Tsunami. The villagers' religious affiliation is mixed. The majority, however, are Buddhists, and between 10 and 30 % are Muslims. The Moken/Moklen, an ethnic minority group, has also lived in the area for more than a century. Their culture and ancestor worship are unique to them; however, some have simultaneously long been close to the Buddhist temples. After the Tsunami, groups of Moken became targets of Christian missionaries, and some of the groups converted to Christianity.

Christian missionaries have operated in the Tsunami-stricken areas, and initially Buddhists converted in exchange for material goods. Before the Tsunami, there were two Christian churches in Phang Nga; by 2007 the number had increased to more than 20.

4 New Settlements

After the Tsunami, there have been disputes over land, and many families have faced threats and being denied to return and rebuild their houses. I have found that overcoming fear and regaining trust have been important in the recovery process. Many of those who live in houses today that are rebuilt at the same place as before the Tsunami are living with the fear that a Tsunami would hit again. They listen constantly to the news and are always prepared to run. Some have found it too stressful and have, therefore, abandoned their houses and moved to safer ground.

A whole village at one of Phang Nga's small islands was wiped out by the Tsunami, and those who survived moved to the mainland. The village had a small temple with three monks of whom two were killed when the Tsunami hit. The young monk who survived had been in Phuket, a nearby province, to collect a Buddha statue. He came back to the island 2 days after the Tsunami and said that nothing was left in the village. The small temple, the school, and all the houses had been smashed to the ground by the waves. During the first days, he helped to collect dead bodies. He explained that it was important to collect the bodies as quickly as possible. They brought the bodies to a temple at the mainland.[2] The villagers decided to move to the mainland and that implied not living close to the sea as they were used to. The monk said that in the beginning, the villagers complained that living on the mainland meant that they had to spend money to an extent that they were not used to. They had difficulties making ends meet. They needed motorbikes to transport fishing gear, something they did not need at the island where the fishing gear was close to their houses on the shore. After living 2 years on the mainland, the villagers seemed to have adjusted themselves to their new environment, and the complaints have decreased. The monk said that the villagers do not look upon themselves as victims, and they did not talk much about the Tsunami. The complaints have changed into a talk about the advantages of living on the mainland and discussions about coping with the new circumstances.[3]

5 Gender and Buddhism

Buddhist temples in Thailand follow an ancient tradition. The Thai Buddhist *sangha* is totally male. The Thai Buddhist nuns, *mae chii*, do not belong to the *sangha* and are excluded from the benefits that their male colleagues enjoy. Monastic life is strictly regulated and creates a sharp boundary between the ordained community and the laypeople. The position outside the *sangha* of *mae chii* makes their position somewhat ambiguous (see Falk 2007).

[2] Interview, April 15, 2006.

[3] Interview, July 23, 2007.

Gender issues are emerging globally in Buddhist communities. Today, Thai women who aspire to go forth have at least two possibilities: either to become a *mae chii* or to become a *bhikkhuni*. *Bhikkhuni* was introduced during the Buddha's time, and the category of *mae chii* is a Thai term used for female ascetics. Both categories are outside the Thai Buddhist *sangha*, which is solely a male congregation, and demonstrates that female ascetics in Thailand have had to create space outside the formal religious structure. Both *bhikkhuni*s and *mae chii*s struggle for recognition of their ordained status. In Thailand, there are several categories of Buddhist women who have renounced the lay life and live according to the ascetic Buddhist principles. The *mae chii*s constitute the largest group of Thai female ascetic. They have a long history in Thailand and have for centuries lived in the Buddhist temples where they have a subordinated position in relation to the monks.

*Mae chii*s' exclusion from the *sangha* implies that women are expelled from Thai society's most prestigious arena. However, being excluded has given some *mae chii*s the opportunity to create space for themselves and establish their own *samnak chii*s, "temples," and thereby better fulfill their roles as ordained persons (see Falk 2007). In recent decades, the *mae chii*s have begun to take advantage of their ambiguous position outside the *sangha*. They have accentuated their religious vocation by refining their practice, upgrading their educational level, and drawing a more distinct boundary between themselves and the laypeople. The recent decades' growth of self-governed "nunneries" and the reports of Thai women's increasing interest in Buddhist monastic life are notable changes in women's behavior in the spiritual field. This connotes a modification of the restricted male religious domain (Falk 2007).

6 Places of Refuge

After the Tsunami, both monastic and laypeople lived at the temples, and dead bodies were also taken care of there. Some temples were destroyed by the Tsunami and could not be used for keeping dead bodies or as shelters, so people brought the dead bodies to the temples that were intact. In the first month, temples were the main places for the identification of dead bodies and the work place for forensic specialists. Temples also provided a place to stay for many of the volunteers who came to help. Moreover, the temples served as centers for information about missing persons.

Dealing with questions about life and death is a special expertise of Buddhist monks and nuns. Buddhism offers detailed and in-depth explanations about how life is constituted, how to deal with personal as well as social difficulties, how to live harmoniously, and how to die peacefully. Most temples in Phang Nga do not host *mae chii*s, and they lack a nuns' section at the temple. Buddhist monks in Phang Nga, like monks in other provinces, are recognized by their followers for individual skills, and the monks are free to specialize if they want to. Some are socially engaged and involved in different social projects, some focus on Buddhist meditation practice, and some are known for their magical skills and for their healing power. Most monks, however, live quiet lives in ordinary village temples, carrying out their daily routines, doing their practices, and performing ceremonies.

7 The Temples in the Affected Areas

Most of the temples in the Tsunami area are small and have about 8–10 resident monks. Several of the small temples (*samnak songs*) have only a few resident monks. The day when the Tsunami struck was a full moon day. The monks and laypeople call it *wan phra yai* (the big *wan phra*), occurring monthly. *Wan phra* is the Buddhist observance day, which follows the lunar calendar and occurs once a week. In Thailand, monks, and also some *mae chii*s, go on alms rounds every morning, and once a week, on *wan phra*, laypeople also bring food to the temple.[4] Most Theravada Buddhist monks eat twice a day. They have their first meal in the early morning and the second before 12 noon. According to their monastic discipline, they are not allowed to eat after noon. Donating food to the ordained community is considered meritorious and part of many Thai Buddhists' daily lives. At the temples on *wan phra*, after the laypeople have donated food to the monks, the monks give Buddhist speeches, conduct chanting, and thereafter give the five Buddhist precepts to the laypeople.

At a small temple at an island in Phang Nga, the head monk said that he sat on the floor in the *sala* when he heard a tremendously loud sound, and he thought that it was a fire in the forest. When the wave reached the temple, it was 6 m high. He said: "At 10:45 the water was very high and at 10:55 very low. High five minutes and low five minutes, and it cost us two million baht." The villagers had come to the temple to donate food, and most of them survived. However, six villagers died in the Tsunami. The monk remarked:

> The villagers who survived were happy and felt encouraged when they saw that the monks were alive. The monks are an encouragement for the people. The temple was damaged and it was impossible to stay at the temple. We could not have any temporary shelter at the temple. We were evacuated to the mainland. When we returned to the island, people came to the temple and helped.[5]

A temple on Phang Nga's mainland in one of the worst-hit villages is located behind a big pond, and the water did not reach the temple ground. At the time of the Tsunami, they had four resident monks, but no *mae chii*s lived at the temple. The abbot said that after the Tsunami, people came running to the temple, and they had about 1,000 people who stayed there. He said:

> The waves had taken their clothes and at first we had to give people clothes and rice. Some people went to stay in other areas, for example in Khao Sok [the national park] up in the

[4] For more information on gender and Buddhism in Thailand, see Falk (2007).

[5] Interview, April 16, 2006.

> mountain, and they returned to the temple when the temporary shelters were set up. This temple had temporary shelters for 80 families. Most of the families stayed for six months and about 10 families stayed for more than a year. The families who stayed longer did not dare to return to their houses. They were scared and some of them said that they could not afford to live outside the temple. They had lost their livelihoods.[6]

Some temples gave shelter to people for a couple of days up to a week. They stayed in the temples' *sala*s, and thereafter many went to stay with relatives, moved to temporary shelters, or returned home. Other temples had people staying for more than a year. However, most people stayed in the temporary shelters for about 6 months. There were villages on islands outside Phang Nga that were completely destroyed, and people who survived came to stay at the mainland. Those people have to cope with totally new living conditions.

A *mae chii* who is from the affected area and now lives and studies in Bangkok told about her experiences after the Tsunami:

> On 26 December 2004 I visited Chonburi province together with another *mae chii*. After lunch, I listened to the radio and people were talking about what had happened in the south. I did not pay much attention to the news. I went back to Bangkok by bus and I went to the chanting at my temple at four o'clock as on other days. The next morning, I went to the university as usual. I heard the news on the bus and at the university the teacher and my classmates talked about what had happened. When I returned to the temple that afternoon, I tried to phone my mother in Phang Nga. I saw that I had several missed calls. One was from a teacher in Phang Nga. I also had missed calls from a student that I had been teaching when I was back in Phang Nga a couple of months earlier. That day, I could not get in touch with anybody in Phang Nga. I watched TV and on the 28th my mother called me. I called the head monk at the temple and he asked me to bring certain things that they could not buy in the market. A teacher asked me to bring milk powder. My friends in Bangkok donated money and I bought what they needed. The same evening, I went by bus to Phang Nga. I arrived at 7 o'clock in the morning and the teacher and students were waiting for me and helped to carry all the things. When I arrived, the temple was packed with people and there was a traffic jam on the one big road. I did not know how many people had died, but I knew that they kept many dead bodies at the temple ground.[7]

After they had carried all the things to the temple, the *mae chii* told the teacher that she wanted to visit the student who had called her when she was in Bangkok. Her mother had brought breakfast to the temple, and her mother wanted her to eat before she went to look for her student, but the *mae chii* said that she did not have time to eat. She went to look for the student along with the teacher. The teacher had a list with names of the students at the school, and she checked whom she could find. Around 11 o'clock, they arrived in the nearby province Ranong where the student lives. The *mae chii* said that everything had been destroyed. She had brought some sweets that she gave to the Muslim students who came to meet her. She also met the student who had phoned her. The student told her that her mother had died, and her father was injured. The family was preparing for the cremation at their village temple. The *mae chii* met other *mae chii*s, and they had lunch together. Before she went back to her village, she also went to visit a hospital. When the *mae chii*

[6] Interview, April 2006.

[7] Interview, February 21, 2007.

arrived at her village in Phang Nga, her family and relatives were preparing for cremations of her relatives who had died in the Tsunami. The *mae chii* said that in the beginning, she spent most of the time participating in cremation ceremonies. Many of the people who had died in the Tsunami in that area were her relatives.

Despite the lack of a *mae chii*s' section, the *mae chii* stayed for many months at the temple and helped out with donations, talked with survivors, and helped them in many ways. She was the only *mae chii* at the temple. Groups of monks and *mae chii*s from other places came to help out for a couple of days and then went back to their temples. The *mae chii* explained that there were so many people at the temple and in the beginning that they could not plan. They had to live hour by hour and day by day.

Some temples were crowded with people seeking refuge, and other temples were overloaded with dead bodies. A monk at a temple that had 1,600 dead bodies at the temple grounds said that:

> The situation at the temple was extremely inconvenient during the time after the Tsunami. At the temple, we were 12 resident monks and three *mae chii*s. Our health became bad and the smell from the dead bodies was almost unbearable. We could not move. We had to stay here because we had to be with the dead bodies and receive all the people who came to visit. From 27 December and the following three months, everything at the temple was dirty and useless. But after another three months, things became better and we received help from monks and many people. Monks from other temples came and helped out with the cremations. We started to cremate the dead at 6 o'clock in the morning and continued the whole day and stopped at 11 o'clock in the night. We got sore throats from all the chanting. We had difficulties to handle the large number of dead bodies. Other temples had other difficulties. We had only dead bodies here. Dead bodies do not eat and do not need all the things that people who lived at the temples for a long time need.[8]

At many temples in the affected area, the crematoriums cracked as a consequence of the constant heat. At some temples, they continued to cremate the dead bodies by using rubber tires, and at other temples they used wood, which is the traditional way of cremating dead bodies in Thailand.

8 Buddhist Teachings After the Tsunami

For most Thai people, Buddhism is the basis of explanations about life and death (see also Chaps. 4, 5, and 28 in this volume). After the Tsunami, people who did not pay much attention to Buddhism before the Tsunami turned to temples for ceremonies, counseling, temporary ordination, and listening to Buddhist teaching, *dhamma*. The head monk at a temple that became the refuge for many villagers who survived from the affected islands off the coastline said that both Thai people and people from other countries came to his temple and searched for family members and relatives:

[8] Interview, January 18, 2007.

> I remember one Australian woman. She was in Thailand to celebrate her honeymoon. Her husband died in the Tsunami and she came here and she cried and cried. I wanted to help her and tried to explain what she could do for her dead husband. I said to her that:
>
> 1. First you must know what has happened. That is important so you must find out what has happened.
> 2. [The] Next step is to accept what has happened.
> 3. After that, you shall try to adjust your mind to be ready for the next day, the next month, and the next year.
> 4. Finally, you must be strong; if you help other people, you will be stronger.
>
> The most important thing is to solve the problems in your mind and try to stand by yourself.[9]

In interviews with monks about how they helped people to recover after the Tsunami, they said that they used Buddhist explanations about life and death. They tried to teach on a level that people would understand. Buddhism teaches why we experience dissatisfaction and suffering in life and how we can overcome it. One monk who is well known in Phang Nga for his teaching and often invited to other temples explained:

> Suffering and dissatisfaction will not last forever and we have to find ways out of suffering. Sometimes we can handle suffering but not always. The best way of solving problems is to do it with wisdom. Some people are wiser than others. For example, we cannot stop the rain. Nobody can stop the rain. But on the other hand, we do not need to stop the rain. We can protect ourselves from the rain by building a roof. We cannot stop the rain, but we can protect ourselves from being wet. Dissatisfaction comes to visit us but does not have to stay with us forever. In some situations, time helps to overcome suffering.[10]

The basic suffering concerns the body. After the Tsunami, it was important to help people to get medical treatment and also to get food, cloths, and other basic needs. In dealing with suffering that concerns the mind, the monk said that in the beginning when people were still in shock, he did not give any explanations; he simply told them that the Tsunami was caused by nature. When the survivors seemed to feel better, he tried to explain and teach about *dhamma* – about cause and effect. He said that:

> If I had talked about *dhamma* from the beginning, people would have thought about the bad deeds they had done and that would not have helped them. Therefore, it was better only to say what happened was done by nature, *thammachaat*. I told them that before the Tsunami we had never experienced anything like this, but it is over now and we must begin to live again. I tried to give them perspectives by talking about how other countries had been hit and I told them that in some countries the situation was much worse. I talked about Sri Lanka and Indonesia, where many more people had died; those countries were worse hit than Thailand. I tried to encourage them to start over again and try to overcome suffering. People who survived wanted to come in contact with their dead family members and relatives. They believe that they can help the dead people to receive merit through monks conducting ceremonies, and they feel happy and content when they have *tham bun* (made merit) and participated in ceremonies. Personally, however, I doubt that we can help dead people by that.[11]

[9] Interview, April 3, 2006.

[10] Interview, July 27, 2007.

[11] Interview, February 28, 2007.

Phra Maha is a monk who lived at a temple on a small island when the Tsunami hit. On that island, 72 people died, and those who survived were evacuated to the mainland. He moved to a small temple close to the temporary shelter where the villagers from the island had taken refuge. He talked with the villagers every day, and they stayed at the shelter about 5–6 months. He said that, in the beginning, the most important thing was to encourage them so they would get some hope. Most of the victims were in shock, and he went to many other places and talked with the survivors. He said: "We shared experiences and I wanted them to relax. Those who had lost family members wanted to understand why they had died." He said that he offered explanations according to how well the victims were. For those whom he considered were in better shape, he referred to the Buddha's teaching by telling the story of Kisa Gotami who lost her child. The focus was not on the death of the child, but the experiences of loss and grief felt by the mother.

> Kisa Gotami was a poor woman who faced many hardships during her life. She had lost all her family members including her only son, who died from an illness. She went to the Buddha and asked him to cure the baby, who by that time was already dead. The Buddha responded that he could cure him with proper medicine. He said he had all the necessary ingredients to make the medicine except for a mustard seed. He would need a very pure mustard seed – so pure that it had to come from a family that had known no death. Kisa Gotami ran to her village to collect the mustard seed, but every home she visited had known the death of a relative at some point. Finally, she understood the real meaning of the mustard seed: it was a spiritual medicine to teach her the deeper meaning of suffering and compassion.

Phra Maha said that he had to be careful about the way he talked to people. He said that he explained about the reality of life and those who have less *bun* (religious merit) would have a shorter life span. Phra Maha and other monks said that it was important for the survivors to transfer merit to their dead family members and relatives. After the Tsunami, *tham bun* (merit-making ceremonies) increased tremendously. All monks and laypeople that I have interviewed said that *tham bun* was the religious activity that had increased most after the Tsunami. Laypeople visited the temples and donated to the monks, with the intention of transferring merit to their dead family members, relatives, and friends (Falk 2010).

9 Communication Through Temporary Ordination

After the Tsunami, Buddhist monks and nuns became important in creating order and meaning and also became vehicles for communication between the living and the dead. Ordination is the ultimate act to make merit. Many survivors who had lost family members received temporary ordination as Buddhist monks or nuns. They said that the main reasons to be ordained were that they wanted to transfer merit to dead family members and to be close to those who had died. Several of the female informants received ordination. The temples organized ordination retreats for children, women, and men. Those who had been ordained said that the ordination made them feel at peace and brought them closer to the persons that they lost in the Tsunami. They experienced that they communicated with their dead family members, and they felt that it was good for their healing and that helped them to recover.

In January 2005, a woman who lost her son and several family members in the Tsunami received lay ordination, as *chii phram*, without shaving her head and eyebrows. A monk from central Thailand had set up a small Buddhist temple, a *samnak song*, close to the temporary shelter where she was staying and organized a 10-day ordination retreat. My informant said that it was a time of "heavy suffering," and those who were worried and sad (not *sabai jai*) were encouraged to receive ordination. About 50 women participated. Most of them received *chii phram* ordination, and five received nuns' *mae chii* ordination and shaved their hair and eyebrows. I asked the woman how she felt during the 10-day ordination. She answered with a big smile that she felt really at peace and that she experienced that she was close to her dead son and family members. She remarked: "It was like I could communicate with them. I felt like I was in a different world." She said that during that time many monks had come to teach, and that made her feel like she was in the "*dhamma* world and not in ordinary existence."[12]

10 From Victims to Survivors

Many of the women I met in the different groups had lost the social support networks they had before the Tsunami and had to create new belongings. They concentrated on their activities rather than relying on outside experts. The emphasis has been on the inside of the individual or group. The internal factor stands out, and in these groups, the survivors have helped each other and regenerated inner strength. Paradoxical as it may seem, giving help has been a way of being helped, and they developed from victims into survivors.

Monks have emphasized the importance of helping others in the process of helping oneself. After the Tsunami, self-help groups emerged, and Buddhist monks initiated some of them. More women than men participated in these groups. Khun Amara was 35 years old when I met her after the Tsunami. She participated in one of the self-help groups. She did not want to talk about the Tsunami, saying that it made her sad to think about what happened the day when she lost her home, livelihood, and people who were precious to her. She said that she was happy to be working together with the other women in the self-help group. She had a small child who was born after the Tsunami who is with her all the time. It has been difficult for her to find a job, and the products that the self-help group produces and sells give her a regular income.

Another member of a self-help group was 28 years old when I met her, but she was not in the same group as Khun Amara. This woman lost her husband and her child in the Tsunami. They were at home, and she was at the temple to pick up her

[12] Interview, February 4, 2007.

mother when the Tsunami hit. Before the Tsunami, her husband and she worked at two of the big tourist hotels. Both hotels were smashed to the ground by the waves. She said that after the Tsunami, she felt depressed, and she did not want to meet or talk with anybody. She took medicine more than 2 years after the Tsunami. She said that it was a neighbor at the temporary shelter who brought her to the self-help group. She told me that:

> Before I joined the group, I felt totally confused. I did not know what to do with my life; I had lost my husband and daughter in the Tsunami. I joined the group because I wanted to work and train to be with other people. I like being together with the other women. I have changed my plans. My goal is to work at a hotel again but I will continue to work here for a longer period. I appreciate my friends here. I feel more relaxed here than working at a hotel. Another reason is that I have to be close to my mother so I can pick her up if there was another earthquake. Perhaps, I will work at a hotel in the future.[13]

11 Conclusion

Basing on a gender perspective, this chapter has focused on the significance of religion in coping with the Tsunami disaster. The survivors' lives in the Tsunami-stricken areas in Phang Nga will never return to how they once were. The experiences of the Tsunami have changed their lives forever, and they are now coping with living with the experiences. Comparing survivors who live in villages that have moved to new land, at a secure distance from the sea, with those who live in houses rebuilt on the same land, the former seem to recover faster. Many of the houses that were rebuilt after the Tsunami are today empty or rented out to newcomers. They were built at the same places as the destroyed houses stood, and the survivors do not dare to live there; some prefer to continue living in temporary shelters; others have moved to other places. After the Tsunami, the temples and the monks became safeguards and tried to moderate the negative consequences. They provided the survivors with a sense of coherence, rendering their traumatic experiences more comprehensible, meaningful, and manageable as a shared challenge. The survivors have adapted local strategies, and they use Buddhism to improve their resilience. For many individual survivors, religion became their lifeline after the Tsunami, and Buddhism has helped them to cope with the very stressful situation. Monks and *mae chii*s have been important in answering questions of life and death and offered the survivors an increased feeling of control in the chaotic situation. The temples provided them with a sense of community, belonging, and direction. The survivors appreciated the monks and the *mae chii*s who came to help out after the Tsunami. The *mae chii*s have proved to be an asset to individual people and to the society, and they have the potential to be as effective as the monks are if they were given the same opportunities as ordained persons as the monks have.

[13] Interview, March 27, 2007.

Acknowledgment This research project is supported financially by the Swedish Research Council, (VR). I would like to acknowledge my informants for sharing their knowledge and experiences with me. I wish to thank Ms Nantana Pidtong for her excellent research assistance.

References

Falk, M. L. (2007). *Making fields of merit: Buddhist female ascetics and gendered orders in Thailand*. Copenhagen/Washington, DC: NIAS Press/University of Washington Press.

Falk, M. L. (2010). Recovery and Buddhist practices in the aftermath of the Tsunami in Southern Thailand. *Religion, 40*, 96–103.

Isalapakdee, P. (2006). *Tsunami: Deaths and injuries in the affected areas*. Paper presented at the 2nd annual conference of population and social research, Asia Hotel, Bangkok, Research Institute of Population and Social Research, Mahidol University, Thailand (in Thai).

Lebel, L., Khrutmuang, S., & Manuta, J. (2006). Tales from the margins: Small fishers in post tsunami Thailand. *Disaster Prevention and Management, 15*(1), 124–134.

Chapter 25
Not Yet Queer Enough: Revising "Gender" in Development

Witchayanee Ocha

1 Gender and Bodies

After the birth of a baby, the first question asked seems almost inevitably to be regarding its sex. From then on, having ascertained the sex, the process of gender forming begins, or at least that is the story of sex and gender as portrayed by theoretical models. Modern Western society distinguishes sex from gender with the argument that whatever biological sex the child appears to be is intractable and gender is, subsequently, culturally constructed. As a consequence, according to Butler (1990: 3), "it becomes impossible to separate out 'gender' from the political and cultural intersections in which it is invariably produced and maintained."

At the center of commonsense, thinking about gender in contemporary Western culture is the idea of bodily difference between women and men. There are, it is usually assumed, two types of bodies, male and female, which are sharply distinct from each other, indeed, opposed to each other. These distinct bodies, it is assumed, give rise to two different kinds of person.

In the 1970s, feminist theorists proposed a sharp distinction between *sex* and *gender* that seemed to dispose of this problem. Sex was the biological fact, the difference between the male and female human animal. Gender was the social fact, the difference between masculine and feminine roles, or men's and women's conditioned personalities. Second-wave feminism tended to universalize men and women so as to make the case for women's liberation. This generated a huge critique by women around the world, suggesting that this second wave did not adequately include those whose identities developed along plural axes. Butler's critique was that second-wave feminism's gender discourse merely reproduces heteronormativity

W. Ocha, Ph.D. (✉)
Rangsit University, International College (Building 11, 2nd Floor) 52/347 Muang-Ake, Paholyothin Road. Lak-Hok, Pathumthani, 12000, Thailand
e-mail: witchayaneeocha@gmail.com

P. Liamputtong (ed.), *Contemporary Socio-Cultural and Political Perspectives in Thailand*,
DOI 10.1007/978-94-007-7244-1_25,

and in doing so, performs a great disservice to nonnormative women. Butler's works (1990) "Gender Trouble" gave rise to third-wave feminism as a critique of the second wave. Earth (2006: 7) writes: "Many exponents of the third wave consider male to female transgenders to be a further category of the female gender and therefore a legitimate inclusion to the women's movement." The gay liberation movement has long recognized the rights of transvestites,[1] transsexuals,[2] and intersex[3] people located on the fringes of the gay movement. The convergence of feminism and the gay liberation movement, essentially through the emergence of third-wave feminism recognizing more marginal sexualities, has resulted in the emergence of "queer" as an inclusive category. Queer includes many diverse and marginal sexualities, intersex people and transgenders. Gender is not a continuum stretching between binary opposites, but a multidimensional space in which a galaxy of possibilities exists. The visible nature of these marginalized sexualities in Thailand has encouraged those who visit to perceive a sexually free culture, whatever the actual truth may be.

2 Medical Technology

Aizura (2011: 144) points out that "Thailand is now known by many as one of the premier sites worldwide to obtain vaginoplasty and other cosmetic surgeries; indeed, many surgeons advertise that Bangkok is the 'Mecca' of transsexual body modification." Winter (2004: 7) too writes that "Thailand probably boasts one of the highest incidences of transgenders worldwide. No one knows for sure how many transgenders there are, but the figures range from 10,000 to 300,000. Even the lowest of these figures would put the incidence way above western countries." Although exact numbers for the transgender population are elusive, "the estimated ratio of transgender to straight men is 1:30,000" (Banyanathee and Piyyopornpanit 1999: 324). Nowadays, Thailand is a popular place for sex-change operations not only for Thais but also for foreigners, because there are many clinics which produce satisfactory results and are less expensive than in the west (Totman 2003).

[1] Transsexual (MTF) male to female transgenders who have had full sex reassignment surgery to be full female (outwardly appearing).

[2] Queer includes many diverse and marginal sexualities, intersex people: "human beings whose biological sex cannot be classified as clearly male or female" (Money and Ehrhardt 1972; Domurat 2001) and transgenders. The convergence of feminism and the gay liberation movement, essentially through the emergence of third-wave feminism recognizing more marginal sexualities, has resulted in the emergence of "Queer" as an inclusive category (Jagose 1996). *Queer theory* studies and has a political critique of anything that falls into normative and deviant categories, particularly sexual activities and identities.

[3] "The term 'transgender' is widely used to encompass transsexual people, cross-dressers or intersex" (Tirohl 2007:287): "to described those who do not conform to the expected roles of either male or female" (Chau and Herring 2002: 333).

Tiewtranon and Chokrungvaranont (2004) note that sex reassignment surgery (SRS), considered as a medical treatment for GID, to change the body to fit the self-image, was established in 1975 in Thailand. However, this specific treatment requires a large budget both before and after the operation. Many transgenders (referred to as *kathoeys* in Thai – see Chap. 26 in this volume) enter the sex trade with the promise of easy money to save for this specific purpose. It does not mean that every transgender has a chance to have this specific treatment. Transgenders who wish to undergo surgical treatments but do not have the financial means to achieve this still maintain a fully male body but continue with their diverse sexual preferences.

3 Thailand's Sex Tourism

According to Gallagher (2005: 1), "sex tourism has received minimal attention in academic arenas and consequently remains under-theorized and restrictively conceptualized as brief sex-for-money exchanges between heterosexual men and brothel-based female sex workers. However, these images are becoming increasingly divorced from the realities of Thailand's sex tourism industry in the twenty first century." Gallagher (2005; cited in Ocha 2013: 202) notes that "alongside female sex workers, burgeoning numbers of male and transgender (*kathoey*) sex workers are now serving male, female and transgender tourists."

Thailand is known as "*the* sex tourist destination" (Gallagher 2005: 4), and although this is still a valid viewpoint, the nature of that sex has begun to shift dramatically in recent years, with male and transgender sex workers now increasing in number to serve in the sex tourism market (Ocha 2012). Gallagher (2005; cited in Ocha 2012: 566) states that "two salient trends in particular have emerged: the growing heterogeneity of sex tourists and the variety of sex workers and, sexual-economic exchanges." The tourism campaign often promotes Thailand as "exotic and erotic" in an attempt to attract tourists. The sex industry appears to be drawn to Thailand as a place for these emerging other sexual forms to flourish and feel welcomed (Ocha 2012). Therefore, the global sex industry is very much the source stabilizing and driving forward the creation of new gender identities that are becoming a more visible element of the sex industry in the contemporary period of Thailand (see also Chaps. 19, 20, 23, and 26 in this volume on sex industry in Thailand).

The study on which this chapter is based was conducted in Thailand's sex tourist industry. It reveals that economic exchange diversifies more sexual practices and performativity (Butler 1990)[4] is maximized. The research shows that the capitalization of the sex industry is opening new possibilities of gender identities, which are

[4] Performativity is the condition of sexuality of a person who has been exposed to certain influencing factors. These factors can never be constant from person to person, and therefore sexualities developing in response to these factors will be different in every case, giving rise to the notion of "endless performativity" by Judith Butler (1990).

influenced by the modernization of sex work as well as the medical technologies, which have superimposed on the Thai transgender identities (Ocha 2012). These make gender concepts even more complex. Finally, the chapter concludes that bodies are plural and very diverse. There are not just two kinds. There are multiple kinds of bodies and lots of differences among them. Even in reproductive biology, human bodies are not strictly dimorphic. There is a complex group of intersex categories, such as people with extra or missing or damaged chromosomes. Connell (2000: 23) says this clearly: "These categories have long fascinated sexologists; they do not correspond in any simple way to behavior or a sense of identity."

4 Gender Performativity

Judith Butler (1990) explains her notion of performativity in simple terms showing that it is in no way related only to stage performances or drag. Performativity implies that a process of iteration of situations and occurrences that constitutes the subjects' condition and shapes and leads the subject down a particular path of behaviors. Accordingly, "iteration implies repetitiveness and this, coupled with the threat of ostracism through threat or taboo; even death can shape the production of behaviors but not fully determine them in advance of current situations" (Butler 1990: 17).

Performativity then is the conditioned sexuality of a person who has been exposed to certain influencing factors. These factors can never be constant from person to person, and therefore sexualities developing in response to these factors will be different in every case and constantly in flux as more iterations play out giving rise to the concept of "endless performativity" (Butler 1990).

Drawing on the work of Judith Butler (1990), a conceptual framework of the study is to explain how the global-Thai sex sector is creating/re-creating under the context of globalization. The sex industry in Thailand has in fact been a key source of proliferation of diverse performativity among sex workers. The research aims to explore areas of "performativity" as producing/reproducing by sex workers as well as the effect of the medical technology resulting in "gender diversification." Gender as a concept has to be accommodated, including all the variations of Thai gender discourse impacted on globalization in the contemporary period. See also Chap. 26 for other interesting theories regarding gender performativity (Fig. 25.1).

5 The Study

Between 2006 and 2009, I interviewed 65 male to female transgender sex workers who were working in the famous tourism hot spots: the cities of Bangkok and Pattaya in Thailand. Within the research framework, the primary method of gathering data was in-depth interviews. The respondents were recruited from those who could provide expert or semi-expert opinions regarding their gender/sexual identities.

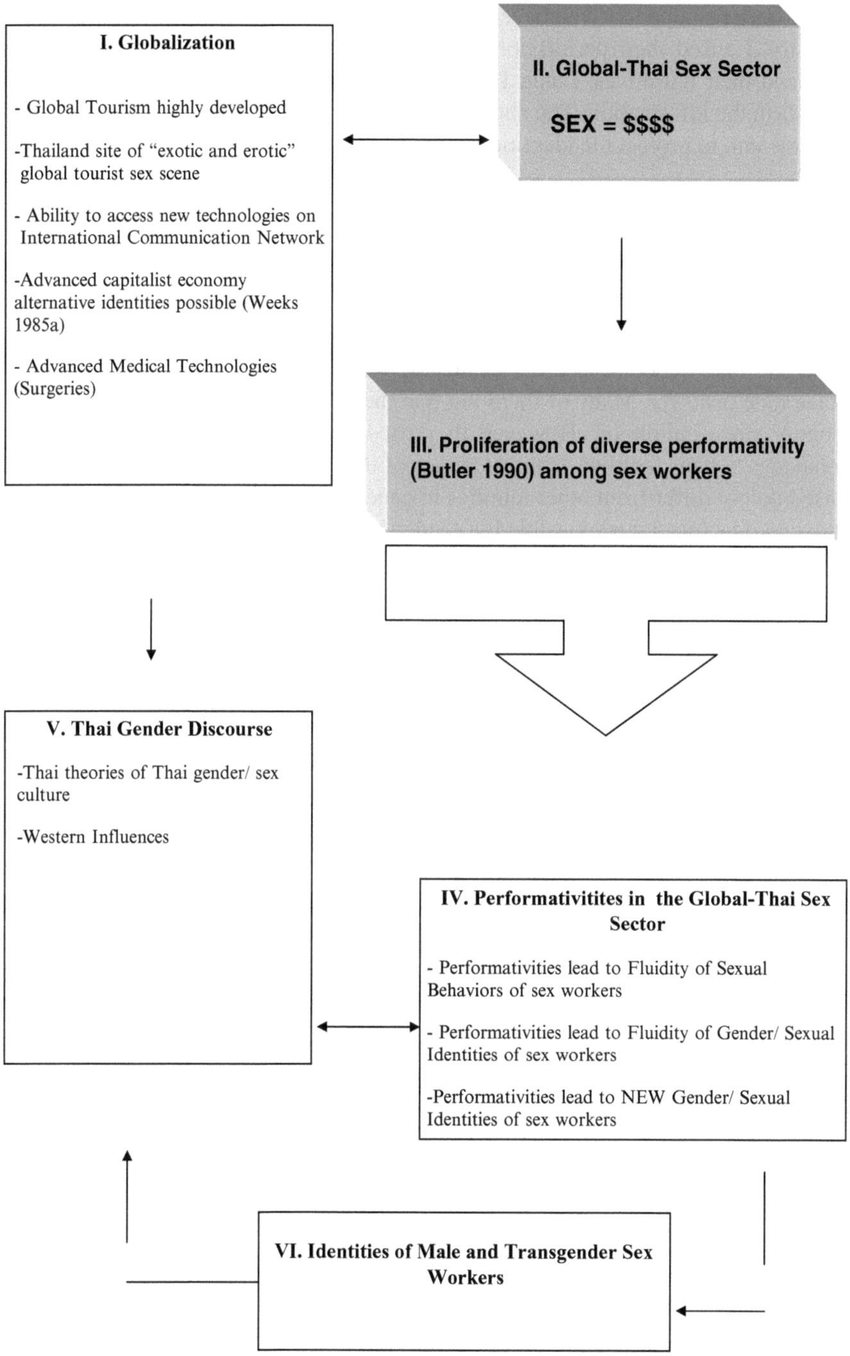

Fig. 25.1 Conceptual framework of research. How globalization shapes gender/sexual identities in the Thai contemporary period?

These were respondents who have more than a year's experience in the sex tourism industry. I asked their permission to interview them and carefully recorded and analyzed their narratives. Later, I returned the conclusions for them to audit and reconfirm the information. The names mentioned in this chapter have been changed with the aim to protect the identities of the respondents.

6 Transsexuals (Full Transformation)

The study finds that the participants have an age range of between 17 and 37 years. Nine had high school education or higher, while the majority had quit school at grade nine or lower. Many of them felt that they wished to have a female physical identity since childhood. However, they tried to avoid showing gender-bending behaviors to their families. Characteristics of their family and how they have been raised do not differ from other families in general. It is not able to confirm that the above two factors are responsible for gender-bending behaviors.

The tourist sex sector is the key to accomplishing a female body both by creating the demand for transsexual sex services and by being the one place where transgenders can access the amounts of money needed to acquire and maintain a female body. All 25 informants entered the sex trade because it was a place that both demanded and paid for a transsexual body. Their self-motivation on sex reassignment surgery was explained in different ways.

> I have been attracted to men so this makes me think I'm probably a woman. (Prim, 27 years old, a sex worker in a Go-Go bar in Patpong)
>
> I feel I am a woman so I think that I have to like men. (Tik, 23 years old, a sex worker in Host Bar in Patpong)
>
> I am not a woman but I just want a female body. (Nok Yung, 30 years old, Nang Show in a Calypso Cabaret Patpong)

These are three samples of transsexual group who received sex reassignment surgery (SRS) in the same year (2002). Nok Yung, Prim, and Tik received their sex reassignment surgery from three different hospitals. Nok Yung was a waiter in the restaurant in Pattaya before the operations. Prim and Tik have been working in the sex industry since they began employment. Nok Yung cross-dressed and appeared to have a feminine identity after undergoing full gender reassignment operations, breast augmentation and vaginoplasty, while Prim and Tik start cross-dressing before undergoing the surgical operations. Their practical experiences and comparisons from before and after the full operation are explained in the following Table 25.1.

The gender transforming ideologies can be explained through the above table. There are various sexual identities among the respondent group, representatives from both before and after the SRS, and it is evident that their sexual preferences do not necessarily correspond to their gender identities. Tik has a transvestite identity before the surgery but performs sexual acts with her clients as a man (vaginal intercourse-top with women). Generally, in the case of male to female transgenders, the gender identity, either female or third sex, develops well before sexual preference,

Table 25.1 Before/after sex reassignment surgery (SRS)

	Nok Yung	Prim	Tik
1. Surgical status	Postoperations	Postoperations	Postoperations
2. Marital status	Divorced with two kids	Never married	Never married
3. Career/education	High school diploma	Primary school	Vocational degree
4. Gender identity realization (coming out)	Neither man nor woman since 13	Third sex (gender-bending behaviors) since 8	Claims feeling trapped in the wrong body since 4–5
5. Gender presentation prior to SRS	Man	Female (hormones, cross-dressing, breast implants)	Transvestites
6. Preferred sexual activities/partner(s) prior to SRS	Anal sex-bottom with men Vaginal intercourse-top with women	Anal sex-bottom with men	Vaginal intercourse-top with women
7. Sexual orgasm prior to SRS	Strong psychological	Male's orgasm but not strong psychological	Male's orgasm
8. Sexual orgasm after SRS	Fake orgasm	Women's orgasm	Mostly psychological
9. Preferred sexual activities/partner(s) after SRS	Vaginal intercourse-bottom with men and lesbian sex (passive role) to women	Vaginal intercourse-bottom with men	Vaginal intercourse-bottom with men
10. Gender presentation after SRS	M to F transsexual	M to F transsexual	M to F transsexual
11. Sexual objectives practice	Everyday (oral/vaginal/anal)	Two to three times a day (vaginal/oral/hand)	Everyday (vaginal/oral/hand)
12. Stability of sexual preferences	Unstable	Stable men	Rather stable
13. Religious practices	Meditation	Visit temples	Donation and reading Buddhist Principle
14. Satisfaction with SRS	Not quite	Satisfied	Quite satisfied
15. Consequences problems after SRS	Not being able to reach women orgasm	Specific treatments and money are required to maintain the body	Not able to reach orgasm as before
16. If they could go back to the phase before operation, would they do it?	No	Yes, but would choose to apply SRS in other hospital	Yes, but would study more in depth for side effects from transsexual side, not from doctor's side!

Source: Compiled from in-depth interviews, 2006–2009

but there are a few, such as Prim, who find that their sexual preferences lead them to develop their own gender identity. This group tends to develop essentially as young women, developing what they see as a heterosexual attraction to men in the same way any natural woman would. From an early age, they feel that they are woman on the inside. Prim adhered strictly to sexual acts with men which she performed anal sex-bottom with men before SRS but now performs vaginal intercourse-bottom with men. Nok Yung was bisexual and performed anal sex-bottom with men and vaginal intercourse-top with women, but after SRS, she usually performs vaginal intercourse-bottom with men and lesbian sex (passive) with women. Tik performed vaginal intercourse-top with women, and after SRS, she usually performs vaginal intercourse-bottom with men and she sometimes can also perform lesbian sex (passive) with women.

7 Subsequent Problems After Surgical Operations

"Human monster" (*a-manut*) is translated from the Thai word "*a-manut*" by transgenders themselves (Ocha 2012). They refer to themselves as "sick human beings" after the surgery turned out badly and made them into something unrecognizable in Thailand. Some transgenders are dissatisfied with the medical technology they undergo as they can suffer unforeseen consequences and side effects. For identity purposes, some male to female transgenders still want to become transsexuals, while others do not think this necessary. Knowledge of the side effects the surgery could bring is passed through the community by word of mouth, generally spread by the older generation of transsexuals to the young generation. This knowledge in some cases does give them cause for concern, and this, coupled with the financial issues, may encourage them not to go ahead with the surgery. This shows that these two groups are different in the form of body.

From the fieldwork, 7 out of the total 25 transsexuals were satisfied with the result of their surgeries, despite the special care, knowledge, and extra money required to maintain the new anatomy. The remaining 18 transsexuals complained about side effects, and their satisfaction with the surgeries varies, depending on the severity of the side effects they experience. Furthermore, ten transsexuals accepted that if they could go back to the phase before the sex-change operation (vaginoplasty), they would not have had the surgery done since a vaginoplasty would generally have more serious side effects than having breast implants, and a vaginoplasty is irreversible.

Tina was one sex worker who has undergone SRS three times within 10 years by three different doctors. She accepted that regular health checks and money are required with specific treatments to maintain the new anatomy. In order to control the long-term effects after surgeries, it means raising more and more money when she gets older. She is now a long-term patient who will require medical treatments forever.

Nira, 32 years old, a sex worker in Patpong, had to remove her silicone breasts when the size and shape did not turn out right 3 years after the surgery. She was performing sexual services with unnatural body (vagina but no breasts) during that time. It took her a year to collect money and once again have breast implants to enable her to look perfectly feminine. She said that many of her transsexual friends experienced unsatisfactory results after surgeries but some did not have money to correct them. These people are living as "human monsters" (*a-manut*), and three of Niras transsexual friends who were suffering from side effects after the surgeries committed suicide 3 years ago, one by stabbing herself and two by jumping from tall buildings.

I contend that important to all transgenders are questions relating to whether or not to undergo a full sex-change operation. Is full sex reassignment worth the risk? Is full transformation the only way to be more fully themselves? Or is it possible to have a compromise? These are current discussions in the subcultures. This might be an exploitation of a growing numbers of "unnatural" bodies in Thailand's sex tourism.

8 Transgenders with Unnatural Bodies (Semi-reassigned State)

This group of respondents is, on average, aged between 20 and 35 years. Most of them did not graduate from high school, generally exhibiting a lower level of education than fully transsexual sex workers. Transgender (breasts, penis and vagina, no breasts) sex workers usually appear feminine identities (cross-dress) in public spheres which are difficult to distinguish from transsexuals. They engaged in sex work as a full-time job. There were some however who work part time when their bodies are not yet ready for sexual services due to medical treatments. They drink and talk with tourists for some hours but do not work full time or provide sexual services. It was difficult for them to gain mainstream employment when their gender identities do not fit with the gender indicated on their identity card. Some transgenders who have "unnatural body" reported experiencing criminal charges for submitting fake identity cards for job applications.

Out of the total of 40 transgenders with a feminine identity (on stage), 32 received breast implants but maintain their natural genitalia. Out of these 32 transgenders, 7 were waiting to receive a vaginoplasty in the near future to become complete transsexuals, while 25 were satisfied with an unnatural body, having breasts and a penis. Eight have received a vaginoplasty but did not have breast augmentation, and from those eight transgenders, five planned to receive breast implants when they have sufficient finance, while three are satisfied without breast implants. Characteristics of the family and the way transgenders have been raised do not differ from other families in general, and this study is not able to speculate on the above two factors being responsible for one becoming a transgender. Some felt that they were actually female from birth, while some felt their physical sex was incorrect once they entered puberty. Other members of the family accept the identity of these transgenders with unnatural bodies gradually and to varying degrees. The various bodies and intentions regarding their bodies are summarized as follows:

9 Transformation of Gender Identities of Semi-reassigned State (Breast with Penis) Transgenders

9.1 *Mint (Type A1)*

Mint (22 years old, an artist in Patpong) is a transgender who called herself a *sao siap* (a woman who can penetrate). Like other transgenders, she dreamed of having a great female figure but after the breast implants, found great pleasure in her ambiguous body.

> I have been wearing female costumes since I was 15 years old. My desire to have full sex reassignment surgery has changed through time. I started with breast implants at the age 18 because I wanted to get a job as an artiste in a cabaret theatre. I felt that I needed breasts, vagina, and beautiful legs to be a success in my career. I have been using the plastic tape to hide my penis but I was very disappointed that I couldn't wear some specific female costumes. It was at this time that I felt that I really wanted to go ahead with a vaginoplasty…
>
> When I was saving money to for the vaginoplasty. I met a boyfriend who liked my penis. I also heard from many of my transsexual friends that they lost their sexual feelings after this operation and felt that having a vagina was not worth losing my sex drive and the pleasure of sex. I want to stay as *sao siap* (a woman who can penetrate). I feel comfortable as *sao siap*.

9.2 *Num Fon (Type B1)*

Num Fon (27 years old, a sex worker in Patpong) is one of the five transgenders who have had a vaginoplasty and rejected to apply breast implants in the near future. Num Fon began to perform all kinds of sex with men in the sex industry before having the vaginoplasty. After the operation, Num Fon had to learn to perform receptive vaginal intercourse which she described as not easy because she had to get used to having new and different genitals and the way that sex feels and makes her feel. Num Fon was one of three transgenders in the respondent group who decided against breast augmentation, while five of the others expect to have breast implants in the near future. Num Fon mentioned in the interview that the fluidity of her sexuality corresponds to her new anatomy. She felt that without the vaginoplasty, she could perform as a homosexual male but was unable to be a fully functioning female. After the surgery, she was limited to performing as a heterosexual female.

> There is no rule governing which part of the body should be operated on first. Some start with the upper part, some start the lower part, some struggle to decide due to insufficient budget or instability of sexual preferences and some are afraid of the side effects. I first

> started my sexual services (all kind of sex) strictly with men tourists but five years later, I had a vaginoplasty with the plan to have a complete female body. When I had enough money for breast implants…I was not sure if I still wanted to do it.
>
> I can always cross-dress and use breast enhancers or push ups for a great feminine feature. I have seen my friends who have had breast implants…they looked far different from nature in terms of size and shape. They need a lot of money to maintain the silicone breasts and to cope with all the consequences and problems when we get older and older. No, I don't think I want breast implants anymore.
>
> The money for the breast implants is saved in my bank account. It is much cheaper to buy just breast enhancers. I perform only vaginal intercourse-bottom/ anal sex-bottom with men at the moment…and my tourists do not mind about my body. My boyfriend is ok with my unnatural body and I have a few sizes of breast enhancers to fit different costumes. Oh Yeah, I do feel comfortable this way.

These are examples of transgenders out of the total of 40. All of them showed different kinds of identities comprising distinct subjectivities and sexuality in distinct way. Num Wan was one of the 32 transgenders in this study who was satisfied with the semi-reassigned state (breast with penis).

Here, his/her transformation of body is followed though the phases. Nok Yung, Prim, Tik, and Num Wan were visitors to the Empower Foundation on the fifth of May 2006. At that time, Nok Yung, Prim, and Tik displayed cross-dressing behavior and appear to the public as feminine, while Num Wan had not yet decided to cross-dress. Num Wan was confused about his/her own identity, and I was interested in examining his/her identity transformation and behaviors. The phases of transformation of Nam Wan will now be analyzed.

9.3 Gender Transforming Ideologies: The Case Study of Num Wan

9.3.1 The 1st Phase (May 2006): "I'm accepted as a man"

Num Wan felt that he/she was accepted as a man in the relationship with his/her female lover; they shared a heterosexual relationship with each other. Num Wan served as both vaginal intercourses-top with women and anal sex top/bottom with men tourists in Patpong. Nok Yung (Num Wan's friend) was the first person Num Wan told that he/she was not happy being a man. It was Nok Yung who recognized Num Wan's confused identity and changed his/her attitude and behavior toward him/her.

9.3.2 The 2nd Phase (Sept. 2006): "I'm not happy to be treated as a man"

In this phase, Num Wan suffered mental conflict and was frustrated at being treated as a man by others; this was exacerbated when his/her lover wanted others to treat him/her as a man. All sexual services provided for both men and women tourists that he/she performed created more pressure for Num Wan when he/she was not sure who he/she was. Nam Wan would ask himself/herself: What is my gender identity and actual preference?

9.3.3 The 3rd Phase (Jan. 2007): "I can't belong to both categories of man and woman"

Num Wan was feeling isolated from others, even his/her own female lover and said: "*Women consider me as a man, and some men feel that I am actually a man but slightly different.*" At that time, Num Wan felt closest to transgender people like Nok Yung, Prim, and Tik. Num Wan started to take female hormones orally and dress up as a woman at times.

9.3.4 The 4th Phase (May 2007): "I discovered that I'm very definite in my perception of the categories of man and woman"

In the 4th phase, Num Wan was suspicious about his/her female lover who warned him/her to behave in a manly fashion. Num Wan felt that this was an attempt to control his/her gender. Eventually, this control by his/her female lover annoyed Num Wan, and the relationship ended when Num Wan decided to dress up as a woman permanently like Nok Yung, Prim, and Tik.

9.3.5 The 5th Phase (Dec. 2008): "It doesn't matter whether people treat me either as a man or a woman"

The 5th phase is divided into three parts. Each part enhances Num Wan's self-narrative: "*I won't be controlled by the treatment of others.*" Num Wan's girlfriend expected him/her to behave in a manly fashion, disregarding how he/she feels inside. Many of Num Wan's clients expected female behaviors, Num Wan's friends consider him/her to be a man but slightly different, and Num Wan felt being pulled in different directions.

Part 1. "I just want a female body"
Num Wan's view changed from wanting to be treated by others as a woman to just wishing to have a female body. At this phase, Num Wan decided to receive breast implants.

Part 2. "I had a boyfriend"
Nam Wan had a boyfriend who was initially just a friend. This had an enormously positive effect, and Num Wan began to consider having sex reassignment surgery. Nam Wan was convinced from this new relationship that he/she probably is a woman.

Part 3. "I haven't ever had 'woman education'"
Num Wan began to realize that the boyfriend liked his/her penis and felt satisfied with the unnatural body. He/she performed both anal sex-top/bottom with his/her boyfriend and men tourists. After some time, Num Wan noticed the fact that women have a "certain aura" which is instilled in them from birth and developed through life and became convinced that he/she could not learn to emulate this aura.

9.3.6 The 6th Phase (Mar. 2009): "I decided to live as a transgender with unnatural body though I'm disconcerted by others' suspicious glances"

Num Wan decided to live as *sao siap* and no longer desired to be treated as a real woman. Num Wan expressed this phase as the "delicate phase."

9.3.7 The 7th Phase (July 2009): "I want to be myself but my feelings vary according to the situation at the time"

Num Wan had a concrete desire that he/she should be treated as a person who is a transgender (breasts with a penis) but realized that his/her feelings varied according to the present situation because he/she was also a person living everyday life. The story of Num Wan demonstrated the concept of fluidity of sexuality; he/she was not sure if the *sao siap* identity was his/her stable identity and accepted that it may change with time and his/her situation at any point in life. The factors which could affect a change Num Wan's gender identity are place, time, situation, clients, and of course, the preferences of his/her own lover.

In the Thai sex tourism's industry, the unique selling point of the transgenders who have unnatural bodies (breasts with a penis) or *sao siap* (a woman who can penetrate) is the ability to perform both anal sex-bottom and anal sex-top in private while outwardly displaying a perfectly feminine identity in public. This allows their male partners to keep up the pretense of a heterosexual status in public (Ocha 2013). There were seven tourists interviewed during the fieldwork who accept that they prefer transgenders with unnatural bodies who cross-dressed, behave with a feminine identity, but maintain a penis.

Transgenders with unnatural bodies have not been well known in society until recently despite the long and gradual process of change undergone to transform from a full male to an outwardly appearing full-female body. The gender identities of these transsexuals must change on a sliding scale between full male and full female from the beginning up to the point of complete transformation. Previously, transsexuals were probably less open about their partially gender reassigned bodies than they are in the present day, and some transgenders are happy to remain in this semi-reassigned state and do not desire the full reassignment surgery. These new gender identities are expressed freely in Thailand's sex tourism industry in the twenty-first century, but was kept hidden in other areas of Thai society in the past.

Presently, transgenders with unnatural bodies especially *sao siaps* have become available in the sex industry alongside transsexuals. These *sao siaps* advertise the fact that they can offer a choice of unique sexual experience. Not only do these new gender identities hope to be recognized in the Thai society, but there are also reports of growing demand in foreign countries (Yamphaka 2007: 13).

The globalization of the sex industry is not only responsible for driving the fluidity of sexual behaviors/identities in Thailand. It is one of the factors responsible for the creation of new gender/sexual identities (Ocha 2012). This driving force of financial gain brought by the global sex trade when coupled with advancing medical technology and the unlimited human imagination allows the argument that new gender/sexual identities are and will continue to be created in order to satisfy the sexual desires of those who can afford to pay for them. The chapter confirms that transgenders who are satisfied with their semi-reassigned state have their own identities, providing a different kind of sexual service than transsexual sex workers. These new gender identities have their own market and their own customers with the sex industry providing the secure environment in which they can flourish. This evidence of transgender with unnatural bodies demonstrating a differing self-identity from that of the transsexual (full transformation) inserts another identity into the scale between male and female, adding evidence for the fluidity of sexuality. These identities would be difficult to differentiate without the now available medical technology to enable a physical demonstration of their differences, but it is unlikely that they are a new phenomenon, just emerging in this world of technology, rather that the technology allows the realization of their inner identity.

10 Discussion and Conclusion

The global tourist-Thai sex sector in Bangkok and Pattaya is large and dynamic, but experiences of gender-variant people are not widely appreciated due to social marginalization. Drawing on the work of Judith Butler (1990) on "endless performativity" concept, the study demonstrates that each person is a product of the situations and experiences that are lived through and that the performativity demonstrated by the sex workers cannot be understood outside of a process of iteration, a repetition of events, or situations experienced through their life in the sex industry. The experience in the commercial sex industry may impact on both new forms of gender/sexual and identities of sex workers. This study fills the "gaps" in the knowledge of body, sex, gender, sexualities, and new subject positions that still need to be understood at national and international levels in order to arrive at an accurate understanding of the concept of gender in Thailand today.

This chapter argues that in order to understand gender as a historical category, it requires a recognition that gender, understood as one way of culturally configuring a body, is fluid and constantly in flux, and that the relationship between anatomy and sex is not rigidly set out as the transgenders have clearly shown. Butler (1990: 63) contends that "gender is a different sort of identity" in which identity is repetitively constituted, "and its relation to body reference is complex." My research has set out to prove this by demonstrating empirically the great diversity of life experiences, which cannot be described as conforming to hegemonic models of masculinity or femininity. The male to female transgenders show that gender is the sort of identities, and that they can mimic or even change nature using medical technologies, opposing themselves from social constructionists (Ocha 2013). Medical technology can respond to human needs in a corrective capacity by helping match the body to the state of mind of transgender people, but they can also be used in a creative capacity, encouraging and providing the means for people to change or create new genders in order to profit from the resulting "unnatural" body in Thailand's sex tourism.

The sex tourism is a major site of new sexual and gender expressions that can inform a more complex concept of gender. Weeks (1985; cited in Ocha 2012: 198) suggests that "the impact of global capitalism may affect life style changes that enable gender and sexuality to diversify." Transgender sex workers (*kathoeys*) are the most visible faces of these diversifying forms emerging, and the "gender diversification" by advanced medical technology suggests that various gender possibilities are open in Thailand. The desire of a unique experience of foreign tourists on holiday is one of the driving forces, encouraging positively tolerated environment on the modification of the human bodies on "transgender" sex workers in Thailand's sex tourism.

Since medical technology allows humans to change their sexual anatomy, the link between gender and performativity must be relearned. The subjectivity/practice unity offers a new formulation for the study of gender diversification which everyone has rights to self-expressions as human beings. The chapter shows that transgenders who are happy to remain in the semi-reassigned state ought to be understood as engaged in a practice of self-determination, an exercise of autonomy. As Cornwall (2007: 76) contends, "if the 'gender agenda' is ultimately about redressing that which is unfair and unjust and challenging unequal privilege, then surely a focus on the changes that those who pursue it wish to see happen- greater fulfillment of human rights, equality, wellbeing and justice," it is time, then, to refocus the "gender agenda" more explicitly not only on women's right but also paying attention to "gender diversification." In the backdrop of these quiet but real stories, the decision of the UN Human Rights Council to pass a historical resolution that seeks equal rights for all regardless of sexual orientation on June 17, 2011 is just a drop of morning dew in a thick forest of marginalization and discrimination (Ocha 2011).

References

Aizura, A. (2011). The romance of the amazing scalpel: "Race", labour, and affect in Thai gender reassignment clinics. In P. Jackson (Ed.), *Queer Bangkok: 21st century markets, media and rights* (pp. 143–162). Hong Kong: Hong Kong University Press.

Banyanathee, W., & Piyyopornpanit, M. (1999). The dynamic of sex tourism: The case of Southeast Asia. In S. Rungetrakul (Ed.), *Tumra Sitawetchasart* [Abnormal psychology]. Banghok: Ruen Kaw Publisher.

Butler, J. (1990). *Gender trouble: Feminism and the subversion of identity*. New York: Routledge.

Chau, P. I., & Herring, J. (2002). Defining, assigning and designing sex. *International Journal of Law, Policy and the Family, 16*, 327–367.
Connell, R. W. (2000). *The men and boys*. Cambridge: Policy Press.
Cornwall, A. (2007). Revisiting 'gender agenda'. *IDS Bulletin, 38*(2), 69–78.
Domurat, D. A. (2001). *Hermaphrodites and the medical invention of sex*. Cambridge, MA: Harvard University Press.
Earth, B. (2006). Diversifying gender: Male to female transgender identities and HIV/AIDS programming in Phnom Penh, Cambodia. *Gender and Development Journal, 14*(2), 258–271.
Gallagher, R. (2005, July 7–9). *Shifting market, shifting risks: Male and transgender tourist-oriented sex work in South-East Asia*. Paper presented at "Sexualities, Genders and Rights in Asia: The first International Conference of Queer Studies," organized by the Office of Human Rights Studies and Social Development at Mahidol University and the Asia Pacific Queer Network, at Ambassador Hotel, Bangkok, Thailand.
Jagose, A. (1996). *Queer theory: An introduction*. New York: New York University Press.
Money, J., & Ehrhardt, A. (1972). *Man & woman, boy & girl: Differentiation and dimorphism of gender identity from conception to maturity*. Baltimore: The Johns Hopkins University Press.
Ocha, W. (2011). Thai transsexual's experiences with discrimination in employment: Migration and commercial sex in Thailand and The Netherlands. In A. Sharon, S. Petcharamesree, & Y. Sumarlan (Eds.), *Breaking the silence* (pp. 227–240). Bangkok: The South East Asian Human Rights Studies Network (SEAHRN).
Ocha, W. (2012). Transsexual emergence: Gender Variant identities in Thailand. *Culture, Health & Sexuality: An International Journal for Research Intervention and Care, 14*(5), 563–575.
Ocha, W. (2013). Identity diversification among transgender sex workers in Thailand's sex tourism industry. *SEXUALITIE. The Study of Society and Culture, 16*(1/2), 195–216.
Tiewtranon, P., & Chokrungvaranont, P. (2004). Sex reassignment surgery in Thailand. *Journal of Medicine Thai, 8*(11), 1404–1405.
Tirohl, B. (2007). A study of the rights of cross-dressers in the UK. *Journal of Gender Studies, 16*(3), 277–289.
Totman, R. (2003). *The third sex: Kathoey – Thailand's ladyboys*. London: Souvenir Press Ltd.
Weeks, J. (1985). *Sexuality and its discontents: Meanings, myths and modern sexualities*. London: Routledge and Kegan Paul.
Winter, S. (2004). Transgender and society: An Asian perspective. *Gender Identity Disorder (GID) Journal, 2*(1), 7–13.
Yamphaka, J. (2007, June 13). Thai kathoeys go international. *Manager Newspaper Daily News*, p. 13.

Chapter 26
Conceptualizing Thai Genderscapes: Transformation and Continuity in the Thai Sex/Gender System

Dredge Byung'chu Käng

1 Introduction

The blockbuster film *Iron Ladies* (2000, directed by Yongyoot Thongkongtoon), based on a true story, about a team of *gay* and *kathoey* players coached by a *tom* that won the national volleyball championship, kick-started an explosion in the representation of transgenderism and homosexuality in mainstream Thai media. At the time of its release, the film was the highest-grossing Thai film ever. Although *Iron Ladies* advocates for the rights of gender minorities, in reality, many of the players were barred from international competition, to maintain the country's reputation. The state, previously self-conscious about the androgyny of its female population, is now discomfited about a male population that is deemed too feminine. Nevertheless, the film also acts to legitimize Thai gender diversity in its portrayal of five genders.

In this chapter, I expand on the notion of "-scape" (Appadurai 1996: 33) in conceptualizing genderscapes in Thailand, which can act as a case study in developing genderscapes elsewhere. I argue for the conceptualization of a Thai sex/gender system, or genderscapes, based on five key gender categories.[1] I explore the cultural logics of naming and transformations in meaning ascribed to gender-variant people and describe the contemporary genderscapes, or the conceptual distribution of gender/sexuality forms in everyday practice as they are conditioned by fields of uneven power. I contend that genderscapes provide an enhanced theorization of contemporary

[1] This research is part of a larger project comparing how class structures *kathoey* and *gay* life opportunities, romantic partner preferences, and risk for HIV. Anthropological fieldwork consisting of participant observation, in-depth interviews, and discourse analysis of media was conducted for 42 months between 2004 and 2011 with approximately 300 *gay/kathoey* informants and their families and friends. Emphasis was placed on class differences and East Asian cultural flows.

D.B. Käng (✉)
Departments of Anthropology, Epidemiology, and Global Health, Emory University,
207 Anthropology Building, 1557 Dickey Drive, Atlanta, GA 30322, USA
e-mail: dredge@alum.emory.edu

P. Liamputtong (ed.), *Contemporary Socio-Cultural and Political Perspectives in Thailand*, 409
DOI 10.1007/978-94-007-7244-1_26, © Springer Science+Business Media Dordrecht 2014

Thai gender categories. The lines between *tom* : woman : *kathoey* : *gay* : man are neither clear nor fixed, but coalesce around these key formations.[2] These categories are grounded via the repetition and ritualization of routine practices in everyday life as they appear to others but also remain fluid in that gender performances exceed their intentions and interpretations.

My aim in articulating the localized field of gender and sexual diversity as "genderscapes" is to integrate prior scholarship in the Thai sex/gender system, which, in turn, destabilizes universal notions of sexual dimorphism and heterosexual compulsion through cross-cultural comparison. I intentionally use the plural Thai "genderscapes" to denote the contextual and perspectival figuration of any given genderscape at a time, such that genderscapes are always plural between people and even within a person given a particular situation or focus. The conceptual configuration of genderscapes shifts depending on the dimension of gender being considered (e.g., self-presentation and desire) or an individual's social position and ideological perspective (e.g., academics, activists, artists, clergy, general actors, political figures, and sexual minorities). I underscore that the contemporary terrain of gender/sexuality is habituated by one's class position and shaped by social evaluation and moral legitimacy.

2 Historical Background and Theoretical Framework

2.1 Transformations in the Thai Sex/Gender System

Thailand is the only country in Southeast Asia that circumvented direct colonization. Without a colonial power, in either direct or indirect senses, Thailand is characterized by its semicolonial status (Jackson 2010). Yet, colonial history is important in understanding Thai gender/sexuality because the threat of foreign encroachment and subsequent nationalist modernization projects reformulated gender and produced unexpected consequences in gender relations. In part, Siam avoided external rule by proffering and employing autocolonial practices to demonstrate its *siwilai* (civilized) status (Winichakul 1994, 2000, 2010). While it would seem that these effects are more indirect since Thailand was never colonized, the consolidation of monarchical power and colonial impulse in the pursuit of *siwilai* actually heightened the ability of the state to recast cultural conventions. Arguably, autocolonial governmentality in Thailand was more direct and stronger a force of change than that imposed in its colonized neighbors by European rule. An intact absolute monarchy followed by a constitutional monarchy provided greater ability of the state to model and legislate gender norms than was possible in the colonies. For Thailand to

[2] Nouns from Thai are not modified to express plural form. That is, like "sheep," the plural of "*kathoey*" is "*kathoey*." Thai transliteration is rendered in a modified version of the Royal Institute system unless a common or preferred rendition exists.

remain free from Western domination, the population was subjected to new forms of rule (Connors 2007). One should not, however, romanticize the Thai past as a place of greater gender pluralism or egalitarianism.

The project of modernization contrasts the traditional Thai system of three sexes with a system that promotes standardization into two gender-normative sexes ideally engaged in monogamous marriage (Loos 2006). Semicolonialism imposed sexual dimorphism and heterosexual matrices that become refashioned in the Thai case of *siwilai*—but this state process of de-androgynizing local genders is a Foucauldian (1990) disciplinary mechanism that is productive of new kinds of thirds, which may or may not be ambiguous, since polarizing binary sex makes their transgressions more apparent. The early twentieth-century interventions, particularly those during the Field Marshal Plaek Phibunsongkhram era, were particularly virulent, legislating gender-specific hair, dress, and behavior (e.g., long hair and pantyhose for women, husbands kissing wives) that would be recognizable to Westerners (van Esterik 2000; Barmé 2002). These changes were not uniformly adopted, with urban elites being most influenced. Van Esterik (2000) notes how working-class women avoided and resisted Thai bureaucratic pressures to conform to ideals of Western femininity. Besides European encroachment and subsequent attempts at modernization, rapid pulses of gender and sexual transformation also followed other key historical, economic, and technological events such as the Vietnam/American War, AIDS, the Asian financial crisis, and the availability of birth control, hormones, and sexual reassignment and cosmetic surgeries. Furthermore, cultural influence from the migration of Chinese immigrants has affected gender relations, particularly among the merchant class (Bao 2005).

A new era of development post-WWII increasingly drove capitalist modes of production and consumption in Thailand (see also Chap. 9 in this volume). These came to be inhabited under the skin and combined with new discourses around economic restructuring, consumerism, development, modern identity, and cosmopolitanism that produced a post-Fordist system of flexible gender identities that modified historical forms but whose contours vary by subject position and moral valence. Involvement with Vietnam as an American ally greatly expanded sex tourism in Thailand and helped develop Thailand's infrastructure and economy (Bishop and Robinson 1998; Jeffrey 2002). Ironically, the expansion of the middle class made possible by prostitution has increased stigma for sex workers among those eager to make novel class distinctions. More recently, the Asian financial crisis and the subsequent recovery have both produced anti-Western sentiment and greater political, economic, and cultural integration with other Southeast and East Asian nations.

Thai biopolitical intervention in the production of modern sex is thus the basis for the production of the current genderscapes. The autocolonial intervention re-articulates a newly localized sex/gender system. Discursive governmentality is the catalyst to create this shift, yet cannot fully account for the variation present. Its erasure of former gender conceptualizations and reconstruction of a system in line with modern Western sexual dimorphism remains incomplete. In fact, hybrid resistances, cosmopolitan engagements, and everyday practices exceed the limitations placed on sex forms. The microstructural adjustments in the performance of gender also provide a degree of fluidity that cannot be accounted for in taxonomic models of the Thai sex/gender system. Nevertheless, these mundane performances are enabled and constrained via socio-moral understandings of appearance. Here, I turn to a theoretical elaboration of these additional processes.

2.2 Globalization and Localization of Gender Transformations

Thai gender and sexuality categories are not given, but rather historically contingent (Scott 1999) and culturally produced locally in dialogue with globalizing forces. Having provided a brief historical overview of Thai biopolitical intervention in the production of modern sex vis-à-vis its autocolonial governmentality, I propose a formulation of Thai genderscapes. This conceptualization of genderscapes, based on Appadurai's (1996) notions of disjuncture and localization, is operationalized through Thai statecraft and everyday concepts of face, appearance, and propriety. First, I briefly outline Appadurai's-scapes in relation to Rubin's (1975, 1984) sex/gender system and Herdt's (1996) discussion of third sexes. Then, I compare Morris' (1994), Jackson's (2000), and Sinnott's (2004) formulations of Thai gender and sexuality and provide additional data about the contemporary Thai situation from the last decade. By examining issues of morality, appearances, and everyday practice, I argue for a Thai genderscape revolving around five major gender/sexuality nodes. Finally, I consider what this means in relation to Altman's (2001) global gay hypothesis.

In Modernity at Large, Appadurai (1996: 33) argues that cultural flows have increasingly non-isomorphic paths along five dimensions (ethnoscapes, mediascapes, technoscapes, finanscapes, and ideoscapes) which he refers to with the suffix "-scapes." Thus, Appadurai proposes that scapes are not objectively given relations but rather deeply perspectival constructs historically inflected through the situatedness and power of different types of social and individual actors. Scapes themselves act as facilitators and constraints on each other, creating unexpected routes and often contentious imaginings of the lifeworld. Flows across national borders are also indigenized and are instrumental in producing locality. For Appadurai (1996: 178), locality is not already given but has a "complex phenomenological quality, constituted by a series of links between the sense of social immediacy, the technologies of interactivity, and the relativity of contexts … which expresses itself in certain kinds of agency, sociality, and reproducibility."

The various processes of globalization are disjunctured and thus require multiple scapes to demonstrate analytically how these unsmooth routes are generative of the new forms that are inherently hybrid and contradictory. But, as these scapes continue to circulate and recirculate unevenly, they are then re-indigenized through processes of localization that filter and mold them into yet another set of forms in an ongoing cycle. This formulation allows for the theorization of complexly interrelated phenomena that do not privilege stability or movement. It also leaves open cultural forms to profound irregularity and unpredictability.

Scape terms highlight the positionality, contingency, and contextual nature of globalizing forces on local processes. Here, I focus on the local phenomenological quality of Thai gender and articulate it as Thai genderscapes attentive to the discursive structures and everyday discourses that produce relative stability. The terrain of the sex/gender system is indigenized and becomes local in the tension between the autochthonous and the global.

I refer to genderscapes as a sex/gender system, a culturally elaborated mode of inhabiting reproductive differences in relation to subsistence, kinship, politics, and so forth (Rubin 1975). While I agree with Rubin (1984) that gender and sexuality should be separated analytically, they are emically intertwined and mutually constituted in Thailand and elsewhere. With the exception of masculine gay men, Thais typically do not distinguish gender and sexuality in their own lives. Sexuality is generally neither necessary nor sufficient to transform one's gender. Thus, following Jackson (2003) and Sinnott (2004), I conceptualize gender and sexuality within the purview of genderscapes as autonomous but related domains of a sex/gender order. Eroticism is corollary to but not necessarily derivative of gender, requiring relational rather than independent analysis.

Conceptualization as a -scape reveals greater possibilities for various genders. Modeling gender in a three-dimensional space rather than as a dualism opens up crosses, unities, mixes, alternatives, and liminalities beyond male-to-female and female-to-male transgenders. Incorporating time, the nodes of gender can shift and need not be fully formed to be recognized. I thus benefit from Herdt's conceptualization of third sexes, although I do not go as far as arguing that the ontology of third sexes requires a "stable social role, that can be inhabited—marking off a clear social status position, rights and duties, with indications for the transmission of corporeal and incorporeal property and rights" (Herdt 1996: 60). Instead, I embrace dynamism within the realm of habituated practice (Bourdieu 1990), as key nodes in the system help to anchor genderscapes. The performance or practice of gender allows for their ongoing rearticulation; yet the possibilities are always shaped through ritualization and regulatory discourses (Butler 2004; Morris 1995).

Currently, I argue for five major gender nodes, which exist in relation to one another based on anatomical differences, presentation of self, socioeconomic roles, desire for certain others, and so on. Each of these nodes has spin-offs or subdivisions, creating a large number of possible categories. However, they coalesce around five forms with significant ontological fixity in public everyday life. These are realized through the repetition of symbolic processes and everyday practices which make them appear to be real and part of the natural and hierarchical order of things (Bourdieu 1990). These processes include the presentation of a gendered self in daily life as well as the dissemination and reinstantiation of these practices via media representations. Face and appearance are key to Thai social norms and the regulation of behavior and propriety (Mulder 1997), especially gender performance and its formation (Barmé 2002). Surfaces (van Esterik 2000) and the gaze (Morris 1997) are technologies for the regulation of Thai gender and sexual relations. Appearances act as a mechanism to discipline idealized social forms, irrespective of interiority, through the fear of losing face. Within this public "regime of images"

(Jackson 2004), private sexual practices are sequestered while gender presentation is brought to the fore. Therefore, public enactments of gender variance become highlighted for their difference at the same time sexuality can, and "should," remain unknown. In sum, the images one projects about the self are more important than identity in public interactions. Such exteriorities are not expected to access an essential truth. Furthermore, the Thai concept of *phet* frames sexuality as an extension of gender. Thus, my focus in constructing Thai genderscapes emphasizes the public performance of gender, and nonnormative gender presentation, rather than sexuality.

3 Thai Genderscapes

Kathoey: a male-to-female transgender person, typically engaging in or desiring relationships with heterosexual men, irrespective of operative status

Gay: a male, masculine or feminine, who engages in or desires same-sex relationships with other males

Tom: a masculine woman who engages in or desires same-sex relationships with a woman

Dee: a feminine woman who engages in same-sex relationships with *tom*

3.1 Contemporary Thai Gender and Sexuality

In this section, I review the literature on the Thai gender and sexuality system and propose conceptualizing it as a "genderscape." Gender/sexuality categories are neither essential nor constant arrangements. They are culturally and historically specific, socially structured and structuring, but also tactically employed, resisted, and manipulated. Gender does not operate in isolation, but interacts with other forms of social difference. Following Jackson and Cook (1999: 23), I emphasize dynamism: "the diversity of ways in which notions of sexuality and gender are manifested and contested in everyday social practices, as well as their rapidly changing nature." Furthermore, as gender pluralism (Peletz 2009) continues to be challenged, albeit in new ways, responding to new concerns, the legitimacy of gender/sexual variance requires assessment. Class, moral status, and experience must be highlighted in understanding Thai gender/sexuality because they shape representations, everyday practices, and the acceptability afforded to various forms.

Every day Thai does not distinguish between sex, gender, and sexuality (เพศ: *phet*). Jackson and Sullivan (1999: 5) suggest that "within Thai discourse, gay and *kathoey* are not distinguished as a sexuality and a gender, respectively. Rather, gay, *kathoey*, together with 'man' (*phu-chai*), 'woman' (*phu-ying*), and the lesbian identities *tom* and *dee*, are collectively labelled as different varieties of *phet*." Academics use specialized terms to differentiate sex, gender, sexuality, and other aspects of *phet*, but these are not commonly understood. Activists also have developed specialized terms. In the last decade, the development of HIV services for males who have sex with males and transgender women has also elaborated new specialized terms, often derived from international NGO, public health, and human rights discourses. In the general operations of *phet*, sex, gender, and sexuality are bound up in metaphorical packages which discourage dissonance between gender presentation and a presumably gendered desire rather than between sex and gender.

The multifaceted nature of *phet* has been conceptualized in two primary ways in the literature: a Westernization model and an indigenization model. In the former, modern Western understandings of gender/sexuality usurp and supplant Thai ones. In the latter, new sexual identities are ensconced within the Thai *phet* system. Morris (1994) contrasts the traditional three-sex system with a modern four-sexuality system. She argues that the Thai ternary of man, woman, and *kathoey* (กะเทย) is increasingly being replaced by four modern Western sexualities based on the two binaries of male:female and homosexual:heterosexual, which create the four positions of female-heterosexual, female-homosexual, male-heterosexual, and male-homosexual. According to Morris (1994), these systems coexist but are incommensurable, and thus the "modern" system is replacing the "traditional" one. Similarly, van Esterik (2000: 218–219) states that "the influence of international gay culture including new media (magazines and videos) may be increasing the numbers of category labels, but is breaking down the diversity in the Thai gender system to stress identity based on object choice, heterosexual or homosexual."

In contrast, Jackson (2000) and Sinnott (2004) argue that Western sexual identities are indigenized through local conceptualizations of gender, thereby multiplying gender categories. Jackson (2003) uses the term "eroticized genders" and Sinnott (2004) uses the term "gendered sexualities." They emphasize that sexual desire is an extension of gender identification rather than separate domains of gender and sexual orientation. Based on the historical analysis of the Thai press and academic texts, Jackson (2000: 412) asserts that there are at least ten gender terms commonly used in contemporary Thai discourse. He charts how the three categories of (1) man, (2) *kathoey* (transgender), and (3) woman have proliferated into ten categories from the 1960s to the 1980s: (1a) man, (1b) *seua bai* (male bisexual); (2a1) *gay king*, (2a2) *gay queen*, (2b1) *kathoey*, (2b2) *kathoey plaeng phet* (transsexual), (2b3) *khon sorng phet* (hermaphrodite), (2c) *tom*; (3a) *dee* and (3b) woman, respectively. These terms refer to seven common *phet* categories: "man," *gay king*, *gay queen*, *kathoey*, *tom*, *dee*, and "woman" (414).

Yet, the categories of salience that I documented in everyday talk are those that are visibly distinguishable by outward appearance: man, effeminate *gay*, *kathoey*, *tom*, and woman. I want to note that the categories of woman and man are not natural, preexisting forms. Nor do they require heterosexuality. For instance, a woman can be a *dee* or a man can have a female, *kathoey*, or male partners while maintaining a gender-normative status. Additionally, the range of acceptable demeanor, dress, and other gender markers is quite wide and has historically shifted. All Thai genders are modern formations that have undergone tremendous transformation over the last century. However, for lack of space, here I focus on individuals who would be considered gender variant and update the contemporary literature (see also Chaps. 25 and 26 in this volume).

In Thai, *kathoey* is a general term encompassing all third-gender categories, theoretically referencing all nonnormative gender presentations and sexualities beyond heterosexual male and female. But in practice, *kathoey* seldom refers to female-bodied individuals, regardless of their gender expression. In cosmopolitan Bangkok, among the middle classes, *kathoey* only refers to male to female transgender persons, that is, transgender women (Jackson 2000; Sinnott 2004; see also Chap. 25 in this volume). *Gay* are typically offended when others refer to them as *kathoey*, although the term is used for in-group joking and accepted when outside Bangkok, as the locals are considered not to know better. People identified as *kathoey* may also be offended by the term as it can be used as a slur. There are numerous words that are considered more polite or respectful. Thus, if a person who is not *kathoey* is in the presence of one, she might use a term like สาวประเภทสอง (*sao-praphet-sorng*: second category woman). Thai academics often refer to gender "fluidity," as identities follow a developmental trajectory and situational positioning. Witchayanee (2008) differentiates between "half and half" (those who have either breast implants or neo-vaginas but not both) and "fully transformed" transgender sex workers (see also Chap. 25). Pramoj Na Ayuttaya (2008) identifies five types of *kathoey*: postoperative transgender, preoperative transgender, drag queen, penetrating girl (active in sexual intercourse), and those who live part time as transgender and part time as men.

In February 2010, the term ผู้หญิงข้ามเพศ (*phu-ying-kham-phet*: transsexual woman) was introduced by Nok Yollada to differentiate a transsexual (who desires or has had gender surgery) from a transvestite. Around the same time, the Rainbow Sky Association of Thailand, a sexual diversity NGO primarily funded to provide HIV prevention services, started using the term สาวทีจี (*sao-thi-ji*: transgender woman), borrowing from the English abbreviation "TG." However, most *kathoey* use the term among themselves or simply use สาว (*sao*: young woman). "Ladyboy" refers to *kathoey* who are cabaret performers, beauty pageant contestants, and bar-based sex workers. Some *kathoey* consider "ladyboy" distasteful as it upholds the stereotype that they are prostitutes and thus inherently indecent and criminal. *Kathoey* are also differentiated by their operative status. But, many *kathoey* consider it offensive to be asked whether they have had sexual reassignment or gender confirmation surgery because they feel their identity does not need to follow their genitalia. While there has been a proliferation of terms around male-to-female transgenderism, I suggest that they coalesce around one commonly understood gender form: *kathoey*.

For *kathoey*, transgenderism is made visible via sartorial practice, cosmetic use, bodily comportment, and language (Thai uses gendered particles that mark the speaker as male or female). Bisexual men, who are labeled based on sexual behavior rather than desire or gender presentation, are generally said to be *gay*, but ashamed (อับอาย: *ap-ai*) to identify themselves. There is no equivalent term for a bisexual woman. *Dee* and masculine *gay* express gender normativity. Thus, *dee* are only discernable when with their *tom* partners and masculine *gay* are said not to "show"

(แสดงออก: *sadaeng-ok*). Importantly, as public display of affection is considered impolite, nonnormative sexuality is generally not apparent while nonnormative gender presentation is. Sexuality is understood as private and thus not subject to social condemnation. However, for gender nonnormative individuals, sexuality is presumed as an extension of gender presentation. Thus, only effeminate *gay*, *kathoey*, and *tom* noticeably do not conform to gender norms; and among them, *kathoey* are the most stigmatized. Though, with the growing use of surgery and other medical technologies, *kathoey* visibility is decreasing, as they increasingly pass as women.

Gay are further characterized by age and effeminacy (ตุ๊ด: *tut*, sissy or queen; แต๋ว : *taeo*, sissy; สาวๆ *sao-sao*, girly; อีแอบ: *i-aep*, a feminine person who presents masculinely in public). These terms are usually not labels of self-identity but are used as insults or for in-group joking. Use of the terms "*king*" and "*queen*" in relation to *gay* is now considered passé (although the terms have been taken up by lesbians in *lesking* and *lesqueen*), perhaps because gender presentation has become more independent of preferred sexual positioning (แบบ: *baep*), and *baep* is often flexible depending on the partner. *Gay* rather matter-of-factly disclose their *baep* (รุก: *ruk*, penetrate; รับ: *rap*, receive; โบ๊ท *bot*, versatile; สลับ: *salap*, reciprocate or alternate) as Thais would their age. These are among the first questions one might be asked upon meeting a stranger in a gay venue or online. However, *baep* does not constitute a public identity.

Along the continuum of *kathoey-gay*, distinction making occurs at both ends (see also Jackson 1997). Masculine *gay* refer to effeminate *gay* as *tut*, *kathoey*, or *i-aep*, individuals who would be *kathoey* given the opportunity. Postoperative transsexuals differentiate themselves from those who have not had surgery. They say they have already become women and often assume they pass (even when they do not), confident in the alignment of their essentially female mind and body. At the same time, there is fluidity between *gay* and *kathoey* categories, both in identity and sartorial practice. *Kathoey-noi* (กะเทยน้อย: little *kathoey* or just a little transgendered), for instance, use makeup like women but dress in men's clothing. *Kathoey-noi* are not transgender; they are not *gay*; they are an in-between category. *Kathoey-noi* are not uncommon. They are generally young, around 16–26 and often said to be transitioning into a *kathoey* lifestyle. There are, however, adult males who fit into this pattern. Some *kathoey* become *gay* and vice versa, although the former conversion is more prevalent. As *kathoey-kathoey*, *gay-kathoey*, and effeminate *gay* pairings become more common, the disgust associated with similar-gender coupling is diminishing. New terms such as *sao-siap* (สาวเสียบ: penetrating girl, referring to *kathoey* who are active in anal intercourse) and *tom-gay* (a *tom*, masculine female, in a relationship with another *tom*) describe variations that incorporate putatively discordant gender expression and sexual practice. These changes point to the breakdown of the heterogender sexual matrix (Peletz 2006), in which only sex between individuals of "opposite" genders is socially acceptable.

In English, we say "gay man," with "gay" sexuality (an adjective) modifying "man" (a noun). But in Thai, "*gay*" is already a noun so that one is either "*gay*" or "man." Thus, one can say "I am a *gay*" or "I am a man." However, these are not exclusive categories and there is a recognition that sexual desire does not have to follow gender identification. For example, one can say the two in sequence, as in ผมเป็นเกย์ ผมเป็นแมน (*phom pen ke; phom pen maen.*) to emphasize that one is a masculine gay man. Bee, who is *gay*, once told me: ผมไม่เป็นเกย์ ผมเป็นแมน (*phom mai pen ke; phom pen maen*: literally "I am not *gay*. I am a man") to stress that he does not see himself as effeminate at all, since the term "*gay*" can invoke effeminacy, as in เกย์มากเกินไป (*ke map koen pay*: too *gay*). In the statement ไม่เป็นรุกไม่เป็นรับเป็นเกย์ (*mai pen ruk, mai pen rap; pen ke*: He is not top/penetrator or bottom/receiver; he is *gay*), the term is referencing sexual versatility. Thus, the term "*gay*" is polysemic in everyday use, contextually referencing effeminacy, masculinity, or sexual versatility. These examples show that while gender and sexuality are linked, they can be distinguished from one another. At the same time, they are conflated in everyday life.

Phet terms are not isomorphic with identities. Neologisms and variants do not necessarily constitute new forms; they can be situationally employed or used to label others and make fine distinctions. Masculine *gay* often refer to themselves as แมนๆ (*maen-maen*: very manly, like a man), although this is more a descriptor of gender presentation than an identity. Similarly, the term เมโทรเซ็กชวล (*me-tho sek-chuan*: metrosexual), while defined in Thai Wikipedia and in many lifestyle magazines as a heterosexual man who appears gay based on his interest in fitness, fashion, and grooming, is typically used in speech to refer to someone who is *gay* or closeted. Indeed, this 'ผู้ชายสายพันธุ์ใหม่' (*phu-chai saiphan mai*: new breed of man) category was popularized by the film *Metrosexual* (2006, directed by Yongyoot Thongkongtoon), in which a group of women tries to prove to their friend that her fiancée, who is too perfect to be heterosexual, must be *gay*. The Thai title is แก๊งชะนีกับอีแอบ (*kaeng chani kap i-aep*: Gang of Girls and the Closet Case). Metrosexuality is marked visibility by being too perfect a man to be straight, just as *kathoey* beauty contestants are often said to possess โอเว่อร์บิวตี้ (*owoe-bioti*: over beauty) in comparison to women. Many new gender expressions are derived from films, songs, and Internet sites, although their usage is typically short-lived and the terms do not constitute identities, though they may be variations upon them.

Female-bodied gender forms are highly visible but have less social presence in Thai society and media (Käng 2011). Like female same-sex sexuality in other parts of the world, it is limited by income differentials, safety concerns, and social proscriptions around propriety. Additionally, female same-sex relationships can also be less challenging to the sex/gender order. Many Thai women are able to circumvent the issue of respectability as being in a same-sex relationship can be morally less damaging than a heterosexual one (Sinnott 2004). In particular, one can avoid unwanted pregnancy and the contamination associated with the loss of virginity. This, however, is more applicable to young women and those from wealthier backgrounds. Compared to women in other regions of the world, Thai women also have relatively high employment and financial independence, allowing many of them to live independently of family and forestall marriage (Mills 1999; Muecke 1984). Thailand has the highest rate of single women in Asia and one of the lowest birthrates in the world. These factors perhaps provide more opportunity for female same-sex relationships than in other geographic areas.

Tom-dee (the terms are derived from the English "tomboy" and "lady") couples are ubiquitous and easily identifiable in mainstream commercial venues such as shopping malls (Wilson 2007). Suburban malls have stores targeted to *tom*, selling men's clothes in smaller sizes (in contrast to stores targeting *kathoey* that provide women's clothes in larger sizes). I suggest that *tom-dee* couples are actually more visible than gay men in Thai public space, where they become legible by learning their social codes. Female couples can be seen holding hands, one sporting short hair and men's clothes, the other with long hair and women's clothes. Sinnott (2004: 142) has referred to the public conspicuousness of these relationships in terms of "visual explicitness and verbal silence." The couples are discernible but unremarkable. Women are also highly active in Thai activism around sexual diversity, with organizations such as Anjaree (founded in 1986) among the most vocal advocates for sexuality rights. However, their work is often overshadowed by an infusion of international HIV prevention funding for *gay* and *kathoey* in the mid-2000s, which has been mobilized to promote the acceptance of sexual minorities and their human rights more broadly.

In *tom-dee* relationships, it is only the former who can be considered misgendered. *Toms* are masculine women. They are biological females attracted to women, but this attraction to women is an extension of their masculinity. Their gender does not match their sex, though their sexuality can be seen as an extension of their gender. *Dees* are their female partners. But, as gender normative or "ordinary women," *dee* identity becomes relevant in relation to *tom*. That is, *dee* are labeled as counterparts of *tom* rather than as another category of women, often being temporary members of the *tom-dee* community (Sinnott 2004). Thus, while *tom* represent a more or less stable *phet* identity in contemporary Thailand, *dee* have a more liminal position. They exist primarily in association with *tom* rather than as an independent category. *Dee* remain peripheral to the nodes of *tom* and woman in Thai genderscapes.

Dee inhabit a relational and situational identity (Sinnott 2007). Sexuality can be tied to temporal gender positions in the life cycle: what is appropriate in youth may not be so in adulthood. Engaging in sexual acts inappropriate for one's status can modify ascribed gender positions. Yet, being *dee* is considered relatively unproblematic. Many women, often married, have told me, without remorse or shame: "I was a *dee* before." From a Western perspective, *dee* are a lesbian sexual identity, women who desire or engage in sexual relations with other women. However, gender difference is more important to *tom-dee* couplings than sexual identity (Sinnott 2004). From the perspective of Thai *phet*, as a feminine woman attracted to the masculinity of another woman, their desire is homosexual but heterogender (Peletz 2006) and thus normatively paired.

In the alternate genders of *tom* and *kathoey*, blending of sex/gender attributes is a more typical feature than the disavowal of a biological sex and the recreation of a newly contrasting gendered persona. *Tom* maintain many characteristics of women (e.g., being good caretakers) as *kathoey* maintain many characteristics of men (e.g., being sexually assertive). Some *kathoey* are more like transsexuals in the classic sense of seeing themselves as an "opposite" sex, and this is essential to the new conceptualization of *phu-ying-kham-phet* (transsexual woman), literally a woman who has crossed sex. But, this is generally not the case for *tom*, who see themselves as masculine women rather than as men. Sinnott (2004: 22) refers to *tom* "in the feminine form ("she," "her") to reflect the common understanding among Thais that *toms* are female, and although they are masculine, they are distinct from males."

3.2 Five Genders?

The proposal of five *phet* categories is reminiscent of Davies (2010) five genders among the Bugis of Sulawesi, Indonesia. Yet, the sex/gender system in Thailand does not follow the same pattern of crossings (i.e., female, female to male, male/female androgyny, male to female, and male). Nor are the spiritual aspects of *bissu* unity at play.[3] The five gender forms I propose are similar to the seven *phet* categories Jackson (2000) states are commonly described in Thai literature. However, rather than representing the categories like a phylogenetic tree, which emphasizes the historical transformations of the categories, I propose a multidimensional -scape. On the one hand, this formation provides greater flexibility in the enactments of gender as they are practiced in everyday life at a point in time. On the other, a -scape model shows the layered relationships between nodes and can shift based on historical transformations, one's social positioning, or ideological perspective.

With the proposed five gender nodes, I have not included *dee*. As Sinnott (2004: 9) notes, "masculine women have long been evident in the Thai system of sex and gender, but the linguistic and social marking of feminine women who are partners of masculine women creates a new and precarious field of identity." Sinnott likens *dee* to the gender-normative partners of *kathoey*, who are simply categorized as men. As women who are feminine in dress, comportment, and speech, they are not marked as gender different. Most *dee* do not refer to themselves as *dee* but as "women." *Dee* is more frequently a label that *tom* use for their feminine partners. Ploy, a neighbor of mine who ran a noodle shop, talking to me about her brother's transition from *kathoey* to *gay*, stated matter-of-factly: "Well, I was a *dee* before I was with him," nodding her head in the direction of the unmarried father of their daughter. Many other women told me that they had been in relationships with women when younger, but typically did not refer to the relationship as *tom-dee*. Instead, the relationship was with another *phu-ying* (girl/woman). The expectation among *tom* is that *dee* will eventually leave *tom* for a man. Similarly, a "real" man

[3] The *bissu* are transgender ritual specialists whose mixture of male and female characteristics identify and represent the undifferentiated nature of the universe. *Bissu* gender unity allows them to access spiritual powers unattainable by males or females. Peletz (2006) notes that this pattern exists throughout Southeast Asia. However, the situation in Thailand is more complex. Transgender and gay ritual specialists are currently increasing in popularity in both the North and Central regions, yet the lack of an historical record makes it unclear whether this is a resurgence of prior practices. Of course, transgender ritual specialists exist in other world areas, with the *hijras* of South Asia perhaps the most well-known case.

is anticipated to leave a *kathoey* for a “real” woman in order to have a family, or keep the *kathoey* as a mistress. A *dee* is thus generally considered ธรรมดา (*thammada*: ordinary or normal) but could shift positions within genderscapes, for example, if one emphasizes sexual object choice over gender presentation.

Additionally, I have not differentiated nodes for masculine and feminine *gay*, which can be thought of as two different categories based on different gender presentation, public visibility, and sense of self. Like *dee*, masculine *gay* are gender normative in presentation or often hypermasculine. However, unlike *dee*, *gay* have a strong sense of identity based on their sexual desires. Sinnott (2004: 29) suggests that “the category ‘gay’ has introduced a third possible kind of masculinity positioned between normative ‘men’ and *kathoeys*, in that gay men are masculine yet desire other masculine men as sexual partners.... [Masculine gay men] are not highly visible, in that they do not match the perception that gayness equals effeminacy—they simply fall off the radar for many Thais.” Masculine *gay* break the rules of the heterogender matrix; they represent a singularity where the traditional three-sex system and the modern four-sexuality systems intersect in Thai genderscapes. Of course, feminine *gay* would provide a fourth male position. Yet, while only the feminine *gay* is visibly identifiable, both masculine and feminine *gay* have a sexual identity that is often an important component of self-concept and lifestyle. They also conceive of themselves as a community using shared social space and having a common identity and transnational ties with other gay communities around the world. The terms *king* and *queen* are rarely used and tend to reference sexual position more than an identity. Thus, while focusing on the appearance of gender-variant performance, which would exclude masculine *gay*, who are relatively invisible, I combine them here as a single node. Indeed, no genderscape nodes are homogenous or consistent. Yet, the gay node has a particularly two-faced characteristic. As Sinnott (2004: 30) notes, “an important difference between gay men and *dees* is that *dees* are only *dees* in relation to a *tom*. The masculine female gives the *dee* her identity, whereas gay men take pains to distinguish their community and identities from *kathoey* identity.” *Gay*, *tom*, and *kathoey* are more like what Foucault (1990) might refer to as a “species” with discursive and ontological fixity. They all have elaborated subcultures with specific social spaces and organization. At the same time, elaborating gender categories as nodes in the Thai genderscapes acknowledges the variation within each in relation to the others.

3.3 Social Position and Ideological Stance

Class, education, geography, and *phet* identification also affect how people conceptualize gender/sexuality categories. In Thailand, geographical regions and urban/rural distinctions are very important and highly associated with class differences. Central Thais, who are culturally and linguistically dominant, conceive of Northerners as “soft.” The women are thought of as more gracile, polite, and lighter skinned. The men are similarly effeminized. Southern men, by contrast, are considered rough, hard, and dark. They are also portrayed as more patriarchal as a result of Islamic conversion or interaction. Northeasterners are often said not to be Thai and, instead, referred to as Lao, and therefore, less developed. For many Central Thais, Bangkok is the *only* city. All other areas are considered ต่างจังหวัด (*tang-changwat*: provincial, upcountry) or, less politely, บ้านนอก (*ban-nok*: the boonies). While rural populations consume the same national media as produced in the capital, interpretations are filtered through their daily experience, which includes the out-migration of many young people, including the gender variant. There is also less access to the consumer products that allow for greater gender differentiation.

One of my best friends, Wan, who is a *kathoey* in her mid-30s from *Isan* (the Northeast region), often makes the statement: "I was the first *kathoey* in my village." This assertion struck me as strange because I imagined there must have been *kathoey* who preceded her since there is a history of *kathoey* in Thailand. I have traveled with her to her home village three times, and people have confirmed that she was the first *kathoey* that they can remember. Before, villagers were quite hostile to *kathoey*, until she and a few others showed themselves as *kathoey*, dressing and living as transgender women.[4] Now there are approximately ten adult *kathoey* in her village, one of whom was married to a man in 2009 in a day-long celebration attended by several hundred guests. Both sets of parents gave speeches about their happiness during the wedding. There are also several *kathoey* children. When I asked a mother of a 10-year-old boy about when the child started expressing herself as a girl, the mother replied: "Since birth. When she/he started talking, she/he used 'ค่ะ'" (*kha*: the female polite particle).[5] But, this increased acceptance has only occurred since around 2000. Wan only began living as a *kathoey* after the death of her father, who was a respected village leader. Others soon followed and transgenderism became a visible part of village life. Thus, Wan feels that the situation for *kathoey* is improving rapidly.

Wan believes that while there is a strong inclination toward being *kathoey*, one can choose to be *gay* instead. When we met with a 16-year-old at a temple fair who was cross-dressing, Wan immediately went to speak with her. "What are you?" she asked. "Are you like me or him [nodding toward me]?" She went on to ask whether her father accepted her cross-dressing, which the young *kathoey* affirmed. She then said: "You have to choose whether you will be like me or him. If you choose to be like me, life will be harder." Wan counseled the youth, acknowledging the fluidity between *kathoey* and *gay* as well as the different opportunities associated with these life trajectories.

Wan notes that the number of *gay* in her village is increasing, although their normative masculinity renders them relatively invisible and uncontroversial. Villagers simply refer to men and women; the distinction between the two is based

[4] As in other parts of Asia, there is not an emphasis on "coming out" in Thailand. However, unlike Confucian Asian societies, there is less emphasis on hiding one's gender/sexual nonconformity. Effeminate *gay* will often state that people know about their sexual orientation, even if they have not been told, because they "show" themselves.

[5] The third person singular pronoun in Thai is gender neutral.

on outward presentation. However, when someone is verbally identified as *gay*, the reaction is often: "I didn't know she/he was a woman." Such comments show that villagers perceive sexuality in terms of a gendered desire that should be an extension of their gender presentation. For most villagers, a *gay* is someone who appears like a man, but is actually a woman based on their จิตใจ (*jit-jai*: mind/heart or inner being), their desire for male partners. One of Wan's friends, who used to be *kathoey* when living in the provinces but has since become *gay* after moving to Bangkok, overheard our discussion. He commented: "Before, things were bad for us, but now it is getting much better." The repetition of an improved situation for the "third gender" has become a refrain among Thais of all genders. But, the increased acceptability of gender variance is neither embraced nor uncontested (Jackson 1995, 1999b; Sinnott 2000). See also Chap. 26 on the Third Gender.

In particular, moral stance can override other classificatory schemes, as was evident from a pile sort exercise I conducted to develop a conceptual map of Thai genders among a diverse group of Bangkok residents.[6] Respondents were asked to think aloud while making their taxonomic decisions. Individuals used a variety of factors in creating groups: anatomy, gender expression on a male-female continuum, romantic attraction, common/normal/natural status, and personal experience. I was not surprised when an early free list by a man in his 50s returned two items: man and woman. I was, however, taken aback when, after elaborating a wide number of gender categories, he created two piles: man and woman in one called "normal" and the rest in another called "abnormal" (ผิดปกติ: *phit-pakati*). I had erroneously assumed that man and woman were counterparts and would remain in separate piles because I failed to account for the moral valence attached to *phet* categories.

Gender classification is not an amoral process. *Phet* are defined by factors which are variously invoked by different people, situationally dependent, and experientially based. Instead of seeing Morris' and Jackson's and Sinnott's interpretations as orthogonal, I suggest the three are complementary. Class, generation, rural/urban upbringing, moral stance, personal experience, and context mediate how the local repertoire of gender/sexuality is practiced, interpreted, and labeled in relation to differential exposure to market mechanisms, bureaucratic institutions, and cultural forms. That is, social stances and life opportunities condition how Thais inhabit and interpret *phet*. Furthermore, I argue that gender forms are interpolated by the moral valence attached to their normativity. These concerns not only expand the terrain of gender/sexuality but also force a reconsideration of their topography. I suggest that *phet* should not be enumerated individually but conceptualized in nodes and clusters. That is, gender/sexuality categories are not fixed to four

[6] Pile sorts are a cognitive mapping procedure to understand how community members think about and attach meaning to different items within a conceptual domain. I began the exercise with a free list to identify the *phet* respondents conceived of as most salient. Up to 22 terms were then sorted based on similarity. If there were more than three initial piles, I asked participants to subsequently sort into three piles and then two piles as I wanted to see if the three-sex system would be reproduced and how genders in the third category, especially *kathoey*, would be categorized as males or females. There were 37 participants.

modern sexual positions. Nor are they proliferating with each new addition of a term. Rather, *phet*, which may or may not be publicly visible, cluster around several key nodes (man, woman, *kathoey*, *gay*, and *tom*), which are renewed through everyday experience. These forms shift over time, often proliferating in punctuated bursts that retreat into refined forms. Furthermore, as Thais use different criteria to assess *phet* (e.g., anatomy, sartorial presentation, desired partner, normality, personal experience), their classifications vary widely and the boundaries between groups overlap. For example, *phu-ying-kham-phet* (transsexual woman) are variously grouped with men (based on anatomy at birth), women (based on postoperative anatomy, social presentation, or desired partner), or *kathoey* (based on their being transgender or "not normal"). The framework Thais use to think about these differences is conditioned by social experience. There are multiple stances and layers to the evaluation and categorization of gender/sexuality. Thus, I argue that the multidimensional nature of Thai *phet* are best conceptualized as a localized genderscape, a terrain of archetypes in which fields of power, morality, and experience shape its continually shifting boundaries over time.

4 Discussion and Conclusion

4.1 The Persistence of Gender Variance

Genderscapes also acknowledge that locality is produced when autochthonous forms interact with the forces of autocolonial governmentality, capitalist expansion, and other globalizing processes. Thais, regardless of gender/sexuality, say that there is a massive proliferation of *gay*, *kathoey*, and *tom*. A precursory *kathoey* form of some kind predates *gay*. However, as Jackson (2009) has argued, the modern *kathoey* is not a predecessor to *gay* but emerged concurrently vis-a-vis the regulation of Thai gender norms, particularly in dress. The Thai state proffered and enforced sexual differentiation as a means to show its civilizational status and to resist colonial encroachment. In particular, the androgyny of Thai women in Western eyes compelled the state to require their feminization in dress, hair, and behavior. This polarization of femininity and masculinity is the very mechanism of biopower that makes cross-dressing and transgendering more legible. That is, the fixing of masculinity and femininity enables greater possibilities for their transgression.

Kathoey today are clearly a different form of transgender personage than what existed in the past. Yet, middle-class urban Thais consider the *kathoey* form an archaic predecessor to *gay* in Thai culture, possessing an indigenous quality of local distinction. In particular, "ladyboy" cabarets are commodified by government and private agencies for tourists to demonstrate the "amazing" character of Thainess, an exotic place with an institutionalized third gender. However, as *kathoey* themselves note, their beauty often requires the utilization of modern medical technology such as hormones, Botox, and surgery. Younger urban *kathoey* refer to themselves as กะเทยสมัยใหม่ (*kathoey samai-mai*: modern *kathoey*) in contrast to กะเทยควาย (*kathoey khwai*: country bumpkin *kathoey*), older, more androgynous *kathoey* who are not as gracile and polished. These comments suggest that a discursive shift is occurring in the way that kathoeyness is construed in popular media and everyday life. Increasingly, *kathoey* are being referred to as new and modern rather than traditional and anachronistic (Käng 2012).

When I started preliminary fieldwork in 2004, middle-class heterosexuals would often refer to *kathoey* as strange and embarrassing. I would often ask people the question: how many *phet* (gender/sex) are there in Thailand? They would look at me as if I just landed from the moon. The response was invariably two. When I followed up with a question about *kathoey*, the response was often, "Oh yes, there are those people, ha, ha, ha." Such discussion would often elicit giggles among women. If I asked for any other *phet*, a short list of gender/sexuality types would emerge, typically including *gay* and *tom*, but not *dee*. Thais readily acknowledged that Thailand is known for having a large transgender population, often citing the North as a region with a particularly large number. Among middle-class Thais, there was some embarrassment about having so many *kathoey*, a sense that kathoeyness was backward compared to being *gay*, another feature that showed Thailand lagging developmentally behind other countries (Sinnott 2000). This attitude is particularly prevalent among those educated in international schools or abroad. In their minds, the presence of *kathoey* literally demonstrated that Thailand had not succeeded in civilizing gender.

For the middle class, modern masculine *gay*ness, which is often said not to "show" because of its normative masculinity, was clearly more cosmopolitan than kathoeyness. *Kathoey* are almost always portrayed as comic, criminal, or tragic in the media, as if those are the only life trajectories. However, since the coup of the Thaksin government in 2006, which attempted to censor kathoeyness on television, there has been an explosion of more balanced and humane representations of *kathoey* (Käng 2011). The increase in depictions of kathoeyness is assumed by most Thais to reflect their increasing numbers in society, although this presence more likely reflects greater openness to alternate gender expressions.

In the Thai context, public surfaces and face are highly valued and regulated without the need to refer to private behavior, interiority, or truth (Morris 2000; Mulder 1997; van Esterik 2000). Ousted Prime Minister Thaksin had many social campaigns to recreate Thai society (see Chaps. 10, 11, 12, and 13 in this volume). In 2004, his Minister of Education stated that the number of *kathoey* on television should be limited. Similar restrictions were proposed in the 1990s (Jackson 2004). Popular media images that do not uphold Thai respectability or values are often suppressed by government censors. In nationalistic discourse, the expansion of alternative genders is linked to an increasingly pathologizing discourse, expressed as a loss of Thainess and the inability of Thai society to reproduce itself. The historical legacy of anticolonial national projects continues to act as a regulatory force of sex normalization. However, now the concern is with the virilization of masculinity.

4.2 Conceptualizing Thai Genderscapes

I argue that the gender-inflected sexualities of Thailand were produced by the very forces of autocolonial governmentality, modernization, and globalization (including the institutionalization of sexual dimorphism, restructuring of kin relations, and the construction of tradition) that tried to erase them. While masculine *gay* represent a gender node where a "modern" sexuality intrudes into a system of multiple genders, *gay* is itself a product of modern *phet* formation that developed concomitantly with the West and in relation to *kathoey* and other local gender configurations. The addition of gay identity forms in Thailand cannot be described as a "rupture" as transgenderal homosexualities both continue unabated and modernize alongside new forms of homosexuality that, at least on the surface, appear modern and Western. That is, gay identity as Altman (2001) describes did not diffuse to Thailand from the West, but developed in parallel dialogue at approximately the same time (Jackson 1999a). While capitalist modes of consumption facilitate such new identities, the conditions are not the same, particularly in relation to a break in kinship relations.

The continued prominence of *kathoey* and their hypervisibility alongside "modern" gay identity attests to the fact that replacement by a Western system based on sexuality is not the only model operating. Jackson (2003) notes that the *kathoey*, while being a traditional gender category, have taken their modern form alongside *gay*. *Kathoey* have developed their current gender/sexual identity and proliferated simultaneously. There is limited evidence on the existence of *kathoey* before the mid-twentieth century. They were likely ritual specialists in the North and theatrical performers. But, their current form, devoid of spiritual power and associated with sex work and, increasingly, beauty, is a modern phenomenon that parallels the timeframe of gay identity development. These dual trajectories, of gay identified and gender-transformed homosexualities, will likely persist into the future, albeit with different implications than the recent reassertion of transgender identities in the West. The putative projection of transgenderism into the premodern past ignores that the very possibility of transgenderism is enhanced by modernist gender differentiation into binary modes. Heterogender same-sex sexuality and gayness in Thailand both articulate modern refashionings of gender logics as they are mapped onto local systems of gendered presentation and identity. Thus, the historical assumption that *kathoey* come prior to *gay,* and that they are a "traditional" form of homosexuality being replaced by a "modern" one via capitalist expansion, is unsupported.

The regulatory discourses of biopower simply have not operated in Thailand as they have in the West. Thus, the decoupling of gender and sexuality, and the replacement of gender-transformed modes of homosexuality by modern *gay,* is not occurring. Transgenderisms in Thailand continue to thrive and are expanding at the same time gayness is, not being displaced. These gender formations are also evident among females. Sinnott (2004) notes that Lesla, a more recent lesbian organization than Anjaree in Thailand, is more supportive of the gendered terms *tom* and *dee*, while Anjaree promotes a more neutral term *ying-rak-ying* (women who love women). Significantly, Anjaree also avoids the term "lesbian" to claim a locally authentic female sexuality rather than one imported from the West. Thus, forms that are "modern" or new in Western contexts are actively resisted. Rather, both "modern" and gendered forms of homosexuality are proliferating simultaneously. The emergence of new categories, for the most part, is subsumed within existing conceptualizations of *phet*.

Sexual desire has not been made independent of gender presentation. However, the field continues to be shaped by the practices of individual actors, often in unexpected ways. On March 19, 2012, the **วีไอพี** (VIP) program produced a talk show called **ทอม แต่งงานกับกะเทย** (*tom* marries *kathoey*). While a heterogender couple, the show was still sensational for its novelty. Such instances of innovation have the potential to revise gender positions in Thai genderscapes. However, they are more likely to pass without sticking, leaving traces but not reconstituting the terrain.

Thai genderscapes are a localized production of gender and sexual differences that negotiate the tensions between local and global gender/sexuality forms. As such, they are hybrid: indigenizing the global and recasting the local for international audiences. The disjuncture or tension arising from the differences of autochthonous and global forms produces local distinction, distinguishing Thailand from many of its Asian neighbors. Furthermore, regardless of whether a gender form is considered "traditionally" Thai or not, they are all constituted via historical transformations interacting within the forces of human, capital, technological, ideological, and other flows. Thai genderscapes are already completely hybrid and globalized. But, they maintain local character as gender/sexuality forms are, for the most part, indigenized through local conceptualizations of *phet*.

I have argued for the conceptualization of contemporary Thai gender and sexuality as genderscapes grounded in five major gender/sexuality categories: *kathoey*, *tom*, *gay*, woman, and man. These categories are not the only ones that exist. Rather, they possess an ontological fixity which comes from their reproduction in the repetition of everyday performances and symbolic practices, which can shift norms over time. Moreover, key historical incidents produce punctuated expansions of possibilities, which may or may not shift the terrain of gender forms. Finally, the social position and ideological stance of an individual shapes how she/he inhabits and interprets *phet*, making genderscapes a perspectival endeavor.

Acknowledgments I would like to thank Nguyễn Tân Hoàng, Mark Johnson, and Evelyn Blackwood, who provided feedback on sections of this chapter. Bene Nightchild was an encouraging Facebook interlocutor. Dr. Pimpawan Boonmongkol of Mahidol University, my local research sponsor, smoothed the way for me when necessary. My research project (Gender Pluralism, Social Status, and Asian Regionalism in Bangkok, Thailand) was approved by the Office of the National Research Council of Thailand. Research funding was provided by the National Science Foundation and the Wenner-Gren Foundation.

References

Altman, D. (2001). *Global sex*. Chicago: University of Chicago Press.

Appadurai, A. (1996). *Modernity at large: Cultural dimensions of globalization*. Minneapolis: University of Minnesota Press.

Bao, J. (2005). *Marital acts: Gender, sexuality, and identity among the Chinese Thai Diaspora*. Honolulu: University of Hawaii Press.

Barmé, S. (2002). *Woman, man, Bangkok: Love, sex, and popular culture in Thailand*. Lanham: Rowman & Littlefield.

Bishop, R., & Robinson, L. S. (1998). *Night market: Sexual cultures and the Thai economic miracle*. New York: Routledge.

Bourdieu, P. (1990). *The logic of practice*. Stanford: Stanford University Press.

Butler, J. (2004). *Undoing gender*. New York: Routledge.

Connors, M. K. (2007). *Democracy and national identity in Thailand*. London: NIAS Press.

Davies, S. G. (2010). *Gender diversity in Indonesia: Sexuality, Islam and queer selves*. New York: Routledge.

Foucault, M. (1990). *The history of sexuality: Vol. 1. An introduction*. New York: Vintage.

Herdt, G. (Ed.). (1996). *Third sex, third gender: Beyond sexual dimorphism in culture and history*. New York: Zone Books.

Jackson, P. (1995). *Dear uncle Go: Male homosexuality in Thailand*. Bangkok: Bua Lunag Books.

Jackson, P. (1997). *Kathoey*>< gay>< man: The historical emergence of gay male identity in Thailand. In L. Manderson & M. Jolly (Eds.), *Sites of desire, economies of pleasure: Sexualities in Asia and the Pacific* (pp. 166–190). Chicago: University of Chicago Press.

Jackson, P. (1999a). An American death in Bangkok: The murder of Darrell Berrigan and the hybrid origins of gay identity in 1960s Thailand. *GLQ: A Journal of Lesbian and Gay Studies, 5*, 361–411.

Jackson, P. (1999b). Tolerant but unaccepting: The myth of a Thai 'gay paradise'. In P. Jackson & N. Cook (Eds.), *Genders and sexualities in modern Thailand* (pp. 226–242). Bangkok: Silkworm Books.

Jackson, P. (2000). An explosion of Thai identities: Global queering and re-imagining queer theory. *Culture, Health & Sexuality, 40*(4), 405–424.

Jackson, P. (2003). Performative genders, perverse desires: A bio-history of Thailand's same-sex and transgender cultures. *Intersections: Gender, History and Culture in the Asian Context* 9. Retrieved June 6, 2004, from http://intersections.anu.edu.au/issue9/jackson.html

Jackson, P. (2004). The Thai regime of images. *Sojourn, 19*, 181–218.

Jackson, P. (2009). Capitalism and global queering: National markets, parallels among sexual cultures, and multiple queer modernities. *GLQ: A Journal of Lesbian and Gay Studies, 15*, 370–395.

Jackson, P. (2010). The ambiguities of semicolonial power in Thailand. In R. Harrison & P. Jackson (Eds.), *The ambiguous allure of the west: Traces of the colonial in Thailand* (pp. 37–56). Hong Kong: Hong Kong University Press.

Jackson, P. A., & Cook, N. M. (Eds.). (1999). *Genders & sexualities in modern Thailand*. Bangkok: Silkworm Books.

Jackson, P. A., & Sullivan, G. (Eds.). (1999). *Lady boys, tom boys, rent boys: Male and female homosexualities in contemporary Thailand*. New York: Routledge.

Jeffrey, L. A. (2002). *Sex and borders: Gender, national identity, and prostitution policy in Thailand*. Honolulu: University of Hawaii Press.

Käng, D. B. (2011). Paradise lost and found in translation: Queer media loci in Bangkok. *GLQ: A Journal of Lesbian and Gay Studies, 17*, 169–191.

Käng, D. B. (2012). Kathoey "in trend": Emergent genderscapes, national anxieties, and the re-signification of male-bodied effeminacy in Thailand. *Asian Studies Review, 36*, 475–494.

Loos, T. (2006). *Subject Siam: Family, law, and colonial modernity in Thailand*. Ithaca: Cornell University Press.

Mills, M. B. (1999). *Thai women in the global labor force: Consuming desires, contested selves*. New Brunswick: Rutgers University Press.
Morris, R. (1994). Three sexes and four sexualities: Redressing the discourses of gender and sexuality in contemporary Thailand. *Positions: East Asian Cultures Critique, 2*, 215–243.
Morris, R. (1995). All made up: Performance theory and the new anthropology of sex and gender. *Annual Review of Anthropology, 24*(1), 567–592.
Morris, R. (1997). Educating desire: Thailand, transnationalism, and transgression. *Social Text, 15*, 53–79.
Morris, R. (2000). *In the place of origins: Modernity and its mediums in Northern Thailand*. Durham and London: Duke University Press.
Muecke, M. (1984). Make money not babies: Changing status markers of Northern Thai women. *Asian Survey, 24*, 459–470.
Mulder, N. (1997). *Thai images: The culture of the public world*. Chiang Mai: Silkworm Books.
Peletz, M. (2006). Transgenderism and gender pluralism in Southeast Asia since early modern times. *Current Anthropology, 47*(2), 309–340.
Peletz, M. (2009). *Gender pluralism: Southeast Asia since early modern times*. New York: Taylor & Francis.
Pramoj Na Ayuttaya, P. (2008, September 14). *The variety of kathoey in Thai society*. Unpublished paper presented at *Kathoey* are not women and don't have to be as beautiful as a pageant contestant seminar, Chiang Mai.
Rubin, G. (1975). The traffic in women: Notes on the political economy of sex. In R. R. Reiter (Ed.), *Toward an anthropology of women* (pp. 157–210). New York: Monthly Review Press.
Rubin, G. (1984). Thinking sex: Notes for a radical politics of sexuality. In C. S. Vance (Ed.), *Pleasure and danger: Exploring female sexuality* (pp. 267–319). Boston: Routledge & Kegan Paul.
Scott, J. (1999). *Gender and the politics of history*. New York: Columbia University Press.
Sinnott, M. (2000). The semiotics of transgendered sexual identity in the Thai print media: Imagery and discourse of the sexual other. *Culture, Health & Sexuality, 2*(4), 425–440.
Sinnott, M. (2004). *Toms and Dees: Transgender identity and female same-sex relationships in Thailand*. Honolulu: University of Hawaii Press.
Sinnott, M. (2007). Gender subjectivity: Dees and Toms in Thailand. In S. Wieringa, E. Blackwood, & A. Bhaiya (Eds.), *Women's sexualities and masculinities in a globalizing Asia* (pp. 119–138). New York: Palgrave Macmillan.
van Esterik, P. (2000). *Materializing Thailand*. Oxford: Berg.
Wilson, A. (2007). *The intimate economies of Bangkok: Tomboys, Tycoons, and Avon Ladies in the global city*. Berkeley: University of California Press.
Winichakul, T. (1994). *Siam mapped: A history of the geo-body of a nation*. Honolulu: University of Hawaii Press.
Winichakul, T. (2000). The quest for "siwilai": A geographical discourse of civilizational thinking in the late nineteenth and early twentieth-century Siam. *Journal of Asian Studies, 59*(3), 528–549.
Winichakul, T. (2010). Coming to terms with the west: Intellectual strategies of bifurcation and post-westernism in Siam. In R. Harrison & P. Jackson (Eds.), *The Ambiguous allure of the west: Traces of the colonial in Thailand* (pp. 135–151). Hong Kong: Hong Kong University Press.
Witchayanee, O. (2008, January 9–11). *Expounding gender: Transgender (male to female) identities in the Thai-global sex sector*. Unpublished paper presented at The 10th international conference on Thai studies, Bangkok.

Chapter 27
The Third Gender as Seen in Thai Fiction

Jenjit Gasigijtamrong

1 Introduction

Empirical research relating to LGBTQ in Thailand – including political, social, and health issues – almost exclusively focus on real people (see Chaps. 25 and 26 in this volume). Studies in the field of Thai literature are rare, and among those available, very few are based on the queer theory or feminist theory. As stated by Sullivan (2007: vi), including pop culture like literature in the discussion of queer theory is crucial "if we are to understand the broader significance of queer theory and the extensive range of ways in which notions of sexuality and gender impact … on everyday life." It is, therefore, essential to look at Thai literary works to add to what has been learned from sociological studies. In this study, I use the term "third gender" instead of LGBTQ although it is less used nowadays in the west, simply because it is widely used by Thai novelists (see also Chap. 26 in this volume).

2 Theoretical Frameworks

This chapter is analyzing the perceptions and portrayal of the third gender characters within the framework of the queer theory, feminism theory, and LGBTQ psychology, which are interrelated. The main concept used to guide the discussion in this chapter is a constellation of sex, gender, and sexuality. Sex is biologically innate (male, female), while gender is socially acquired (feminine and masculine). Regarding sexuality, Sullivan (2007: 1) states that "sexuality is not natural,

---

J. Gasigijtamrong (✉)
South East Asian Institute for Global Studies, Payap University,
Muang, Chiang Mai 50000, Thailand
e-mail: jenjit.iseas@gmail.com

P. Liamputtong (ed.), *Contemporary Socio-Cultural and Political Perspectives in Thailand*,
DOI 10.1007/978-94-007-7244-1_27,

but rather, it is discursively constructed. ..., experienced, and understood in culturally and historically specific ways." In addition, some queer theorists have discussed normativity, especially heteronormativity or the denaturalization of heterosexuality (Berten 2001; Clarke et al 2010; Jagose 2000; Spargo 1999; Sullivan 2007). Normativity is a type of operation of power that promotes a set of norms, which tends to be morally established. The normativity of current understandings of sex grants heterosexuality the status of a norm, defined against abnormal practices and desires.

Heteronormativity specifies the tendency in the sex-gender system to view heterosexual relations as the norm and all other forms of sexual behavior as deviations from this norm (Spargo 1999: 73). Clarke and colleagues (2010: 121) posit that queer theory discusses the social privileging of heterosexuality and the assumption that it is the only natural and normal sexuality. Heterosexuality is viewed as compulsory in which women's social, emotional, and sexual needs are subordinated to ensure men's privileged sexual and emotional access to women's bodies.

This chapter will examine how the third gender characters in Thai contemporary novels are marginalized by the concept of heteronormativity, especially the institutionalization of heterosexuality. First, it explores how the third gender is perceived and portrayed in three Thai novels published in the 1980s. Second, it investigates if those perceptions have changed after more than a decade later by looking at a novel published in 2004. Third, it discusses what influences such perceptions and portrayal of the third gender characters.

3 Portrayal of Third Gender Characters in the 1980s

Earlier Thai novels tend to portray the third gender characters, especially male homosexuals, as funny, almost absurd characters – trying to imitate women but overdressing and overacting, thus cannot pass as women. By the 1980s, however, authors began to change their perceptions. Third gender characters are portrayed differently although the clown stereotype can still be seen in many works.

In the book, *Chloe Plus Olivia,* Faderman (1995: xiii) classifies the literature of lesbians into six categories: kindred spirit (romantic friendship), a man trapped in a woman's body (sexual aversion), carnivorous flowers (exotic and evil lesbians), in the closet (lesbian encoding), amazons (lesbian feminism), and flowerings (post-lesbian feminist). This chapter uses Faderman's concepts together with the categories which emerged from the analysis to categorize third gender characters portrayed by Thai novelists. Consequently, seven categories are found: the sexual aversion, the carnivorous, the amazons, the identity searchers, the ideal woman, the earth mother, and the weak links. Table 27.1 lists the four novels and ten characters analyzed in this study and the categories of how third gender characters are portrayed.

Table 27.1 Portrayal of Characters in Four Novels

Year published	Novel	Character	LGBTQ	Category
1981	*Reflection of the Moon*	Phanee	Lesbian	Sexual aversion
				Carnivorous
1982	*The Third Path*	Kaew	Transgender	Ideal woman
		Jan	Transgender	Earth mother
		Chat; La-ong Dao	Transgender	Weak links
1989	*The Golden Chair*	Ajana	Gay	Identity searcher
		Phanida	Lesbian	Sexual aversion
				Carnivorous
2004	*The Heroine*	Kanya	Lesbian	Sexual aversion
				Carnivorous; amazon
		Phim	Lesbian?	Identity searcher

3.1 The Sexual Aversion

Faderman (1995) explains that sexual aversion is lesbian literature telling stories about a man who is trapped in a body of a woman. In this chapter, however, the term is adopted to refer to both males and females trapped in the opposite sex. This idea is widely depicted in most Thai literary works about the third gender during the 1980s. Suwan (1981) describes Phanee as "looking more like a man than a woman" (p. 76), including her clothes (p. 79) and her room decoration (p. 116). The way she treats other characters is also "like a man treating a woman" (p. 87). Phimphilai's fiancé feels like he and Phanee "are competing for one woman – a competition between men" (p. 486). Furthermore, Phanee dislikes being a woman and a mother. She has one child from her brief marriage. The boy is very weak, yet Phanee abandons him. She tells Phimphilai that she wishes that he had not been born (p. 481).

Like Phanee, Phanida is always described as male-like both in the way she dresses and the way she acts, "she has big bones; her manner is like a man" (Ladaawan 1989b: 334). The way she greets an acquaintance is "like a man greeting another man" (Ladaawan 1989a: 166), and she is always compared to a ruffian (Ladaawan 1989b: 42, 58). Similarly, Kaew, a transgender in *The Third Path*, is delineated as female-like:

> … the way he holds a ticket holder in his clean, white hands and his long fingers clearly reveals his tenderness. His face is white, smooth, and clean. His sad eyes mirror the sensitivity of the owners. Kaew is skinny, and what Jan always admires is his smiling. Whenever Kaew smiles, the femininity that is hidden in his male body and clothes is invisible right before the eyes of those who witness his grin. (Chanaa 1982: 5)

Apparently, these appearances are not positively delineated. The characters are made fun of and oftentimes laughed at. Jan describes "… the painful fact.… to know that you were born in the body that you do not want to … the pain, loneliness, melancholy …" (Chanaa 1982: 3–4).

3.2 The Carnivorous

Faderman (1995: 297) explains that the carnivorous lesbian is exotic and evil … "in whose seductive embrace 'the victim' is gleefully destroyed." This is true in Thai novels. In *Reflection of the Moon*, Phanee is portrayed as exotic and almost always evil. She gets involved with two women, Mayura and Phimphilai, since they were in school. However, she is possessive and jealous. Many times, she would verbally harass Mayura and Phimphilai especially when it involves men. She physically abuses Mayura when her jealousy goes uncontrollable. She strategically manipulates both women by playing upon Mayura's weakness which is financial need and upon Phimphilai's weakness, which is her optimism. Phanee's anger is compared to heavy storms (Suwan 1981: 249). Other characters see her as a "lunatic" (p. 251). She successfully destroys Phimphilai's first heterosexual relationship by lying to Phimphilai's fiancé that she and Phimphilai previously had an affair. She once threatens Phimphilai with a knife, and at the end she shows that she can kidnap Phimphilai's son if she wants to. All of these are simply to express her anger because Phimphilai does not return her love.

Like Phanee, Phanida is jealous of Ann, the woman she considers her girlfriend (Ladaawan 1989b: 48). Her jealousy and possessive behavior is apparent to all other characters. These feelings lead to anger and hatred toward men, especially Lakaan, Ann's boyfriend. Her anger is so uncontrollable that she ends up shooting him.

3.3 The Amazons

The idea of the amazons is based on the lesbian-feminist thought, which believes that homosexuality is superior to heterosexuality (Faderman 1995: 548). They reject the idea of lesbian women as men trapped in women's bodies or carnivorous flowers. If lesbian love fails, it is not because of their sickness or sin, but rather due to the difficulties placed in their way by the sick world. In their opinion, lesbianism is the relationship of "harmony and happiness, an escape from the horrors of heterosexuality, a promise of self-fulfillment and healthy independence" (Faderman 1995: 549).

Both Phanee and Phanida openly express this idea. Phanee tries to persuade Phimphilai to live with her. She believes that "men only take physical happiness from women; it is women who have to get pregnant, have the pain. And when men have had enough of us, they will abandon us" (Suwan 1981: 883). Similarly, Phanida does not find anything wrong in her relationship with Ann, although Ann shows her interest in a man and keeps telling Phanida that their romantic friendship is a mistake and should end once they leave school. Phanida believes that men just take advantage of women. She puts the blame on Lakaan, the man with whom Ann is in love.

3.4 The Identity Searcher

Most third gender characters have already come out of the closet, especially when they are among friends and acquaintances. They may sometimes have to pretend to be straight when they are with parents and relatives or at work to cover up their true identity. However, Ajana in *The Golden Chair* is different. His behavior is what Linla, the female protagonist, calls half/half. The author describes him as "unnatural" (Ladaawan 1989a: 116). He himself articulates that he is "not exactly like that" (Ladaawan 1989a: 58). He does not want to show his weakness by crying, which is Thai patriarchal perception of "boys don't cry." However, he believes that he prefers men more than women, especially when he meets Lakaan. All through the book, he keeps searching for his identity, hoping that Lakaan, whose name means a sailing boat, can help guide him to the right shore.

3.5 The Ideal Woman

In *The Third Path,* Kaew, whose name means crystal, is portrayed as an ideal Thai lady, that is, being a good daughter, a good wife, and a good mother. Readers initially meet Kaew as a cute boy of 16, a transgender, who "was born as a biological man, but identifies internally and socially as a woman" (Marinucci 2010: 118). Kaew begins cross-dressing after he moves to Bangkok, dreaming of having a sex change. Kaew reluctantly falls in love with a man, who confesses that he loves Kaew, but cannot go as far as to marry Kaew. Two other men also fall in love with Kaew. Kaew rejects one of them because that man is already married and also rejects the other because Kaew does not want to hurt her friend. After the surgery, Kaew decides to work for children in a small village instead of living in Bangkok. Kaew's thought is shaped by a typical heteronormative idea of Thai society that only a heterosexual relationship is natural and acceptable; hence Kaew's reluctance to "love" her first boyfriend.

3.6 The Earth Mother

Besides depicting Kaew as an idealistic woman, the author also narrates about five transgender characters. One of them is Jan, meaning the moon, who is like a mother figure to Kaew. Jan helps Kaew from the very beginning; he supports and encourages Kaew to come out of the closet, to cross-dress like a girl, and to be proud of being a transvestite. Jan is with Kaew at every stage of Kaew's life – fighting with Kaew's abusive homophobic ex-classmate, accompanying Kaew to his military enlistment, and so on. The only time Jan is not at Kaew's side is when he has his dream surgery because Jan cannot afford to accompany Kaew to the United States where he has his surgery. True to his name, Jan is like the moon shining his kind, cool, and comforting light to guide Kaew's life and always being there when he is needed. Like Kaew's mother who passed away when he was a child, Jan's love and care for Kaew is non-conditioning.

3.7 *The Weak Link*

Two other characters in *The Third Path* are La-ong Dao and Chat, who are portrayed as weak links, the ones that contaminate Thai transgenders' images. La-ong Dao – meaning stardust – has a love-hate relationship with Jan though they are close friends. La-ong Dao comes from a family that cannot accept the fact that he is a cross-dressing, so he has to pretend that he is straight and has to come to Jan's house whenever he wants to dress like a woman. He was kicked out of the house when his father finds out, so he has to support himself by being a prostitute and a gambler. Jan believes La-ong Dao is a degradation of Thai transvestites. He uses La-ong Dao as a sample to warn Kaew not to lead such a shameful life although Jan himself never abandons this friend of his. According to the author, La-ong Dao can be the only stardust that can never shine brightly in the sky.

Chat, meaning a big umbrella, is another transgender that is created to be contrasted to Kaew, highlighting Kaew's idealistic and perfect personality. If Kaew is a crystal, the light, Chat is a shade, the dark side. Like Kaew, Chat wants to have a sex change, yet the similarity ends there. While Kaew views the surgery as the completion of her womanhood, Chat wants the sex change for the sexual purpose. Chat thinks the surgery will enable him to have a penis-vaginal sexuality like a female prostitute so that he can make more money. While Kaew works hard to save money for the surgery, Chat goes for shortcuts like stealing, prostituting, and drug dealing. Ironically, Chat is arrested right after his sex change and is put in prison. He is gang-raped when other prisoners learn that he has had a sex change, and eventually he is dead. The author has made his point clear that it does not matter whether one is a homosexual or a heterosexual; what matters is to live a kind and decent life.

Kaew's quest for transforming from a man to become a "complete" woman is based on the author's true experience. Growing up in Thailand during the post-Vietnam war period, the author was obviously familiar with an ideal image of good women and the importance of heterosexuality. Kaew and Jan are, thus, portrayed as feminine ladies: faithful, loyal, gentle, decent, and kind. They see sexuality as nonessential. The novel is about love, not sexuality, although the main character is a transgender.

4 Perceptions of Third Gender Characters

Thai novelists present nature and nurture as two important elements that lead to LGBTQ. First, the third gender is depicted as unnatural (see Chaps. 25 and 26). The author of *The Golden Chair* explains that only the love and sexuality created by God (heterosexual love) is natural; others are not. Homosexual relationship is unnatural, unlike Adam and Eve in the Bible (Ladaawan 1989a, 52). This allusion to heterosexual relationship apparently reveals the author's perception that only heterosexual relationship is acceptable. That is why the story ends with the victory of heterosexual relationship. Ajana turns out to be straight although he and other characters initially believe that he is gay.

These unnatural appearances and behavior are judged and oftentimes laughed at by other non-LGBTQ characters. Phanee's sexual need is described as "unnatural" (Suwan 1981: 277). One of the characters says that she feels "disgusted" by Phanee's behavior (p. 94). Others criticize and sometimes make fun of her appearance and behavior behind her back. Similarly, Kaew and Jan are oftentimes laughed at and teenagers in their neighborhood made fun of them. Ajana and his gay friends are often criticized by people around them; Frank's gardener wonders, "Man and man, how could it be fun?" (Ladaawan 1989a: 62). Linla judges Ajana when they first meet, "Well, your look tells what kind of a 'man' you are!" (p. 6). According to Phimphilai's mother, a lesbian like Phanee can only be the reflection of the moon in the water, never able to shine as brightly as the authentic one upon the sky. Apparently, the author compares homosexuality to shadow, something unreal and unequal to the authentic one – heterosexuality.

Additionally, some characters express that the third gender is the result of karma. Phaen says that Phanee must have done something bad to someone in her past life, so in this life, she is "abnormal, unlike other women" (Suwan 1981: 752). Similarly, Jan and Kaew also accept that being born a transgender is because of karma done in their past lives.

Furthermore, the third gender is perceived as being sick. Phanee is the character that is openly described as mentally ill and needs professional help. Her former husband tries to persuade and eventually forces her to see a doctor. But, Phanee does not cooperate; she sees her sexual preference as normal, and it is others who are sick. However, she has to "act" to cover up her true identity. Similarly, Lakaan also sees Niphat as "mentally sick" when he tries to convince Ajana that he is not (Ladaawan 1989a: 280).

All three novels present the idea that the ways human beings are nurtured, including family and a coed school, are the main factors that will lead to homosexuality. First, the family is believed to play the most important role. Phanee is the only girl in the family. Her parents have their business to tend to, and all her male siblings are, according to Phanee, badly spoiled. "They would do or buy whatever they want; they also sexually harassed our female servants" (Suwan 1981: 122–123). Besides, her father has a mistress though he does not leave the family. Her father's and her brothers' behaviors lead to Phanee's perception of men as "up to no good."

Like Phanee, Ajana's childhood has an influence on his behavior. His father hates women. He has a very manipulative mother and sister, which leads to a failure in his marriage. After Ajana's mother leaves, his father turns to alcohol and keeps telling Ajana how evil women are and how they destroyed his life. Therefore, Ajana grows up believing that women are his enemies. Similarly, Niphat, one of Ajana's acquaintances, grows up in a very strict family. His childhood evolved around conservative adults, who deny sexual needs of boys. His elder male cousin taught him about it, but "it is not natural, unlike what is stated in the Bible that God created Adam and Eve to spend their lives together naturally in this world" (Ladaawan 1989a: 52).

Second, most novelists claim that a coeducational school is one of the major factors that nurture the third gender. Phanee and Phanida go to coeducational schools. Both of them have a romantic relationship, to state in Faderman's term (1995: xiii), with their female schoolmates, a behavior that most adults think will disappear after they leave schools. However, the author of *Reflection of the Moon* states that it is "the beginning of dangerous thing for a girl's life" (Suwan 1981: 100).

Third, the author of *The Golden Chair* states that the third gender is not permanent; it is more of a trend among high society people (Ladaawan 1989a: 5). "They simply want to try and experiment with this sort of life" (p. 51). She presents a group of gay men led by Frank, a bisexual, who "the older he gets, the more he is interested in men only" (p. 58). Three other men turn queer simply because they want to experiment with it. Even a straight man like Lakaan sees no harm in it since he is "born in the era in which things are chaotic and the world turns upside down" (p. 84).

Whatever leads to the third gender, Thai novels present it as curable. Two ways for healing are heterosexual relationship and medical care. The first approach is mentioned in most novels. Phanee's mother insists that she marries Phaen although no other characters think it will work. Phimphilai's mother criticizes that "she probably thinks that if Phanee gets married, the problem will be gone. But I'm not sure that a person, who is as mentally ill as she is, will be able to adjust herself to a normal, natural life" (Suwan 1981: 371). This foreshadowing proves to be true because Phanee tells Phimphilai later that she hates every minute of her marriage life.

On the contrary, *The Golden Chair* seems to show that this method works. Ajana does not like women mainly because he believes that he is always defeated by them. He sees women as arrogant and annoying enemies. He especially dislikes a woman who is strong and successfully relies on herself – a very patriarchal idea. For him, women like Linla seem to always beat him for the golden chair – a symbol of success about which he always dreams but is never able to achieve.

Ajana attempts a heterosexual relationship with Linla, the woman he used to dislike, after Lakaan insists that he himself is straight and does not like Ajana in a sexual way. Lakaan tries to convince Ajana that he is not gay; he is only weak and dislikes women. If Ajana controls himself and changes his thought about women, he will be able to overcome whatever feeling he thinks he has for Lakaan (Ladaawan 1989b: 198–200). Ajana goes to a bar and spends a night with a prostitute. Finally, he tries to woo Linla because he just finds "the beauty of love between men and women. Though it involves sexuality, it is normal" (Ladaawan 1989b: 324).

Phanee is the only character that is portrayed as seriously ill. Her marriage to a man fails. No one believes that it will work (Suwan 1981: 396), except her mother who is in denial. Therefore, her husband looks for professional help. He attempts to take her to consult a doctor, hoping that she can be cured from this sickness. However, Phanee is incorrigible.

5 A Decade Later

A novel written almost two decades later, *The Heroine,* has changed a little in terms of the portrayal of third gender characters. For instance, it does not depict a lesbian as looking or dressing like a man. Instead, Kanya, whose name means "a beautiful woman," is portrayed as graceful, elegant, and stunning, but her femininity stops there. As stated by Faderman (1995: xiii), a lesbian heroine is "an outsider, a monster, a self creation in a hostile world." Kanya fits this description. Everyone who works under her thinks she is "fearful, having great leadership, serious, honest, investigative, and powerful" (Wiwatthanachai 2004: 15–19). She is always compared to diamonds in which she is an expert (p. 74). Kanya is successful in the world of business; she is truly self-created. Her expertise in diamonds puts her at the top of her field. Her boss relies on her knowledge for the company's success. Most male colleagues envy her and do not like her; some even attempt to come on to her sexually. She is an outsider in a man's world, a true amazon.

Kanya once told Phim about her love and sexual experiences with men when she was young and attempts to have a heterosexual relationship. She describes that she felt as if she was having sex with her brothers or her close friends (pp. 162–163). She is definitely a male trapped in a woman's body. Her feminine beauty is compared to a tumor, unwanted and needed to be eradicated (pp. 170–171). In addition, Kanya is also portrayed as a sadistic and evil person – a carnivorous flower – who tries to devour Phim, her victim. She would not stop at anything. To reach her goal, Kanya fires one of her workers, breaks up with her girlfriend, and rapes Phim.

Although there are not many differences between the first three novels and *The Heroine*, the trace of what Faderman (1995: 689) calls "flowerings" literature can be found. Faderman articulates that flowering literature is "likely to focus exclusively on women's sexual passion for each other." The main theme of this novel is just that. Kanya is madly in love with Phim and tries to persuade Phim to spend the rest of their lives together, but Phim denies this. Unlike Kanya, Phim is not ready. She wants to marry a man, to have a family, and to have children like any "normal" women. The heteronormative idea planted in her while growing up is too strong.

Of all characters analyzed in this study, Phim is the most sympathetic. Like Ajana, Phim is on a journey in search of her own identity. Phim is a young and naïve woman, newly graduated from college, who is raped by her female supervisor. Growing up in a warm and supportive family, Phim is shocked. She cannot believe that a beautiful, elegant, and graceful woman is a lesbian and is doing that to her. The horrifying part is Phim realizes that she does not object to what Kanya does. Worse than that, she seems to enjoy it. She resigns from work to avoid seeing Kanya. She goes so far as to sleep with her fiancé to cleanse herself and to prove to herself that she is not a lesbian. When Kanya persuades Phim to live with her as part of a couple, Phim, although does not deny that she likes Kanya, runs away to ask for help from a shopkeeper near her house. Like Ajana, she has made her decision to live a socially acceptable normal life and to have a heterosexual relationship.

Clarke and colleagues (2010: 154) state that many third gender characters are caught in an identity comparison "between perception of self as homosexual and others' perceptions of her homosexuality which result in feelings of alienation from peers and a sense of self as not belonging or being different." The heteronormativity causes Phim to deny her identity as a lesbian. She seeks physical help from a bystander to save her from the carnivorous Kanya and mental help by having a heterosexual relationship. For Kanya, although she openly expresses her true identity to Phim and a few of her lovers, she hides it from others. At home she is a good daughter and a good granddaughter taking great care of her mother and grandmother. She cooks and cleans the house for them when she does not go to work. But, they do not know about her sexual preference. She, too, is affected by heteronormativity.

In sum, after almost two decades, third gender characters are still perceived and portrayed in the same way and under similar assumptions. What is different is only the surface – an appearance – and that is because the characters want to hide their identities from the whole world, the world set by heteronormativity.

6 Discussion and Conclusion

There are three factors that influence the belief of Thai novelists and lead them to portray third gender characters the way they do. First, the belief influenced by psychological theories, which are adopted among Thai academics during that time. All empirical studies reveal this and one novel goes into details explaining how nurturing a child can affect them. Second, heteronormative ideas play very important roles, and probably this is the most significant factor. Thais strongly believe that only heterosexuality is natural; others are not.

Third, publisher and peer pressure is another factor that plays an important role in shaping the authors' thought. Faderman (1995: xii) states that "publishers also would have pressured writers to present their subject in a way that was consonant with public knowledge and expectations – which were formed by earlier male representations." This is another possible factor among Thai novelists. Kisana Asoksin, one of Thai renown novelists who wrote a few books on the third gender, once mentions that one of her fellow authors told her not to write in a way that encourages homosexuality, and her answer is "Trust me, I won't" (Asoksin 1991: Introduction). She explains that she sympathizes with third gender characters but she has the duty of an author that she has to perform, a duty to keep the world in its heteronormative frame.

All third gender characters in the four novels have goals that they are looking for. In *The Third Path*, Kaew and Chat are obviously traveling for the same destination – sex change, although with different reasons. Jan is satisfied by being a cross-dressing protector godmother of Kaew; he has completed his own journey as a transgender and keeps on performing the role of the earth mother. Phanee looks for someone with whom she can love and spend her life. To the end, she still keeps searching. Rebellious as she is, Phanee does not dare to confront her mother and inform her mother that she herself is a lesbian. She even agrees to marry a man as her mother insists. Therefore, Phanee's quest never ends.

Ironically though, the author of *Reflection of the Moon* names the hero who comes to save Phimphilai from the evil lesbian, Phaen. This is the name of a hero in a Thai classical literary work called *Khun Chaang, Khun Phaen*. This hero is well known among Thais as a womanizer. In that classical work, Phaen has five wives, some of whom he betrays, seduces, kidnaps, and murders. Though in *Reflection of the Moon*, Phaen is a good policeman who divorces Phanee and tries to help save Phimphilai. The question is whether the author implies anything in naming this character like that womanizer hero. Is she saying that it is acceptable if the seducer, the abuser, or the womanizer is a man? Does it mean that the author, though unintentionally, expresses her acceptance of heterosexual male's power of having more than one lovers, being jealous of his lover, and protective of the woman he "owns" whereas Phanee, the carnivorous lesbian, cannot have more than one lover, cannot be jealous of a person she loves, and cannot abuse her girlfriend? Of course, I do not mean that abusing anyone is right. Yet, it is almost impossible not to see the double standard and the influence of heteronormative idea implied here, unconsciously though it is.

In conclusion, the third gender was mainly perceived and presented through the dichotomy lens of heterosexuality. Being the third gender is not socially accepted; it is perceived as unnatural and a sickness that needs to be cured. Family influence and coeducation are depicted as the main causes of such behavior. Heterosexuality is the main hope for curing it, while professional help is the second choice.

References

Asoksin, K. (1991). *Nam soh sai*. 4th edn. Bangkok: Chokchaithewet.

Berten, H. (2001). *Literary theory: The basics*. London: Routledge.

Chanaa, K. (1982). *The third path* (2 vols). Bangkok: Wannakam Phua Cheewit.

Clarke, V., Ellis, S. J., Peel, E., & Riggs, D. W. (2010). *Lesbian, gay, bisexual, trans and queer psychology: An introduction*. Cambridge: Cambridge University Press.

Faderman, L. (1995). *Chloe plus Olivia: An anthology of lesbian literature from the seventeenth century to the present*. New York: Penguin.

Jagose, A. (2000). *Queer theory: An introduction*. New York: New York University Press.

Ladaawan, S. (1989a). The golden chair [*เก้าอี้ทอง*] (Vol. I). Bangkok: Ruamsaan.

Ladaawan, S. (1989b). *The golden chair* [*เก้าอี้ทอง*] (Vol. II). Bangkok: Ruamsaan.

Marinucci, M. (2010). *Feminism is queer: The intimate connection between queer and feminist theory*. Chiang Mai: Silkworm Books.

Spargo, T. (1999). *Postmodern encounters: Foucault and queer theory*. New York: Totem Books.

Sullivan, N. (2007). *A critical introduction to queer theory*. New York: New York University Press.

Suwan, S. (1981). *Reflection of the Moon*. Bangkok: Banluesan.

Wiwatthanachai, A. (2004). *The heroine* [*นางเอก*]. Bangkok: Praphans.

Part V
Contemporary Health Concerns

Chapter 28
Theravada Buddhist Temple Taking Care of People Living with HIV/AIDS in Thailand: A Case Study of Phrabatnampu Temple

Yoshihide Sakurai and Kazumi Sasaki

1 Introduction

In Japan, Wat Phrabatnampu, a Theravada Buddhist temple located in Thailand, is famous not only in its origin but also as a hospice for AIDS patients. The activities of this temple are considered examples of the efforts of development monks, who have a history of engaging in social services and community development in Thailand (Soucanh 1996; Noda 2001; Urasaki 2004; see also Chap. 5 in this volume). Moreover, this temple has recently accepted students who study nursing and welfare in Nihon Fukushi University and Koyasan University and provided them with training programs on spiritual care (Yasuda and Oshita 2007; Yasuda 2008).

This temple is known as an excellent example of a hospice for AIDS patients and social engagement of Theravada Buddhist monks, but this understanding is only one side of the whole story. What we also know from this example is that it is actually possible for many HIV patients to live with their families in community, and this approach seems more appropriate when we talk of the normalization of AIDS patients' lives.

If the responsibility of providing medical services and community care were well fulfilled by the government, the Buddhist temple would soon have completed its role as a hospice. And monks engaged in community development from the 1970s to the 1980s could finish their missions and return to the realm of religious activities (Sakurai 2008; Pinit 2009).

Y. Sakurai (✉)
Graduate School of Letters, Hokkaido University,
kita 10 nishi 7, Sapporo 060-0810, Japan
e-mail: saku@let.hokudai.ac.jp

K. Sasaki
NPO Tobe Bath chair, minami 8 nishi 2, Sapporo 064-0808, Japan
e-mail: kazumi_thorpe@yahoo.co.jp

P. Liamputtong (ed.), *Contemporary Socio-Cultural and Political Perspectives in Thailand*,
DOI 10.1007/978-94-007-7244-1_28,

However, to this day, this is not the real case. Wat Phrabatnampu is continuing its supports for AIDS patients and is going to further develop its project to help more people. What are the social backgrounds and management methods of this hospice? Here, we wish to show (1) the social context in which people living with AIDS could not sufficiently receive community health and familial care and finally they had to come to this hospice and (2) the cultural and economical context in which Wat Phrabatnampu has accepted patients and functioned as a hospice for healing and terminal care. In other words, the purpose of this chapter is to understand how the temple has attempted to receive socially excluded people and helped to integrate them into community life. We shall then offer an evaluation of the activities held by the temple.

2 HIV/AIDS Problem and Buddhist Temple in Thailand

2.1 Health Care and Traditional Medical Treatments

Thailand has attained a high rate of economic growth as a fairly developed country, allowing the country to further improve and strengthen its medical welfare system. However, there are still many people suffering from social exclusion, for example, hill tribe people and migrant workers who are not permitted citizenship, children who can receive neither suitable education nor parental care, women and youths who are exploited by human trafficking or sex industry, and people living in areas where socioeconomic inclusion has not progressed for political reasons (Sakurai and Michinobu 2010; see also several chapters in Parts I, II, III, and IV of this volume). People living with HIV/AIDS (PLWHA) also tend to suffer from social exclusion because of the intractable nature of the illnesses, stigma, and discrimination in neighborhoods, offices, or hospitals. They also have difficult access to medical facilities (see Chap. 30 in this volume).

The first AIDS patient was diagnosed in Thailand in 1984. However, due to the lack of appropriate medications, the government just conducted an inspection and prevention campaign targeting some high-risk groups, such as homosexuals, sex workers, and drug addicts, who were in the chain of infection and more susceptible to HIV. Since then, the fear of infection and the moral stigma of being an HIV/AIDS patient have proliferated among the general public, and patients have suffered from discrimination and prejudice up to the present (Liamputtong et al. 2009, 2012; USAID 2012).

Since 2002, antiretroviral (ARV) treatment has become available in Thailand following the establishment of "comprehensive continuous care centers" based in regional national hospitals (Ministry of Public Health Thailand 2008). Prior to this, PLWHA patients, with the supports of local resident organizations, health centers, and doctors, formed self-help groups through which they could try various health-care treatments. They coped with the illness using traditional therapies, such as prayer, Thai traditional treatment, Buddhist meditation, and Thai massage. They also built the care communities based on the network of the sick and supporters (Tanabe 2008).

Patients who are isolated from their own communities and human relations have complemented the insufficiency of "cure" with "care," which corresponds to the movement found in advanced nations where PLWHA have also formed self-help groups in addition to receiving medical treatments in hospitals (Konishi and Onizuka 2004). Simultaneously, this movement also concurred with the idea of community-based alternative development advocated in the North and Northeast Thailand from the second half of the 1980s to the 1990s (Sakurai 2005).

But, even if PLWHA have a strong will to live or can obtain family care after the development of symptoms, some critically ill patients are struggling to survive (Irie 2000). For the welfare of these people, the temple opened the hospice in the 1990s. In what follows, we will discuss the activities held by this hospice.

2.2 *Buddhist Hospice*

In 1989, "the widow's meeting" was formed in the Doi Saket Temple which aimed to take care of the women who had been infected with HIV from their husbands (Tanabe 2008). In 1993, "*suun phuan chiwit*," a center affiliated with the *samnaksong* of Phra Phongthep in Chiang Mai, accepted ten AIDS patients and relieved their fear of death through reciting sutras every day (Urasaki 2002).

These temples provide spiritual care to PLHIV as well as to bereaved families. Before ARV was invented, HIV/AIDS was a fatal and incurable illness with obvious physical symptoms. It was the monks who provided spiritual and moral supports which could not be easily obtained elsewhere. In this regard, these monks were, unexpectedly, practicing terminal care which is prevailing in advanced nations. Moreover, it was medically proved that mental strength is positively related to autoimmune power (Nagata 1993).

Wat Phrabatnampu established its hospice in 1992 and expanded its capacity to 400 beds in 2001 (Urasaki 2002). The hospice has operated and continued its support to HIV/AIDS patients and families to the present. Although Wat Phrabatnampu has accepted and helped people who have been failed by the current medical system, accommodating PLWHA at a hospice may be, paradoxically, criticized as a form of isolation and exclusion of patients from society. Recently, however, the functions of hospices have changed from places where one goes to die to providing home care to patients whose symptoms are alleviated during treatment. Are such functional changes found in the Wat Phrabatnampu?

Before answering this question, we will first briefly introduce the backgrounds and methodologies of this study.

As part of the fieldwork for her MA thesis, Kasumi Sasaki worked as a volunteer in Wat Phrabatnampu in 2009. Through assisting in the changing of used diapers, massage, and so on, she was able to conduct participant observation from August 7 to 17 in 2009 and worked as a volunteer again from July 16 to August 16 in 2010. At that time, Juthathip Sucharikul, a lecturer from Rajapak University, helped her to conduct interviews. Yoshihide Sakurai and Teraopl Kulpranton, a part-time researcher of Hokkaido University, also visited the temple and conducted supplementary investigation on January 25, 2012.

3 Temple as AIDS Hospice

3.1 Phra Alongkot Dikkapanyo

Wat Phrabatnampu is located in the base of east mountain range, several kilometers from Lopburi city. This Mahanikhai denomination temple was founded in Namchan, Khao-sam-yot, in 1976, and was a small temple until Phra Alongkot Dikkapanyo moved into in 1988.

Phra Alongkot was born in Potaram, Racha-buri, on December 9, 1953. After graduating from the faculty of technology of Kasetsart University, he earned his master's degree in mechanical engineering at Australian National University and began to work at the Agency of Cultural Affairs in 1984. In 1990, he was ordained as a Buddhist monk at the age of 35 and started to visit HIV patients in hospitals. Realizing how serious this problem was, he initiated the project in 1992 to help these patients. Because of this, he received many honorary degrees for his efforts in social engagement (Sommitr et al. 2002).

In 2001, Phra Alongkot, together with 21 monks and 1 novice, set the four objectives for future development of the temple: (1) to ease corporal and mental anguish for terminal AIDS patients and protect the dignity of patients, (2) to guide patients in their study of Buddhism and meditation, (3) to dispel discriminations and prejudices against patients with AIDS in Thai society, and (4) to support not only patients but also AIDS orphans (Noda 2001: 187–204). Phra Alongkot preached: "If a person is always worried about the whereabouts of afterlife, one would suffer more. Recollecting good memories and discovering Buddha nature of oneself would calm down your hearts" (Uuda 2000: 221).

The spiritual care performed by chaplain and vihara priests in the ward of terminal care had drawn worldwide attention (Tamiya 2007). Some medical- and welfare-related persons and organizations even visited and conducted studies on Wat Phrabatnampu. Indeed, a number of peculiar features can be found in their spiritual care. For instance, in Japan, where many people acknowledge themselves as irreligious and nonbelievers, spiritual case workers (SCW) are strictly prohibited from teaching and practicing particular religions on their clients. In Western countries, however, where religion pluralism is highly respected, responding to patients' spiritual needs is considered very important by many religious organizations and denominations. The patient's spirituality is protected by the caregivers and the related help groups. But, in Wat Phrabatnampu, HIV/AIDS patients do not need to be practitioners of a particular spirituality, and the temple aims at offering care to all

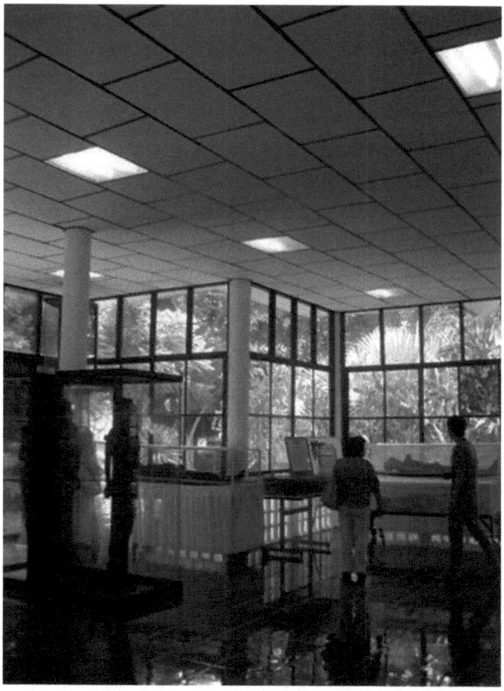

Fig. 28.1 Exhibition of AIDS patients' mummies

eligible patients based on Buddhist religiosity, regardless of their religious identities. Furthermore, this community requires patients to play the role of caregivers before they themselves enter the terminal stages and become care-receivers. So, what kind of spirituality could the patients gain in this community? And what are the characteristics of this temple?

3.2 Temple Facilities

The total area of Wat Phrabatnampu is 53 rai (approximately 8.48 ha). Visitors usually enter the auditorium first, where they can see the sentence "To gaze at plain death (memento mori)." Approximately 12 mummies of AIDS patients and 2 child mummies are displayed in this hall. The mummification of the corpses of AIDS patients and the public display of them have raised controversies over human rights both inside and outside Thailand. However, we heard that the temple has allegedly received consent from related people to run the exhibition for the purpose of HIV/AIDS education and prevention (Fig. 28.1).

Inside the precinct, there are offices for administrative works, residential cottages for infected persons, a convenience store with ATM, and an office which attracts and receives donations. Donors will be given a certificate of donation, a photograph of Phra Alongkot, and a pendant with his image. The notice board shows the names of the contributors and the amount of their donations, for example, the Thailand Honda foundation 3,459,367 baht in 2010 and Bangkok University 50,000 baht in 2011.

Patients who are seriously ill are received in the Walailak ward which is named after HRH Princess Chulabhorn Walailak, and its construction was sponsored by the Queen Sirikit Foundation. On January 25, 2012, the temple, with a total capacity of 130 beds, received 123 patients in which 35 were in serious condition. In addition to this ward, there is also a hospital where slightly ill patients stay on the third and fourth floors. There are also accommodation facilities for patients' relatives who stay.

3.3 *Organizational Operation*

Basically, doctors do not reside permanently in the hospice. Instead, as of January 2012, a volunteer doctor from a prefectural hospital visited the hospice regularly and each time spent half a day there to conduct periodical medical examinations of patients. Three nurses who graduated from nursing school with the Phra Alongkot's Scholarship were required to work in the hospice for 4 years as one of the terms of the scholarships. Their duties include distributing ARV to 500–600 visiting infected persons, medical consultation, and medical checkups.

The hospice has accepted short- and medium- to long-term volunteers locally and globally since its establishment. As of January 2012, two volunteers have arrived from Germany and the Netherlands. Since 2006, the Dutchman (64 years old) has been to the hospice every year and each time he stayed for 3 months. He said: "I was seriously ill 15–16 years ago and I lost my work and partner. When faced with death, I decided to participate in the AIDS project in the Netherlands."

Several volunteers are needed to assist in massage, diaper change, and meal care for patients in the Walailak ward which has a total capacity of 35 beds. It is a hard work from the morning to the evening. In January 2012, there were 10 full-time and 28 part-time workers with daily wages of 100–200 baht. One young person from Nong Khai Province, who graduated from a college with the Phra Alongkot's Scholarship, worked there. His brother has also worked with the Phra Alongkot. The number of clerical staff is higher than medical workers owing to the management considerations of the Phra Alongkot's enterprise and foundation. This issue will be examined in the following section.

3.4 *Operating Funds*

Wat Phrabatnampu is open to visitors in order to promote HIV/AIDS education and prevention and to attract more donations from the public. The running costs stated in the Thai brochure (Table 28.1) are very different from that on the English

Table 28.1 Running cost of the temple (Thai brochure)

Income	Baht/month
Donations	1,200,000
Official subsidy	100,000
Total	1,300,000
Expenditure	
Food	300,000
Medicine	300,000
Staff compensation	350,000
Cremations	150,000
Electricity	60,000
Telephone	10,000
Transportation	30,000
Miscellaneous	50,000
Total	1,250,000

Source: AIDS: What we should know to protect children

Table 28.2 Running cost of the temple (English brochure)

Income	Baht/month
No description	
Expenditure	
Office supplies	300,000
School supplies	300,000
Food	500,000
Medicine	300,000
Staff compensation	400,000
Cremations	100,000
Electricity	300,000
Telephone	60,000
Transportation	350,000
Miscellaneous	400,000
Total	3,010,000

Source: Temple website URL: http://www.phrabatnampu.org/brochure/br3L.jpg. 2012/02/11

brochure (Table 28.2). Members of the management advisory board of this hospice include medical workers, Lopburi governor, Lopburi provincial education board, the Thailand army, Lopburi hospital director, and the head of the Lopburi monastic order. The provincial government provided the building for meetings and the Thai government also subsidized approximately one million baht per year.

In addition, there are huge donations from the general public and supporting groups both inside and outside Thailand. Two or three visiting groups study on weekdays and more on weekends. The manager told us that "visitors came to the temple and wrote their study experience on the Internet. Now the Internet is another information tool."

Table 28.3 Change of the patients' number

Year	Hospitalized	New comers	Discharged	Fatality	Total
1996	1,622	589	189	364	1,658
1997	1,355	662	348	351	1,318
1998	1,154	833	253	547	1,187
1999	1,540	941	270	668	1,543
2000	1,772	816	215	558	1,827 (12 unknown)
2001	1,523	636	137	427	1,595

Source: Winai et al. (2002: 28)

Table 28.4 Sex

Year	Male	Female	Total
1996	1,785	425	2,210
1997	505	157	662
1998	880	234	1,114
1999	1,589	617	2,206
2000	1,817	771	2,588
2001	1,038	557	1,595

Source: Winai et al. (2002: 88–93)

Table 28.5 Original source

Year	Sex	Drug injection	Others	Total
1996	1,839	322	51	2,212
1997	589	69	4	662
1998	968	96	27	1,091
1999	2,090	279	46	2,415
2000	2,248	309	43	2,600
2001	1,211	263	131	1,605

Source: Winai et al. (2002: 88–93)

3.5 *Change of the Hospice and Patients' Life*

According to the statistics of HIV/AIDS patients in this temple (Tables 28.3, 28.4, and 28.5), many infected persons and patients entered this shelter from 1996 to 2001. The number of male patients was the double of female. Every year, 300–500 deceased persons were cremated, and the bags filled with their bone ashes were piled up in the backyard because they would not be returned to patients' relatives.

Those who observed "the battle field" of this hospice and wrote journalistic and academic reports preferred to evaluate these activities from the perspective of social work (Suda 2000; Noda 2001; Taniguchi 2006). However, an ambivalent evaluation of the hospice was found in the notes of Paul Yves Wery (2005), a French man who

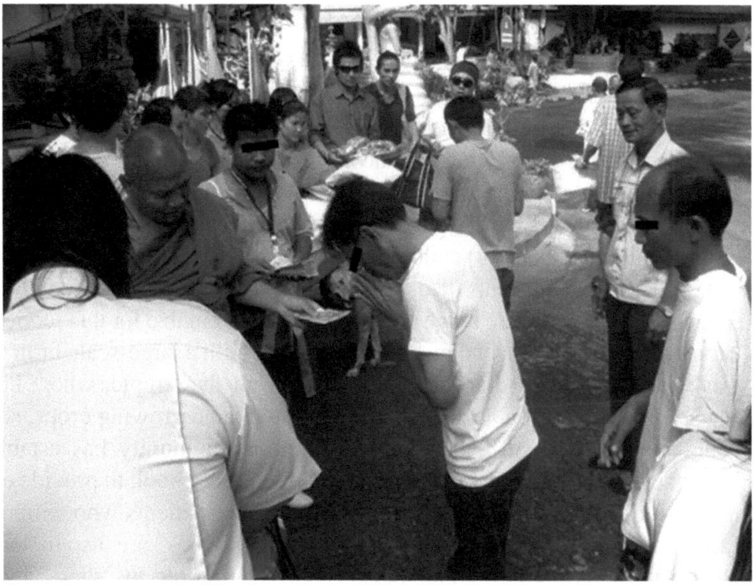

Fig. 28.2 Patients receive 60 baht from Phra Alongkot every Sunday

had worked as a volunteer doctor in this hospice for five and a half years between 1997 and 2005. Although he did his best to reduce patients' pains, he certified the death of several patients every day and sent their corpses to the crematory. He had some contradictory feelings regarding the hospice management. First, patients with mild symptoms took care of serious patients, and Wery considered it as a kind of slavery. Second, although consent was obtained, the dead, including children, were exhibited as mummies and used for prevention education as well as attracting donations from visitors. Third, Phra Alongkot was busy expanding his enterprise and left the operation of the hospice to patients and the volunteers.

If human and economic resources were sufficient in the Wat Phrabatnampu temple, Wery's distress could be dispelled. However, the reality is that the temple could not respond to so many patients who suffered from HIV/AIDS. Moreover, this hospice could not be financially maintained without Phra Alongkot's deification and creativity.

Since the middle of the 2000s, this shelter has gradually changed to a hospital with a capacity of 130 beds and has been able to accommodate 500–600 visitors. The duration that an infected person with mild symptoms has to take care of a serious patient has increased because their lives have been prolonged by the use of ARV drugs. In fact, the lives of many mild and serious patients have markedly improved.

Every Sunday, Phra Alongkot distributes 60 baht in cash and a chocolate drink to every participant in an open space. He also makes the rounds of the wards where serious patients stay. People expect his coming and appreciate his mercy. To Phra Alongkot, they all say with one voice: "I am warm and glad." (Fig. 28.2)

3.6 Social Inclusion by "2000 rai *(320 ha) Project"*

Confronted by the lack of human resources, Wat Phrabatnampu has explored the way to achieve self-reliance, that is, to rely on a group of infected persons who still have self-help capabilities and the skills to manage the hospice. People who are approved to stay in the hospice and community are (1) AIDS terminal patients; (2) the second-term patients of AIDS who do not have relatives; (3) parents infected with HIV, their children, and all other family members; (4) children infected with HIV or in the early stages of AIDS; (5) orphans whose parents died of AIDS; and (6) elderly whose caregivers are AIDS patients. Arguably, a wide range of target groups are eligible for this service.

In "project 2" alias "2000 *rai* plan," Phra Alongkot built a large-scale farm on the forests-and-fields background several kilometers from the temple, where he provided one *rai* to each household for breeding livestock and growing crops, so residents could become self-sufficient. Nowadays, this community has established educational facilities, ranging from nursery school to high school, to provide education opportunities to unfortunate orphans. Moreover, the patients who temporarily recovered in the hospice but still held "psychological wounds" are also included in this project. As of 2010, 150 infected persons and 89 children live there, and they practiced farming as well as Buddhist meditation. The total number of staff including nurses and noninfected persons was 34. Infected persons were responsible for looking after the yard, dogs, and cats, as well as cleaning, elderly care, and construction works. Their daily allowance was 60 baht per day, and 150 baht in the case of special business. About 80 infected persons were engaged in these kinds of works. Six monks, who were also patients, worked in "the project 2."

Since the social stigma against infected persons and patients of HIV/AIDS was strong, they were seen as passive recipients of care. In this project, however, everyone will be given the roles suitable to their abilities until one day they go to the Walailak ward. In this way, they could develop a stronger sense of self-recognition and self-esteem through working to the fullest of their abilities. According to the manager, "the enterprise of Wat Phrabatnampu is to set up a community that gathers people who are considered useless in society, and let them become useful persons again."

Next, we will discuss how PLWHA can "restart" and what kind of "self values" they can rediscover in the community.

4 People Living with HIV/AIDS (PLWHA)

4.1 Grounded Theory Approach

This chapter draws insights from Cathy Charmaz's grounded theory approach (1997) and analyzes the life stories of PLWHA. Through her caseworks in hospital, Charmaz was able to clarify the time sense (or recognition of time) of patients who are living with chronic disease (Charmaz 1997).

Patients suffering from chronic diseases are different from those with usual illnesses and/or injuries because the former have no or little hope of recovery by medical treatments. They also suffer from physical pain and mental anguish for the rest of their lives. Living with a lifetime of pain and extreme inconvenience, they can hardly imagine their recovery, let alone their futures. Chronic illnesses affect all aspects of everyday life, and patients might easily develop a sense of worthlessness when they think of their healthy past. It is found that patients who have been living with chronic diseases for several years and healthy people show substantial differences in their sense of time consciousness. "Living one day at a time" is the reality faced by chronic patients. Those who fail to develop a strong faith in the midst of distress can hardly find meaning and purpose in their lives.

From the viewpoint of "living with health impairments," a group of clinicians have investigated how patients who are HIV-infected hemophilia victims in Japan have reconstructed their lives after infection. The four factors that facilitate this reconstruction process include more working experience, social participation, intimate relation with others, and reduction in discriminatory experiences (Mizota 2010: 136–142). In this regard, Wat Phrabatnampu is considered to be a good example of a hospice because it provides a platform for patients to achieve these important goals. The following section verifies this point through analyzing the narratives of Wat Phrabatnampu patients. Their sense of time and self-identity are also investigated here.

4.2 Career of the AIDS Patients

Table 28.6 shows the details of informants with whom Kazumi has built close relationships through her volunteer experience in the hospice. Having been diagnosed with HIV infection, Sakchai (a fictitious name) entered the hospice before somatic symptoms emerged. On the contrary, Orawan, Anuwat, and Kanokporn entered there after their health worsened and symptoms appeared. Orawan's health condition improved after receiving treatment in the hospice, and she could walk around and help with cleanup and table setting for meals. "There is no salary. I would like to help those who are not fine. This makes me feel happy" (Orawan). Orawan also regained her vitality there, saying "I can do my best because I have the desire to live," and "I would like to help Phra Alongkot. If we don't do so, he will have to pay for outsourcing. I will do what I am able to help." When being asked about the reason of becoming healthier, Kanokporn said "I thought I was going to die, but now I am alive, so I am glad." Other patients were sent there when their bodies became partially paralyzed and because their families could no longer take care of them.

Sakchai, a Chinese, crossed the Thai-Chinese border and married a Lahu woman, an HIV carrier. Facing strong discrimination in China, he decided to return to Thailand. After entering the hospice, he met a woman named Thapanee who had Basedow's disease and stayed there as a volunteer worker. Neither her family nor

Table 28.6 Respondents' personal data

Name (pseudonym)	Sex	Age	Hometown	Education	Job	Infection route	Condition
Orawan	Female	25	Lopburi	Middle school	Factory worker	Boy friend	Advised by her father to enter hospital and has stayed for a year in the temple as a caregiver
Anuwat	Male	54	Chonburi	No statement	Police	Remarried wife	Came here after watching TV news about this temple and has stayed for 8 years as a guardsman
Boomchu	Male	44	No statement	Middle school	Salesperson	Sex industry	Suffered from partial paralysis and his family could no longer take care of him
Kanokporn	Femalee	27	Korat	High school	Accountant	No statement	Has stayed for 2 months as a caregiver
Sakchai	Male	44	Shanghai	No statement	Guide	Divorced wife	Came by himself and married with T. After temporal leave they came back due to discrimination
Thapanee	Female	29	Bangkok	University	Kindergartener	Uninfected	Wife of Sakchai with Basedow's disease and worked as a caregiver
Yoksapon	Male	58	Lopburi	University	Military personnel	Sex industry	Suffered from partial paralysis and abasia
Urairak	Female	54	No statement	No statement	No statement	Divorced husband	Has stayed for 2 years with partial paralysis
Nopporn	Male	28	Lopburi	Middle school	No statement	No statement	Suffered from partial paralysis and his family could no longer take care of him. Has stayed for a month

Source: Survey

her friends were happy when they knew she married an HIV-infected person. Thapanee said: "The others tend to say, being a college graduate I was too foolish to do that. But I would not mind them, because it is my way. Infected persons are pitiful. Why do people still bully them?"

Anuwat and Yoksapon could not live together with their families, although they did not show any AIDS physical symptoms. Fifteen years ago, Yoksapon knew about his infection with HIV when he received medical inspection before donating blood. In order to overcome the disadvantages as a result of insufficient education he experienced in the military, he resigned his service and entered Kasetsart University. Unfortunately, soon after he earned his Bachelor degree at the age of 53, AIDS symptoms began to emerge. Young women like Orawan and Kanokporn became infected by their lovers from whom they eventually separated. Although Orawan was asked by her family to be a *mae chi* (a Buddhist nun), she devoted herself to dancing. Kanokporn was looking for a new lover in the hospice.

Urairak was partially paralyzed and unable to worship despite being a Muslim, but she believed that she would probably be forgiven by God because of her poor health condition. She was infected by her first husband, and without knowing she has become an HIV carrier, she remarried again. Very regrettably, she said: "If I had known that I was infected, I would not have married again. I would rather die of AIDS alone." Nopporn also suffered from partial paralysis, but he never gave up his hope of returning to home after medical treatments. He said: "I will go home next week" and "I want to go home immediately. I want to meet my child so bad." Although he could only use his right hand, he was able to do some light work and take care of serious patients. Another female patient added, "I can work because I am fine. I have decided to work in a supermarket in Bangkok in order to live together with my child."

While this temple is a hospice for serious patients, PLWHA who can still work and receive familial support will leave when their conditions have stabilized. Their decisions are highly respectable. The participants in this research are patients who stayed for medium-to-long period. So, how were their mental conditions when they were diagnosed with HIV/AIDS and their symptoms started to emerge?

4.3 Mental State Before and After Development of HIV/AIDS Symptoms

The mental state of patients when diagnosed with HIV is, in a simple word, confusion (see also Liamputtong et al. 2012). When patients talked about their past, they seemed to be happy. "I was working in the dressmaking factory. Since I had many friends there, my workplace was enjoyable" (Orawan). "I enjoyed seeing people demonstrating on Rachadamnoen Street. I did not join, but just watched" (Boomchu). When asked "Did you go out and have fun at night?" K said "I often did." But they were perplexed when they were diagnosed with HIV by blood tests and symptoms suddenly appeared. If they could not receive appropriate medical treatments, the illness would progress irreversibly to the advanced stages. Suddenly, they realized they were living toward the end of their lives.

When people encounter misery and misfortune in life, they tend to give certain meanings and explanations to them (Berger 1967). Why me but not the others? Even if there is no religious meaning and it is just merely an accident, in the case of medical harm, it seems morally acceptable for these HIV-infected patients to show their anger to the medical systems and administration and to drug companies. And their sufferings earn the sympathy and support from the general public. However, stigma against HIV/AIDS patients is still deep rooted in the society (Liamputtong et al. 2009: see also Chap. 31 in this volume). For instance, male patients are believed to become infected because they "buy" sex from others, while for unmarried woman, it was through premarital sexual relations.

Such moral anguish has been accelerated by the popular merit-making virtue of Theravada Buddhism in Thailand. According to this Buddhist percept, a person with good fortune is believed to have accumulated his/her merits in previous lives and this world, whereas bad fortune is the result of the lack of virtue (*bun*). Nowadays, such discourse is not openly preached by monks, but HIV/AIDS patients who are influenced by this belief might still feel a sense of indebtedness (see Liamputtong et al. 2012). Therefore, they tend not to assert their rights of medical treatment like ordinary sick people. A sense of isolation is also strong among the patients who are distant from their family and community. How did the patients overcome this sense of moral inferiority and isolation as a result of discrimination and prejudice, and then could finally regain their self-esteem?

4.4 Regaining Mental and Physical Stability in the Hospice

Wat Phrabatnampu has been playing the role of a shelter. Orawan told us that "Since all the members here are infected people, I feel a sense of security staying here. Even though sometimes I am allowed to leave the temple temporarily, I just stay inside my house and will never go out. I am wavering on whether I should leave the hospice even if my condition improves because I wonder if people outside will accept me. I feel uneasy."

Since the appearance of red spots on Kanokporn's face, and Yoksapon's body paralysis became obvious traits of the disease, both of them would be vulnerable to discrimination if they leave the temple. Kanokporn asked Kasumi, the interviewer, "Do you discriminate AIDS? Some volunteers discriminate AIDS. Even the patients themselves do the same to each other." When Kasumi replied, "some of the people I worked with in Japan are also PLWHA. I do not discriminate you," Kanokporn appeared to be so relieved.

Admittedly, discrimination against patients still exists within the hospice. For example, a patient kindly advised Kasumi not to approach the patients with many festering wounds, saying "that patient is suffering due to bad karma. If you have to touch her, you must be careful about infection and wear gloves." On the other hand, there are some patients who are not regarded as having bad karma although they have opportunistic infection as well as partial paralysis. As will be discussed in details later, whether patients are said to be having bad karma or not depends heavily on if they have accumulated virtue through merit-making with the right attitudes in their daily lives (see also Chap. 31 in this volume on Merit-Making in Thai Culture).

Additionally, a new female patient (28 years old) who came to Wat Phrabatnampu after being hospitalized said that "in that hospital a doctor and a nurse did not want to go near me because I have AIDS. I could not receive much care." The infected persons and patients who have experienced various kinds of discrimination in the society can feel freer in the hospice because they do not need to hide and worry too much. And probably because of these changes in living environment, their physical conditions have also improved with the loss of psychological stress.

4.5 Recovery of Self-Esteem Through Merit-Making in Hospice

There are two roles that infected patients have to play in the temple. Firstly, they have to work as guards, salesperson in the shop, sanitation staff, as well as providing personal care and meal care for bedridden patients who are seriously ill. Another role is to share their illness experience with visitors. Patients with good physical conditions work more, while those bedridden ones talk about their experiences to visitors who come to visit them.

In this hospice, food, clothing, accommodation, and medical treatment are all free. However, patients do not want to be dependent and prefer to work when their health conditions still allow them to do so. Being taken care of by others, patients also learn that even a sick person could still accrue merit through helping others. Based on "the Commandment for Caregivers" preached by Buddha, the merit of caring for others is identical to devoting to Buddha, and this virtue leads people to the "eight merit paddy field" (punyakasetra) (Sugita and Fujita 2004: 22).

Anuwat respects Phra Alongkot and wishes to help him. Orawan and Nopporn also hope to help without expecting anything in return as long as their health conditions allow. Such devotional services and attitudes are regarded as virtues and meritorious, and therefore these kinds of patients, including those in serious conditions, are highly respected. Moreover, instead of being annoyed by visitors or tired of entertaining them, many patients actually enjoy sharing their experiences and thereby increasing people's understanding and awareness of HIV/AIDS. They could not talk about their sufferings or stories until someone visits the temple. HIV/AIDS is something not to be divulged, and when it is disclosed, people may receive sympathy at best but also discriminatory treatment in lives. In this hospice, however, they can talk about HIV/AIDS and share their own experiences with ordinary people, through which they gain deep respect as well as sympathy. They can even talk to people with high social status

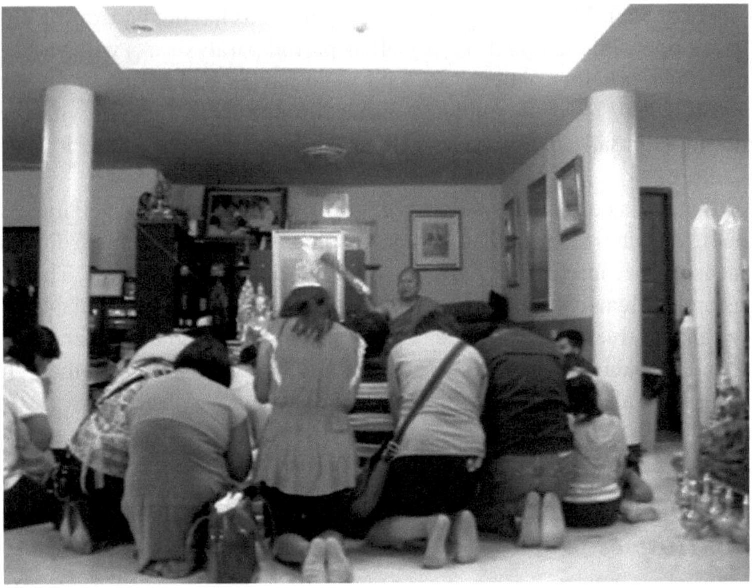

Fig. 28.3 Visitors listening to Phra Alongkot's preaching

and celebrities. Inside this temple, it seems that the feeling of moral inferiority among HIV/AIDS patients has disappeared

Moreover, this hospice is recognized as a place for merit-making not exclusively for HIV/AIDS patients. A male vice-nurse (24 years old) who has problems with his liver also works to accrue merit while at the same time, he receives medical treatment. A volunteer woman (in her 30s) who was apparently running away from debt collectors also accumulates her merit in the temple.

4.6 *Patients as the Objects for Merit-Making*

Temples and priests are the objects through which people can earn merit. Therefore, the general public visit temples run by renowned monks like Phra Alongkot, listen to Buddhist preaching, and obtain holy water to purify their spirit simply for the purpose of accumulating more merit. Spending time with patients who are enduring unimaginable pain and waiting for their final days, invoking Buddha's protection and blessing, or making donations are also ways to make more merit. "I was told by a fortune-teller something bad about my life, so I came here for merit-making" (a female visitor, 30 years of age). Moreover, a remark like "I come here to contribute because there are many people having trouble here" (a male visitor) was frequently made by visitors (Fig. 28.3).

One female visitor often comes to the hospice at supper time to help distribute meals and look after bedridden patients. Consequently, as a caregiver, she accumulates the merit. Among the visitors, there are also celebrities such as models, actors, and singers who would lean on patients and take pictures with them as proof of their visits. People who have wealth, political power, and publicity may think that they can gain more social prestige as consequences of their virtue.

As shown in this case, the purpose of many visitors is to make more merit rather than to care for HIV/AIDS patients. This phenomenon can be explained by the fact that this hospice is attached to a Buddhist temple. In Wat Phrabatnampu, the object of merit-making is HIV/AIDS patient rather than Buddha statue, and the former is seen as "the paddy field of merit." The temple is a medium through which patients become merit paddy field while visitors become merit-makers. And these three actors, the temple, patients, and visitors, are the financial backbones of Wat Phrabatnampu. We could not know to what extent Phra Alongkot and his staff intend to utilize the exhibition of mummies and storytelling by patients. However, their real intention to maintain the hospice and project 2 is probably understood by people living with HIV/AIDS.

5 Conclusion

Although the HIV/AIDS problem in Thailand was aggravated in the 1990s, the situation has improved, because new medical developments, in particular ARV, and the ever-improving medical care system have allowed the disease to gradually change from a deadly illness to an intractable chronic disease called AIDS. Wat Phrabatnampu, which initiated the Hospice for AIDS patients in 1992, has also changed its function from caring for the dying to looking after people who live with AIDS. Based on these changes in HIV/AIDS treatments, it is necessary to reexamine the existing studies on Phra Alongkot which evaluate him as a "development monk" engaging in spiritual care as well as terminal care.

Through participant observation and interviews in the Wat Phrabatnampu from 2009 to 2012, this study has attempted to understand the spirituality of people living with HIV/AIDS from their own angles, through studying the reconstruction process of their lives, and also the structures and systems that make this process possible.

Infected people and patients of HIV/AIDS who enter Wat Phrabatnampu were persons that cannot be healed only by family or community care or medical welfare. The extent of physical, mental, moral, and relational torments as a result of infection or development of symptoms may vary among patients. However, the conditions under which HIV/AIDS patients can live with dignity are not yet available in the community. In the hospice, many infected patients who recover with the help of medication and care can live without hiding their illnesses anymore, thereby relieving their mental distress. The great deal of working opportunities provided by the temple and the tacit rule of merit-making have encouraged infected persons and patients to help each other through which they also improve their self-identity. Those who are perplexed by the unreasonableness of life and a sense of moral inferiority realize the importance of "living one day at a time" and show their gratitude to others after listening to the lectures of monks and doctors and participating in many Buddhist ceremonies conducted at the temple.

A large amount of money is needed for the maintenance of the hospice and the project 2 which serve infected persons and patients, orphans, and old men. Apart from the support from the government and private sectors, various mechanisms to facilitate fundraising are also important for the long-term development of the temple. Donations from visitors are indispensable to Wat Phrabatnampu. As a merit paddy field, the hospice has storytelling patients and patients' figures (in the form of mummy) to attract visitors.

In the 1990s, this hospice served as a shelter for dying AIDS patients. Mummy is a symbol of death, reminding us the fact that life is transient and everyone must die. Now, people living with HIV/AIDS have converted this hospice into a place of care where patients can reconstruct their lives. The symbolic meaning of mummy has changed; it is now an integral symbol to attract visitors to make more merit.

References

AVERT. (2012). *HIV & AIDS in Thailand*. Retrieved February 15, 2012, from http://www.avert.org

Berger, P. (1967). *The sacred canopy: Elements of a sociological theory of religion*. New York: Doubleday & Company, Inc.

Charmaz, K. (1997). *Good days, bad days: The self in chronic illness and time*. New Brunswick: Rutgers University Press.

Liamputtong, P., Haritavorn, N., & Kiatying-Angsulee, N. (2009). HIV and AIDS, stigma and AIDS support groups: Perspectives from women living with HIV and AIDS in central Thailand. *Social Science & Medicine*, Special Issue: *Women, Mothers and HIV Care in Resource Poor Settings, 69*(6), 862–868.

Liamputtong, P., Haritavorn, N., & Kiatying-Angsulee, N. (2012). Living positively: The experiences of Thai women in central Thailand. *Qualitative Health Research, 22*(4), 441–451.

Ministry of Public Health Thailand. (2008). *Thailand health profile 2005–2007*. Bangkok: Ministry of Public Health.

Mizota, Y. (2010). Yakugai HIV Keiken kara imamadeni Eta mono. In H. Inoue, M. Ito, & Y. Yamazaki (Eds.), *Kenko Higai wo ikiru: Yakugai HIV sabaiba to sono Kazoku no 20 nen* [Experience from AIDS caused by contaminated blood products: Living with health hazard: HIV survivors and their families in Twenty Years] (pp. 115–133). Tokyo: Keiso Shobo.

Nagata, N. (1993). Sutoresu niyoru Menekinou no Henka to No/Menekirenkan [Change of Brain and Immunity Cased by Stress in Relation to Disease]. *Journal of Engineering and Health University, 15*(2), 161–171.

Noda, M. (2001). Tai Kindaika/Toshika niokeru ShinBukyoundo to Kaihatsuso/niso [New Buddhist movements and development monks and nuns in the modernization and urbanization of Thailand]. In J. Nishikawa & M. hen Noda (Eds.), *Bukkyo/Kaihatsu/NGO: Tai Kaihatsuso ni Manabu Kyosei no Chie* [Buddhism, development, and NGO: Wisdom of symbiosis learned from Development Monks]. Tokyo: Shinhyoron.

Phavady, S. (1996). *Psychosocial factors affecting the coping behavior of people living with HIV/AIDS at Phrabat Nampu Temple, Lopburi, Thailand*. Unpublished MA thesis, Health Care Management, Mahidol University, Salaya.

Sakurai, Y. (2008). *Tohokutai no Kaihatsuso: Shukyo to Shakaikoken* [Development monks in northeast Thailand: Religion and social engagement]. Tokyo: Azusa Shuppansha.

Sakurai, Y., & Michinobu, R. (2010). *Gendai tai no Shakaiteki Haijyo: Kyoiku, Iryo, Shakaisannka no Kikai wo Mezashite* [Social exclusion in modern Thailand: Searching for education, healthcare, and social participation]. Tokyo: Azusa Shuppansha.

Sommitr, W., Tipspapkul, B., & Ruennakarn, P. (2002). *khwamsamret nai karpdibatipharkit khong wat:sueksa chepha krni wat phrabatnampu amphomueang changhwat lophburi* [The success of the mission of temple: A case study of Wat Prabatnampuin Lopburi]. Bangkok: Samnakngan kanakammakan kansuksa haengchat Samnaknayokratthamonti, Khrongkan pattana kanchad-kansuksa Samnakngan kanakammakan kansuksa haengchat.

Suda, O. (2000). *Robyoshi no Tera* [The temple takes care of aging, illness, and dying]. Tokyo: Kawabeshorin.

Sugita, K., & Fujiwara, T. (2004). *Ima Naze Bukkyo Igakuka* [Why is the Buddhist healthcare needed now?]. Tokyo: Shibunkaku Shuppan.

Tanabe, S. (2008). *Keano Komuniti* [Caring community]. Tokyo: Iwanami Shoten.

Taniguchi. Y. (2006). *Ima Sokoni aru Tai no AIDS Nihon no AIDS* [Thai AIDS and Japanese AIDS now and here]. Tokyo: Bungeisha.

Urasaki, M. (2002). Tayokasuru Kaihatsuso no Yukue: HIV/AIDS kea nikakawaru Kaihatsuso no Shutzugen wo Jirei toshite [Varieties of development monks in future: A case study of the development monks who engaged in HIV/AIDS care]. *Religion and Society, 8*, 79–92.

USAID. (2012). *HIV/AIDS health profile*. Retrieved February 15, 2012, from http://www.usaid.gov/

Wery, P. Y. (2005). *Chronicle of a Thai hospice: Secret door to the mystery of Thai culture*. Retrieved February 15, 2012, from http://www.stylite.net/MMB/livres/originalfileschronicles/Chronicle_en.pdf

Yasuda, Y. (2008). Kaigai Jijyo Wat Phrabatnampu AIDS hosupisu ni miru Tai no Shiseikan to Shumatuki kea [Oversea report: Vale of life and death of Thai and terminal care in AIDS hospice of Wat Prabatnampu]. *Palliative Care, 18*(3), 231–233.

Chapter 29
Authoritative Knowledge, Folk Knowledge, and Antenatal Care in Contemporary Northern Thailand

Pranee Liamputtong and Somsri Kitisriworapan

1 Introduction

The concept of "authoritative knowledge" has been a focus of discussion among medical anthropologists who engage in the critical analysis of the social production of knowledge (Kaufert and O'Neil 1993; Lindenbaum and Lock 1993; Rapp 1993). These writers have focused their attention on "the privileged status of biomedicine as a realm of knowledge, which is separate from other cultural or social domains and which is seen as objectively valid" (Sargent and Bascope 1996: 214; see also Rhodes 1990; Lock and Scheper-Hughes 1990). Discussion of authoritative knowledge in childbirth was initiated by Brigitte Jordan, and since her first publication in 1978, there have been several researchers applying this concept in different childbirth domains (see Davis-Floyd 1992; Lazarus 1994; Davis-Floyd and Sargent 1997; Whittaker 2000; Root and Browner 2001; Liamputtong 2007a).

In this chapter, we examine the extent to which authoritative knowledge is prevalent among women in contemporary Northern Thailand. We also present the experience of pregnancy, folk knowledge, and antenatal care among women in Northern Thailand. Specifically, we look at what middle class and rural poor women have to say about their antenatal care and the extent to which they adhere to the hegemony of Western medical discourse and whether women, within the Thai context, have choices or control over their pregnancy.

P. Liamputtong (✉)
School of Public Health and Human Biosciences, La Trobe University,
Kingsbury Drive, Bundoora, VIC 3086, Australia
e-mail: pranee@latrobe.edu.au

S. Kitisriworapan
Kasetsart University's Demonstration School, Kasetsart University,
Paholyotin Road, Bangkhen, Khet Chatuchak, Bangkok 10900, Thailand
e-mail: somsri_kus@hotmail.com

P. Liamputtong (ed.), *Contemporary Socio-Cultural and Political Perspectives in Thailand*, DOI 10.1007/978-94-007-7244-1_29,

This chapter is based on a larger study on the cultural construction of childbearing and motherhood among women in Chiang Mai, Northern Thailand. An in-depth interviewing technique (Liamputtong 2013: Serry and Liamputtong 2013) was employed to elicit information. Thirty Thai women who are living in Chiang Mai were individually interviewed. Fifteen women were recruited from Chiang Mai City and fifteen from the Mae Chantra (a fictitious name) subdistrict, 49 km from the municipality of Chiang Mai. This was to ensure that women from different socio-economic backgrounds would be selected. Women from Chiang Mai City were mainly from urban and middle class backgrounds with a higher educational level, while women from the Mae Chantra subdistrict were from a peasant background and have lesser educational attainment and income. The majority of the women in this study had recently given birth, but only a few women were pregnant at the time this study was being conducted.

2 Authoritative Knowledge and Antenatal Care: Conceptual Framework

Brigitte Jordan (1997: 56) convincingly argues that in any social situation, there exist different kinds of knowledge, but some kinds of knowledge may have more weight than others. And this becomes known as "authoritative knowledge" (Jordan 1997). The reason for this, as Jordan (1997: 56) argues, may be due to its "efficacy" because it may "explain the state of the world better for the purpose at hand." It may also be due to "structural superiority"; that is, it is associated with a stronger power base. Under most circumstances, however, it is usually both. Drawing on Jordan's concept of "authoritative knowledge" (1997), we examine the experiences of antenatal care of Thai women in Northern Thailand in this chapter.

All too often, in order to legitimize one kind of knowledge as authoritative, other kinds of knowledge are either dismissed or devalued (Armstrong 1983; Jordan 1997; Lupton 1995; Turner 1995; Whittaker 2000). Alternative knowledge such as embodied or folk knowledge may be "correct" but is regarded as "backward, ignorant, naïve, or simply trouble makers" (Jordan 1997: 56; see also Ehrenreich and English 1978). Therefore, this alternative knowledge does not "count," as Jordan (1997: 58) succinctly puts, "the power of authoritative knowledge is not that it is correct but that it counts." As we shall show in this chapter, very often women possess embodied knowledge about the stage of their pregnancy but this knowledge is dismissed as naïve. Only knowledge gained from pregnancy tests would "count" as legitimate. As well, folk knowledge relating to safe pregnancy and childbirth has been subscribed by women, but it has been subjugated as backward and ignorant within the domain of Western biomedicine (Cohen 1989; Liamputtong 2007a). As we have seen in the Thai society, traditional midwives and other healers have been subjugated and do not hold similar privileged status as those from biomedical backgrounds (Cohen 1989; Whittaker 2000; Suwankhong et al. 2011a; see also Chap. 31 in this volume). Folk knowledge similarly does not count.

According to Michel Foucault, power relations are "produced and reproduced through the everyday activities and social encounters" (Lupton and Fenwick 2001: 1012; see also Foucault 1980; Lupton 1997; Turner 1997). Jordan (1997: 56) too sees authoritative knowledge as constructing through "an ongoing social process that both builds and reflects power relationships within a community of practice." Eventually, she argues, all those involved in the process learn to "see the current social order as a natural order, i.e., as the way things (obviously) are." Through this social process, the patients come to see the knowledge of medical professionals as authoritative.

In clinical encounters, authoritative knowledge is constructed through unequal power relationships between the medical professions and the patients (see Ehrenreich and English 1978; Porter and Macintyre 1984; Rapp 1993; Browner and Press 1996; Lupton 1995, 1996, 1997; Georges 1997). As implied in Foucault's genealogies of power/knowledge (Foucault 1980) that "power is possessed by … a class, a people and power is centralized in the law, the economy and the State" (Sawicki 1991: 52), those who possess more knowledge also possess more power, and in many cases, as in the medical domain, we argue that they also possess authority. While Jordan (1997: 58) indicates that she does not consider authoritative knowledge as "the knowledge of people in authority positions," in this chapter, we follow the argument put forward by Carolyn Sargent and Grace Bascope (1996: 214), who suggest that authoritative knowledge indeed "reflects the distribution of power within a social group." By this, we mean the power between the doctors and the pregnant women. In Sargent and Bascope's study (1996: 232), they show that "the social status and cultural authority of biomedicine created through discourse and embedded in the status of physicians maintained its ideological dominance." To Andrea Whittaker (2000: 124), authoritative knowledge "involves differential power relations between differing knowledge systems and different groups in society." Hence, authoritative knowledge is seen as what Pierre Bourdieu (1977) refers to as "cultural capital"; knowledge that is distributed unevenly among different social classes in a society, and this knowledge allows the holders to possess the status of dominance. Almost all Western-trained doctors in Thailand are those from higher social status with more wealth, education, and power. As we shall show, to our women, doctors' authoritative knowledge incorporates their authorities as well. Our position in this chapter, hence, departs from Jordan's theoretical background at this particular point.

Childbearing including pregnancy in any society is a biological event, but the childbearing experience is also socially constructed (Hoban 2007; Liamputtong 2007b; Selin and Stone 2009). It takes place in a cultural context and is shaped by the views and practices of that culture. Therefore, there exist numerous beliefs and practices relating to the childbearing process that the woman and her family must adhere to in order to ensure the health and well-being of not only herself but also that of her newborn infant (Laderman 1983; Steinberg 1996; Jordan 1997; Liamputtong Rice 2000; Hoban 2007; Liamputtong 2007b). Taking Jordan's argument (1997), if folk or cultural knowledge is constructed through a consensus of "what is thinkable and unthinkable" (Georges 1997: 91–92), folk knowledge, we argue, can then be construed as authoritative knowledge in the context of our study. Folk knowledge has been incorporated into the lives of Thai people (Suwankhong et al. 2011a; see also Chaps. 30 and 31 in this volume) and in childbirth in the forms of traditional beliefs and practices (Liamputtong 2004; Liamputtong et al. 2005; Liamputtong 2007a, b, 2009). In childbirth, women are instructed to follow dietary and behavioral regimes to ensure safe pregnancy and childbirth (Muecke 1976; Mougne 1978; Liamputtong Rice 2000; Whittaker 2000; Hoban 2007; Liamputtong 2007a, 2009). In this chapter, we shall show that women regard some folk knowledge as authoritative and they would incorporate this knowledge into their pregnancy care. However, in some cases, folk knowledge may clash with biomedical knowledge and it may mean that folk knowledge has to be surrendered.

Since authoritative knowledge is consensually constructed, it is, therefore, persuasive. Authoritative knowledge then has the possibility of "powerful sanctions." Individuals may be able to move between different forms of knowledge (see Root and Browner 2001), but in certain boundaries and at certain times, they may have to surrender to knowledge of those in authority. In situations of structural inequality, such as in clinical care, often medical knowledge gains authority and hence sanctions and devalues and delegitimizes others in doing so (Browner and Press 1996: 1420). Often, it also "serves as grounds for action" (Sargent and Bascope 1996: 213). We shall show in this chapter that, in antenatal care, women posses embodied knowledge and may wish to follow folk knowledge but they may eventually give in to sanctions and authoritative knowledge of their medical professions, making them adhere to biomedical care of pregnancy.

In antenatal care, as in childbirth, there is evidence that women tend to accept medical knowledge as legitimate. In Brigitte Jordan and Susan Irwin's study (1989: 20), they found that "most women willingly submit themselves to the authority of the medical view" and the women believe that their physicians act "in their own…best interests." Maureen Porter and Sally Macintyre (1984) too show that women in Aberdeen see doctor's advice as legitimate, as they believe what the doctor recommends has been well thought out and, therefore, it must be the best options for them. Although there are women in Robin Root and Carole Browner's study (2001: 208) who resist antenatal norms, those who comply have strong faith in authoritative knowledge of their medical professionals. These women consult and seek advice from their doctors regarding diet and behaviors. The women not only "privilege biomedical know-how" but also "relegate the non-bio-medical to the realm of non-credible."

How does this phenomenon come about? In many parts of the world, childbirth has been seen as a medical event and controlled by the medical professions (Ginsburg and Rapp 1991; Lukere and Jolly 2002; Hernandez 2007; Hoban 2007; Liamputtong 2007a, b, 2011). This medicalized view sees childbirth as "potentially pathology" and that "something can go wrong at anytime" (Lazarus 1994: 27–28). This has put women under the control of the medical professions. As Lazarus (1994: 27) succinctly puts, if women do not do "everything" like following the advice of doctors, it is their responsibility if the mothers do not have a "perfect" birth, or a healthy baby, and they must be blamed for it. This is a powerful message that pregnant women receive. It is not too surprising then that women come to believe that their doctors know best about their childbirth, and they have to rely on medical knowledge to ensure that they have done everything possible to ensure a healthy birth (Lazarus 1994; Liamputtong 2007a, b).

3 Pregnancy and Embodied Knowledge

Embodied knowledge, according to Carole Browner and Nancy Press (1996: 142), is referred to as "subjective knowledge derived from a woman's perception of her body and its natural processes as these change throughout a pregnancy's course." Accordingly, women possess knowledge about the changes in their bodies and they often are able to diagnose their pregnancies long before other means may confirm it (Davis-Floyd 1992; Martin 1992; Jordan 1997). This embodied knowledge is equalized to the concept of "haptic" in Root and Browner's writing (2001: 201). Women adopted "haptic" including "emotions, fatigue and hunger" as a means to acquire and access knowledge of their pregnant bodies during the early months in their pregnancies. Similar to women throughout history and cultures, women in our study used their embodied knowledge to diagnose their own pregnant state. Although not all women subscribed to this, the most common of all was that they missed their period, and that they started to notice a change in their bodily parts, particularly the enlargement or soreness of their breasts. Some noticed their bodily weight as they became thinner and the loss of their appetite as a phenomenological indicator of pregnancy.

Despite their embodied knowledge, some urban and educated women wished to be sure about their pregnancy by having a pregnancy test, as Patanee, an urban woman, remarked:

> I wanted to have a child and had been waiting for it, so as soon as I felt that it must be, I had a pregnancy test to see if I really became pregnant. And, it was positive.

It is important to note that to all women, including the women who learned about their pregnancy from a pregnancy test kit (a technological means), however, their embodied knowledge was not sufficient enough for them to be certain about their pregnancy. All women wished to have their pregnancy confirmed by a medical professional, most often a doctor at a local hospital or an obstetrician at a private clinic. The women's attempts clearly point to their trust in the knowledge of their medical professionals. Sira, an urban woman, said:

> My breasts become bigger and my menses came late, so I went to buy a pregnancy test from a pharmacy shop to test if I was pregnant. It was positive so I went straight to a hospital to have my pregnancy confirmed.

4 Antenatal Care and Authoritative Knowledge

As soon as their pregnancy was confirmed, all women sought antenatal care (*fak tong*). Women, who were older who believed they were more "at risk" due to their advanced age and women with a first pregnancy, were particularly eager to do so. Women believed that having put themselves under those who have authoritative knowledge such as their doctors, they could at least avoid any negative situations that might arise during pregnancy (see also Root and Browner 2001). Siriporn, an urban well-educated woman, explained:

> I *fak piset* (had special care) with a private obstetrician for both of my pregnancies. As soon as I knew I was pregnant I went to *fak tong* [register for antenatal care]. I was an older woman and I knew that I might be at risk.

All attended antenatal checkups throughout their pregnancy. It is noted that none of the women, both rural and urban, ever missed any antenatal appointment. They all made particular efforts to attend their appointments. Malai, a rural woman, said she never missed any antenatal checkup, as she was afraid that the doctor would be angry at her if she did and, hence, she did not dare to miss any appointment. The experience of Srinang, a rural woman who had her antenatal care in a public hospital in Chiang Mai City as I have given at the beginning of this chapter, clearly showed authoritative knowledge of a medical profession.

Some women kept the appointment on schedule due to their concerns about their doctor's medical knowledge. This is what Warunee, an urban educated woman, remarked:

> I never missed the appointment. I tried to make sure that the doctor would see me on time. I felt considerate as I had *fak piset* with him and he did not really charge me that much, so I went according to the appointment. Also, I did not want to see that any problem happened. Say for example, the appointment was on the 10th, but I went on the 14th, the doctor's prognosis/diagnosis would be wrong. I was worried about that, so I went on the time we had made.

Other women said that they were more concerned about the health and well-being of their fetus. By having a regular checkup, the doctor's knowledge would help them to look after their pregnancy better.

> I never missed an appointment… because I was afraid if there was anything wrong with the baby. Sometimes, I couldn't feel the baby movement in my abdomen. Because I am a new mother, I often could not feel it, so I panicked. So, when it was a time to go for a checkup I would go and talk with the doctor about my concerns… I went every month. (Pimpilai, an urban woman)

Kesara, a rural uneducated woman, too remarked that:

> I never missed an appointment. I was there exactly whenever the doctor had made the appointment for my baby. It would be good for the baby because if I let the doctor check it, then I would know if the baby is healthy or not.

A vaginal examination, a common practice in many countries, was also carried out in the Thai antenatal care. But, not all women were subjected to a vaginal examination. For those who underwent the examination, they expressed their fears and said they could feel the pain when the doctor was performing and also afterward. Despite this, women were happy to "go along" with the flow and follow their doctor's authoritative knowledge, as Warunee, an urban woman, said:

> I had a vaginal examination… The doctor wanted to do it, so I gave him my consent. I thought it was a normal way of medical care, it was the way that doctors do for a pregnant woman. So, it should not be any bad consequences and so I agreed.

The gender of a doctor seems not to be an issue among the women who went through a vaginal examination. In the mind of many women, all doctors, males or females, possess medical knowledge, and, hence, they have authority to perform a vaginal examination, and as patients, they should not feel too concerned about it. Malai, a rural woman, explained when she was asked about her concern:

> When the doctor did the vaginal examination, I did not really feel anything. I did not feel shy or ashamed even though the doctor was a male doctor. He is a doctor, so I should not feel shy about it. When he wanted to do, it I just went along with it.

Authoritative knowledge of a doctor was more obvious among women who had prior negative pregnancy outcomes (cf. Root and Browner 2001). This was true for both the rural poor and urban educated women in our study. Somehow, these women believed that because they did not follow medical or folk knowledge strictly enough that the pregnancy went wrong. Ruchira, a rural woman, miscarried with her previous pregnancy. With her present baby, she would welcome whatever the doctor told her to do. She had a vaginal examination so that the baby would be safe.

> The doctor did a vaginal examination on me but I did not feel shy because I wanted my baby to be safe. I lost my first one through a miscarriage so I wanted the doctor to take care of me with this pregnancy.

Wilai, a middle class and well-educated woman from Chiang Mai City, also lost her first child through a stillbirth. Due to this, she too subjected herself to medical knowledge. She attended all antenatal checkups. She also requested and insisted on having all prenatal tests including ultrasound and chorionic villus sampling (CVS) to ensure the well-being of her baby, despite the fact that her private obstetrician did not recommend any. Due to her persistence and also her advanced age, eventually her doctor ordered three ultrasounds and performed CVS.

> After I had CVS, I felt good about it because I had a test to ensure me that the chromosomes were normal. I felt that I had done the best for this baby because I lost the last one.

By putting themselves under the authoritative knowledge of their doctors, women felt that they had done the right thing. When Saijai, an urban middle class woman, was asked how she felt when a doctor was performing an antenatal checkup, she said:

> I felt happy when the doctor told me that the baby was strong and healthy. So, when the doctor was doing a checkup I felt good inside myself.

5 The Culture of Antenatal Care: *Fak Piset* versus *Fak Thamada*

Most women from Chiang Mai City in this study had a special care (*fak piset*) with their obstetricians or gynecologists. These women were mainly from a middle class background, well-educated, employed in a secure employment, and had a secure financial situation (cf. Riewpaiboon et al. 2005). Those from Mae Chantra district, except for a few women, tended to have a general antenatal care (*fak thamada*). They were poor and had a lower level of education. Most of them worked their farms or stayed at home. Financial constraints were common among these women. As there were costs associated with *fak piset* including medical consultation fees and the cost of transportation, poor women did not have the same access to *fak piset* as did the women in the city. In our study, twenty women received antenatal care from private obstetricians or gynecologists, and the majority of them were women from Chiang Mai City. Ten women received care from nurses or midwives and sometimes local doctors at local health centers and most of them were from Mae Chantra district. Kesara, a rural woman from Mae Chantra district, said she had antenatal checkups with local health personnel at her local health station (center) and she only saw any doctor or midwife who was on duty. Similarly, Srinang, a rural woman also from Mae Chantra, only had her antenatal care at a public hospital in Chiang Mai City. She said: "I went to have antenatal care as a public patient where most poor women go. I didn't have *fak piset* or anything. I saw any doctor according to my turn." This is in the opposite of Sinjai, an urban middle class woman, who had her antenatal checkup with her obstetrician/gynecologist at his clinic or at the hospital when he was on duty. For Sinjai, a continuity of care was then ensured throughout her pregnancy.

The well-being of their fetus seems to be the central concern of women who chose *fak piset* as a means of antenatal care. To a degree, the women in our study believed that by adhering strictly to antenatal care and the advice of their doctors, their fetuses would be healthy and safe, and in some ways, might even prevent undesirable pregnancy outcomes such as physical and mental abnormalities in the fetuses. Patanee, an urban well-educated woman, contended that she had *fak piset* with her private obstetricians, as she was worried about the health and well-being of her fetus.

> At the beginning, I was so worried and afraid; would the baby be normal or not! I was so worried because I have seen crippled children and I felt so pity for them. I thought if they were my children, it would be difficult for the children and it would be a long time burden for parents too… So, I wanted special care from my private doctor and never missed the appointment.

For some women, issues of choices and controls become apparent. There were few middle class women who would actively seek doctors whom they could trust to take care of them during pregnancy. Pimpilai, an urban educated woman, elaborated:

> My menses were late, so I went to buy a pregnancy test to make sure that I was pregnant. Then I asked my aunt whom should I go to see, as this is my first pregnancy and I did not know a good doctor. My aunt recommended Dr [X] as he has a very reputable work history… He has a good reputation of taking care of a mother and a baby. So, I felt relieved that I could trust someone who would take good care of me.

Warunee, an educated woman from Chiang Mai City, said she selected her own doctor if he or she could match with what she wanted. This is what she said:

> I chose this doctor because I know him, but I did seek information about him prior to going to see him. I would look for the doctor's reputations, such as this doctor prefers a natural birth and wants a woman to help herself more, or that doctor likes giving a woman a caesarean and likes blocking woman's back or not, and so on. After all the information about these doctors, I chose my own.

Sinjai, an urban woman, had difficulty with conceiving. Hence, she actively sought information about a gynecologist who could help her. Through a brother of her husband, she learned that there was a new doctor who had just graduated from the USA and had a good reputation in assisting women to conceive. In her case, she believed that a good doctor would enable her to have children.

> It was necessary for me to have a good doctor because this doctor would advise me about the safety of the fetus. He would have to control my weight and constantly provide me with medication and so on. And he was very good, indeed.

6 Prenatal Screening and Diagnostic Test and Doctors' Recommendations

Women were also recommended by their doctors to undergo prenatal screening such as ultrasound to screen for any abnormality or check the progress of the fetus. But, this recommendation was not given by all doctors. Some doctors did not recommend even though they provided a special care (*fak piset*) to a woman. It appears that doctors, in at least the Northern part of Thailand, are not all prepared to use medical technology. Sirin's doctor did not recommend her to have an ultrasound, as:

> The doctor said it was not really necessary. Also it was expensive to have this test too. He said it was not necessary because the baby was healthy and strong and he usually did a routine antenatal checkup anyhow. (Sirin, an urban middle class woman)

Pimpilai, an urban middle class woman, did not have an ultrasound either. She said her doctor did not recommend it. However, it was also her own concern about the safety of the fetus that she did not ask the doctor to recommend one.

> My doctor did not tell me to have it, and I did not want to have it either. I could have a girl or a boy, this did not matter. From what I have heard, why should we subject our baby to any tests. Why should we interfere with the baby who is lying peacefully in our womb? … I think this was my first pregnancy and I should not have any problem, and my doctor did not recommend it. I was only 28 then and very healthy. I didn't have any problem with my pregnancy either. So, I did not have one.

For those doctors who advised the women to have an ultrasound, in the minds of the women, there were good reasons for it. Saijai, an urban woman, for example, said that her doctor organized three ultrasound scans for her because she had a frequent abdominal pain. The doctor wanted to make sure about the condition of the fetus, hence, ultrasounds were organized. Kesara, a rural woman, had an ultrasound when she was 5 months pregnant, as she became pregnant soon after she had a vaccination for German measles.

> The doctor wanted to make sure that my baby is normal because of the vaccine I had prior to my pregnancy. The doctor told me not to become pregnant soon after the vaccine, but I did. So, he gave me an ultrasound just to check if the baby is okay.

Siriporn, an urban middle class woman, was over 36 when she became pregnant for the first time. She was classified as an "at risk" mother. Hence, her doctor recommended an amniocentesis test.

> The doctor said he would like me to undergo an Amnio because I was over 35. However, he also said that it was up to me, but he would like me to do it. So, I did go along.

Siriporn also had an ultrasound when she was 4 months pregnant due to a sudden bleeding. The doctor thought she might miscarry, so an ultrasound was organized. Fortunately, her cervix was not totally opened. And so, he ordered her to have a total rest, and the baby was safe.

Prapaporn, an urban woman, had an ultrasound when she was 5 months pregnant. Her doctor advised that the fetus seemed to be too big and he was concerned that she might have a twin pregnancy. Prapaporn said she was worried about undergoing an ultrasound, as she thought it might be dangerous. However, her doctor used his authoritative knowledge to reassure her that he only wanted to "have a good look" at her pregnancy. So, she agreed.

Pimpan, a rural woman from the Mae Chantra district, had her second child after 35 and her doctor wanted her to have amniocentesis as she was in the "at risk" group (over 35). She agreed as he recommended. However, at the local hospital there was no facility for the doctor to do a test, so it was arranged for her to travel into the town. When she turned up at the town hospital, the doctor did not do the test, but just conducted a routine antenatal checkup. She was puzzled about the change, but did not question.

> Because the doctor thought it was all right for me not to have it, then it should be ok. He did a regular checkup on my pregnancy, so I thought it should be ok too. I trust my doctor.

7 Authoritative Knowledge and Instructions During Pregnancy

Authoritative knowledge of medical professionals became very clear when women talked about their diet and behaviors during pregnancy.

7.1 Diet During Pregnancy

According to tradition, women are advised to be cautious about certain foodstuffs during pregnancy (cf. Laderman 1984; Nichter and Nichter 1996; Liamputtong Rice 2000; Whittaker 2000; Liamputtong 2007a, b, 2009). Most often, women are warned to avoid any foodstuff referring to as *khong salaeng* (allergic foodstuff) (see Liamputtong Rice 1988; Liamputtong 2007a). Thai people take *khong salaeng* seriously, as it is said that the consumption of *khong salaeng* can cause health problems and perhaps death in the mothers. During pregnancy, *khong salaeng* may have a negative impact on the health and well-being of a fetus. In the context of pregnancy, *khong salaeng* include pickled and fermented food such as pickled cabbage, spicy hot food, bamboo shoots, egg plants, and anchovies. Women are told to consume only half of a banana, as eating a whole banana may result in a birth obstruction. Consuming shellfish and Northern Thai relishes during pregnancy will prevent the perineum from drying out properly after giving birth. Similarly, the consumption of Thai eggplant during pregnancy will cause anal pain after giving birth or during a confinement period.

But, very often when asked if there is anything they should eat or should avoid during pregnancy so that the baby will be strong and healthy, women would first refer to the authoritative knowledge and advice of their doctors as a way to follow rather than tradition. Pimpilai, an urban woman, told us that:

> My doctor kept telling me that I should not eat too much, that I should eat good food, like milk and fruit, so that I would not have digestion problem, and that I should avoid tea, coffee and soft drinks. If I felt like a soft drink, he said I could have some but not too much.

Saijai, an urban middle class woman, similarly explained:

> When I saw my doctor, he would ask me how many cups of milk I drank per day. I said just one, and he would ask me to take two cups, one in the morning and one in the afternoon... I don't really like milk because I always feel that I will vomit after drinking it, but I tried my best to drink some milk as the doctor told me to do.

Prapaporn, another urban middle class woman who followed her doctor's advice strictly, said:

> I mainly ate according to my doctor's advice. I asked my doctor if I needed to take any extra medication, but the doctor said I was healthy so I did not need any medication to nourish my body, only eat good and right food and never miss any antenatal checkup. This would be substantial to ensure my pregnancy.

Medical advice about diet during pregnancy was taken very seriously by women who had experienced a miscarriage or those who desperately needed to have children. This is what Ruchira, a rural poor woman who lost her previous child through a miscarriage, said:

> I must drink milk and eat good food so that my body and the baby would be strong. When I was pregnant I would eat according to my doctor's advice. I would not touch a soft drink, cigarette or alcohol as the doctor told me because I desperately wanted to have children.

Authoritative knowledge and doctor's advice regarding diet was somewhat problematic for poor women. As most doctors recommended drinking milk and consuming good food as a means to improve the health of their fetus, it was difficult for poor women due to their financial constraints. Srinang, a poor woman from Mae Chantra, had this to say:

> Women living in my situation [being poor] would not be able to afford too much good food during pregnancy. We could only eat according to our meager means. At most, we can afford some milk. But, to eat like women in the city do, it is impossible for us.

Traditionally, Thai women may consume some traditional medicines to ensure the health of their fetus and prepare for an easy birth. One common herb used by

Thai women in the north is *pu loai* or *plai* – a ginger-like plant. Traditionally, its root is boiled with water and this is consumed by a pregnant woman. However, most women in the study did not wish to take any herbal medicine during pregnancy due to their fear of harming their fetus. But, they would take whatever their doctor prescribed them.

> I never used traditional medicines during my pregnancy, but took only what the doctor prescribed for me. We should not use a traditional medicine because it may have a harmful affect on the baby. We should use only medicines recommended by our doctor; just take whatever the doctor advises. (Ruchira, a rural woman)

7.2 *Behaviors During Pregnancy*

Tradition dictates that pregnant women must take many precautions for the safety and well-being of their fetuses (Liamputtong Rice 2000; Liamputtong 2007a, b, 2009). These include avoidance of rigorous activities and sexual intercourse. Traditionally, pregnant women are cautioned to avoid sexual intercourse as the activity is believed to cause a miscarriage in early pregnancy and stillbirth in late pregnancy. However, women sought advice from their doctor if they should have sex during pregnancy. Pimpilai, an urban educated woman, elaborated:

> My doctor advised that we could have sex during pregnancy but he said it should not be too vigorous. He said we should not have it in the first one to three months, as the fetus is in the process of getting attached to the womb. Having sexual intercourse may disconnect the fetus from our womb [a miscarriage]. But, after four months we can have sex, but not too vigorous as the fetus may be affected [miscarry]… Also, the doctor said that if we have sex, we may pass on some diseases to the baby. So, my husband was afraid and he stopped having sex since I was seven months pregnant.

In the mind of Kesara, a rural woman, if there was no danger in having sex during early and late pregnancy, why should the doctor tell them not to have sex during these periods. Siriporn, an urban woman, too said that she did not have sex during her pregnancy although her doctor said that it was all right in the middle trimester. She and her husband understood that the doctor's advice must have some good reasons, and so they decided to have total abstinence during pregnancy.

Wilai, an urban educated woman who lost her first child through a stillbirth, was very cautious about sexual intercourse during pregnancy. She sought advice from her obstetrician and was told that it was all right to have sex only in the middle trimester.

> I consulted my doctor if we should have sex, and he advised me that we could have some but he also advised what to do to ensure that the baby would not miscarry. He said we could have some, not to avoid it at all.

Although women tended to follow their doctor's advice, in some situations they might not. Ruchira, a rural woman, said her doctor advised her to take some exercise during pregnancy. However, due to her history of a miscarriage, she did not do so, as she feared that she might miscarry again. It seems that women only follow authoritative knowledge if it makes sense to them and does not threaten the well-being of their fetus.

8 Authoritative Knowledge and Folk Knowledge

As in other parts of Thailand (Golomb 1985; Jirojwong 1996; Whittaker 2000), other forms of knowledge continue to influence pregnancy care of women in Northern Thailand. Pregnant women in the North are given advice by their mothers or people of older generations about the preparation derived from Northern Thai folk knowledge for the birth of their baby. One notable cultural belief and practice which almost all women mentioned was the advice to consume *pak plang*, a vine-like green vegetable which is believed to make women give birth easily.

The vegetable is rather slippery in its texture. Being "easy slipped" symbolically indicates having an easy birth. However, women believed that the vegetable would make the baby's body slippery, hence facilitating an easy birth. Some said that they consumed this vegetable throughout their pregnancy but others mentioned that it is only taken toward the end of their pregnancy. The vegetable can be prepared in a soup form with chicken meat or stir-fried with pork mince.

> I ate a lot of *pak plang* during pregnancy. *Pak plang* is a soft vegetable and we make into hot soup, a Northern style hot soup... We eat all the leaves and the water because it is slippery and this makes the baby slip out easily. (Isara, a rural woman)

Also a common practice is to gather *pak plang* and *maiyarab* plant (another vine-like green plant) and make them into a loop and then boil them with water. A pregnant woman then showers with this herbal water. When she is taking a shower, the loop will be put on her head. This is believed to facilitate an easy birth. Women who were told to do so had no problem in following this cultural practice, as it did not interfere with their pregnancy or harm their fetus.

Another common advice given to pregnant women was to drink *nam maprow* – fresh juice from a young coconut. It is believed that if a mother drinks fresh coconut juice during pregnancy, the baby is born without fatty stuff on its body and scalp; hence, the baby will look clean and beautiful. This belief seems to be pervasive regardless of the woman's social background. Pimpilai, a woman from Chiang Mai City, explained:

> Older people tell me to drink fresh coconut juice from seven months onward. They say when the baby is born its scalp will have no fatty stuff and it is clean. They say fresh coconut juice is pure. My husband would buy me fresh coconut juice... Ironically, the baby was still born with fatty stuff anyhow, even though it was not too much. However, I followed what older people told me for their sake. They have more experiences than me, so I wanted to follow their advice. My husband would buy me one coconut each day and I would drink it.

To buy a fresh coconut each day throughout pregnancy seems to be feasible for women who are financially sound. For some, particularly poor women, this became difficult and in some cases impossible. Malai, a poor woman from Mae Chantra, said that she believed that drinking fresh coconut juice would make her baby beautiful at birth, but she could not afford to drink it too often.

> I only had fresh coconut juice on and off; did not have it throughout pregnancy because I did not have enough money to buy them. One coconut costs me about 15 baht and my husband had to go into town to buy it. We could not really afford it.

Women were also told to keep doing light exercised such as walking or doing light household chores throughout pregnancy to facilitate easy birth. As this cultural practice seems to coincide with their daily life, most women had no difficulty in following the advice.

> Most often people would tell me to do some light work and walk. They say do not just sleep or lie down all the time. If you do some work it will be easy to give birth. I walked a lot during pregnancy. (Pimpilai, an urban woman)

However, any rigorous or heavy work is not advisable during pregnancy, as this can lead to a miscarriage. Most women were cautioned about this and tried to avoid rigorous activities. But for some women, particularly poor women, this would be difficult for them to follow or even impossible. Malai, a rural poor woman, remarked:

> People told me not to lift heavy things because they said the baby would be harmed. But, I still had to do it. We work in a farm and I often have to lift an engine to draw water into the farm. Even when I was eight months pregnant, I still had to help my husband doing that.

Isara, another rural poor woman, also commented on the difficulty in observing this cultural knowledge.

> My parents told me that I should not do too much heavy work and that I should rest more … so that I won't miscarry… But, talking about women in our situation [being poor], not to work hard or not to work at all is impossible. We have to continue working throughout pregnancy for survival.

Another strong cultural knowledge that women were cautious during pregnancy was not to prepare anything including nappies and clothes for their baby. Advance preparation would result in the death of the unborn baby. As Saijai, an urban woman, explained:

> I did not prepare anything for my baby. It is a taboo in this region. They say if you prepare anything for your baby, you won't get the baby [meaning the baby will die]. The baby will not have a chance to be born, so people would tell me not to prepare anything.

When asked what she did with things that the baby needed, she said:

> Well people would buy things for you before you gave birth, but they would keep them until they were sure that the baby was born and the baby was safe, then they would bring them to you. Also, my mother would prepare most things for me and she would bring them into the hospital for me.

Most rural poor women in this study tended to follow cultural beliefs and practices, as they believed in the wisdom and knowledge of older generations. Pimjai, a rural woman from Mae Chantra, did not prepare anything for her newborn baby.

> If you are talking about a Northern Thai cultural practice, we cannot prepare anything in advance. People believe that something will happen to the baby if we prepare things for it.

> The baby will be in danger [die]. I did not prepare anything for my baby. When older people tell you anything, you need to believe them and follow their advice. They know better, and it is not good for us if we do not follow their advice.

However, folk knowledge was seen to be less relevant to their pregnancy among urban women in Chiang Mai City. Women stated that they had become more modernized than their older generations. Tradition and modernity is a dichotomy of being in the old days and new times (Mills 1999). Andrea Whittaker (2000: 5) suggests that this dichotomy is captured in the way that Thai people at all level refer to "perceived differences" between past and the present. For Mary Beth Mills (1999: 13), modernity points to "a break between past and present as distinctive ways of life, contrasting the achievements and forward-looking potential of modern life against the failings or disadvantages of backward-looking 'tradition.'" The tradition/modern dichotomy is also a perceived disparity between "the status and prestige of images and practices" between the urban middle and upper classes and rural communities. According to Whittaker (2000: 5), this dichotomy is best seen as disparity "in the distribution of wealth and power as matters of having (or lack of) knowledge and experience of 'modern' ways rather than as inequalities of class."

Being modern, in the mind of some women, meant an abandonment of traditional knowledge. Araya, an urban woman, for example, remarked that she did not follow any folk knowledge regarding safe pregnancy given by her mother, as this knowledge belongs to the old day (*samai khon*). A modern person (*khon samai mai*) need not observe the traditions belonging to old beliefs. Similarly, when asked about traditional beliefs and practices concerning a preparation for an easy birth in the North, Pimpilai, an urban woman, answered that she no longer believed in traditional knowledge.

> I don't know about it because I am a modern person. I don't really believe in the old way. This does not mean that I look down on traditional beliefs and practices, but I don't really hear about them either, so I don't know much about them. Now, whatever a woman does in pregnancy is not relevant, as if she has a difficult birth, she just has to go into hospital and she has an operation [caesarean].

Often, women received two sources of authoritative knowledge: medical and folk. Lakana, a woman from Mae Chantra district, said her doctor advised her to drink a lot of milk, to eat food containing the five food groups, and not to consume pickled food or smoke or drink alcohol. Her mother, however, told her to observe traditional food such as consuming *pak plang* for an easy birth and take only half a banana so that she could avoid an obstructed birth. Isara, a rural woman, provided a logical explanation of why she followed any authoritative knowledge:

> I followed what other people told me to do because I wanted to make sure that the baby would be fine. I was afraid that the baby would be abnormal. If I didn't follow their advice, and if something was wrong with the baby, it would be difficult for me as a mother and it would be difficult for the crippled baby. If the baby was abnormal, then I had to find money to cure him and that would be difficult for me. The baby would also be looked down on by others in society because a crippled person is not valued in the society.

More often, women could incorporate both systems without difficulty. But occasionally, folk knowledge clashed with medical knowledge. Pimpilai, an urban woman, talked about her experience of diet during pregnancy:

> People of older generations would always tell me to eat for my baby too, but Dr X would say it was not necessary. He said I didn't have to eat for my baby. He said what I ate would go to the baby, so I didn't have to eat two serves because I would put too much weight on.

In some cases, women chose to only observe medical knowledge rather than traditional knowledge. Sinjai, an educated woman in Chiang Mai City, said about her diet during pregnancy that:

> People advised me to take Chinese herbs or Thai traditional medicines … so that the baby would be strong and clever, but I did not believe in it. I mainly consumed good food like milk, egg and other foodstuffs which provide all sorts of good things rather than taking Chinese herbs or Thai herbs, as I was afraid that these would be dangerous to my baby.

9 Conclusion

Brigitte Jordan (1997) and Michel Foucault's insights (1973, 1980) into the unequal power relationships between those who possess medical knowledge (such as medical professionals) and those who lack it (such as pregnant women) are particularly apparent in this study. The women in our study perceive that medical professions have authority and legitimate authoritative knowledge. As Jordan (1997) notices, in certain situations, such as in antenatal care, some forms of knowledge count and others do not, regardless of "truth value." This is clearly mirrored in this study. Although women suspected that they became pregnant and although they sought a pregnancy test to confirm it, they would still seek confirmation from medical professionals. Women come to trust authoritative knowledge more than their own embodied knowledge. In the minds of these women, authoritative knowledge seems to "count" more than their own "bodily experience." But, for some women, their embodied knowledge encourages them to follow authoritative knowledge. As illustrated in Carole Browner and Nancy Press's study (1996), women who have experienced a miscarriage, for example, would eagerly incorporate medical advice into their everyday lives. This is, for these women, the way to ensure a safe pregnancy and the well-being of their fetuses. This can also be clearly seen in the women's narratives in Robin Root and Carole Browner's study (2001). The women who complied with authoritative knowledge expressed their ideas that their miscarriages were caused by not following the advice of their doctors. The women in our study, who have prior adverse pregnancy outcomes too, eagerly do so for the well-being and safe journey of their fetuses.

The medicalization of childbirth in Thailand health care, like childbirth in many Western societies, makes medical knowledge "supersede" other kinds of relevant sources of knowledge such as the woman's prior experience and the knowledge she has of the state of her body (see Ehrenreich and English 1978; Duden 1993; Root and Browner 2001). The woman herself comes to believe that the professional's medical knowledge is the best for her (Jordan 1997: 61). It seems, as Maureen Porter and Sally Macintyre (1984) have pointed out in their study of antenatal care in Aberdeen, women see that whatever is recommended by their doctor must be "best" for them.

Jordan's assumption that authoritative knowledge is more pervasive when it is related to technology (1997) is not contested in the Thai context (at least in this study). As Eugenia Georges (1997: 92) points out, most kinds of technologies have authoritative power due to their "symbolic (and practical) value" and "their association with experts." Carole Browner and Nancy Press (1996: 141) point out in their study that few US women refused the offer of ultrasound or other forms of antenatal diagnostic screening. This is because the women see "information derived from technology as inherently authoritative knowledge" (see Davis-Floyd 1992, 1994; Rapp 1987, 1999). Some urban women in our study too seek a pregnancy test kit to confirm their embodied knowledge, and they willingly accept prenatal screening and diagnostic tests recommended by their doctors. However, not all women and medical professions in Northern Thailand totally succumb to medical technology.

We find that the class background of the women determines the extent to what women can do as well as their wishes to follow medical advice during pregnancy (see also Martin 1992; Davis-Floyd 1994; Lazarus 1994; Zadoroznyj 1999). Only those who have better education and employment are in a better position to seek a special care from their own medical professionals. Unlike their urban middle class counterparts, to rural poor women access to a special care is denied and they have to rely on public health care. To these women, issues of choice are not an option for them. As a public patient, they only receive care from a doctor who is on duty. Poor women are, therefore, as Ellen Lazarus (1994: 26) puts, "constrained by the conditions under which they have babies and the kind of care open to them."

Despite the fact that rural poor women do not have as good access to good care as those urban middle class women, it is noted that the acceptance of authoritative knowledge is more prevalent among these women than urban women. What can account for this? Authoritative knowledge is derived from the power structure of the medical profession. As Lazarus (1988: 45) argues "the control of medical knowledge, [and] technical procedures... creates a world of power for the medical profession." The lack of medical knowledge does not enable women of any background to challenge power/knowledge of their doctors or other health-care providers. With little or no education, rural poor women are further pushed under medical dominance. Power structure can clearly be seen from the fact that women fear offending their health-care providers, particularly their doctors, as they may not be helped if anything happens. And this may explain why they do not miss any appointment made for them. Rural poor women are even more cautious about this, although they have to travel a long distance to see their doctors. To offend their doctors is unthinkable.

But, we also notice that although some rural poor women accepted authoritative knowledge of their doctors, in reality many recommendations could not be easily incorporated into their everyday lives. A recommendation of taking "good food" such as milk, for example, was impractical and unrealistic to many poor women due to their financial constraints. It is too costly for them. Medical advice is all too often offered without sufficient regard of the realities of women's lives (Browner and press 1996: 150; Root and Browner 2001).

Similarly, although folk knowledge tended to be observed by rural poor women, to follow this may pose some difficulties for some of the women. To drink a fresh coconut each day throughout pregnancy, for example, seems to be feasible for women who are financially sound. But, particularly for poor women, this becomes difficult and in some cases impossible. In addition, any rigorous or heavy work is not advisable during pregnancy as this may cause a miscarriage. For poor women, this caution may be difficult to heed if at all, as they still have to perform their heavy routines throughout pregnancy.

Although folk knowledge has been utilized by women and men alike in Northern Thailand (and other parts), it has become structurally inferior to Western biomedicine (Lee 1982; Golomb 1985; Cohen 1989; Sermsri 1989; Brun and Shumacher 1994; Hoban 2007; Suwankhong et al. 2011a; see also Chaps. 30 and 31 in this volume). Folk knowledge is largely and gradually losing its authoritative status in the urban Thai context. This is because birth in urban Thailand, as in many other parts of the world, has been medicalized, and this has placed pregnant women under medical authoritative knowledge. But even so, folk knowledge is still prevalent among those in rural and remote areas where modern medicine has not totally penetrated. As we have shown, some women in this study still observe Thai traditional practices during pregnancy. Rural poor women in particular adhere more to their folk knowledge than urban middle class women. The practices are passed on by those who possess traditional knowledge. Although there is evidence in other contexts that folk and medical knowledge can coexist and complement each other (Golomb 1985; Sermsri 1989; Whittaker 2000; Liamputtong Rice 2000; Suwankhong et al. 2011b; see Chap. 31), within the context of this study, women can only follow folk knowledge which is not sanctioned by, or clashes with, medical knowledge. In certain circumstances, women have to surrender to the authoritative knowledge of their doctors.

According to the Foucauldian perspective, power relationships often fluctuate and are not always one way (Foucault 1980; Lupton and Fenwick 2001; Root and Browner 2001). We do see some middle class women in this study, although they are in the minority, wanting to have some control over their pregnancy and having an active say in their antenatal care. They do seek the authoritative knowledge of the medical professionals, but they also make sure that they have their own choices regarding from which they should seek care. They actively gained knowledge about a "good doctor" on whom they could rely. Such women are able to challenge the power of their doctor by asserting that they are not a passive patient but a knowledgeable consumer. But, as Lazarus (1994: 29) points out, "taking control of one's life and body is a middle class perspective." In this study, the women's class, education, and financial positions enable them to do so. This is denied to those rural poor women, who are restricted by limited knowledge and overwhelmed with economic problems. Hence, they have limited choices and control over their pregnancy (cf. Whittaker 2000 in her writing about poor women in northeastern Thailand).

Our findings have implications for quality antenatal care and further research in Thailand. First, women from different social class backgrounds may receive different clinical services. The possible consequence of *fak piset*, for example, is that it may discriminate against quality of antenatal care of those who cannot afford such special care; those who have to conform to *fak thamada*. This culture of antenatal care practices, hence, may create a two-tiered system where urban middle class women receive better quality of care including the choices of perceived "good" doctors and continuity of care, and rural poor women can only access a second-class care (cf. Riewpaiboon et al. 2005). This reinforces inequality among social classes in health care.

Second, our findings show that authoritative knowledge is less likely to be detrimental, but rather, it does not take into account the social positions of women and their living circumstances (cf. Root and Browner 2001). It may be more appropriate if a doctor spends time discussing with the women their needs and constraints prior to making any advice so that his or her recommendations to the pregnant woman may be more pragmatic. And third, our findings apply mainly to authoritative knowledge of medical professionals, particularly obstetricians and gynecologists, in antenatal care. As nurses and midwives also play a major role in the provision of antenatal care in Thailand, it may be important to examine the role of authoritative knowledge of a nurse or midwife or other health personnel dealing with pregnancies so that sensitive and appropriate antenatal care may be achieved. Unfortunately, it is beyond our capacity to discuss this issue in this study.

In conclusion, in the minds of many Thai women in this study, the cultural authority of biomedicine pervades. Our data clearly show that the construction of "legitimate health knowledge" (Abel et al. 2001: 1145) has resulted in the marginalization of other kinds of knowledge including embodied experience and cultural knowledge. And, if medical hegemony continues to be constructed through the social process of unequal power relationships between those who possess knowledge and those who lack it, authoritative knowledge continues to be the discursive practice that shapes the lived experience of many pregnant women. This will make an attempt to improve the cultural relevance and sensitive care amidst the mainstream of dominant culture of Western medicine and medicalization a challenging task indeed.

References

Abel, S., Park, J., Tippene-Leach, D., Finau, S., & Lennan, M. (2001). Infant care practices in New Zealand: A cross-cultural qualitative study. *Social Science & Medicine, 53*, 1135–1148.

Armstrong, D. (1983). *Political anatomy of the body: Medical knowledge in Britain in the twentieth century*. Cambridge: Cambridge University Press.

Bourdieu, P. (1977). *Outline of a theory of practice*. Cambridge: Cambridge University Press.

Browner, C. H., & Press, N. (1996). The production of authoritative knowledge in American prenatal care. *Medical Anthropology Quarterly, 10*(2), 141–156.

Brun, V., & Shumacher, T. (1994). *Traditional herbal medicine in Northern Thailand*. Bangkok: White Lotus.

Cohen, P. T. (1989). The politics of primary health care in Thailand, with special reference to non-government organizations. In P. T. Cohen & J. Purcal (Eds.), *The political economy of primary health care in Southeast Asia* (pp. 159–176). Canberra: Australian Development Studies Network, ASEAN Training Centre for Primary Health Care Development.

Davis-Floyd, R. E. (1992). *Birth as an American rite of passage*. Berkeley: University of California Press.

Davis-Floyd, R. E. (1994). The technocratic body: American childbirth as cultural expression. *Social Science & Medicine, 38*(8), 1125–1140.

Davis-Floyd, R. E., & Sargent, C. F. (Eds.). (1997). *Childbirth and authoritative knowledge: Cross-cultural perspectives*. Berkeley: University of California Press.

Duden, B. (1993). *Disembodying women: Perspectives on pregnancy and the unborn*. London: Harvard University Press.

Ehrenreich, B., & English, D. (1978). *For her own good: 150 years of the experts' advice to women*. New York: Anchor.

Foucault, M. (1973). *The birth of the clinic. An archaeology of medical perception*. London: Tavistock.

Foucault, M. (1980). The politics of health in the eighteenth century. In C. Gordon (Ed.), *Power/knowledge. Selected interviews and other writings, 1972–1977* (pp. 166–182). Brighton: The Harvest Press.

Georges, E. (1997). Fetal ultrasound imaging and the production of authoritative knowledge in Greece. In R. Davis-Floyd & C. F. Sargent (Eds.), *Childbirth and authoritative knowledge: Cross-cultural perspectives* (pp. 91–112). Berkeley: University of California Press.

Ginsburg, F., & Rapp, R. (1991). The politics of reproduction. *Annual Review of Anthropology, 20*, 311–343.

Golomb, L. (1985). *An anthropology of curing in multiethnic Thailand*. Urbana: University of Illinois Press.

Hernandez, P. (2007). Sensing vulnerability, seeking strength: Somali women and their experiences during pregnancy and birth in Melbourne. In P. Liamputtong (Ed.), *Reproduction, childbearing and motherhood: A cross-cultural perspective* (pp. 195–208). New York: Nova.

Hoban, E. (2007). Celebrating safe childbirth. In P. Liamputtong (Ed.), *Reproduction, childbearing and motherhood: A cross-cultural perspective* (pp. 99–112). New York: Nova.

Jirojwong, S. (1996). Health beliefs and the use of antenatal care among pregnant women in southern Thailand. In P. Liamputtong Rice & L. Manderson (Eds.), *Maternity and reproductive health in Asian societies* (pp. 61–82). Amsterdam: Harwood Academic Publishers.

Jordan, B. (1997). *Birth in four cultures: A crosscultural investigation of childbirth in Yucatan, Holland, Sweden, and the United States* (4th ed.). Prospect Heights: Waveland Press Inc.

Jordan, B., & Irwin, S. (1989). A close encounter with a court-ordered cesarean section: A case of differing realities. In B. Hans (Ed.), *Case studies in medical anthropology: A teaching and reference source* (pp. 185–199). New York: Gordon and Breach.

Kaufert, P., & O'Neil, J. (1993). Analysis of dialogue on risks in childbirth: Clinicians, epidemiologists, and Inuit women. In S. Lindenbaum & M. Lock (Eds.), *Knowledge, power, and practice: The anthropology of medicine in everyday life* (pp. 32–55). Berkeley: University of California Press.

Laderman, C. (1983). *Wives and midwives: Childbirth, and nutrition in rural Malaysia*. Berkeley: University of California Press.

Laderman, C. (1984). Food ideology and eating behavior: Contributions from Malay studies. *Social Science & Medicine, 19*(5), 547–559.

Lazarus, E. S. (1988). Poor women, poor outcomes: Social class and reproductive health. In K. L. Michaelson (Ed.), *Childbirth in America: Anthropological perspectives* (pp. 39–54). South Hadley: Bergin & Garvey.

Lazarus, E. S. (1994). What do women want? Issues of choice, control, and class in pregnancy and childbirth. *Medical Anthropology Quarterly, 8*(1), 25–46.

Lee, R. L. (1982). Comparative studies of health care systems. *Social Science & Medicine, 16*, 629–642.

Liamputtong, P. (2004). Yu duan practices as embodying tradition, modernity and social change in Chiang Mai, Northern Thailand. *Women & Health, 40*(1), 79–99.

Liamputtong, P. (2007a). *The journey of becoming a mother amongst women in Northern Thailand.* Lanham: Lexington Books.

Liamputtong, P. (2007b). Situating reproduction, procreation and motherhood within a cross-cultural context: An introduction. In P. Liamputtong (Ed.), *Reproduction, childbearing and motherhood: A cross-cultural perspective* (pp. 3–34). New York: Nova.

Liamputtong, P. (2009). Pregnancy, childbirth and traditional beliefs and practices in Chiang Mai, NorthernThailand. In H. Selin & P. K. Stone (Eds.), *Childbirth across cultures: Ideas and practices of pregnancy, childbirth and the postpartum* (pp. 175–184). New York: Springer.

Liamputtong, P. (2013). *Qualitative research methods* (4th ed.). Melbourne: Oxford University Press.

Liamputtong, P. (2011). Childbearing, culture and social conditions: The experiences of South East Asian immigrant women in Australian health care. *Diversit-e*, 2, 16–17. Available from www.dhi.gov.au/clearinghouse

Liamputtong, P., Yimyam, S., Parisunyakul, S., Baosoung, C., & Sansiriphun, N. (2005). Traditional beliefs about pregnancy and child birth among women from Chiang Mai, Northern Thailand. *Midwifery, 21*(2), 139–153.

Liamputtong Rice, P. (1988). *Health and sickness: The influence of cultural knowledge and commonsense interpretations Among Thai schoolchildren.* PhD thesis, Faculty of Education, Monash University, Melbourne.

Liamputtong Rice, P. (2000). *Hmong women and reproduction.* Westport: Bergin & Garvey.

Lindenbaum, S., & Lock, M. (Eds.). (1993). *Knowledge, power, and practice: The anthropology of medicine in everyday life.* Berkeley: University of California Press.

Lock, M., & Scheper-Hughes, N. (1990). A critical-interpretive approach in medical anthropology: Rituals and routines of discipline and dissent. In T. Johnson & C. Sargent (Eds.), *Medical anthropology: A handbook of theory and method* (pp. 47–73). Westport: Greenwood Press.

Lukere, V., & Jolly, M. (Eds.). (2002). *Birthing in the Pacific: Beyond tradition and modernity?* Honolulu: University of Hawai'i Press.

Lupton, D. (1995). *The imperative of health: Public health and the regulated body.* London: Sage.

Lupton, D. (1996). Your life in their hands: Trust in the medical encounter. In V. James & J. Gabe (Eds.), *Health and the sociology of emotions* (pp. 102–120). London: Blackwell Publishers.

Lupton, D. (1997). Consumerism, reflexivity and the medical encounter. *Social Science & Medicine, 45*, 373–381.

Lupton, D., & Fenwick, J. (2001). 'They've forgotten that I'm the mum': Constructing and practicing motherhood in special care nurseries. *Social Science & Medicine, 53*, 1011–1021.

Martin, E. (1992). *The woman in the body: A cultural analysis of reproduction.* Boston: Beacon.

Mills, M. B. (1999). *Thai women in the global labor force: Consuming desires, contested selves.* New Brunswick: Rutgers University Press.

Mougne, C. (1978). An ethnography of reproduction: Changing patterns of fertility in a Northern Thai village. In P. A. Stott (Ed.), *Nature and man in South East Asia* (pp. 68–106). London: School of Oriental and African Studies, University of London.

Muecke, M. (1976). Health care systems as socializing agents: Childbearing the north Thai and western ways. *Social Science & Medicine, 10*, 337–383.

Nichter, M., & Nichter, M. (1996). The ethnophysiology and folk dietetics of pregnancy: A case study from South India. In M. Nichter & M. Nichter (Eds.), *Anthropology and international health: Asian case studies* (pp. 35–69). Amsterdam: Gordon and Breach Publishers.

Porter, M., & Macintyre, S. (1984). What is, must be best: A research note on conservative or deferential responses to antenatal care provision. *Social Science & Medicine, 19*(11), 1197–1200.

Rapp, R. (1987). Moral pioneers: Women, men, and fetuses on a frontier of reproductive technology. *Women & Health, 13*(1–2), 101–116.

Rapp, R. (1993). Accounting for amniocentesis. In S. Lindenbaum & M. Lock (Eds.), *Knowledge, power, and practice: The anthropology of medicine in everyday life* (pp. 55–76). Berkeley: University of California Press.

Rapp, R. (1999). *Testing women, testing the fetus: The social impact of amniocentesis in America*. New York: Routledge.
Rhodes, L. (1990). Studying biomedicine as a cultural system. In T. Johnson & C. Sargent (Eds.), *Medical anthropology: A handbook of theory and method* (pp. 159–174). Westport: Greenwood Press.
Riewpaiboon, W., Chuengsatiansup, K., Gilson, L., & Tangcharoensathien, V. (2005). Private obstetric practice in a public hospital: Mythical trust in obstetric care. *Social Science & Medicine, 61*, 1408–1417.
Root, R., & Browner, C. (2001). Practices of the pregnant self: Compliance with and resistance to prenatal norms. *Culture, Medicine and Psychiatry, 25*, 195–223.
Sargent, C., & Bascope, G. (1996). Ways of knowing about birth in three cultures. *Medical Anthropology Quarterly, 10*(2), 213–236.
Sawicki, J. (1991). *Disciplining Foucault: Feminism, power, and the body*. New York: Routledge.
Selin, H., & Stone, P. K. (Eds.). (2009). *Childbirth across cultures: Ideas and practices of pregnancy, childbirth and the postpartum*. New York: Springer.
Sermsri, S. (1989). Utilization of traditional and modern health care services in Thailand. In S. R. Quah (Ed.), *The triumph of practicality: Tradition and modernity in health care utilization in selected Asian countries* (pp. 160–179). Singapore: Institute of Southeast Asian Studies.
Serry, T., & Liamputtong, P. (2013). The in-depth interviewing method in health. In P. Liamputtong (Ed.), *Research methods in health: Foundations for evidence-based practice* (2nd ed., pp. 39–53). Melbourne: Oxford University Press.
Steinberg, S. (1996). Childbearing research: A transcultural review. *Social Science & Medicine, 43*(2), 1765–1784.
Suwankhong, D., Liamputtong, P., & Rumbold, B. (2011a). Existing roles of traditional healers (*mor baan*) in southern Thailand. *Journal of Community Health, 36*, 438–445.
Suwankhong, D., Liamputtong, P., & Rumbold, B. (2011b). Traditional healers in southern Thailand: The barriers for cooperation with modern health care delivery. *Journal of Community Health, 36*, 431–437.
Turner, B. S. (1995). *Medical power and social knowledge* (Rev. ed.). London: Sage.
Turner, B. S. (1997). From governmentality to risk: Some reflections on Foucault's contribution to medical sociology. In A. Petersen & R. Bunton (Eds.), *Foucault, health and medicine* (pp. ix–xxi). London: Routledge.
Whittaker, A. (2000). *Intimate knowledge: Women and their health in north-east Thailand*. Sydney: Allen & Unwin.
Zadoroznyj, M. (1999). Social class, social selves and social control in childbirth. *Sociology of Health & Illness, 21*(3), 267–289.

Chapter 30
Moral Aspect and the Effectiveness of Local Healing in Northern Thailand

Yongsak Tantipidoke

1 Introduction

Studies on local healing mostly explain their effectiveness through either their instrumental or their symbolic aspects. In anthropological studies, symbolic, performative, and persuasive dimensions of specific rituals and healing events are naturally taken into account. Little attention has, however, been given to local morality and its effects on the everyday practices of the secular healing process. In this chapter, I investigate the process of local healing to show how local morality can create effectiveness of healing. I will describe stories of two folk healers in Chiang Mai. The concept of local world and moral sensibility will be used to analyze the narratives created by these key informants.

2 Sympathy and Humanized Healing

It took me more than 1 h to drive from the center of Chiang Mai to the house of the 44-year-old *mor* Som.[1,2] This was not due to the distance but to my unfamiliarity with the area—a *tambon* in Mae Sa district. I was invited to the second floor of his house. A conversation then started. "We were sitting on the floor which once was stained with blood and pus of many HIV/AIDS patients," *mor* Som said. "At that

[1] *Mor* is used to call persons who have special skill in their careers such as doctor (*mor rak sa rok*), fortune teller (*mor du*), and lawyer (*mor khwam*). In this context *mor* is a title given to a person who is respected as a doctor or healer in the community.

[2] All cases are presented with fictitious names.

Y. Tantipidoke, Ph.D. (✉)
Society and Health Institute, Ministry of Public Health, 3rd Floor, Building on Public Health Lane 6, North of Health Park, Tiwanon Road, Nonthaburi 11000, Thailand
e-mail: yskpidok@yahoo.com

P. Liamputtong (ed.), *Contemporary Socio-Cultural and Political Perspectives in Thailand*, DOI 10.1007/978-94-007-7244-1_30, © Springer Science+Business Media Dordrecht 2014

time, the villagers feared AIDS and hated HIV/AIDS patients. My wife could not continue her small noodle business here. She had to change to sewing since then."

Mor Som has provided care and cure for HIV/AIDS patients for nearly two decades. It is quite an ordeal for an ordinary villager to persist with such a risky and objectionable task for such a long period. *Mor* Som himself never had imagined before the extent to which he had to involve himself in this hard job. To better understand the motive that urged him, we need to explore his life history in more detail.

Like any ordinary rural lad in Thailand, *mor* Som finished his study at grade four and then ordained as a young novice (young monk) for 7 years. During the period of ordainment, novice Som was attracted by the ancient knowledge regarding charms, amulets, and magic. This interest even remained when he left his noviceship to marry and to work as a motorcycle repairman. Family life with his wife and a lovely daughter could not distract him from practicing magic. *Noi* Som continued to try out whether the amulets he had made himself had the expected magic power.[3] "I had to control strictly my personal conduct in accordance with the way to make powerful amulets that was taught since generations. Sometimes, I made them in the night at the village cemetery, where I could perform intently meditation and incantation," *mor* Som recalled his boldness.

When *noi* Som was 28, his motorcycle repair business met difficulties. At the same time, Yot, his nephew, who lived in the same village, fell sick from an unknown disease. He was discharged from a district hospital even though he still coughed up blood. The doctor only said that his blood was positive due to an incurable disease. Yot had no other choice than to ask assistance from *noi* Som, in the hope that he could discover a way to cure the disease. *Noi* Som decided to set aside his career and to spend his time to help his ill nephew.

From information of the hospital and the mass media, *noi* Som learned that his nephew might be ill from HIV. He looked again at the knowledge of medicinal plants he had learned during his ordainment and searched in old medical scriptures for traditional drugs that could eradicate AIDS-related symptoms. He dispensed some traditional drugs he had found in old medical scriptures to treat the disease.

After a year of treatment, the major symptoms disappeared, only some skin papules were left. Yot was able to do his work as usual. Thinking that he had already recovered, his nephew ate grilled meat and spirits during a party at a building site. This caused him to have acute fecal blood for 10 days and then he died. *Noi* Som learned from this case that AIDS is a new disease. The traditional drugs from his medical scriptures alone could not cure this disease.

The second HIV/AIDS patient who sought help from *mor* Som is San.[4] He devoted himself to becoming without any condition the object of *mor* Som's trial. San was also a native of the same village as *mor* Som and was 2 years younger. San and his wife, a Burmese immigrant worker with whom he had lived since 1990, had

[3] *Noi* is a title given to a person who has ever been a Buddhist novice in Northern Thailand. It is used to express the respectable status of persons who have devoted themselves to learn Dharma and are expected to succeed the Buddhist tradition in their mundane life.

[4] From now on, I will use *mor* (doctor) Som instead of *Noi* Som since he became acting as a healer.

moved to another district where they found jobs. In 1993, something unusual happened to them. After his wife had an annual checkup at the factory where she worked, she did not get the results from them, and no explanation was given.

One afternoon San fainted and lost consciousness after he had eaten pickled wild boar meat as lunch. He was taken to a hospital and treated until he recovered. Before he was released from the hospital, a doctor told him to have blood tests again at a hospital close to where he lived but the doctor did not explain why. Not long afterward, his wife became chronically ill with a lot of coughs and weight loss. When she died, San knew that he himself had AIDS and thought of committing suicide. But the thought of his children and parents changed his mind, and he decided to fight the disease.

When San came to see *mor* Som, to whom a relative had recommended him, the sick man asked the healer not to feel constrained to prescribe him any medicines for experimentation because he would die from AIDS anyway.

After trying a number of folk medicine recipes for 1 year, *mor* Som and San finally found formulas which could cure illnesses caused by eating the wrong food. Together, they compiled a list of forbidden foods that AIDS patients should avoid if they want to improve their conditions. Additionally, they experimented with recipes that consisted of blood tonics and with recipes that rebalanced elements. They found that these medicines could lessen the negative effects of wrong food. After 3 years of these trials, San became healthy again although the results of his blood tests from the hospital showed he was still infected with HIV.

Meanwhile, San took a second wife, but the couple had a troubled relationship which worsened when she ran away with another lover. San went after them and brought her back. The woman was also infected with HIV and treated by *mor* Som, but she was hardly cooperative in the treatment. The couple often had quarrels, and the healer had to mediate between them. There was a time when San got himself into trouble with a neighbor. The man, seeing that San helped with cutting the meat that had to be cooked for the village's merit-making activity, lashed out at him: "You have AIDS. What is your business chopping meat here?" San was enraged and punched him in the mouth. When the neighbor filed complaints with the village chief, again *mor* Som had to intervene to settle the dispute.

To help San reduce his stress and prevent him from becoming suicidal, the healer asked him to work as his assistant. San proved to be very useful and was able to share his mentor's workload. He helped with all sorts of work from harvesting medicinal plants in the forests, washing, cutting, and drying to grinding them into powder, until he was familiar with those herbs. Whenever *mor* Som earned some money, such as well-off patients paid for the medicines, or study tour groups visited his practice or when Som was invited to be a resource person, *mor* would give half of the money to San. If San had no money left for buying rice, the healer would share his meal with him. *Mor* Som also had San's old pickup truck overhauled and paid for the gasoline when it was used for his work. When the two were going off to the forests to collect herbs, the healer would buy fresh food and ask his assistant's wife to prepare food for the trip. San had been both a patient and the assistant of *mor* Som for 8 years when another disaster befell him.

San's wife took her own life by hanging herself in the bathroom. Deeply depressed, San took to drink, and for 2 months he stopped eating food and taking medicines. His condition deteriorated, and *mor* Som could do nothing to save his life. San once told his healer that when he died, he wanted to be cremated with wood that made such an intense heat that it would destroy even his bones and leave nothing but ashes, because the torment he suffered from the disease was so great that he did not want to be reborn.[5] But at his last moment, San grasped *mor* Som's hands and said with his dying breath: "See you in the next life, *mor*."

Since San's death, *mor* Som went every year to pay respect to San's mother. On special occasions—the start of the Buddhist Lent, the local New Year's Day, and *Tan Khao Mai* Day[6]—the healer would make merit and dedicate it to San to show his gratitude to the man who had been his helper as well as his "teacher." *Mor* Som said San was a "living school" from which he learned how to treat the deadly disease and that his late patient gave his own life to prolong the lives of other HIV patients. This has given the healer strength to continue in his dedication to people with HIV and AIDS.

Besides learning from his patients, other events made clear that *mor* Som is an enthusiastic learner. In 1996, he participated in a class conducted in the district hospital to provide knowledge of traditional Thai medicine. The course intended to prepare the students for the national license examination. *Mor* Som was one of the successful students who passed the examination. He told me that he wanted to understand better the principles of traditional medicine so that he was able to formulate the proper traditional drugs for his patients. He learned how to differentiate hot and cold quality of materia medica and their effects according to taste and quality. He also learned from the other healers who had more experience to identify medicinal plants in the jungle. All these learning activities occurred after he was inspired by his inner calling to search ways to help his patients.

During the period of fieldwork in 2008, I learned that only eight HIV patients still had contact with *mor* Som. The number of patients had gradually decreased after the advent of antiretroviral drugs. This change lessened the time *mor* Som spent to his healing activities because he kept close contact with only a few HIV patients. Although some patients had changed to taking antiretroviral drugs, they still had a good relationship with the healer.

On the basis of the story of *mor* Som and his patients, and what I have learned from the observation of his healing activities, I will analyze how the sensible nature of the healer became associated with a moral value and led to the beginning of a healing process.

---

[5] Thai belief about rebirth is based on the belief of Buddhism and Brahmin. Every being is traveling in the continuous flow of life, samsara—the cycle of birth, life, death, rebirth, or reincarnation. From this point of view, life is not considered to start with birth and end in death, but as a continuous lifetime from past to present and extending beyond.

[6] *Tan Khao Mai* Day is, according to the lunar calendar, the full moon day of the fourth month when the in-season rice is already harvested. Northerners celebrate this traditional event by donating cooked rice and other food on behalf of the deceased ancestors who once possessed the rice fields and by feeding the monks as well.

In this chapter, the concept of local world (Kleinman 1995, 1999) will be used to address the location in which healers and patients intersubjectively participate in a healing process. A local world is an intersubjective medium—a world which is constituted from the outcome of cultural categories and social structures that interact with psychophysiological processes (Kleinman 1995, 1999). Kleinman uses the concept of local world to interfuse collective processes of particular social, cultural, historical, and political forces with subjective processes. Since a local world is a sphere where experience takes place, moral value in the local world upon which the subjective experience bases can therefore be considered as a value that mediates what are thought as important things and what are really practiced by the people (see also Chap. 31 in this volume).

Folk healers in Northern Thailand in the old days always considered helping patients as a kind of merit-making. For the present days, some healers still hold this as a core value of being an ideal healer. This traditional value has dissolved from the local world of the villagers when it is contested by the new values attached to modern society. The AIDS epidemic is a crisis that is perceived as a danger that threatens the villagers' ways of life. HIV people are so frightened that they isolate themselves from the normal relationship with their neighbors. Many villagers are scared and refused to help others, even family members who are HIV-infected. This situation calls for a reflection about the villagers' engagement with the local world and shaped a great deal the ways they relate to each other. But, at the same time, it urged some people to do something in order to correct the distorted moral life in the villages.

Mor Som was a person who was sensible to the divided local world and the despair of people with HIV living around him. It may be said that the AIDS epidemic, in Kleinman's words, ordered the course of the moral process with which *mor* Som was involved (Kleinman 1999: 362). In this process, the moral value that helping others is an activity of merit-making was unconsciously adopted. This value became apparent again because HIV/AIDS patients were perceived as persons who were at risk. Demanding healing fees from these persons might therefore, from the perspective of healers, be an improper action (see also Chap. 31).

However, a question still remains. Why was *mor* Som sensible to the divided local world and has he devoted himself to this task? I found that the idea about sympathy of David Hume (1711–1776), the most outstanding proponent of the moral theory of sentimentalism, is appropriate to this case. According to Hume, sympathy is the predisposition to feel what other people are feeling, even those people to whom we are totally unrelated (Brown 2005: 1505). A person's sympathetic link resonates him with the pleasures and pains of others (Norton 1993: 165). Only when we do so, we will share a common point of view with other persons and let moral sensibility evolve.

The case shows that sympathy arose from the intimacy between the healer and his patients either through kinship, neighborhood, or collegiality. It also grew from the moral training during the ordainment and the moral dispositions which were automatically internalized through learning from the conduct of his grandfather who also was a healer. This demonstrates the significance of intimate relationships and moral socialization for the growth of sympathy of the healer. To a great extent, sympathy accounts for the ability of *mor* Som to feel other people's emotions, especially when they suffer, and urged his internal calling to perform moral practices. In this case, healing is seen as a practice of merit-making.

Sympathy potentially leads to the growth of other moral dispositions. I learned from this case that compassion has appeared vividly during the healing course of his second patient. I also discovered the emergence of other moral dispositions, which were apparently nurtured inside the healer and continually guided him to complete his healing tasks. They consist of the will or ambition to help his patients, the efforts to search from traditional medical scriptures, possible ways to help patients and to do trials, the thoughtfulness to observe and analyze the results, and the reflection in order to improve the healing procedures.[7] Other moral dispositions that should also be mentioned are hospitality, gratitude, and the feeling that one has to reciprocate the person who has given some benefit.

Another important point from this case is the fact that sympathy enables the healer to go beyond the realm of disease treatment. The healer entered the realm of caring not only as a healer but also as neighbor and fellow human being. The shift from viewing "a patient in the healing setting" to considering him as "a being in the samsara" broadens the scope of sickness in a way that it encompasses other aspects than physical suffering. From this point of view, healing requires from the healer to sympathize with their patients' feelings and to care for them as fellow beings in the world where all inescapably face suffering from birth, aging, sickness, and death. This was especially shown when *mor* Som helped San to enable him to fight for his life by providing any possible kind of support. Despite San's death, *mor* Som still was active in giving spiritual support for a good next life of his patient.

However, the scope of the actions resulting from sympathy and its consequent moral dispositions were limited by burdens the healer and his family had to bear—both material and nonmaterial ones. His material limitations were the lack of outside financial support and his inability to exploit his healing commercially. *Mor* Som depended on the help of patients who paid full respect to him. In nonmaterial respect, the stress from difficult cases also limited his healing activities since it often disturbed his mental status. I observed that the healer often immersed himself in the suffering of his patients and developed feelings of tension. For example, he felt sad when he received a call from an HIV patient who encountered the problem of having to disrupt her family life. Sensitivity to the tragedies of his patients made him vulnerable for stress. The healer had therefore to limit the amount of patients so that he could treat them well. The ability to limit his healing activities was, therefore, the result of the self-reflexivity that *mor* Som practiced to adjust himself in a situation of mental constraint and of limited support for his healing activities.

From this analysis, I contend that in difficult times sensibility, which is nurtured by sympathy, serves as an internal starting point and essential part of a moral process, a process in which a moral value from the local world is reified into moral

[7] In Buddhist teaching this set of mind qualities is named *Itthibat Si* or the Four Paths of Accomplishment.

practices and a person's moral dispositions are developed so that moral practices can be appropriately performed to achieve the purpose of the person. The course of the process is not only ordered, as Kleinman (1999: 362) explains, by the perceived threat—in this case the divided local world resulting from the AIDS epidemic—but also relies on into what extent the person can arrange the related moral dispositions in a proper manner to conduct suitable practices. It also rests on the ability of the person to reflect on oneself and the ongoing circumstances. Since this intrapsychic process is experiential, interpersonal engagement also takes part in the development of persons' moral dispositions.

In what follows, I will refer to some outcomes of the moral process that can be considered as core components of local healing and apparently affect its effectiveness. They are *khun* and *bun*.

3 *Khun*

Both folk healers and their patients, whose worldviews are shared in the same local world, see folk medical knowledge as something that belongs to the healer teachers who have passed it down through generations. Therefore, when any healer applies this knowledge to healing, he acts as a medium of the healer teachers. Moreover, the medicines he dispenses have to be blessed for *khun*, power of virtue or power of moral goodness.[8] In this respect, successful healing can be ascribed not only to the healer's treatments and the medicines he prescribes but also to the power of virtue for which they have received when they were blessed.

To express their gratitude for the *khun* they receive by recovering from illnesses, patients should pay respect and deference to the healer teachers as the source of medical knowledge, to the healer as the medium through which the knowledge was transmitted, and to the medicines originated by the teachers. The patients whose lives are saved should regard the healer teachers, the healers, and the medicines as their benefactors and life givers, to which they should be grateful for the rest of their lives. In some communities, when an annual ceremony is conducted by a folk healer to show respect to the healer teachers, many locals will attend as they consider it an auspicious occasion. It is part of a tradition that has made folk healers the central figures of the circles of their pupils and former patients. I found this tradition still alive in the folk healing practiced by some Buddhist monks in lower Northern Thailand.

This study found, however, that in Chiang Mai nowadays such rituals draw mostly only the pupils of the healer who want to absorb his way of life and the arts

[8] I translate *khun* as power of virtue or power of moral goodness. This translation differs from the one given by Mulder (1979) since he separates power (*decha*) from moral goodness (*khuna*). In the context of healing, *khun* or *khuna* expresses their effects in the form of power. Therefore, when villagers mention *khun* of something, they intend to mean simultaneously both power and moral goodness.

of folk healing, but very few former patients participate. Among the people gathering at a ceremony of a folk healer in Hang Dong, I found just one of his former patients and an apprentice who studied massage with him; the rest were his family members. At the ceremony held by another healer, the crowd included his fellow healers, family members, and pupils. Another healer's ceremony was attended by groups of similar people and by youth members of the Northern Folk Healers Network.

From my own observations, the Northern ritual is evidently more significant for healers than for their patients, probably because it is a requisite for every healer to show respect for his teachers. Healers generally hold that a failure to perform the ceremony reflects disrespect for their teachers, and as a consequence they will not be successful. Or worse, they could fall gravely ill, and only when they perform a ritual to ask for forgiveness from their teachers that they will recover. The ritual is also significant as it reminds the healers that they must exercise more restraint in their conduct and behavior than others because their healer teachers are above humans. The purity and virtues the healers gain from observing this code of conduct have established their moral authority over ordinary people and made their healing power superior to the malevolent forces of evil spirits that are believed to cause sickness.

The power of the healer teachers in healing is recognized, although not directly, through the mediation of the healer's behavior toward his teachers. If he treats his teachers respectfully, his practice will produce good results for the patients. And, vice versa, improper behavior toward the teachers can have adverse effects on them. Therefore, the patients themselves are expected to take part in the rituals to express their gratefulness to the healer teachers. If the patients are not present, the healer will do it on their behalf to maintain proper relationships among the healers, the patients, and the healer teachers.

The belief in *khun* of the healer teachers, the medicines, and their effects on the effectiveness of healing can still be found among middle-aged Northerners. These people were born and grew up in times when local cosmology as embedded in customs and traditions still influenced their ways of thinking and living, and *khun* belongs to that reality. In contrast, patients of younger generations, residents migrated from other areas, or visitors from other parts of the country were not familiar with this belief; and *khun* meant little or nothing to them. The latter did not appreciate the connection between the healer's morality and conduct and the virtue of the teachers and the medicines. For instance, they would not keep their medicines on the shelves for Buddha images or pray for the healing power of the medicines as the former did. Rather, they believed in the potency of the substances in herbal medicines. Spiritually, they would meditate to ease their minds rather than pray to sacred beings or objects.

From the perspective of healers and patients who share this belief, medical knowledge, morality, and the effectiveness of healing are inseparable. *Khun*, which is culturally constructed, has been instilled in the people of Northern Thailand through rituals and traditional ways of life. The concept of *khun* as in the power of virtue of the teachers and sacred things allows people involved in local healing to make the connection between morality and sacred power. The folk healer, who leads a moral conduct, acts as a medium for channeling that healing power. That is to say, moral behavior strengthens the ability of the healer to deal with sacred power and harmonize this power with his medical knowledge to achieve the effectiveness of healing.

I state that *khun* emerges as the outcome of the healing process when the healer and the patient practice what can associate the healing with the virtue of healer teachers and other sacred things. It is evident that respect is paid to the healer teachers in the ritual and in the process of preparation of medicines when the power of medicines and healing are requested by the healer in front of the shrine of the healer teachers and other sacred objects. It is believed that the demand can be answered only when the healer is confident that he leads the moral conduct which is translated from the moral values of his healing tradition. The request is also done by the patient, but mostly in front of the Buddha statues in his or her house. Reciting mantras[9] and holding religious precepts[10] are also recommended to cultivate the mind of the patient so that the Buddha's *khun* and the *khun* of other sacred objects as well as the result of this merit-making can protect the patient from bad things and help him or her to recover from the illness.

4 *Bun*

Studies of ritual healing have revealed that the effectiveness of those ritual processes for healing illnesses caused by social conflicts is made possible through the participation of the entire communities (Turner 1975; Waldram 2000). In this study, no field data was collected to support this supposition.

Most activities at the healing center of *mor* Chan, a folk healer in another district where I did my fieldwork, for example, construction of the building, the ceremony to install a Buddha statue in the shrine hall, its opening ceremony, vocational training, Thai massage training, and a free lunch for orphans with HIV, were accomplished due to the participation of villagers and communities through volunteered labor and donations. With this support, the beneficiaries of the center knew they were not neglected, and this reassured them of their own worthiness and strengthened their will to live. *Mor* Chan's initiative illustrates that in modern society, where health problems may give rise to social conflicts such as the stigma of AIDS, healing activities led by folk healers and supported by the communities can keep the

[9] Mantra is a word or phrase repeated by a priest, a healer, or a person who performs a ritual and other religious practices. Each mantra is considered competent in producing change for specific purpose. Buddhist mantras are formulated by compilation of the words that is viewed as the heart of Buddhist teachings. It is therefore a way to remind person who recites the mantra of the Buddhist teachings.

[10] The precepts in Buddhist tradition are commitments to abstain from doing things that are considered as the obstacle of the progress toward spiritual development. The basic precepts for all Buddhists are the five precepts which consist of abstaining from harming living beings, stealing, sexual misconduct, lying, and intoxication.

function of ritual healing in resolving social conflicts stemming from illnesses such as AIDS and thus alleviate the patients' suffering.

These activities were made possible because they revolved around *bun* or merit.[11] Believing that helping others was a means of making merit, *mor* Chan has proved it with his actions, and thus he gained in stature as a trustworthy folk healer. To implement his project, the healer appealed to the Northerners' benevolent disposition derived from the belief in *bun* and he succeeded in rekindling the spirit of mutual help in the community for the benefit of people in distress. Through his healing, *mor* Chan educated his patients and the people in the community, and he corrected their misinformation on HIV and AIDS. They learned that having the disease did not necessarily lead to death; AIDS patients could recover and continue to live healthily. Gradually, the healer was able to dispel the fear of contracting the disease from the patients as the villagers began to understand how the disease was actually transmitted. In caring for AIDS patients, he came into closer contact with them than anyone in the village and considered it as a proof of his family's belief that merit would protect people against deadly diseases:

> In former times, people didn't go to McCormick Hospital. They came to [my grandfather] *por* Ui to be treated for chicken pox or smallpox. The house was thronged with patients. But no one in our family caught smallpox. In my father's time, there was an outbreak of cholera. He treated those who had cholera, but again no one in our family suffered from it. It seemed as if *bun* protected us.

Moreover, *mor* Chan's healing center was invariably linked to *khruba* Siwichai[12]—his grandfather was once the personal doctor of *khruba*, *Mor* Chan's dream about *khruba* had inspired the project, and the medicines he prepared from formulas found in the manuscript of *khruba* Khaopi, an important follower of *khruba* Siwichai. All these connections were believed to draw sacred power from the merit and virtue of that great spiritual teacher and give protection to the patients seeking refuge there.

One may contend that establishing the role of *bun* at the heart of all healing activities is simply a ploy to raise funds and promote community participation, and that *bun* has no bearing on the results of the healing. It is not unusual to take this position because in consumer society, this belief has been used to lure people into merit-making that will guarantee them good fortune in the future or the next life. But, there is a significant difference between *bun* as a commodity and self-development. The latter aims to rid of selfishness and makes oneself helpful to others, the former has the opposite effect. The question as to whether *bun* affects the result of healing is more difficult to answer because it involves the complexity of karma, the law of cause and effect, a Buddhist principle which explains that there are causes for all phenomena.

---

[11] *Bun* is a thing that when it happens in any person can lead to good qualities of mind. The mind of person who has *bun* is clear, unfettered, calm, and pure, as well as an absence of defilement, namely, greed, anger, covetousness, prejudice, confusion, jealousy, and conceit.

[12] *Khruba* Siwichai was a Buddhist monk who lived from 1878 until 1938. His moral teachings were based on the Northern traditional style of Buddhism which was appreciated by most Northern people in the revolutionary period of the inclusion of the North into the Kingdom of Siam.

If one attempts to determine the effectiveness of healing on the basis of *bun* and karma,[13] one will realize that the possibilities of the outcome are infinite. When *bun*, karma, the healer, medicines, healing methods, the patient, and so on are included in the equation, the problem is too complex for humans to solve. Instead of trying to analyze the impossible, those who are involved in the healing process—the healer, the patients, and relatives—can try their utmost to do noble deeds, make merit, and produce causal conditions for relieving and healing sickness. Then let the law of karma take its course and accept whatever comes.

From this perspective, the patient's noble actions committed prior to and during the healing are relevant to its effectiveness. The happiness from doing good deeds could lessen the anxiety and agitation a patient might experience as a result of physical suffering. While it is difficult to refute the effects of meritorious actions and good deeds on healing, the extent to which they can produce positive results for each patient is conditional upon his own actions, past and present.

The belief in *bun* was instilled in Somsri, a person with HIV, although she was not a native of the North. Somsri survived in her struggle with AIDS after losing her husband and daughter to the disease between 1995 and 1996. She gave a few reasons for her recovery: her will to live for her remaining twin sons, the use of herbal medicines, and merit-making by means of practicing meditation and helping other AIDS patients. She was a volunteer in a district hospital in Chiang Mai, paying visits to the patients' houses: "I feed them water and foods till their ends, one by one," she said. It was, to her, "*bun* extending *bun*," which means the merit she made by helping the patients had kept her alive so she could take care of her two sons and keep on offering her help to others. She worked at night embroidering clothes to support her family. Hard work had weakened her health, and doctors asked her to start taking ARV to prevent complications.

In this case, the belief in *bun* played a significant role in the healing process. However, it was not imposed by the folk healer since the belief has permeated Thai society for a long time. When in trouble, many Thais will naturally think of making merit. Generally, people will choose to make merit by various forms of giving, among them are offering alms to monks and freeing captive animals (see also Chap. 28 on merit-making in this volume). A form of merit-making that is more concerned with mental development is to stay at a temple or a meditation center for activities as observing the precepts, praying, and practicing meditation. Although merit-making is considered as part of the healing, the healers usually focus on the medical treatment and rarely apply religious practices. However, since most folk healers have the experience of entering the monkhood for a certain period, they are able to give instructions to their patients on how to meditate.

In sum, due to the fact that *bun* extends the capability of the healer to protect and care for his family and patients, the moral process that involves the healer most in

[13] Karma literally means action or doing. Any kind of intentional action whether physical, verbal, or mental is regarded as karma. In its ultimate sense, karma means all moral and immoral volition. Involuntary, unintentional, or unconscious actions do not constitute karma. In its popular sense, karma is the result of our own past actions and our own present deeds.

his career revolves around moral values that aim to amass *bun*—that is, helping others without expecting returns, offering things, teaching and support that can relieve patients' suffering, and training himself in a religious way to strengthen his mental and spiritual capacity. For the patients, who believe that the person who is going to die spent all his *bun* in this present life, the moral process in this difficult time is always concerned with making new *bun* to extend their lives. These ongoing moral processes influence the process of healing in the strong hope that its outcome—*bun*—will function in the end according to the law of karma. This explanation is still alive among the healers and the patients who value merit as a thing that matters to their lives, not only in this life but also in the next ones.

5 Conclusion

This chapter demonstrates the role of sensibility as an internal starting point of the moral process in a difficult time. This becomes clear during the AIDS epidemic when a healer appears sensible to a local world that is divided by stigma and discrimination related to AIDS (see Liamputtong et al. 2009, 2012; Chap. 28 in this volume). It shows that the sympathy of the healer, which developed as the result of an intimate relationship and moral socialization, is the significant moral disposition that facilitates the fact that moral sensibility occurs. This chapter demonstrates that sympathy, together with the consequent compassion and other related moral dispositions, enables the moral process of the healer to perform humanized healing which components can potentiate the effectiveness of healing.

This chapter also concludes that the moral behavior empowers the healer to deal with the power of virtue, which belongs to the healer teachers and sacred objects and exposes it to their patients in the healing process. The moral experiences of the healer and the patients, which aim to make merit, come however from the same religious foundation, but they have different objectives. For the healer, making merit is to accumulate *bun* so that the healer can protect and support his family and patients more extensively. But for the patients, the objective is to extend their lives which, they believe, are nearly ended.

Acknowledgments I would like to thank Professor Annemiek Richters, Dr. Han ten Brummelhuis, and Dr. Komatra Chuengsatiansup for important comments and feedback offered during the writing and editing of this article.

References

Brown, C. R. (2005). Moral sense. In M. C. Horowitz (Ed.), *New dictionary of the history of ideas* (Vol. IV, pp. 1504–1507). Detroit: Thompson Gale.

Kleinman, A. (1995). *Writing at the margin: Discourse between anthropology and medicine*. Berkeley: University of California Press.

Kleinman, A. (1999). Experience and its moral modes: Culture, human conditions and disorder. In G. B. Peterson (Ed.), *The Tanner lectures on human values* (pp. 357–420). Salt Lake City: University of Utah Press.

Liamputtong, P., Haritavorn, N., & Kiatying-Angsulee, N. (2009). HIV and AIDS, stigma and AIDS support groups: Perspectives from women living with HIV and AIDS in central Thailand. *Social Science & Medicine*, Special Issue: Women, Mothers and HIV Care in Resource Poor Settings, *69*(6), 862–868.

Liamputtong, P., Haritavorn, N., & Kiatying-Angsulee, N. (2012). Living positively: The experiences of Thai women in central Thailand. *Qualitative Health Research, 22*(4), 441–451.

Mulder, N. (1979). Concepts of power and moral goodness in the contemporary Thai worldview. *Journal of the Siam Society, 67*(1), 111–131.

Norton, D. F. (1993). *The Cambridge companion to Hume*. Cambridge: Cambridge University Press.

Turner, V. (1975). Symbolic studies. *Annual Review of Anthropology, 4*, 145–161.

Waldram, J. B. (2000). The efficacy of traditional medicine: Current theoretical and methodological issues. *Medical Anthropology Quarterly, 14*(4), 603–625.

Chapter 31
Phum Panya Chao Baan (Local Wisdom) and Traditional Healers in Southern Thailand

Dusanee Suwankhong and Pranee Liamputtong

1 Introduction

Many countries worldwide utilize local wisdom as a resource in their health-care systems (Sermsri 1989; Raekphinit 2009). Although modern knowledge has partially replaced traditional wisdom, local wisdom still remains and people in the local communities prefer using this resource to care for their health. Many sources of local wisdom are available in communities, including traditional healers and traditional materials. These local resources play a part in encouraging communities to rely on their own stores of wisdom (Sringanyuang et al. 2001; Chokevivat et al. 2005; Chuengsatiansup 2007a).

The development paradigm of Thailand has shifted to promote local wisdom because of failing rural development; something which has caused suffering for many people. The promotion of local wisdom is important so that society can recapture previous lifestyles in which local resources were relied upon for healthy living. This can encourage people to maintain a balance of life, even if rapid social or economic changes occur, people will not be significantly affected. They will have sufficient resources to deal with such adverse changes (Nathalang 1990; Antweiler 1998). A reliance on local wisdom appears to be the root factor in strengthening communities and protecting people from suffering because it enables them to achieve balanced living (National Economic and Social Development Board 2000).

D. Suwankhong, Ph.D. (✉)
School of Public Health, Thaksin University, Baan Prao,
Papayom, Phatthalung, 93110, Thailand
e-mail: dusanee.s@tsu.ac.th

P. Liamputtong
School of Public Health and Human Biosciences, La Trobe University,
Kingsbury Drive, Bundoora, Melbourne, Vic 3086, Australia
e-mail: pranee@latrobe.edu.au

P. Liamputtong (ed.), *Contemporary Socio-Cultural and Political Perspectives in Thailand*, 501
DOI 10.1007/978-94-007-7244-1_31, © Springer Science+Business Media Dordrecht 2014

Thailand has had negative experiences from its efforts to become part of the industrialized world. The lifestyles of Thai people have shifted from a reliance on local wisdom to a desire for economical living (Nathalang 1990; Raekphinit 2009). King Bhumibol Adulyadej formulated and expanded the philosophy of a sufficiency economy to reduce his people's sufferings (News Division 2007). The central concept of a sufficiency economy is to produce sufficient resources to live and consume by relying on local wisdom and local resources (Krongkaew 2003). The conceptual purpose of this philosophy is to encourage the Thai people to modify their economic philosophy and provide them with ways of coping with any economic insecurity that occurs. Its aim is to provide people with a new way of thinking to contribute to the holistic idea of balance between consumption and production (National Economic and Social Development Board 2000). See also Chaps. 9 and 32 in this volume.

This new concept encourages all levels of family, community, and society, but especially the grassroots level, to seek self-sufficiency while at the same time participating in the globalized economy. Its implementation could possibly guard against the negative effects of globalization and any rapid changes which arise in the outside world. King Bhumibol Adulyadej's words were initially drafted in the Ninth National Economic and Social Development Plan (2002–2006), and all national policy sectors are now following this philosophy as the major guideline for Thailand's national economic and social development (Nathalang 1990; Krongkaew 2003).

The principle of self-sufficiency is key vision applied for Thai health-care reform, aiming to build sufficient health system for Thais. This philosophy was initiated by the Thai government during the economic crisis in 1997. Thai experience is that the services of traditional healing practices and medical supplies are less expensive than the resources used by modern health systems. Traditional healing has been a local health-care resource for Thai people and remains so today despite the fact that biomedical services are accessible even at the village level. Thus, indigenous healers have been beneficial sources in Thai health, and their own wisdom in this regard should never be ignored (see also Chap. 30 in this volume).

Thai national health policy has adopted the World Health Organization priorities in seeking to strengthen the sufficient health-care system policy. The local wisdom is seen as an important input to the success of this mission. TM has been integrated in the Western-based biomedical health systems. The important aspect of this health reform is the adoption of the primary care approach which emphasizes the promotion of multi-sector and community contributions and the need for individuals to take responsibility for their own health. The Bureau of Policy and Strategy in the Thai Ministry of Public Health (2009) expects that this approach would decrease health-care cost and increase health-care resources for the Thai people. The integration of local healing treatments with Westernized medicine is an increasing trend because of the evidence that such integration provides local people with an optimal care. It is suggested that this integration enables the system to meet patients' individual situations and their needs (Petrakard et al. 2008; Chokevivat et al. 2010).

2 *Phum Panya Chao Baan*: Local Wisdom

Local wisdom has been referred to as local, traditional, indigenous, folk, native, cultural (Read and Behrens 1989), and indigenous environmental knowledge (Briggs et al. 2007). Although local wisdom is the most widespread term, it applies to all grassroots power and is defined as "local knowledge and the respective knowledge systems are rooted in local or regional culture and ecology, the respective social contexts and their economies" (Antweiler 1998: 469). Read and Behrens (1989) define local wisdom in its broader aspect as the knowledge of a certain culture that is deep and well embedded. Local wisdom includes not only information that is stored in people's minds but also encompasses the process of applying information to benefit people's lives.

Local wisdom, therefore, is referred to as a birthright in many countries and it has historically existed to make available various health benefits for their citizens. The current trend in modern health-care development is the return to use the resources that are locally available whenever possible. In Thailand, local wisdom is preserved and valued as a unique resource for sufficient country development, even extending to the public health field. Thai health policy is to continue integrating local wisdom of indigenous medicine into the official health service systems. Because it is accepted that the principles and practices of traditional healing have originally arisen from lay knowledge and local wisdom, it becomes a possible way for promoting a modern and effective health system, returning the health benefits to lay people.

Local wisdom is created and used by lay people, but not modern professionals. In the earlier times, it is rarely recorded in the formal texts but communicated by oral traditions. This knowledge is culturally specific and is mainly rooted knowledge of the local communities or the group of people (Brush 1996; Amen 2007). Any areas of innovation created by lay people to maintain their balance of living and promote well-being are recognized as local wisdom. The products developed by lay people using traditional resources are accepted as the property of all the local people. On the other hand, Western wisdom is systematic and is preserved in the textbooks. Its principles do not apply to specific cultures, whereas its innovation relies on modern technology and expensive research. It is then often not suited to indigenous contexts and indigenous peoples (Brush 1996; Raekphinit 2009).

Lay people play an important role in creating a body of local wisdom in the community because local wisdom is created by the way people interact with each other, the relationships between people and the environment, and the relationships between people and supernatural powers. Such interactions help people to live better, solve problems, share information, exchange ideas, and collaborate to maintain a good quality of life, based on environmental and sociocultural contexts and their belief systems. This learning process always brings about new local wisdom and skills (Raekphinit 2009). Although knowledge can change from generation to generation, over times, a local body of knowledge is developed from the experiences of lay people. Due to its elements of factual knowledge, capabilities, and skills, local knowledge serves as the practical guidelines which individuals adopt into their lives (Nathalang 1990; Antweiler 1998; Raekphinit 2009). New generations can add new knowledge to the existing body of indigenous knowledge to suit the social contexts of each period (Briggs et al. 2007).

Each community is able to create its own body of wisdom. Because each community has different cultural situations and contexts, this uniqueness has influenced the differences in knowledge that have developed in communities. New knowledge soon becomes assimilated into the internal wisdom of a community (Briggs et al. 2007). However, differences in local wisdom may impede the transfer of wisdom between communities. Although some elements can be transferred between localities, generalization of knowledge between communities is limited, and usually only involves some empirical facts (Nathalang 1990; Antweiler 1998).

All nations realize the importance of local wisdom as a key resource in national development. This realization has happened in part due to socioeconomic changes. Modern development has limited the ability of many people to manage their lives. This has affected the quality of life in many communities (Blackwell and Colmenar 1999), and many have turned to the use of localwisdom as a way to support sustainable community development. Because local wisdom is a local resource, it has great value when adapted as a tool for community development. This development strategy is inexpensive, and it may possibly reduce the negative effects of current socioeconomic problems in many societies (Briggs et al. 2007; Raekphinit 2009).

The scientific knowledge has come to govern large areas of the world. Scientific knowledge, however, has some weaknesses; it tends to discount or ignore other disciplines, especially the practice of local healing (Antweiler 1998; see also discussions on authoritative knowledge and health care in Chap. 29 in this volume). The use of scientific knowledge as the main form of development has had a negative impact at many levels because its conceptual nature creates limited and imbalanced practices in many situations. Lay people, however, recognize that their local wisdom may work better in some circumstances and contexts (Phongphit 1982; Williams and Popay 2006; Raekphinit 2009). Antweiler (1998) confirms that local wisdom has innate strength and is fairly flexible in meeting the life circumstances of people.

It is agreed that grassroots health-care resources are both capable and competent. The local wisdom and natural methods these providers employ are valuable in the health-care development (Office of the National Culture Commission 1991). The application of local wisdom in health care involves less modern technology but encourages community participation and decentralized decision-making. It also utilizes resources available within the community. The communities can share and exchange local resources to benefit the life situations of their inhabitants in various ways. It is expected that this practice will lead to community self-reliance, which is acceptable for many countries, both Western and non-Western. If grassroots health care can achieve success in building its capacity, it can be an enduring factor in the development of a country. Such countries have less need to import expertise from abroad (Phongphit 1982; Antweiler 1998; Raekphinit 2009).

Traditional medicine (TM) is one form of local wisdom and its knowledge about healing methods for illness is accumulated by an indigenous community. This discipline commonly involves the use of natural resources and the knowledge of local people, especially traditional healers (Sringanyuang et al. 2001; Timmermans 2003; Chokevivat et al. 2005; Jiang 2005; Chuengsatiansup 2007b; Liamputtong et al. 2012). Although local wisdom is acquired from previous generations and passed on orally, it can also include current knowledge that may be the result of purposeful experimentation and observation and is integrated with the old knowledge to increase the effectiveness of the healing methods (Correa 2002). TM is accepted as an important resource in the formal health-care sector. It plays a crucial role in the provision of health care in both developing and developed countries (Timmermans 2003; World Health Organization 2002; Liamputtong et al. 2012).

The health practitioners who use local wisdom and natural resources to provide health care are recognized as traditional practitioners. Such healers are accepted as a key group in the retention of the knowledge of a community (Sermsri 1989; Timmermans 2003). Local wisdom created and used by traditional healers should be protected to benefit future generations. This knowledge must not be allowed to disappear when the traditional healers pass away (Timmermans 2003). Numerous developing countries have agreed to promote the roles of traditional healers in the primary level of health service systems, including Thailand (Phongphit 1982; Mahler 1983; Raekphinit 2009).

3 Traditional Healers in Southern Thailand

Traditional healers specialize in different areas of health. Their specialization often overlaps with other illness categories so that they can effectively deal with many types of illnesses. Some herbalists, called *mor samoon prai*, for example, not only specialize in *tom ya samoon prai* (stewed herbal medicine) but they also practice the skills of *mor du* (fortune teller), *mor nuat* (massage healer), and *mor wai phom* (ceremonial healer or faith healer). The massage healers are well known for alleviating pain and enhancing well-being. They also focus on the technique of *mor tom ya* (herbalist), *mor wai phom*, and *mor du*. Some ceremonial healers also have expertise in *mor nuat* and *mor du* to manage various causes of illness. With their specialized skills, they can do so much more successfully because most health problems need an integration of several specializations for effective management. Traditional healers, therefore, need to further develop their knowledge and skills so that they can work across many areas, thus providing customers with a wider range of services.

The services provided by traditional healers have distinctive features when compared with standard professional practice. Traditional healers allow their customers to visit them at any time with no concern about office hours: the *mor* (doctor) offers people help 24 × 7. Although the homes of the traditional healers are the main health-care centers, they may also offer help at their customers' homes. This shows the healer's concern for a customer's situation rather than his or her own convenience. If any customers have severe health problems, or are unable to travel to the traditional healer's place, the traditional healers can travel to provide customers with treatment at their home. During our fieldwork, we found that there were many patients who could not travel to seek treatment because of a disability, most of them suffering from disorders such as paralysis, strokes, and bone fractures. For these customers, and in the case of emergency illnesses such as fainting, dizziness, and dyspepsia, the traditional healers would often travel to the patient's home as these patients cannot travel to the healer's house.

Traditional healers provide services where people are. People can call upon healers in the street should they see them. If this occurs, healers offer help in that vicinity. However, the customers who rely on this type of service usually have only minor illness or discomfort, so they can wait for the treatment or they can receive it when they encounter the healers. This pattern is a normal practice among customers in this community and it is very convenient for them.

Because of the holistic approach taken, family members, relatives, and friends are allowed to participate in the healing process. The service provided to customers is not just diagnosis and treatment, followed by departure. Traditional healers are greatly concerned with their customers' health problems and with sharing their sufferings. It also gives the customers and relatives more time to discuss their problems and related issues. In addition, if there are any complications or the illness is getting worse, they do not hesitate to advise customers to seek further help from modern doctors. The customers can also seek help from other traditional healers when needed.

People can seek the help of traditional healers for a range of medical conditions such as muscular and bone disorders, chronic symptoms related to the cardiovascular system, and other categories of chronic illnesses. These customers require long-term treatment. Many clients with paralysis or who have suffered a stroke seek help from traditional healers because they believe in the healers' treatment, which includes massage and herbal medicine. However, the healers may informally refer patients to other local traditional healers or health-care centers for some health problems for which they may not be able to offer much help (Photographs 31.1 and 31.2).

4 The Perceptions and Experiences of Patients of Traditional Healers

Patients seek help of traditional healers for many reasons. Unsatisfactory experiences and mistrust of the help provided by modern medicine make customers turn to traditional healers. Among the many causes that made customers displeased and mistrustful of the services of contemporary medicine were the beliefs that modern treatments are not safe or can aggravate illness, as well as the negative side effects from prolonged treatment.

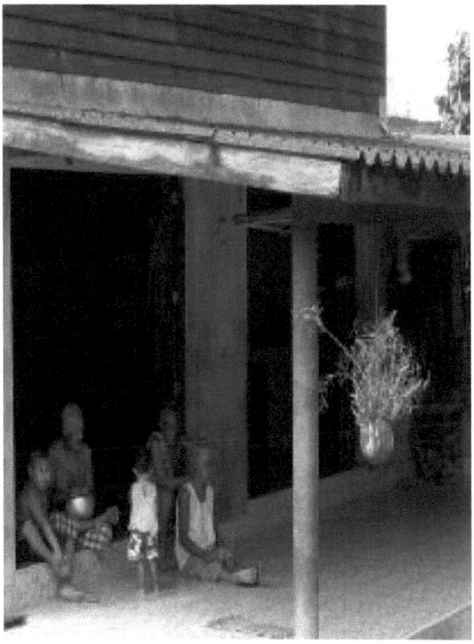

Photograph 31.1 Performing traditional massage at patient's house

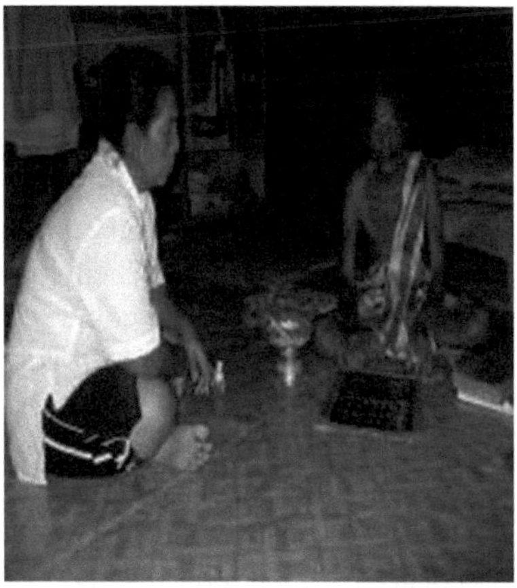

Photograph 31.2 Telling patient the fortune relating to her health

Patients with muscular discomfort are regular customers of traditional healers. A large proportion of the population are farmers, fishermen, and laborers, occupations which make them susceptible to muscular disorders. Muscular dysfunction is also caused by physical pathology. Muscular discomfort is found in both males and females, predominantly in the middle-aged group, even if their jobs do not involve manual labor. It diminishes people's work capabilities and limits their lifestyle. The participants in our study viewed muscular discomfort not as a serious health condition but as a "minor" illness, called *rok boaw boaw* or *rok por dee por rai*, which did not require Western medical attention. Rather, it could be healed by traditional treatments. Thus, they tended not to seek help from modern medicine.

The data from our participant observation showed that there were other health problems that local people included in the category of *rok boaw boaw*, including dyspepsia, *tor nuea*,[1] headache, dizziness, fainting, dysmenorrhea, and lower abdominal disorder. People tended to put more trust in the wisdom of traditional healers than in modern medicine. Although some patients might not recover under the care of traditional healers, these healers could provide basic help and support before the patient sought further assistance at a hospital.

People with bone fractures also often turned to traditional healers rather than rely on modern medicine. This practice was reinforced by family members, friends, and relatives who might have had similar problems in the past. Many participants reported that they were unhappy with the treatment of modern doctors because it did not ease their pain. Rather, the treatment created more suffering. The damaged area could not function as before and this affected their lifestyle.

Cardiovascular patients, who were at high risk of muscle paralysis, were another group who often sought treatment from traditional healers. One participant, Pee Kularb, pointed out from her experience that, "the effects on the body caused by a stroke cannot be healed by modern medicine but they can be healed by traditional healers." Modern medicine provided help for the initial state of emergency and then discharged patients to recuperate at home. Although modern health-care practitioners followed up with regular checking of the patients' condition and gave them tablets, patients and family members often asked traditional healers to help with their rehabilitation.

People suffering from mental disorders were another group who sought help from traditional healers. Patients with anxiety and stress could not be completely healed by modern medicine and often came to depend on drugs to control their conditions for the rest of their lives. Alternative help was sought from traditional healers in the hope that it could relieve them of their illnesses. Often, modern doctors do not understand the patients' situation and circumstances. Sometimes, patients might only need someone to listen to them so they could lift their burdens and relieve their stress and anxiety.

People suffering from unknown illnesses often asked for help from traditional healers who specialize in sacred or ceremonial forms. This sort of illness is closely associated with cultural beliefs in spiritual powers or the supernatural. Usually, this type of ailment is either not detected, or if detected not completely cured, by modern medical treatments as doctors cannot identify a biological cause of the illness. But lay people know who can manage this kind of illness, even if they do not know the exact cause. Although some patients in our study initially sought help from modern doctors, they were diagnosed with a mental illness and treated with modern medicine. Patients would finally be taken to traditional healers by their relatives and family members.

[1] It is an eye disorder involving the growth of medial conjunctiva to form a thickset mass on the cornea area. *Tor nuea* or pterygium mostly grows from the nasal side of the sclera in triangular shape. Sunlight, ultraviolet, dust, wind, or dry air contribute to this eye problem.

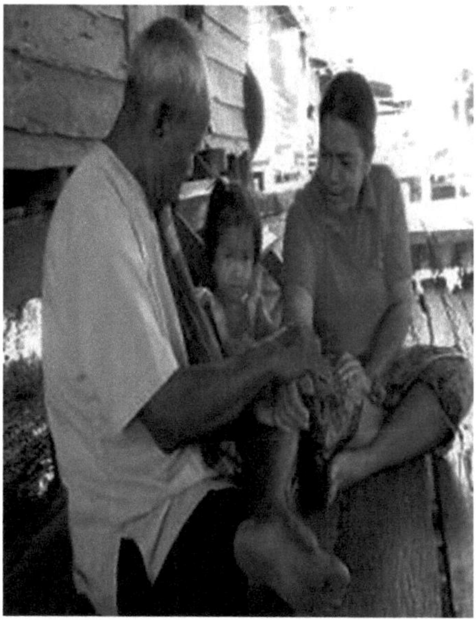

Photograph 31.3 Patient receiving massage to recover wrist sprain

We observed that mysterious illnesses were often identified by traditional healers using spiritual forces. Almost all such unknown illnesses were understood to be related to harm inflicted by the spirits of ancestors or unknown spirits who had been disparaged. Patients fell ill with unusual symptoms and were perceived by people around them as suffering from some form of mental illness. Most such patients lost control of their bodily functions and were unable to recognize things around them or to remember places, times, and dates. They had to rely entirely on carers. The traditional healers would try to restore their health using spiritual powers and by conducting ceremonies. All of the customers experienced an improvement in their symptoms after receiving help two or three times from traditional healers.

Hence, traditional healers are a key group playing a beneficial role for Thai people. Because of these contributions, they are widely recognized as providing basic health care in country areas. The possibility of cooperation with modern health-care providers elicits varied views. Almost all participants seem to agree that it would be possible because it is clearly reflected by participants that this model can produce various advantages to Thai people such as a decrease in health-care costs, an increase in access of people to care, and the provision of health-care choices.

However, the integration between traditional and modern medicine has been promoted in the Thai health-care system. But many barriers to make smooth cooperation between two worlds, traditional and modern health care, are the concern of all participating groups. The barriers that existed mainly included the acceptance of modern doctors, resistance of traditional healers themselves, unclear policy guidelines of promoting cooperation, and license required for traditional healers (Photographs 31.3 and 31.4).

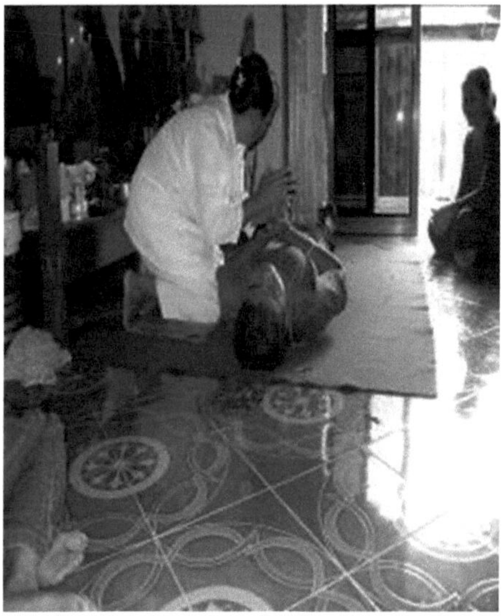

Photograph 31.4 Treatment to dispel an evil ghost

5 The Cooperation Between Two Systems and Barriers

Traditional healers are still viewed as healers who have less knowledge and practices in many areas of health compared to modern doctors who have trained systematically over many years through the academic system. The healers are legally assigned to act as health-care providers in the health-care system. But traditional healers are helping people with their local wisdom that was passed down from previous traditional healers. The knowledge and experience are naturally gained by giving people treatments. The reluctance of acceptance stems from the lack of sufficient empirical evidence to prove effective healing of the traditional healers. Their knowledge stands outside the realm of sciences. It cannot provide the evidence-based clinical practice. Because of this weakness, modern health-care workers do not have a strong trust in the healing but carefully choose some therapeutics to be implemented in the health-care service. Some participants in our study, particularly the community heads were unsure whether traditional healers could play a role in the Thai health care or should they keep to their role providing for their local community as in the past.

On the other hand, many customers that we interviewed seemed to be confident that traditional healers could cooperate with modern health-care workers. This is because, for a long time, the healers have demonstrated their craft in the Thai health system. They agreed that if both mainstreams could cooperate, they would like to see the cooperation happen. This optional help could provide customers with maximum benefits of care seeking. But they had never seen such cooperation between modern and traditional healing. They did not know whether modern health-care providers could or would accept traditional healers as their partners. At the same time, some customers did not agree with traditional healers working together with modern health-care providers. They believed that the traditional healers have a simple lifestyle and their work does not concern systematic management.

The resistance of traditional healers is one barrier of cooperation between the mainstream health-care system. Many traditional healers with whom we talked perceived that it is difficult for cooperation if individual healers are not willing to do so. The majority of traditional healers in our study were not interested in formally working alongside modern health-care staff. They preferred a simple working style in the same way which is already familiar to them. Helping people in their homes, their unique patterns, and informal styles allow them to practice without the need to change their lifestyles. They have more independence in their work and there are no systems to control their life. Also this original pattern has been followed since traditional healers first began healing people.

Traditional healers tended not to trust people from other disciplines. Most of the traditional healers still preserved their knowledge and did not want to share their knowledge with the public, especially with modern health-care providers. This factor created a barrier to cooperation between the two mainstreams as well. The traditional healers did not want to be registered formally. They could not see the benefit of cooperation due to prior negative experiences from the government health service. This led them to have little or no trust in this sector and made them reluctant to cooperate. Nearly all of them complained that the government had never sincerely supported their roles. On the other hand, this sector tended to take their knowledge and retrained them in new wisdom. They considered that even if they attended the training or work cooperatively, it would do nothing to improve their profession and their roles in Thai health. Rather, it would try to change their style to the modern world. However, although the government institutes did not recognize their contribution, they still existed because their customers supported their very existence.

The policy level still has not clearly stated how the traditional healers could legally cooperate with modern medicine. This is despite them being recognized as a primary health-care resource which has provided a beneficial role to Thai people for a long time. Rather, the policy seemed to control and limit their roles. The policy makers always said that they intended to encourage traditional healers in Thai health care to increase people's access to care and preserves Thai TM, but implementing guideline to support role of traditional healers has not been processing through. All traditional healers consulted remarked that they did not understand the policy makers and whether the policy workers would want to promote their role. From their experiences, they said that policy makers seemed not to promote them sincerely.

Many health-care providers and health-policy workers claimed a similar viewpoint, that the current policy does not promote cooperation between the two mainstreams continually; it is occasionally promoted instead. Almost all of them also stated that because their work relies on annual budgets, if the budget is used up before the project is complete, work on the project has to either finish or be stopped until the new budget is received. Although a particular project or activity might be able to continue, they have to wait for the next budget round before they can proceed.

6 Discussion and Conclusion

Traditional healers in this study provide a multiplicity of treatments. All traditional healers have practiced more than one area of specialties. Some are known for the techniques they use for healing while others gain a reputation for specializing in a specific health problem or disease. According to Wongkumdang (2007), some traditional healers may acquire high-level healing skills pertaining to certain illnesses, whereas others may have limited skills in treating particular health problems or disorders. Being able to switch between various therapeutic modes, however, is a useful skill. Patients expect to receive comprehensive care from traditional healers (Oppong 1989; Ovuga et al. 1999). Hence, gaining several specialized skill sets would allow traditional healers to attend to patients with a broader range of health problems and diseases. Folk healing uses a holistic approach and acknowledges traditional practice (Kleinman 1980; Sermsri 1989). Helman (2007) notes that traditional practitioners do not only focus on treating symptoms or physical disorders but also use methods designed to eliminate the causes of illness at their roots. Their treatments always integrate several strategies, drawing upon both visible and supernatural powers, to manage the different illnesses of their customers. There are extensive studies of the experience of folk treatment and its service system. For example, traditional healing uses integrated therapy to defend against invisible causes of illnesses and to increase individual health (Baskind and Birbeck 2005). The Bureau of Indigenous Thai Medicine (2003) supports the notion that the use of integrated treatment is a unique practice of traditional healing and that it can contribute positively to promoting the overall health of individuals.

Cultural beliefs play a salient role in patients' understanding of illnesses and their corresponding treatment (Kleinman 1980; Chuengsatiansup et al. 2004; Helman 2007). The majority of participants consider symptoms such as muscle strain, dizziness, headache, and fainting to be readily treated by traditional healers. They perceive these symptoms to be manifestations of *rok boaw boaw* (minor illnesses) because they do not interfere with their lifestyles or ability to work. From their experience, such symptoms could not be completely cured but only relieved, even if they took a lot of modern drugs. They believe that the more they are treated by traditional healers for these symptoms, the better it will be for them. This concurs with Golomb's assertion (1985) that the main purpose of traditional healing practice is to provide care for individuals with non-life-threatening illnesses. The data in our study also show that patients with bone fractures have greater faith in traditional healing than modern medicine. This belief has been passed down over the generations. Although some are treated by modern medicine, concurrently they seek traditional healers' help because they believe that modern medicine alone will not be able to make the fractured bone function normally again.

Many societies integrate specific types of traditional healers for collaboration with their modern hospital systems. Such healers are expected to share in the workload of the modern doctors and provide people with more choices of care (Courtright 1995; Ovuga et al. 1999; Bureau of Indigenous Thai Medicine 2009). But no single traditional healer in this study who has cooperated with modern doctors formally is found. Some modern health-care organizations at the community level experimented with efforts at cooperation with traditional healers. However, the authority and structure of community health-care organizations is not designed to accommodate cooperation with traditional healers. Many researchers, such as Antweiler (1998), Phongphit (1982), and Chuengsatiansup and associates (2004), are in support of the development of health-care resources at the grassroots level in order to build the self-reliance of communities. These grassroots resources are available to promote the health of Thais, and they are in alignment with Thai culture and beliefs.

The supporting roles which traditional healers provide are consistent with the recent and future direction of the national health development plan for Thailand, which promotes the utilization by communities of existing local wisdom to achieve health-care development. Sermsri (1989), Golomb (1985), Kulsomboon and Adthasit (2007), and Chuengsatiansup (2007a) state that the supporting roles of healers at the grassroots level definitely help with promoting communities' self-reliance agendas because this strategy allows the communities to rely on their own valuable resources for their people's health needs, rather than importing remedies. Moreover, this study provides support for and expansion on previous studies which agree that serving as primary health-care resources is a salient role of traditional healers).

In reality, modern health-care teams have mistrust in the knowledge and roles of traditional healers because they have no recognized medical licenses. As Sermsri (1989) points out, modern health providers view traditional healers as illegal healers whose medical knowledge and treatment methods are questionable. This stigmatizing of traditional healers makes doctors hesitate in referring patients to them. Modern doctors would rather promote the use of modern medical services, especially since these facilities are more available to lay people at the community level than ever before. These findings are mirrored in studies of other societies (Kale 1995; Nelms and Gorski 2006).

Acknowledgments We are grateful to all customers of traditional healers who have provided us with deep understanding of their care-seeking behavior. We would also like to thank the Faculty of Health and Sports Science, Thaksin University, Thailand, and the School of Public Health, La Trobe University, Australia, for the scholarship to support the first author in carrying out the fieldwork in rural Thailand. Additionally, we would like to thank Department for Development of Thai Traditional and Alternative Medicine, Ministry of Public Health, Phatthalung Provincial Health Office, and all local government organizations and their staff who gave the first author their sincere support during the process of our data collection.

References

Amen, M. M. (2007). Different ways of creating knowledge. *Journal of Theory Construction & Testing, 11*(1), 38–39.

Antweiler, C. (1998). Local knowledge and local knowing: An anthropological analysis of contested "Cultural Products" in the context of development. *Anthropos, 93*(4–6), 469–494.

Blackwell, A., & Colmenar, R. (1999). Transforming policy through local wisdom. *Futures, 31*, 487–497.
Briggs, J., Sharp, J., Yacoub, H., Hamed, N., & Roe, A. (2007). The nature of indigenous environmental knowledge production: Evidence from Bedouin Communities in Southern Egypt. *Journal of International Development, 19*, 239–251.
Brush, S. B. (1996). Whose knowledge, whose genes, whose rights? In S. B. Brush & D. Stabinsky (Eds.), *Valuing local knowledge: Indigenous people and intellectual property rights* (pp. 1–21). Washington, DC: Island Press.
Bureau of Indigenous Thai Medicine. (2003). *Thai indigenous medicine: The Thai intellectual property*. Bangkok: Thai Royal.
Bureau of Indigenous Thai Medicine. (2009). *Effectiveness of traditional doctors in treating patients with fractures in 9 areas*. Retrieved November 1, 2009, from http://www.dtam.moph.go.th/intranet/doct/forum/index.php?showtopic=34
Bureau of Policy and Strategy Ministry of Public Health. (2009). *Health policy in Thailand 2009*. Retrieved August 14, 2011, from http://whothailand.healthrepository.org/handle/123456789/589
Chokevivat, V., Chuthaputti, A., & Khumtrakul, P. (2005). *The use of traditional medicine in the Thai health care system*. Retrieved January 29, 2010, from http://www.searo.who.int/LinkFiles/Meetings_document09.pdf
Chokevivat, V., Wibulpolprasert, S., & Petrakard, P. (Eds.). (2010). *Thai traditional health profile 2009–2010*. Bangkok: The War Veterans Organization.
Chuengsatiansup, K. (2007a). Indigenous health system in the rural Thailand. In K. Chuengsatiansup & Y. Tantipidoke (Eds.), *Thai health Thai culture* (pp. 113–144). Bangkok: Nungsurdeeone.
Chuengsatiansup, K. (2007b). Trend of local wisdom in Thai health: Concept and strategy for knowledge management in the area of Thai traditional medicine, indigenous medicine, and alternative medicine. In K. Chuengsatiansup & Y. Tantipidoke (Eds.), *Thai health Thai culture* (pp. 205–214). Bangkok: Nungsurdeeone.
Chuengsatiansup, K., Muksong, C., Tongsinsat, N., Pinkaew, R., Petkong, W., Sirisathitkun, M., et al. (2004). *Dynamic of self-reliance (rural sector)*. Bangkok: Foundation Okml Gold Tweezers.
Correa, C. M. (2002). *Protection and promotion of traditional medicine implications for public health in developing countries*. Geneva: South Centre.
Courtright, P. (1995). Eye care knowledge and practices among Malawian traditional healers and the development of collaborative blindness prevention programmes. *Social Science & Medicine, 41*(11), 1569–1575.
Golomb, L. (1985). *An anthropology of curing in multiethnic Thailand*. Urbana: University of Illinois Press.
Helman, C. G. (2007). *Culture, health and illness* (5th ed.). London: Hodder Arnold.
Jiang, W.-Y. (2005). Therapeutic wisdom in traditional Chinese medicine: A perspective from modern science. *Trends in Pharmacological Sciences, 26*(11), 558–563.
Kale, R. (1995). Traditional healers in South Africa: A parallel health care system. *British Medical Journal, 310*(6988), 1182–1185.
Kleinman, A. (1980). *Patients and healers in the context of culture: An exploration of the borderland between anthropology, medicine, and psychiatry*. Berkeley: University of California Press.
Krongkaew, M. (2003). *The philosophy of sufficiency economy*. Retrieved July 8, 2009, from http://kyotoreview.cseas.kyoto-u.ac.jp/issue/issue3/article_292.html
Kulsomboon, S., & Adthasit, R. (2007). *The status and trend of research in local wisdom for health*. Bangkok: The War Veterans Organization.
Liamputtong, P., Suwankhong, D., & Rumbold, B. (2012). Traditional, complementary and alternative medicine (TCAM): A review of healing practices outside the formal health care system. In Y. Motto (Ed.), *Traditional medicine: New research* (pp. 59–82). New York: Nova Science Publishers.
Mahler, H. (1983). Foreward. In R. H. Bannerman, J. Burton, & C. E. Wen-Chieh (Eds.), *Traditional medicine and health care coverage: A reader for health administrators and practitioners* (pp. 7–8). Geneva: World Health Organization.

Nathalang, E. (1990). *The wisdom of Thai farmers: Contemporary efforts for cultural reproduction.* Paper presented at the 4th international conference on Thai Studies, Kunming, Yunnan.
National Economic and Social Development Board. (2000). *Sufficiency economy.* Retrieved July 7, 2009, from http://www.sufficiencyeconomy.org/en/files/4.pdf
Nelms, L. W., & Gorski, J. (2006). The role of the African traditional healer in women's health. *Journal of Transcultural Nursing, 17*(2), 184–189.
News Division, Department of Information. (2007). *The philosophy of sufficiency economy.* Retrieved July 7, 2009, from http://www.us-asean.org/Thailand/C95.pdf
Office of the National Culture Commission. (1991). *Lay local wisdom and promoting culture for developing rural areas.* Bangkok: Office of the National Culture Commission.
Oppong, A. C. K. (1989). Healers in transition. *Social Science & Medicine, 28*(6), 605–612.
Ovuga, E., Boardman, J., & Oluka, E. G. A. O. (1999). Traditional healers and mental illness in Uganda. *Psychiatric Bulletin, 23*, 276–279.
Petrakard, P., Chantraket, R., & Limpananont, J. (2008). *The integration of Thai traditional medicine: The situation of its service.* Bangkok: Dawn of Printing.
Phongphit, S. (1982). *Back to the root.* Bangkok: Teanwan.
Raekphinit, C. (2009). *Local wisdom.* Phattalung: Thaksin University.
Read, D. W., & Behrens, C. (1989). Modeling folk knowledge as expert systems. *Anthropological Quarterly, 62*(3), 107–120.
Sermsri, S. (1989). Utilization of traditional and modern health care services in Thailand. In S. R. Quah (Ed.), *The triumph of practicality: Tradition and modernity in health care utilization in selected Asian countries* (pp. 160–179). Singapore: Institute of Southeast Asian Studies.
Sringanyuang, L., Wattanapa, A., Peawking, J., Toungratanaphan, S., & Lertmanorat, S. (2001). *Self-care development in family and community.* Nonthaburi: Health Systems Research Institute.
Timmermans, K. (2003). Intellectual property rights and traditional medicine: Policy dilemmas at the interface. *Social Science & Medicine, 57*(4), 745–756.
Williams, G., & Popay, J. (2006). Lay knowledge and the privilege of experience. In D. Kelleher, J. Gabe, & G. Williams (Eds.), *Challenging medicine* (2nd ed., pp. 122–145). London: Routledge.
Wongkumdang, S. (2007). *Knowledge management of Pga K'nyau folk healers in Ban Chan sub-district, Mae Chaem district, Chiang Mai province.* Unpublished master's thesis, Chiang Mai University, Chiang Mai.
World Health Organization. (2002). *WHO traditional medicine strategy 2002–2005.* Retrieved August 15, 2009, from http://whqlibdoc.who.int/hq/2002/WHO_EDM_TRM_2002.1.pdf

Chapter 32
Patronage, Dominance, or Collaboration? Thailand's NGOs and the Thai Health Promotion Foundation

Atchara Rakyutidharm

1 Introduction

The relationship between donors and NGOs has been a critical subject of debate. Thai nongovernmental organizations (NGOs) and people's organizations (POs) have claimed that their identities as nonprofit and independent organizations are free from the domination of both state power and business interests. In recent years, however, the level of official funding for NGOs in development efforts has increased dramatically. Not only funding but the cooperation between Thai NGOs and state agencies in development is increasing. According to a report by the National Institute of Development Administration (NIDA) and Chulalongkorn University Social Research Institute (CUSRI) in 2009, the key source of Thai NGOs' funds was from domestic sources with more than half of the NGOs in Northern Thailand being funded by government agencies (Warunpitikun and Ruengjit 2010).

Thailand's NGOs increasingly obtain financial support from Thai Health Promotion Foundation (THPF), from 22,551,910 THB in 2001 to 1,262 million THB[1] in 2010. Established in 2001, THPF describes itself as "an autonomous state agency which outside the formal structure of government.[2]" THPF's source of fund is "sin taxes" collected from producers and importers of alcohol and tobacco. In order to receive financial support, NGOS have to follow a strict administrative system and receive project advice from THPF. The relationship appears mutually beneficial: development NGOs view the cooperation with state agencies as the way

This chapter is from the research "The Politics of Depoliticization: the Transformation of NGOs-State-People Relations" granted by the Thailand Research Fund (TRF).

[1] This is a total budget to foundations and regional organizations which included NGOs.

[2] http://en.thaihealth.or.th/

A. Rakyutidharm (✉)
Department of Social Sciences, Faculty of Arts,
Silpakorn University, Nakornpathom 73000, Thailand
e-mail: atchara@su.ac.th

P. Liamputtong (ed.), *Contemporary Socio-Cultural and Political Perspectives in Thailand*,
DOI 10.1007/978-94-007-7244-1_32,

to sustainable development and an effective method to participate in government decision-making processes with a view to influencing rather than conforming, while THPF claims its role is to strengthen civil society (THPF 2011b).

The issue of power relations between donors and NGOs has been at the center of critical debates in the development arena, including NGOs in Thailand. Many studies indicate the asymmetrical relationships between the two parties, although the donors often refer to their grantees as "partners" implying a degree of equality (Parks 2008). Despite obtaining funds from THPF or government agencies, it is risky to assume that NGOs are under the patronage of, or being dominated by, THPF or the state. In examining the development concepts and practices of THPF and NGOs, this chapter posits the relationship of THPF and NGOs as collaboration, not just because both parties stand to benefit from, and contribute to, each other, but they also share a common development ideology. In particular, they commonly subscribe to the concept of "self-reliance" that encourages individuals and local communities to rely on themselves rather than to push for efforts at social structural transformation. In this exercise, the state's power is depoliticized and remains critically unexamined, and NGOs merely become the state's "partner" to make local people docile and consensual of the state.

2 Theoretical Framework

Civil society is an ambiguous and problematic concept. In the liberalist perspective, civil society is a diversity of spaces, actors, and institutional forms which are distinct from the force-backed structures of the state. Strengthening civil society means the dismantling of the roles and structures of the state since the actors in civil society will constantly struggle for political power with the assumption that the society is threatened by the abuse of power of the state (Loathammatas 2007; Kitirianglarp 2009). In this sense, the state is opposite to civil society, and the state's intervention could undermine the strength of civil society. At present in Thailand, however, many social activists and intellectuals voice their preference for the civil society's cooperation rather than confrontation with the state (Shigetomi 2000; Kanittachart 2008). Government agencies are also increasingly involved in cooperating with NGOs to strengthen civil society networks. This brings about heated debates about the proper roles of, and relationship among, the state and civil society.

The term "state" is also problematic. The debates in Thailand about the meaning and relationship of the state to society are very broad and varied. On the one hand, state is understood as a concrete political institution comprising different state officials and mechanisms. It establishes a set of rules that apply uniformly to all its constituent societies, claiming to safeguard "public interest." On the other hand, the state is understood as a source of power existing inside and outside formal institutions. According to Bourdieu et al. (1994), the state can exercise its power through social and cultural domination as well as physical forces. For cultural domination, the state constructs a "bureaucratic field" as "a field of power" into which social actors are drawn to interact under the state's rule. The state thus can exert control over the people through a "symbolic violence" that becomes natural without it being recognized as violence.

In so doing, the state incarnates itself in the form of both specific organizational and mental structures. The people in society voluntarily apply the many categories of their perception and thought to all things in their social world and never doubt that it emerged from the influence of the state. They also act as an arm of the state by enforcing the state's order and discipline upon the others. Although they negotiate with the state, this is only because the state made them do so. The field of struggle is a construct as is the construction of the state monopoly over power. In this sense, it is not necessary for state power to inhabit any official institution but other organizations and people.

In this chapter, I view THPF as a "bureaucratic field" of the Thai state that draws nongovernment agencies to play in the field under the state's rules with the financial support of the state. In this field, development NGOs are no longer antagonistic to the state, but collaborate with the state to direct the people's behavior and perspectives. In the modern state, development is a field in which the state's symbolic violence is rendered. As Escobar (1995) and Ferguson (1990) point out, the state identifies the people as "underdeveloped" so that it can derive legitimacy to impose its own forms of social control upon them, discipline them, or educate them in order to change their behavior, attitudes, values, and desires. In Ferguson's term (1990), the development discourse is an "antipolitics machine" that transforms social problems brought about by unequal power relations into technical problems. In the development process, development experts are constituted from scholars, NGO activists, and government officials as "the trustees" who claim to know what is best for the others and how the others should live. This is the way in which the government and nongovernment development agencies impose "symbolic violence" upon the people who are under their cultural domination (Mosse 2005; Li 2007).

In Thailand, NGOs claim that their role is representative of, and also as coordinator among, the different actors in civil society. Many development NGOs also find it preferable to seek to share public resources from government agencies and participate in government decision-making processes. Through examining the relationship between some of Thailand's NGOs and the THPF, this chapter will illustrate how THPF is perceived by the NGOs and whether or not they see THPF as a "bureaucratic field" of state power (Bourdieu et al. 1994).

3 State vs. NGOs in Thailand Context

3.1 Thai Health Promotion Foundation as an Arm of the State

Thai Health Promotion Foundation (THPF) is categorized as an autonomous state agency or an independent organization according to Thailand's Constitution (1997). However, its source of funding is from the government with the Prime Minister as the Chairman of the Board of the THPF, and their policies and fund administered under the instruction from the government. According to THPF's annual report, in the 2010 fiscal year, THPF approved 1,262 million THB or 35 % of its total budget to support various projects related to nonprofit foundations and religion organizations which included NGOs (THPF 2011a).

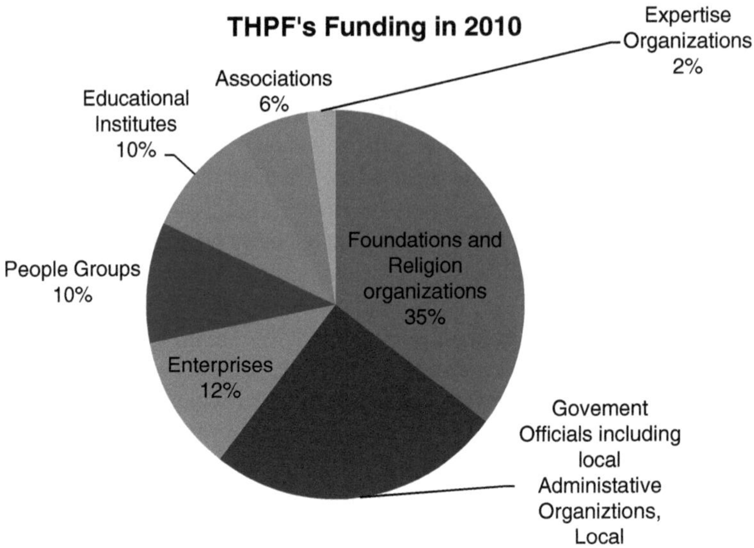

Source: THPF (2011a: 55)

As its name implies, THPF aims at promoting health care in Thai society. Most of its consultant and executive committee members are medical scientists, while some are social development experts. Several kinds of work in the development area including natural resource management, social development, social justice, and community strengthening can be interpreted broadly as health concerns. Not only NGOs but also other types of organizations including government officials, local communities, educational institutions, and businesses have been funded by THPF. The THPF claims that it is attempting to cooperate with and establish networks among businesses, nongovernmental organizations, and civil society.[3]

Since its establishment, THPF has funded 8,569 grantees. In 2010, it funded a total of 822 grantees, of which 67.8 % of them had never received THPF grants previously (THPF 2011a: 55). Several studies point out that power relations between donors and NGOs are usually asymmetrical (Parks 2008). However, as I have mentioned above, it is risky to assume that receiving funds from state agencies like the THPF causes NGOs to come under the patronage or domination of the state. I argue that the cooperation between THPF and NGOs is progressive because both parties share some common development agendas.

I interviewed NGO activists whose organizations are funded by THPF.[4] Their organizations work on different issues such as sustainable agriculture, labor rights,

[3] http://en.thaihealth.or.th/plans/health-community

[4] For example, Witoon Lianchamroon and Kingkorn Narintrakul of Bio Thai; RojarekWatanapanit of Community Forest Support Group; Adisorn Kerdmongkol from the Project for Well-being of Migrant Workers, Ethnic Minorities, Refugees, and Stateless Persons; and Noppan Promsri of Human Settlement Foundation.

natural resource management, and knowledge management. Most of these NGO activists perceived THPF as a state official according to THPF's bureaucratic administrative system, while some of them viewed THPF as a donor just like any other donor with whom NGOs had to negotiate for funding. For Thai NGOs, their categorizations of the key actors with whom they usually interact are not complicated. They are the government, government officials in local and policy levels, donors, business actors, middle-class people, and grassroots people. In general, the term "*rath*" in Thai is usually equated to a grouping of the government (*rathabaan*) and government officials (*rachakarn*) but often includes other state mechanisms such as laws and policies that establish state power. In other words, "*rath*" is simply used to mean a monolithic entity that establishes and employs a set of rules to exert power over the people. For most development NGOs in Thailand, "*rath*" is antagonistic to "*chao bann*" or villager (a term often equated to the grass roots, the rural, or the "local") as they perceive that all state mechanisms are designed to exert control over, and regulate, especially rural people in order to exploit natural resources for profit. The perception of "*rath*" in this sense is framed as a development state that has strong and extensive regulation as well as planning for economic development oriented toward markets, businesses, and capitalism. However, some government officials are viewed as an exception when they support the NGOs' development approaches that are against big business or capitalism.

Like many NGOs in Asia, NGOs in Thailand have experienced funding shortfalls when international donors have either reduced or pulled out funding (Parks 2008). During the late 1960s and until the 1990s, their key sources of funding were from donors in the northern countries such as Sweden (SIDA), Canada (CIDA), the USA (USAID), and the Netherlands (NOVIB) (Kantawit 2008). After the mid-1990s, there was a decline in foreign donor funding for Thailand's NGOs as a result of Thailand's progress in social and economic benchmarks such as GDP used in measuring national development (Parks 2008: 215). Since then, domestic funding such as from THPF has become increasingly important to Thailand's NGOs.

Some Thai activists noted that receiving funds from state agencies was a reason that Thai NGOs were dominated by the state or under the state's patronage system.[5] Some said that NGOs became the extended organs of the state as they helped the state to work rather than empowering and strengthening local people.[6] However, the cooperation between state agencies and many NGOs has developed over a long time. For example, one of the objectives of the NGO Coordinating Committee for Development since it was established in 1985 was "to enhance the understanding and cooperation between NGOs and involved state agencies" (Deesutjit 2000: 66).

The Local Development Institute (LDI), established by a group of senior NGO activists and scholars, is said to be the organization that initiated the cooperation between NGOs and state agencies (Shigetomi 2006). The cooperation has been developed from the idea of "people participation" that NGOs sought to participate in the government decision-making process and has later on spread to other

[5] http://www.youtube.com/watch?v=fhN-6CnJ8LI&feature=related

[6] http://ww.youtube.com/watch?v=nnfbVyOYU8w

administrative activities (Shigetomi 2000: 137). During 1984–1990, Local Development Assistance Program (LDAP) employed a "new working alternative" – promoting the participation of the government, people, and NGOs for encouraging self-reliance of rural communities. This approach was said to be the "supplementation of the state's role" (Kantawit 2008: 21). The LDAP was funded by Canada International Development Agency (CIDA) through the facilitation of the government of Thailand. In 1991, after the LDAP ended, the former LDAP committee members, such as Prawes Wasi, Saneh Chamarik, Anek Nakabutra, and Akin Rapeepat, established the LDI and raised funds from various government agencies and the business sector including the Environment Fund of the Ministry of Science and Technology, Thailand Research Fund, Wanapruek Foundation, and Social Investment Fund (SIF) (Jansomwong 2008).

During 1995–1998, LDI continued LDPA's goal in furthering cooperation between civil society and the state. LDI named this working approach as the "civil society" strategy, which was newly introduced in Thailand at that time in the context that people's organizations and networks were also dramatically expanding (Jansomwong 2008). Prawes Wasi, an intellectual leader of LDI[7] who has been promoting the "civil society" strategy, describes civil society as the social structure that bridges the state and individuals in order to free Thai society from the cycle of karma and solve not only social and economic but also mental, cultural environmental, and political problems (Wasi 1999, cited in Kanittachart 2008: 214). As this strategy was aimed at cooperating with the state, it brought about a gap between LDI and other more militant social movements, despite their previous close relationship (Boonchai 2008). However, since 1995 when "people's participation" became a key means to achieve sustainable development, state agencies have drawn together representatives of the people's sector to participate in the government's policy-making. Cooperation between civil society and state has been gradually developed and adopted by most militant movements as one of the strategies in negotiating with state power.

Dr. Prawes is significantly involved in the policy-making of both government and nongovernment agencies, including in THPF and NGOs.[8] However, the practical cooperation between different NGOs and state agencies is diverse. Despite state funding, the NGO activists I interviewed insisted that they were "independent" from the donors and had full autonomy to design their own projects. Many NGOs claim that they deserve to share THPF's budget because it is from the taxes collected from society. In other words, NGOs claim their share of the public resources from THPF to work for the benefit of local communities. Besides money, some NGOs said that cooperating with state agencies is their "new" strategy replacing radical movements such as protest and demonstrations that are perceived as no longer effective. The "cooperation" in this sense means not only to receive funding from THPF but also

[7] He was the President of Local Development Foundation since 1991.

[8] In the drafting process of the Eighth National Economic and Social Development Plan (1997–2001), he was the Chair of a subcommittee for rural, local, and environmental development planning. He was in the consultant committee of THPF during 2000–2006.

to share opinions, collaborate in planning, join some activities, and support each other for achieving a common goal. They believe that by this new strategy, it is possible to gain positive responses from the state than militant strategy.[9] Some government policies and programs are claimed by NGOs as a result of their activities, for example, THPF's support of food sovereignty advocacy, the government policy on communal title deeds, and the national policy on sustainable agriculture promotion. Once government agencies begin to support people's demands or the policies advocated by NGOs, Chatchawan Thongdeelert, a senior NGO activist in Northern Thailand, said that "there is no longer a reason to oppose the state.[10]"

My interviews with many NGO activists reveal that most NGOs granted funds by THPF willingly and increasingly cooperate with the THPF and other state agencies. Like other donors, THPF refers to grantees as "partners" or "owners of the issues" and positions itself as "supporters." NGOs prefer the term "network" or "alliance" to describe their relationship with THPF because they believe that they can always discuss and negotiate with THPF and other state agencies fairly. Most NGOs satisfy the role claimed by THPF that THPF is creating and strengthening the networks among state, business, civil society, and local community sectors, although they have realized that THPF is a state agency. It is obvious that the NGO activists interviewed for this paper pay less attention to the politics of the construction of THPF and its political projects and act as if the structure and work of THPF emerge naturally without politics.

The cooperation between THPF and NGOs is not considered the achievement of NGOs but also points to the ability of THPF in drawing NGOs to work with a state agency with its own mission which is to cooperate between civil society and government agencies. Although THPF claims that it considers all funding requests from any group, community, or organization fairly and objectively, its funding decisions are actually highly selective based on its yearly framework. This bias is evident from this paper's NGO interviewees[11] who mostly accepted that, apart from the reputation or work experience of the organization seeking support, the personal relationship between THPF staff and an NGO or referee played an important role in approval of funding from THPF. Although THPF positions itself as a "supporter," it has its own specific agendas before funding, and it is the duty of grantees to make the funding proposals fit with these agendas. For large budget projects (usually over one million baht), the THPF will first make a survey of the key groups or organizations working on THPF's concerned issues. The representatives of these organizations will then be invited for a meeting in which THPF presents its specific aims and encourages the representatives to submit a proposal for funding. Some organizations with networking potential are appointed to be the head of a group of NGOs so that they can attract more partners to THPF funding and coordinate with these

[9] Interview with DechoChaitap of Sustainable Development Foundation, May 2, 2011.

[10] Interview with Chatchawan Thongdeelert, May 7, 2011.

[11] Such as Witoon Lianchamroon and Kingkorn Narintrakul of Bio Thai, Rojarek Watanapanit of Community Forest Support Group, and Adisorn Kerdmongkol from the Project for Well-being of Migrant Workers, Ethnic Minorities, Refugees, and Stateless Persons.

organizations to work together under the same THPF umbrella. THPF will grant an organization funding for three phases as maximum (1–3 years for a phase).[12]

Although the THPF funding is highly selective, NGO activists I interviewed did not mention this angle and the depoliticization of state power brought about by THPF. The cooperation between THPF and grantee NGOs makes both sides happy as it seems to be a win-win relationship for them. This contrasts to the claim by Hume and Edwards (1997, cited in Parks 2008: 217) that the relationship between donors and grantees is somehow marked by coercion from the donor. Nevertheless, the win-win relationship between THPF and NGOs might not be a win-win for the people who are the intended beneficiaries of their projects. The next section will illustrate some intended and unintended consequences of the collaborative development approaches of NGOs and THPF.

3.2 *The Collaborative Development and Common Ideology of THPF and NGOs*

THPF's self-described character as a health promoter supposedly frees it from politics. But, the converse situation is true: THPF is involved in politics from the upper policy level to people's everyday lives. Encouraging self-reliance in a collaborative work is the approach of THPF, and many Thai NGOs claim to work toward sustainable development. THPF's philosophy as stated in its website is that "all Thais can attain better lives, in a self-reliant way, through increase in cooperation."[13] It says that one way to encourage self-reliance is to strengthen local communities. The Healthy Community Strengthening Sector, one of THPF's 11 sectors, directly supports capacity building of local communities through the support of the cooperation among organizations working with local communities.[14] This sector was established by the attempt of Dr. Prawes Wasi, a well-known academic mentioned in the previous section. A few years ago, this sector granted funds to the Alternative Agriculture Network (AAN), which promotes sustainable farming to build small-scale farmers' self-reliance. Besides, many other sectors of THPF also support Thai NGOs working on different issues related to community strengthening. For example, the Heath Factor Control supports Bio-Thai, an NGO working on biodiversity and sustainable agriculture, and the Open Grant and Innovative Projects supports the Human Settlement Foundation working with the homeless people's network.

For the modern-nation state, constructing an "imagined community" (Anderson 1991) is aimed at claiming state power over the population. The state constructed village community in order to create a system of control of the countryside

[12] My personal communication with THPF's staff and some NGO activists.

[13] http://en.thaihealth.or.th/about#policy

[14] http://en.thaihealth.or.th/plans/health-community

(Kemp 1981) and an image of peaceful rural life, bountiful nature, and livelihoods (as has been portrayed in the song "In the fields, there is rice; In the rivers, there is fish"[15]). This "imagined community" is created in order to herd people into an imagined identity of "Thainess" (see also Chaps. 1, 8, and 15 in this volume). In the present context, which is called an age of individualism, Thai families, national culture, its institutions, and communities are said to be threatened by capitalism. The Thai state, therefore, pays a lot of attention to strengthening local communities in order to reconstruct the "peaceful livelihoods" of Thai society so that Thailand can overcome the fierce competition that is economic globalization (cf. Chap. 9 in this volume).

Thai NGOs have promoted local communities' self-reliance since the late 1960s. They thus appreciate the support of THPF in this working approach, and the collaboration between THPF and Thai NGOs is welcomed by both the partners. The Director of Bio-Thai pointed out that Dr. Prawes is very "progressive" in integrating community development and health issues. It can be said that Dr. Prawes is a key person who bridges THPF and NGOs to work together, and community-based development is a concept that enhances this cooperation between NGOs and state agencies like the THPF.

In fact, "self-reliance" is a radical concept. Although the understanding and application of the concept has changed over time, it aims at empowering local people to challenge the state and the business actors and their economic monopolization and to determine their own way of life. During the late 1960s until the late 1990s when Thailand began to embrace capitalism, the concept of traditional community and culture was fairly widespread among Thai NGOs who mostly aimed to "liberate" village communities from the domination of what they perceived was an elite-driven profit-based market economy. Since the late 1990s to the present, community economy and community-based resource management has been promoted as a parallel concept against capitalism (Nartsupa et al. 2005, cited in Boonchai 2008: 34). Nowadays, self-reliance becomes another tool to discipline local people rather than to help them negotiate with the state and business sector. This is obvious when the government and NGOs collaboratively promote "sufficiency economy" emphasizing the poor rather than the rich (see also Chaps. 9 and 31). The implication is that the poor can be encouraged to live happily, although they suffer hardship. The risk of this campaign is that if the poor are satisfied with their poor living conditions, they might become inactive in participating in economic and political decisions and structural reform (Ganjanpan 2001). In this regard, self-reliance is favorable to the Thai state because it will enable the state's attempt to reduce state services and welfare.

Focusing on Thai NGOs advocating sustainable agriculture and community-based natural resource management, the literature produced consistently points to the numerous problems in Thai society that emerged after the First National Economic Development Plan (NEDP) was launched in the mid-1950s that spelled out Thailand's new direction toward capitalism. The plans are still seen as an

[15] *Nai Nam Mee Pla Nai Na Mee Khao* is a song's name composed in 1932 by Luang Vichit Vichitvatakarn to serve the construction of Thai nationalism.

attempt to undermine rural, subsistence-based livelihoods and traditional culture of "local" communities. Since then, Thai NGOs have attempted to strengthen local communities through reconstructing social bonds among community members and recovering "community culture" while aiming to build sustainable livelihoods and protect the natural resources of local communities. The self-subscribed terms of self-reliance proposed by Thai NGOs such as community sovereignty, self-help, self-reliance, and independence form the basis of their work. Here, I shall give two examples of NGOs' advocacy in order to show how "self-reliance," which is the collaborative approach of NGOs and the THPF, is actually quite problematic.

3.3 *Sustainable Agriculture Advocacy*

Sustainable agriculture programs are supported by many sectors of THPF. Safe food is said to be a key factor in staying healthy, and safe food production and consumption are a way to reduce health risks. Alternative Agriculture Network (AAN) got funds by the Heath Promotion in Community sector, and Bio-Thai Foundation received funds of 50 million baht[16] by the Heath Risk Factors Control sector of THPF. Despite specific objectives and different working approaches, NGOs working on sustainable agriculture issues collaborated to promote sustainable farming, advocate sustainable agriculture policy, and oppose mono-cropping and chemical farming. Bio-Thai, an NGO under the AAN, builds the self-reliance capacity of farmers and consumers by supporting them to have land to farm, to establish alternative markets, and to create community enterprises. These strategies work under the assumption that to reduce local communities' dependence on "outside" factors is to liberate them from capitalist domination and exploitation. At the policy level, NGOs advocate the government to have policies and programs that support sustainable agriculture, such as banning the use of agrochemicals, to proclaim official laws to protect farmlands and farmers, provide financial and other support to small-scale farmers, and so on. At the community level, the farmers who have good farming practices are supported, and they are formed into groups of villager intellectuals. Numerous public campaigns, lectures, training programs, and study trips are organized by NGOs and government agencies so that other farmers learn from these groups of intellectuals who can showcase and discuss good farming practices. From these efforts, sustainable farmland, and agriculture, the farmers are slowly growing in number. Moreover, urban consumers are increasingly concerned about their health and environment. These consumers also demand safer and chemical-free farm products. Witoon Lianchamroon[17] of Bio-Thai points out that NGOs have not yet achieved their actual goals in empowering local farmers and enforcing structural reform.

---

[16] This fund is for a 3-year program consisting of 14 projects.

[17] My interview, June 3, 2011.

One of the activities supported by the Health Risk Factors Control sector is mental and spiritual health promotion: "to enhance compassion, selflessness, and wisdom."[18] Similarly, in sustainable agriculture promotion by NGOs, to have good farming practices means not only agricultural techniques but also proper economic and social way of living, including a belief in the sufficiency economy, Buddhist ways of living, and strong bonds to the motherland and the local community. The polarized perception about "good" and "bad" farmers has recently proliferated in Thai society as reflected through several television programs. The more the self-sufficiency economy is promoted, the more the farmers who practice commercial or market-oriented farming are condemned both directly and indirectly as hungry for money, selfish, uneducated, or even unenlightened while at the same time dismissing without sympathy and understanding the hard conditions that these farmers face in making their commercial farming livelihoods. This paradox was clear in a 90-s TV advertisement of THPF which compares the situations of a mono-cropping farmer and that of a sufficiency economy farmer's life. The mono-cropping farmer grows only sugarcane and gets short-term profits but takes the long-term risk that his life will be unhappy and insecure, while the sufficiency economy farmer has sufficient food, has contented livelihood, and is shown as happy in the long term. This advertisement reflects that the sufficiency economy farmer is smart, rational, and responsible. The opposite characteristics are the representations of the farmers who practice market-oriented agriculture.

As the new alternative farming becomes fashionable in Thailand, many middle-class people and elite people are now turning to rural areas to practice "sustainable agriculture" as a hobby, business, or an alternative way of life. They are shown on covers of magazines and are interviewed in television documentaries: they are always clothed in simple often dark navy blue cotton apparel which is the traditional image of rural farmers. They appear tired but apparently happy and contented with their new lifestyle. These stories and images are widely disseminated through magazines, TV programs, and other public media in appreciation of their attempt at conserving the identity of "Thainess" and true Thai culture.

In a reality show TV program "I will be a farmer," a famous actress who grew up in Bangkok learned to practice organic rice farming on her newly bought land in a rural community. This actress is admired by the director of Bio-Thai Foundation that she has changed the perception of "farmer" and "farming" as "being foolish, poor, and sick" to be wise, dignified, and healthy. In other words, it is a cultural contest over the meanings of farmer and farming. However, farming in the show is represented as the systematic and knowledgeable farming of an elite who is well-educated, is rich, and, more importantly, has other alternative ways to earn a living. Before practicing farming, the film showed how she learned to farm from many intellectual farmers, NGO activists, and scholars. Although she had only a short time for learning and preparation, she employed her social and financial capital to farm. She could therefore afford to buy a fertile piece of land, machines, and also hired labor. She also had a fan club that contributed voluntary labor.

[18] http://en.thaihealth.or.th/plans/healthrisk

Therefore, farming by this actress was completely different from the real farming by small-scale farmers whose living conditions and economic situations are vastly different from hers.

3.4 Communal Land Title Deed

THPF does not directly grant funds for advocacy work on "community land title deeds.[19]" But, it has funded some NGOs indirectly working on this issue. Although land rights seem to be far from health, land tenure security is interpreted as a means to long-term security and happiness. Recently, the Land Reform Network, which is a network of landless people and small farmers who cannot gain access to land, demanded that the government issue communal land title deeds as a mechanism for acquiring and distributing land to farmers whose lands were declared as state property and for other landless people who do not have access to land for farming. However, communal land title deeds are also perceived as a mechanism to control landless people, preventing them from transferring land ownership to the community outsiders, and as a motivation to the community to prevent clearing of forests. Strengthening local communities in this sense is aimed at enforcing local control over community members. In NGOs' view, the poor are seen as the victims of capitalism. However, it is inadequate to control only local people, while the economic structures related to land rights and land distribution remain unchanged.

In NGOs' advocacy of community control, "community" is represented as a bounded space independent from the rest of the world. Local communities are promoted to rely on only local resources or products of their own farms, a strategy which does not help them to cope with global economic structures, which in reality needs wider economic and political structural reforms. Moreover, local communities are often ideally represented as a homogenous community, while in reality a community can be heterogeneous where the community members are different and do not equally participate in the "commons" of the community. Not all community members have "good practices" of farming and natural resource management. THPF clearly states its goal in this sense that it will fund the projects that "change values, lifestyles, and social environments…."[20] Buddhist ideas and philosophy are also applied liberally in this development approach as it focuses on the change of humans from the "inside" of their mind rather than the "outside" factors.

THPF, like Thai NGOs, seeks to support some exemplary communities and intellectuals so that the others can learn from them. The communities that cannot practice like the "showcases" find it difficult to gain support from THPF and NGOs,

---

[19] Community land title deed is a concept proposed by scholars and social movements for enforcing land redistribution. The land under community title deeds still belongs to the state, but eligible communities are given the right to access land to farm or harvest natural resources under the control of community. The title deeds cannot be sold or mortgaged.

[20] http://en.thaihealth.or.th/about

unless they can prove that they have the potential to develop sufficiency economy farming. These communities and people are not only excluded from funding; they are also labeled by constructed values as "weak communities," "unenlightened people," and even "immoral farmers" through the public campaigns of THPF and NGOs. In fact, THPF and NGOs also realize the underlying problems of the political and economic system that conditions the livelihood of these individuals. However, to challenge the social structure and dominant ideologies is certainly much harder than to control powerless people. Hence, these groups spend their efforts to create local mechanisms for transforming individuals' mind and behavior rather than working on policy reforms. Moreover, it is notable that the improvement in morality is encouraged more for the poor people than for the rich. This brings about the question of equality in society. Several years ago, these questions were not raised much in Thai society, while nowadays they have become more important because social equity and double standards are seen as problems that have brought about increasing tensions between "rural people" and "urban elites" in the current context of Thailand.

4 Discussion and Conclusion

Many of Thailand's NGOs have changed their working approach from challenging state power to cooperating with state agencies. This chapter has illustrated that one of the reasons for NGOs cooperating with state agencies such as the THPF is not only funding but also that both groups share some common development ideology and approaches. Some NGOs claim success in sharing public resources of THPF and pushing THPF to accept and support the ideas of NGOs through this "new" working approach, while THPF equally claims similar success in its efforts at promoting civil society networks or achieving sustainable development. Similar to THPF, many new state agencies are established in Thailand as an autonomous agency outside the formal structure of government. Most NGOs I interviewed appear likely to accept and cooperate with these agencies as new windows for gaining funds and advocating policy. NGOs insist that they have been negotiating with the state for the sake of sustainable development, and they continue to remain "free" from state domination. Nevertheless, some NGO activists accept that they have not been successful in efforts to empower local people. Although NGOs have been negotiating with the state, the establishment of the incarnated forms of the state can be viewed as the state's success in constructing a "bureaucratic field" (Bourdieu et al. 1994). NGOs are drawn to play in the field under the state-applied rules. Moreover, as the state's partners, many NGOs assist and collaborate with the state for cultural and social domination which is a form of symbolic violence.

Promotion of "self-reliance" and methods of community strengthening that are illustrated in this paper are examples of symbolic violence. They are collaboratively employed by both THPF and NGOs in their approach to development. In fact, these approaches are not problematic per se, but their implementation brings about cultural domination that reproduces inequality among the people. THPF encourages the poor to develop and discipline their mind so that their physical body and society will be healthy. NGOs encourage rural people to learn to live "sufficiently" under the tough social and economic conditions so that they have good farming practices and natural resource management. Hence, development through these approaches leads to pressure and moral control over local people rather than empowering them in struggling with structures of power and domination. These development approaches also reproduce a romantic, imagined "Thainess" in both economic and cultural dimensions and push rural people to preserve it, while unfair social and economic structures are not acknowledged as deserving of their attention. Development in this sense brings about discrimination between the rich and the poor. This is similar to Walker's (2008) notion of the sufficiency economy advocated by government and nongovernment agencies as a tool of elites in morally controlling rural people.[21]

Despite their good intentions, the collaborative development between THPF and NGOs does not guarantee the well-being and satisfaction of the people who are their intended beneficiaries. In contrast, development can be the symbolic violence imposed upon them people who are being "developed." Development agencies usually claim to know what is best for the others and how the others should live, a problematic notion as they cannot be the representative of, or speaking for, all the people. But, to claim such a status is actually an exercise in power as it results in trying to determine another person's choices in developing his/her own way of life.

This chapter has illustrated the relations between NGOs and THPF, an "incarnated" form of state agency (Bourdieu et al. 1994). The relationship has significant effect on the positioning and role setting of NGOs in the development arena. At the same time, the relationship reflects how NGOs currently position their role in society. In this chapter, NGOs no longer play a key role in challenging the state, but are cooperating with the state. This "new" working strategy blurs the boundary between the state and civil society. I find it difficult to jump to conclusions whether or not this relationship is completely appropriate or not. But, it cannot be denied that the cooperation brings about several advantages to local people and helps to shape government policies for the sake of the so-called common good. However, this cooperation is also problematic as it becomes a technology of power of many NGOs and state agencies in depoliticizing development and rendering it as merely a technical problem. Although many of Thailand's NGOs and the state collaboratively construct win-win relationships, it might not be entirely possible to have a win-win relationship between the state and people.

Acknowledgment Thanks to colleagues from Thai Social Movement Watch for sharing the ideas and Rajesh Daniel for editing the paper.

[21] http://www.prachatai.com/english/node/746

References

Anderson, B. (1991). *Imagined communities: Reflections on the origin and spread of nationalism*. New York: Verso.

Boonchai, K. (2008). Local development foundation's concepts and foundation. In P. Pinprateep (Ed.), *Community strength and civil society: Twenty years of local development foundation* (pp. 31–44). Bangkok: Local Development Foundation.

Bourdieu, P., Wacquant, L. J. D., & Farage, S. (1994). Rethinking the state: Genesis and structure of bureaucratic field. *Sociological Theory, 12*(1), 1–18.

Deesutjit, N. (2000). Coordinating committee of Northern NGOs. In C. Thongdeelert (Ed.), *NGOs' secret note* (pp. 65–101). Bangkok: NorthernernDevelopment Foundation.

Escobar, A. (1995). *Encountering development: The making and unmaking of the Third World*. Princeton: Princeton University press.

Ferguson, J. (1990). *The anti-politics machine "development", depoliticization, and bureaucratic power in Lesitho*. Cambridge: Cambridge University Press.

Ganjanpan, A. (2001). *Complexity conception in community research: Dynamics and capacity of community in development*. Bangkok: Thailand Research Fund.

Jansomwong, A. (2008). LDI and the contemporary organization administration. In P. Pinprateep (Ed.), *Community strength and civil society: Twenty years of local development foundation* (pp. 234–261). Bangkok: Local Development Foundation.

Kanittachart, P. (2008). Promoting politics of citizens and examining state power exercise. In P. Pinprateep (Ed.), *Community strength and civil society: Twenty years of local development foundation* (pp. 208–231). Bangkok: Local Development Foundation.

Kantawit, K. (2008). LDAP: Origination of local development foundation. In P. Pinprateep (Ed.), *Community strength and civil society: Twenty years of local development foundation* (pp. 16–30). Bangkok: Local Development Foundation.

Kemp, J. H. (1981). Legal and informal tenures in Thailand. *Modern Asian Studies, 15*(1), 1–23.

Kitirianglarp, K. (2009). *Community intellectuals and the construction of historical bloc of community-nationalism under the leadership of the King after 1992* (pp. 250–399). In Ratasartsan 30th Anniversary 1.

Li, M. T. (2007). *The will to improve: Governmentality, development, and the practice of politics*. Durham: Duke University Press.

Loathammatas, A. (2007). *Politics of citizens to the New Millennium*. Bangkok: Kobfai.

Mosse, D. (2005). *Cultivating development: An ethnography of aid policy and practice*. London: Pluto Press.

Parks, T. (2008). The rise and fall of donor funding for advocacy NGOs: Understanding the impact. *Development in Practice, 18*(2), 213–222.

Shigetomi, S. (2000). Thailand: A crossing of critical parallel relationships. In S. Shigetomi (Ed.), *The state and NGOs in Asia: A comparative study of fifteen countries* (pp. 125–144). Tokyo: Institute of Developing Economies.

Shigetomi, S. (2006). *Bringing non-governmental actors into the policy making process: The case of local development policy in Thailand* (Discussion Paper No. 69). Institute of Developing Economies, JETRO. Retrieved May 23, 2010, from: http://ir.ide.go.jp/dspace/bitstream/2344/149/3/ARRIDE_Discussion_No.69_shigetomi.pdf

Thailand Health Promotion Foundation (THPF). (2011a). *Annual report 2010*. Retrieved May 23, 2010, from: http://documents.scribd.com.s3.amazonaws.com/docs/471g4fqfy8yyec2.pdf?t=1305868557

Thailand Heath Promotion Foundation (THPF). (2011b). *10 years trend, direction, goals, and strategies (2012–2022)*. Retrieved May 23, 2010, from: http://info.thaihealth.or.th/library/academic/13320

Walker, A. (2008). *Sufficiency economy, sufficiency democracy, and rural constitution*. Retrieved August 9, 2008, from: http://www.prachatai.com/english/node/746

Warunpitikun, Y., & Ruengjit, S. (2010). *Thai NGOs*. Bangkok: 21th Century Ltd.

About the Editor

Pranee Liamputtong is a medical anthropologist and holds a Personal Chair in Public Health at the School of Public Health, La Trobe University, Melbourne, Australia. Pranee has previously taught in the School of Sociology and Anthropology and worked as a public health research fellow at the Center for the Study of Mothers' and Children's Health, La Trobe University. Pranee has a particular interest in issues related to cultural and social influences on childbearing, child-rearing, and women's reproductive and sexual health. She has published several books and a large number of papers in these areas.

Her recent books in the health and social science areas include: *The Journey of Becoming a Mother Amongst Women in Northern Thailand* (Lexington Books, 2007); *Community, Health and Population* (with Sansnee Jirojwong, Oxford University Press, 2008); *Infant Feeding Practices: A Cross-Cultural Perspective* (Springer 2011); *Motherhood and Postnatal Depression: Narratives of Women and Their Partners* (with Carolyn Westall, Springer, 2011); and *Health, Illness and Well-Being: Perspectives and Social Determinants* (with Rebecca Fanany and Glenda Verrinder, Oxford University Press, 2012). She has currently edited two books on HIV/AIDS for Springer including *Women, Motherhood and HIV/AIDS: A Cross-Cultural Perspective* and *Stigma, Discrimination and HIV/AIDS: A Cross-Cultural Perspective*. Both were published in 2013.

Pranee is a qualitative researcher and has also published several method books. Her most recent method books include: *Researching the Vulnerable: A Guide to Sensitive Research Methods* (Sage, 2007); *Performing Qualitative Cross-Cultural Research* (Cambridge University Press, 2010); *Focus Group Methodology: Principles and Practice* (Sage, 2011); *Qualitative Research Methods, 4th Edition* (Oxford University Press, 2013); and *Research Methods in Health: Foundations for Evidence-Based Practice, 2nd Edition* (Oxford University Press, 2013).

P. Liamputtong (ed.), *Contemporary Socio-Cultural and Political Perspectives in Thailand*,
DOI 10.1007/978-94-007-7244-1,

About the Contributors

Diane Archer holds a Ph.D. from the Department of Land Economy, University of Cambridge. Her thesis focused on social capital in Thailand's participatory slum upgrading program, the Baan Mankong program, with a particular emphasis on Bangkok slums. Following this, she worked at the Asian Coalition for Housing Rights in Bangkok, a regional coalition of grassroots groups and NGOs active in improving the living conditions of the urban poor in 18 countries around Asia. She is now based at the International Institute for Environment and Development in London.

Adcharawan Buripakdi is a faculty member of English department, School of Liberal Arts, Walailak University, Thailand. Her areas of interests include World Englishes, Postcolonial discourse and identity, second language writing, media literacy, business English communication, and human and language rights.

Dredge Byung'chu Käng is a Ph.D./M.P.H. candidate in anthropology and global epidemiology at Emory University. He conducted ethnographic research in Thailand on gender pluralism, social status, and Asian regionalism with a focus on transnational relationships. Dredge also participates in HIV organizing with transgender women and sex workers in Thailand.

Chantanee Charoensri is Lecturer in Sociology at Thammasat University, Bangkok, Thailand. She has recently completed her Ph.D. in Sociology from University of Essex, UK. Her previous publication includes Postmodernism and Sociology (2001, published in Thai).

Pei-Hsiu Chen is a Professor at the Graduate Institute of Southeast Asian Studies-*GISEAS* and Secretary General of Taiwan Association of Southeast Asian Studies-*TASEAS*, National Chi Nan University, Taiwan. Pei-Hsiu obtained a Ph.D. in Political Science from National Chengchit University, Taiwan, in 1999, and his research interests include Southeast Asian studies.

Monica Lindberg Falk received her Ph.D. in Social Anthropology from Gothenburg University, Sweden. She is the Vice Director and Senior Lecturer at the Centre for East and South-East Asian Studies at Lund University, Sweden. Her

P. Liamputtong (ed.), *Contemporary Socio-Cultural and Political Perspectives in Thailand*, 535
DOI 10.1007/978-94-007-7244-1, © Springer Science+Business Media Dordrecht 2014

research interests include gender, Buddhism, anthropology of disaster, religious movement, and social change in Southeast Asia. Her scholarship includes extensive fieldwork in Thailand. She has published a monograph and several articles on themes related to gender and Buddhism, socially engaged Buddhism, and Buddhism and crises. One of her current research projects is gender and Buddhism's role in the recovery process after the 2004 tsunami catastrophe in Thailand; another of her research projects is about gender and education mobility within Asia. Both projects are funded by the Swedish Research Council, VR.

Jenjit Gasigijtamrong completed a B.A. (Honor) in teaching English at Chiang Mai University and an M.A. in English Literature at Central Connecticut State University, USA. She graduated with an Ed.D. in Reading from Northern Illinois University in 2003. She also received a certificate in teaching poetry from Oxford University, UK. In 1995, she received a grant offered by USIA to be a visiting scholar in teaching contemporary American literature. Her research interests focus on Thai Literature and Film and foreign language reading.

Athip Jittarerk received M.A. in Anthropology from Thammasat University in 2011. His master's thesis is about the economic transformations of heavy metal music production in Bangkok from 1970 to 2010. His previous published academic works, all in Thai, include an analysis of the differences between the first generation of punk in New York and London, a review of the works on music and politic being produced in English speaking world, the history of heavy metal musicians in Bangkok from professional musicians at the beginning to amateur musicians in the present, and the elaboration of the idea of parricide in Slavoj Zizek's works.

Matthew R. Juelsgaard is a doctoral candidate in the Department of Educational Foundations at University of Hawaii at Manoa. He is married to a Red Lahu woman (Natcharat Juelsgaard), and together they work for the educational development of Lahu in Thailand.

Erin Kamler is a doctoral student at the University of Southern California's Annenberg School for Communication and Journalism, where she studies culture and human rights issues in Thailand. She has conducted research in partnership with the US Department of State, published in academic journals, and participated in conferences around the world. An award-winning composer, musician, and playwright, Erin's forthcoming work will focus on using the arts as a tool for political communication in the developing world.

Patcharin Ketjamnong is currently an M.A. student of Medical Anthropology in the Culture and Development Program, Mahidol University, Thailand, and a research assistant of the Communication and Development Research Cluster, Research Institute for Languages and Cultures of Asia, Mahidol University. Obtaining a B.S. degree in Social Psychology from Ramkhamhaeng University, Thailand, she has engaged in such research areas as local health communication, folk media for the youth well-being, care of the elders with chronic diseases in the communities, AIDS, and drugs.

Somsri Kitisriworapan is an Associate Professor at the Kasetsart University's Demonstration School, Thailand. Somsri teaches social science, history, and Thai language at both primary and secondary levels. Her main interests are on the health and psychology of children, and her research has involved children's understanding of health and social issues. She has published several book chapters, journal articles, and textbooks.

Megan Lafferty is a doctoral candidate in Anthropology at the University of Melbourne, Australia, where she is researching western migration to Isan, Thailand. She obtained an M.A. degree in Political Science from San Diego State University. Her research interests include masculinities, transnational marriage, migration, and political economy.

Allan Lee graduated from National University of Singapore with a B.Soc.Sci (Hons) in Sociology and went on to pursue his M.Soc.Sci in the same university. His research interests include political sociology, social movements, social memory, and religion.

Kristen Hill Maher is Associate Professor of Political Science at San Diego State University. She has published work on women's international migration in the contexts of both Chile and the USA, focusing particularly on the everyday geographies of identity and power shaping the experiences of women working in social reproduction economies. She is currently working on a book about the representation of place in the US-Mexican borderlands.

Morakot Jewachinda Meyer is a lecturer at Pridi Banomyong International College of Thammasat University, Bangkok. She has received her Ph.D. in European History from the European University Institute in Florence, Italy. Her current research focuses on contemporary Thai history. She is particularly interested in popular culture, nationalism, and conceptual history.

Suangsurang Mitsamphanta is a researcher at the Department of Public Administration, Faculty of Political Science, Chulalongkorn University, Thailand. She was a Lecturer in the School of Liberal Arts at Mae Fah Lung University, Thailand. She earned her master's degree in Gender and Development Studies from Asian Institute of Technology. She finished her Bachelor's degree in Political Sciences from Chulalongkorn University. Her areas of interest are public policy, gender and development, and women and politics.

Andrea Katalin Molnar is Professor in the Department of Anthropology and an Associate of the Center for Southeast Asian Studies at Northern Illinois University, DeKalb, IL, USA. Besides her ongoing research on women's political participation in southern Thailand, her areas of specialization include Indonesia and Timor Leste.

Witchayanee Ocha is a full time university lecturer at International College, Rangsit University, Thailand. In 2012, she has completed her Ph.D. in Gender and Development Studies at Asian Institute of Technology (AIT), Thailand. Her Ph.D. dissertation focuses on gender, sexualities, and rights. Her works have been published in *Culture, Health and Sexuality; Sexualities Journal; Gender, Technology and Development;* and *'Human Rights in Southeast Asia' Academic Book (SEAHRN)*. In 2009, she worked as a consultant at United Nations Office of the High Commissioner for Human Rights, Regional Office for Southeast Asia (OHCHR), in which she previously received a 6-month internship program. In 2010, she was an Asian Graduate Student Fellow at Asia Research Institute, National University of Singapore, Singapore.

Mayumi Okabe has a doctorate from the Graduate University for Advanced Studies (National Museum of Ethnology, Japan) and is currently Research Fellow of the Japan Society for the Promotion of Science. Her research interests are in Theravada Buddhism, NGOs movement, and new communities in contemporary Thailand.

Kosum Omphornuwat is a lecturer in the Women, Gender, and Sexuality Studies Programme (WGSSP), College of Interdisciplinary Studies, Thammasat University. Her research interests lie in an understanding of women's lived experiences and everyday practices in relation to their bodies. She teaches media representation and the politics of the body. Kosum completed her Ph.D. in the Department of Social Sciences at Loughborough University, UK.

Saowapa Pornsiripongse is currently Associate Professor in Medical Anthropology at the Research Institute for Languages and Cultures of Asia, Mahidol University, Thailand. She has published three books on Knowledge of 'Lanna' Folk Healers, Cultural Physiology of 'Esan' Folk Massage, and Cultural Mapping of Ethnic Groups Along Thai-Cambodian Border and many articles on medical anthropology, namely, social capital and noncommunicable disease prevention, religious syncretism in healing noncommunicable diseases: the role of folk healer monks, religious organizations, and preparing for an aging society.

Suwilai Premsrirat is a Professor of Linguistics at the Resource Center for Documentation, Revitalization, and Maintenance of Endangered Languages and Cultures, Research Institute for Languages and Cultures of Asia (RILCA), Mahidol University, Thailand. She has been researching and writing on ethnic minority languages in Thailand and mainland Southeast Asia since 1975, specializing in Mon-Khmer languages. Suwilai is the founder of the Research Center of Documentation and Revitalization of Endangered Languages and Cultures. She is now a member of the UNESCO MLE working group and has been nominated as SEAMEO MLE fellow.

Atchara Rakyutidharm is a Lecturer at the Department of Social Sciences, Faculty of Arts, Silpakorn University. Currently, she is doing a research on "The Politics of De-politicization: The Transformation of NGOs- State – People Relations" (June 2011 to April 2013) granted by Thailand Research Fund. The chapter which is included in this book forms a part of this research.

Yoshihide Sakurai is a Vice Dean and Professor of Sociology at the Graduate School of Letters, Hokkaido University, Japan. He obtained Ph.D. in Development Studies of Thailand at Hokkaido University and published his book Regional Development in Northeast Thailand and the Formation of Civil Society (Khon Kaen University Press, 2003). He has also been publishing many books about contemporary religion in Japan. His English paper is included in the Hokkaido University Collection of Academic Papers: http://eprints.lib.hokudai.ac.jp/dspace/index.jsp?locale=en

Kazumi Sasaki obtained M.A. in Development Studies of Thailand at Hokkaido University and now is the secretary general of the NPO that supports young disabled people in Asia by distributing second hand order-made wheelchair which are donated by grown-up disabled Japanese.

Kwanchit Sasiwongsaroj serves as a Lecturer of Research Institute for Languages and Cultures of Asia, Mahidol University, Thailand. Her bachelor degree is in Science in Nursing. After receiving an M.A. in Cultural Studies, she earned a Ph.D. in Demography from the Institute for Population and Social Research, Mahidol University. Her field research experiences are mainly on health and cultural issues, as well as other related fields of medical anthropology. Her specific research interests are in the following areas: ethnic diversity, cross-cultural studies, religion and health, and well-being of the elderly.

Aim Sinpeng is a Ph.D. candidate in Political Science at the University of British Columbia. She also serves as a visiting fellow at Thammasat University, a scholar at the Liu Institute of Global Issues and an associate at the Institute of Asian Research, UBC. Aim has published work on the Red-Yellow Shirt political conflict, social movements, and party politics in Thailand as well as Thailand-ASEAN relations. She contributes to New Manadala, provides commentaries on Thailand to various media outlets in Canada, and is an independent consultant on Thai politics.

Sophana Srichampa is Associate Professor at the Research Institute for Languages and Cultures of Asia (RILCA), Mahidol University, Thailand. She was the director of the institute between 2006 and 2009. Her fields of interest include: Vietnamese language and culture; language and cross-cultural communication; language and culture, syntax, and semantics; Southeast Asian sociocultural studies; Vietnamese language and cultural studies; and Indian studies.

Sumittra Suraratdecha is a Lecturer at Research Institute for Languages and Cultures of Asia (RILCA), Mahidol University, Thailand. She graduated with a Ph.D. in Linguistics from University of Hawaii at Manoa, USA. Her research interests are sociolinguistics, anthropological linguistics, and second language studies.

Dusanee Suwankhong is currently a Lecturer at School of Public Health, Faculty of Health and Sports Science, Thaksin University, in Phatthalung province, Thailand. She has published a number of articles and book chapters using data from her Ph.D. research. She has her interests in traditional medicines, lay understanding of Hepatitis C, primary health care, and community health.

Yongsak Tantipidoke is a Ph.D. candidate at the Amsterdam Institute for Social Science Research, University of Amsterdam, where he is researching the effectiveness of indigenous healing of HIV/AIDS in Chiang Mai, Northern Thailand.

He also serves as a researcher of the Society and Health Institute, Ministry of Public Health, Thailand. Yongsak hold a B.Sc. in Pharmaceutical Science from Chulalongkorn University and an M.A. in Medical and Health Social Science from Mahidol University. He was a staff of a nongovernmental organization and has contributed to the development of traditional medicine in Thailand for three decades.

Ratana Tosakul is a senior lecturer of cultural anthropology teaching at Thammasat University in Bangkok Thailand. Her research interests include rural agricultural community studies, diaspora and transnationalism with gender sensitivity. She has conducted her anthropological field research primarily in northeastern Thailand, Laos and Burma. Recently, she has studied Thai diaspora in Japan. She holds a Ph.D. in sociocultural anthropology from the University of Washington, Seattle.

Alexander Trupp is Assistant Professor at the Department of Geography and Regional Research, University of Vienna, Austria, and deputy editor-in-chief of the Austrian Journal of Southeast Asian Studies (ASEAS). His research focuses on ethnic tourism, migrant entrepreneurship, and qualitative research methods, especially in the context of Southeast Asian Studies.

Serhat Ünaldi is a doctoral candidate at Humboldt-University in Berlin, where he is researching the sociopolitical functions of Bangkok's modern city center, Siam/Ratchaprasong. He holds a B.A. degree in area studies from Humboldt-University and an M.A. in international studies from the University of Leeds.

Willard G. Van De Bogart earned his M.F.A. degree from the California Institute of the Arts in Design in Los Angeles, CA, and did master's work in Information Science at the University of Pittsburgh in Pennsylvania in Information Counseling and Database retrieval. His early research on indigenous cultures was with Native American Indians, first with the POMO Indians of Northern California and then with the Esselen Indians on the Central California coast at Big Sur. After moving to Thailand in 2001, he began researching the influence of India on Southeast Asia and specifically on the Khmer Empire. His work continues with the influences of the Hindu religion on the cosmology of the Brahmans in Thailand and their use of an ancient swing still used in royal ceremonies. The history of ancient rituals and their origins in antiquity is his current research project. He teaches in the Language Institute at Bangkok University in Bangkok.

MIX
Papier aus verantwortungsvollen Quellen
Paper from responsible sources
FSC® C105338

If you have any concerns about our products,
you can contact us on
ProductSafety@springernature.com

In case Publisher is established outside the EU,
the EU authorized representative is:
Springer Nature Customer Service Center GmbH
Europaplatz 3, 69115 Heidelberg, Germany

Printed by Libri Plureos GmbH
in Hamburg, Germany